Foundations of Robust Control, Plants, III, 432–432

with 7 reflections, estimates are figures,
unpredictable and whalues, and values [41–]

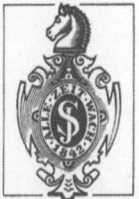

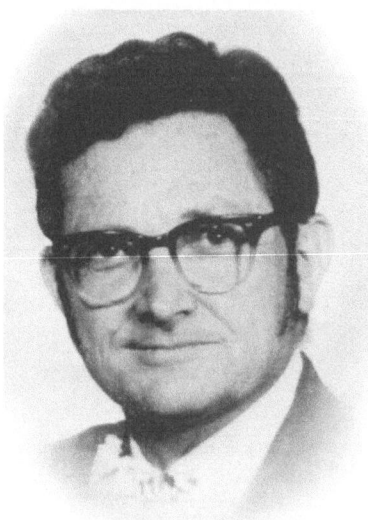

To the memory of Robert L. Peters MD, 1927–1985,
"bench" pathologist, renowned investigator,
inspired teacher and scholar, and warm friend.

Kunio Okuda   Kamal G. Ishak   (Eds.)

Neoplasms of the Liver

With 347 Figures

Springer Japan KK

Prof. KUNIO OKUDA, M.D., Ph.D.
First Department of Medicine
Chiba University School of Medicine
Inohana, Chiba, 280 Japan

Prof. KAMAL G. ISHAK, M.D., Ph.D.
Department of Hepatic Pathology
Armed Forces Institute of Pathology
Washington, DC 20306, USA

ISBN 978-4-431-68351-3   ISBN 978-4-431-68349-0 (eBook)
DOI 10.1007/978-4-431-68349-0

Typesetting: Asco Trade Typesetting Ltd., Hong Kong

Preface

Primary liver cancer is a rather unusual malignancy in that the incidence varies tremendously from one geographical area to another. While relatively uncommon in Western countries, it is the most prevalent malignant neoplasm in Southeast Asia, South Africa, and many other regions; in all, the countries in which primary liver cancer is very prevalent account for more than two-thirds of the world's population. In China alone, approximately 100 000 people die every year from primary liver cancer, mostly hepatocellular carcinoma. The incidence is rising in some countries, especially Japan, where it has doubled among males in the past 15 years or so, a staggering and puzzling trend.

Since the demonstration of an etiological relationship between hepatitis B virus infection and hepatocellular carcinoma, intensive research has been conducted in an effort to elucidate the role of the virus in hepatocarcinogenesis. Though much progress has been made, a full understanding of the molecular events leading to malignant transformation of the hepatocyte will probably require many more years of rigorous investigation. Chemical carcinogens and several industrial pollutants may also be involved in the etiopathogenesis of neoplastic liver disease.

In 1976, the late Prof. Robert L. Peters and one of the editors of the present volume (Okuda) edited a monograph entitled "Hepatocellular Carcinoma," published by John Wiley, New York; this was a milestone in hepatocellular carcinoma research. During the ensuing 10 years, much new information has accumulated, particularly in the molecular biology of hepatitis viruses and oncogenes and in their potential etiological role in hepatocarcinogenesis. Concurrently, remarkable progress has been made in the diagnosis and management. This progress is particularly evident in the diagnostic imaging of liver tumors with the advent of new modalities such as computed tomography, real-time ultrasonography, and magnetic resonance imaging. A 1-cm liver mass can now be detected and differentiated from benign lesions such as hemangioma. We are entering the stage where the "doubling time" (as a measure of the speed of tumor growth) can be determined and the therapeutic modality "tailored" to the needs of the individual patient. New approaches, radically different from previous methods, have been adopted in several countries for the early detection of hepatocellular carcinoma in patients with chronic liver disease.

More recently, a number of new problems have emerged, for example, the indications for liver transplantation in patients with advanced cirrhosis complicated by hepatocellular carcinoma, the risk of liver cancer in seroconverted hepatitis B virus carriers, the clinical and morphological identification and biological behavior of preneopalstic lesions, and the possibility of chemoprevention of malignant transformation in patients at high risk for development of hepatocellular carcinoma.

It is our belief that a new book encompassing authoritative discussion and recent data on various aspects of liver cancer is necessary, both for investigators interested in basic aspects of liver cancer and for physicians directly involved in patient care. The present volume contains 33 chapters contributed by an international group of investigators and clinicians who are leaders in their respective fields. The editors are deeply grateful to the authors for their outstanding contributions.

KUNIO OKUDA
KAMAL G. ISHAK

Table of Contents

Part I
Basic Aspects

Chapter 1
Epidemiology of Hepatocellular Carcinoma

Nubia Muñoz and Xavier Bosch[1]

1 Introduction

This chapter will deal only with hepatocellular carcinoma (HCC), the most frequent malignant tumor of the liver. Worldwide, HCC is the seventh most common form of cancer in males and the ninth in females [1]. There are variations in its frequency in different geographical areas; thus, it is the most common malignant tumor among males in western, middle, and eastern Africa, the second most common in southern Africa and Southeast Asia, and the third most common among males in China. It is a relatively rare tumor in most parts of America, Europe, northern Africa, and middle and eastern Asia [1].

During the last decade, a series of epidemiological and laboratory investigations have established an association between hepatitis B virus (HBV) and HCC. The association is restricted to chronically persistent forms of HBV infection and is strong, specific, and consistent. The evidence indicating that this association is most probably causal will be reviewed. Laboratory and epidemiological studies indicating that aflatoxin plays an important role in the development of HCC in certain areas of the developing world will also be discussed. Data indicating that tobacco smoking and alcohol consumption might be etiological factors in certain areas of the world will be reviewed. The relative contribution of these various risk factors will be estimated for different geographical areas. Finally, the perspectives for prevention will be discussed in the light of the risk factors considered.

2 Geographical distribution

HCC is one of the most common malignant tumors in sub-Saharan Africa and in Southeast Asia. It is also relatively frequent among Chinese who migrated to the United States and in some European countries such as Rumania, Switzerland, Poland, Spain, Italy, and Greece. This geographical distribution is illustrated by three different kinds of data.

2.1 Relative frequencies

Relative frequency is the proportion or percentage of each type of cancer from a total series. It is used when the population from which the cases are drawn is not known. In some areas of the developing world, these are the only data available. The series from which they are drawn are usually selected. Special care in the interpretation of these data should be exercised. For example, a high proportion of one specific cancer may be due either to a really high frequency of that cancer or to a low frequency of other types. Since the relative frequencies of the different cancer types vary considerably with age, an age-standardized cancer ratio (ASCAR) has been used. Table 1.1 summarizes the ASCAR for a series of African, Asian, and Latin American countries included in the IARC publication "Cancer Occurrence in Developing Countries" [2]. The high ratios in east and west African countries and among Malaysian and Chinese groups in Malaysia, and the low ratios in Tunisia, Bangladesh, Sri Lanka, Argentina, and Uruguay are noteworthy.

2.2 Incidence rates

Age-adjusted incidence rates (AAIR) calculated using the world standard population were extracted from "Cancer Incidence in Five Conti-

---

[1] International Agency for Research on Cancer, 150 cours Albert Thomas, 69372 Lyon Cedex 08, France

Table 1.1. Age-standardized cancer ratios (ASCAR)

Registry	ASCAR (%)		Type of registry
	Males	Females	
Africa			
Uganda			
West Nile	21.0	9.2	Hospital
Kampala	12.8	3.7	Histopathology
Zambia			
Lusaka	15.9	17.0	Hospital
Ndola	16.0	0.8	Histopathology
Liberia	11.5	3.5	Hospital
Kenya			
National Registry	8.8	4.7	Histopathology
Mombasa	6.2	1.9	Histopathology
Angola, Luanda	8.0	2.5	Histopathology
Rwanda, National Registry	7.3	0.8	Histopathology
Malawi	6.5	1.8	Histopathology
Sudan	6.4	2.6	Histopathology
Gabon, Libreville	4.2	0.9	Histopathology
Madagascar	1.8	0.3	Histopathology
Tunisia	0.6	0.2	Histopathology
Asia			
Malaysia, Kuala Lumpur			
Malaysians	13.8	0.4	Histopathology
Chinese	12.9	3.6	
Indians	6.0	0.0	
Vietnam, Ho Chi Minh City	3.8	0.7	Hospital
Iraq, Baghdad	2.1	1.1	Histopathology
Bangladesh	1.3	1.3	Hospital
Sri Lanka, Colombo	0.8	0.5	Hospital
Latin America			
Argentina, Santa Fe	1.3	1.3	Hospital
Uruguay, Montevideo	0.2	0.2	Histopathology

All figures taken from Cancer Occurrence in Developing Countries [2]

nents" [3–6] and "Cancer Occurrence in Developing Countries" [2]. The AAIR calculated for hospital- and histopathology-based registries should be considered minimal incidence rates. Table 1.2 summarizes the most recent available data for selected registries of countries in each of the five continents. In Africa, the high rates for African populations in the south, west, and east contrast with the low rate for Algeria. In Latin America, the relatively high rates in Argentina are thought to be due to the inclusion of metastatic liver tumors together with the primary ones (Iscovich J, Castelleto R, personal communication, 1986). In North America, the Chinese populations in the San Francisco Bay area and Los Angeles and the Eskimos in Canada have relatively high rates. In most of Europe, the rates are low; exceptions are Rumania, Switzerland, Poland, Italy, and Spain, which have intermediate

rates. In Asia, high rates are reported from China, Hong Kong, Korea, the Philippines, Indonesia, certain areas of Japan, Singapore, Thailand and Burma. The rates fall abruptly in India, Pakistan, and most Middle-Eastern countries with the exception of non-Kuwaitis in Kuwait. In Oceania, relatively high rates are reported for Melanesian population groups.

2.3 Mortality data

Although mortality is a good indicator of incidence, considering the very poor survival in HCC, it also has serious limitations, particularly as a considerable proportion of cases are registered in national records as liver cancer of unspecified origin. Using WHO data [7], the combined age-standardized death rates (primary plus unspecified liver cancer) and the world standard population were calculated for those countries

Table 1.2. Age-adjusted incidence rates (AAIR) of liver cancer per 100 000 of population

Registry	AAIR		Volume of "Cancer Incidence in Five Continents" or type of registry[a]
	Males	Females	
Africa			
Mozambique, Lourenço Marques	112.9	30.8	I
Zimbabwe, Bulawayo	64.6	25.4	III
South Africa			
Natal			
African black	28.4	6.9	II
Indian	9.5	3.8	
Cape			
Bantu	26.3	8.4	II
Colored	1.5	0.7	
White	1.2	0.6	
Senegal, Dakar	25.6	9.0	IV
Nigeria, Ibadan	15.4	3.2	Hospital
Swaziland	10.5	3.0	Hospital
Tanzania, Kilimanjaro	9.2	1.6	Histopathology
Algeria	1.6	1.4	Histopathology
Latin America			
Argentina			
Tandil	9.9	5.8	Population
Province de la Plata	6.0	2.5	Histopathology
Jamaica, Kingston	6.1	2.1	IV
Costa Rica	5.0	2.5	Population
Cuba	4.1	3.4	Population
Peru, Lima	4.0	2.9	Hospital
Puerto Rico	3.9	2.2	IV
Brazil			
Fortaleza	3.8	3.8	Population
Recife	2.9	3.5	Hospital
São Paulo	1.2	0.3	IV
Paraguay	3.1	2.6	Hospital
Netherlands Antilles	2.9	0.6	IV
Bolivia, La Paz	2.8	4.1	Population
Panama	2.3	1.6	Histopathology
Colombia, Cali	1.9	1.5	IV
North America			
USA			
San Francisco			
Chinese	18.1	3.6	IV
Black	3.9	1.8	
Japanese	3.0	0.4	
White	2.9	1.1	
Los Angeles			
Chinese	12.0	3.8	IV
Spanish	4.1	1.4	
Black	3.9	0.9	
Japanese	2.7	1.6	
White	1.8	0.8	
New Orleans			
Black	4.2	2.0	IV
White	3.3	0.9	
Connecticut	2.0	1.0	IV
Hawaii			
Hawaiian	10.3	7.2	IV
Filipino	9.5	1.8	
Chinese	7.8	3.1	
Japanese	5.7	2.2	
White	2.7	1.4	

(*Table continued on following page*)

Table 1.2 (*continued*)

Registry	AAIR		Volume of "Cancer Incidence in Five Continents" or type of registry[a]
	Males	Females	
Canada			
Eskimos	6.9	3.7	Histopathology
Saskatchewan	1.5	0.6	IV
Alberta	1.3	0.5	IV
Europe			
Rumania, County Cluj	11.8	7.9	IV
Switzerland			
Geneva	9.7	1.3	IV
Vaud	6.3	1.9	IV
Poland			
Warsaw	8.3	4.9	IV
Cieszyn	7.5	4.4	IV
Cracow	5.9	4.3	IV
Italy, Varese	6.9	2.7	IV
Spain			
Zaragoza	6.9	5.1	IV
Navarra	0.5	0.6	IV
France			
Bas-Rhin	4.9	0.7	IV
Doubs	1.9	1.1	IV
FRG, Hamburg	3.6	1.6	IV
German Dem. Republic	3.6	1.5	IV
Sweden	3.4	1.8	IV
Finland	3.2	1.7	IV
Czechoslovakia, Slovakia	3.1	2.6	IV
Denmark	2.9	1.6	IV
Hungary			
Szabolcs	2.9	1.2	IV
Vas	2.9	1.4	IV
Yugoslavia, Slovenia	2.0	0.9	IV
UK			
East Scotland	2.1	0.8	IV
West Scotland	1.3	0.7	IV
Birmingham	1.4	0.4	IV
Oxford	1.1	0.4	IV
Asia			
Hong Kong	34.4	8.9	IV
People's Rep. China, Shanghai	31.7	9.1	IV
Singapore			
Chinese	32.2	7.1	IV
Malay	17.1	3.1	
Indian	14.0	4.8	
Burma, Rangoon	25.5	8.8	Population
Philippines, Manila	19.9	6.2	Population
Korea, Nat. Reg.	13.8	3.2	Hospital
Japan			
Nagasaki	11.9	2.9	IV
Fukuoka	7.2	2.2	IV
Osaka	5.6	1.2	IV
Miyagi	2.5	0.9	IV
Kuwait			
Non-Kuwaiti	9.6	1.8	Population
Kuwaiti	1.9	1.0	
Indonesia, Semarang	9.5	2.8	Histopathology
Thailand, Nat. Reg.	6.8	2.3	Hospital

(*Table continued on following page*)

Table 1.2 (*continued*)

Registry	AAIR		Volume of "Cancer Incidence in Five Continents" or type of registry[a]
	Males	Females	
India			
Bangalore	4.7	1.6	Population
Bombay	2.7	1.0	IV
Madras	2.1	0.7	Population
Poona	1.3	0.8	IV
Israel, Jews	2.9	1.3	IV
Iran, Fars	2.8	1.1	Hospital
Pakistan, all centers	0.7	0.8	Hospital
Turkey, Nat. Reg.	0.7	0.3	Hospital
Oceania			
New Caledonia			
Melanesian	18.7	5.7	Hospital
European	7.9	1.1	
Vanuatu (New Hebrides)	9.4	3.0	Histopathology
New Zealand			
Maori	8.7	2.5	IV
Non-Maori	1.9	1.0	
Fiji			
Fijian	7.8	4.8	Histopathology
Indian	1.0	0.4	
Australia			
New South Wales	1.1	0.4	IV
South	1.3	0.4	IV

[a] All figures taken from Cancer Incidence in Five Contients [3–6] or Cancer Occurrence in Developing Countries [2]

for which no incidence or relative frequency data were available; they are summarized in Table 1.3. Relatively high rates for Greece, Bulgaria, and Chile are observed.

The variation in mortality for HCC within a country has also been reported in China. A 3-year mortality survey (1975–1978) was completed in the People's Republic of China, covering a population of 840 million people. The geographical distribution of 15 malignant tumors by province and county was summarized in "Atlas of Cancer Mortality for the People's Republic of China" [8]. In males, liver cancer is the third most common cancer after gastric and esophageal cancers. Very high mortality is observed in the northeastern province of Jilin, in the southeast coastal provinces of Jiangsu, Zhejiang, Fujian, and Guangdong, and in the southeast in Guangxi Autonomous Region.

2.4 Time trends in HCC incidence

Statistics on HCC are particularly susceptible to classification errors and this should be kept in mind when assessing the time trends. In the four

Table 1.3. Age-adjusted combined death rates of HCC in males for selected countries

Country	Death rates per 100 000 population
Greece	17.0
Bulgaria	13.5
Chile	10.9
Venezuela	8.9
Austria	8.7
The Netherlands	6.0
Ireland	3.7

Rates adjusted to the World Standard Population. Combined rates include primary and unspecified liver cancer

volumes of Cancer Incidence in Five Continents [3–6], 73 population groups have incidence data for HCC on at least two different intervals (average 3.4) and were selected for time-trend analysis. It is worth noting that of these 73, only three populations in Singapore and two populations in Africa are high-risk ones. Consequent-

Table 1.4. Time trends of HCC in males and age-adjusted incidence rates for all ages

Country	AAIR	Country	AAIR
Populations showing a significant increase			
German Democratic Republic		Denmark	
1964–66	2.28	1953–57	2.68
1968–72	3.17	1958–62	2.18
1973–77	3.57	1963–67	3.14
		1968–72	2.85
Hungary, Szabolcs—Szatmar		1973–76	2.91
1962–66	0.85		
1969–71	0.93	UK, Birmingham	
1973–77	2.87	1960–62	0.80
		1963–66	0.80
Finland		1968–72	0.95
1959–61	1.39	1973–76	1.42
1962–65	1.22		
1966–70	2.12	Canada, Alberta	
1971–76	3.16	1960–62	0.41
		1963–66	0.76
Norway		1969–72	1.40
1959–61	1.01	1973–77	1.19
1964–66	0.95		
1968–72	1.51	Israel, Jews	
1973–77	1.56	1960–66	1.79
		1967–71	2.50
Sweden		1972–76	2.90
1959–61	1.79		
1962–65	2.45	Israel, Jews born in Europe and USA	
1966–70	2.91	1960–66	1.45
1971–75	3.38	1967–71	1.95
		1972–76	3.08
Japan, Miyagi			
1959–60	6.01	Puerto Rico	
1962–64	1.25	1962–63	2.74
1968–71	1.75	1964–66	2.48
1973–77	2.48	1968–72	3.26
		1973–77	3.90
India, Bombay			
1964–66	0.48		
1968–72	1.44		
1973–75	2.72		
Populations showing a significant decrease			
UK, southwestern		USA, Connecticut	
1960–62	1.95	1960–62	2.37
1962–65	1.71	1963–65	4.15
1966–70	1.15	1968–72	1.95
		1973–77	1.98

ly, the present analysis will mainly reflect the trends of HCC incidence in low-risk populations. Special attention was paid to sudden changes which could have been due to changes in diagnosis and registry, and more weight was given to trends from registries for which data for at least three time periods were available.

With these considerations in mind, 13 populations were identified for which a significant increasing trend in male HCC incidence was identified (ignoring the first time period of the Miyagi

Registry in Japan; Table 1.4). In only five of these was an increasing trend in women also found. The age-adjusted incidence rates for these populations was on average very low (2.9 ± 1.2). Two registries showed a decline over time which was also statistically significant and corresponded again to areas at very low risk for HCC. In one of these registries, a decline was also seen in women.

A third group of 49 populations showed no clear trend in either direction. These were the majority of the registries in Europe, the Americas and some rather select populations in Africa and Asia (i.e., Israeli non-Jews, Singapore Malays or Indians, New Zealand Maoris and non-Maoris).

Finally, a group of nine populations showed a statistically significant trend (in either direction), but the changes were so sudden that they could have been due to registration artefacts.

Female trends tended to follow the male pattern; however, the number of cases registered was usually smaller and therefore their rates were even more unstable.

The above data show that the majority of the countries or populations for which a decreasing trend or no change in the HCC rates has been observed during the last two decades belong to the Western industrialized world. Therefore, any hypothesis concerning the etiology of HCC in Western industrialized countries has to accommodate the fact that virtually no change in HCC incidence has occurred during the last 20 years.

2.4.1 HCC incidence trends in high-risk countries

In sub-Saharan Africa, available data tend to suggest that a decline in HCC incidence rates is occurring. In Johannesburg, a decrease in the estimated incidence of HCC at a major hospital was documented between the intervals 1953–1955 and 1958–1962 [9]. An update of the studies on cancer incidence among black goldminers in southern Africa confirmed a rather steep and continuous downward trend in crude HCC incidence among miners from Mozambique. The estimated figures were 80.5/100 000 in 1964 and 30.8/100 000 in 1979 [10, 11]. A consistent decline has also been found among miners from parts of southern Africa. Van Rensburg et al. [12] documented a decline in HCC incidence rates of 43% between 1968 and 1975 in the general population of the Inhambane Province of Mozambique. The reasons for this decline are still unknown. It has been suggested that improvements in living conditions and more specifically safer handling of crops and diets with concurrent reduction of aflatoxin exposure might have played an important role [10, 12].

2.5 Sex and age distribution

In general, males are more prone to develop HCC than females. A higher proportion of males than females is especially evident among high-risk groups, such as the Chinese populations in China, Hong Kong, Singapore, and the United States and in African countries. The male

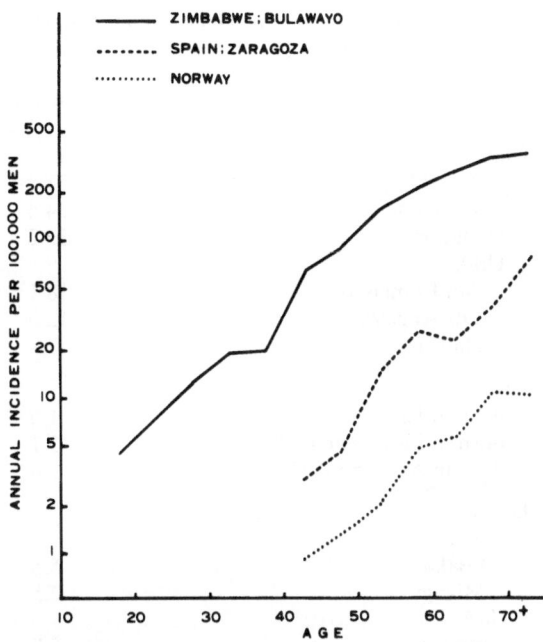

Fig. 1.1. Age distribution of HCC in population at high, intermediate, and low risk

predominance is less marked in the low-risk populations of America and Europe (Table 1.2). The high occurrence of HCC in males in most populations could be explained by a higher susceptibility, genetic or acquired, or by a higher exposure to the environmental factors associated with HCC, as will be discussed below.

In all populations, independently of the risk, the incidence rates increase progressively with age with a tendency to level off in the older age-groups. In the high-incidence areas, such as Zimbabwe, there is a shift toward the younger age-groups. In these high risk populations, the tumor is not infrequently seen in people under 40 years of age, but it does not occur at this age in populations with low or intermediate rates (Fig. 1.1). Thus, in Mozambique, the male incidence in the 25- to 34-years age-group was approximately 500 times that of the equivalent white population of the United States or the United Kingdom, but in the 65 + age-group it was 15 times that observed in the USA or UK [3].

Age at exposure to suspected risk factors might explain the higher differential in risk observed in the younger age-groups between high- and low-incidence populations.

2.6 Studies on migrants

Table 1.5 summarizes the latest available age-adjusted incidence rates for three population

Table 1.5. Age-adjusted incidence rates for HCC among male migrants

Population	AAIR
Chinese	
People's Rep. China, Shanghai	31.7
Hong Kong	34.4
Singapore	32.2
USA	
San Francisco	18.1
Los Angeles	12.0
Hawaii	7.8
Jews	
Born in Israel	1.5
Born in Europe and USA	3.1
Born in Asia and Africa	3.6
Japanese	
Japan	
Osaka	5.5
Miyagi	2.5
USA	
Hawaii	5.7
San Francisco	3.0
Los Angeles	2.7

From Cancer Incidence in Five Continents, vol. IV [6]

groups in their home and host countries [6]. The Chinese populations who migrated to Hong Kong and Singapore have similar rates to the Chinese in Shanghai, but those who migrated to the USA have lower rates. This decrease could be real or alternatively it could be due to the fact that those who migrated to Hong Kong and Singapore came from high-risk areas of China in the southeastern provinces of Fukien and Kwangtung, whereas those who migrated to the USA might have come from intermediate or low-risk areas. Recent analysis of Singapore data indicates that the risk among Singapore-born Chinese is similar to that of Chinese born in China [13]. Among Jews, a higher risk for those born in Africa, Asia, Europe, and the USA than for those born in Israel is consistently observed in three different time periods. Among Japanese, no large differences between the rates in the home country and those outside Japan are observed. In addition, Europeans who migrated from low-incidence areas to high-risk areas in Africa retained their low rates. It can then be concluded that population groups who migrate to other countries in general retain the risks of their home countries, at least for the first two generations. This suggests that exposure during early life to the suspected risk factors is one of the main determinants of the risk for HCC in later life.

3 Risk factors

3.1 Hepatitis B virus (HBV)

Several epidemiological studies and laboratory investigations have established that there is a strong and specific association between HBV and HCC. The association is restricted to the chronically persistent forms of HBV infection characterized by the presence of hepatitis B surface antigen (HBsAg) in the serum as shown by the following data.

3.1.1 Epidemiological studies

Three types of epidemiological study have been conducted.

Correlation studies. In general, correlation studies have demonstrated that there is a positive correlation between the incidence or mortality of HCC and the prevalence of HBsAg carriers [14, 15]. Thus, Southeast Asia and sub-Saharan Africa have very high HBsAg prevalence rates (over 10%) and also have the highest rates of HCC, but most populations in America and Europe that have low rates of HCC also have low prevalence rates of HBsAg carriers [14, 15]. However, there are some exceptions to this general pattern. For example, a high prevalence of HBsAg carriers and a low incidence rate of HCC have been reported for Greenland Eskimos [16].

Case-control studies. In high-risk populations of Africa and Southeast Asia and in populations with an intermediate risk for HCC, such as Greece, case-control studies have shown that the relative risk (RR) associated with the presence of HBsAg ranges from 10 to 20 [17–22]. In the low-risk populations of the USA, where the prevalence rates of HBsAg in the control population are very low, the RR is higher [23, 24]. Table 1.6 summarizes some of these studies. Relative risks and attributable risks were estimated from the published data.

Cohort studies. Cohort studies have compared the occurrence of HCC among HBsAg carriers with that of a noncarrier control population. The cohort studies so far reported are summarized in Table 1.7 [25–29] (Beasley RP, personal communication, 1986). The RR varies from 7 to over 100 with 95% confidence limits ranging from 2 to 212. These prospective cohort studies provide unequivocal proof that the HBV infection precedes the development of HCC.

As seen in Tables 1.6 and 1.7, the estimates of RR in case-control studies are not so different from those reported in cohort studies with the

Table 1.6. Case-control studies on HBsAg and HCC

Study population	No. of subjects		HBsAg + (%)		Relative risk (95% CI)	Attributable risk (%)
	HCC	Controls	HCC	Controls		
High-risk areas						
Senegal [17]	165	328	61.2	11.3	12.4 (7.7–19.3)	56.3
South Africa [18]	289	213	61.6	11.3	12.6 (7.7–20.1)	56.7
Hong Kong [19]	107	107	82.0	18.0	21.3 (10.1–45.9)	78.5
People's Rep. China [20]	50	50	86.0	22.0	17.0 (4.3–99.4)	77.9
Philippines [21]	104	84	70.0	18.0	10.83 (5.3–20.9)	63.9
Intermediate risk area						
Greece [22]	194	451	45.9	7.3	10.7 (6.8–16.6)	41.6
Low-risk area						
USA [23]	34	38	14.7	0.0	(1.5–∞)	—
USA [24]	86	161	17.9	0.0	(10.0–∞)	—

Table 1.7. Cohort studies on HBsAg carriers

Study population	Cohort		HCC risk	
	Total	HBsAg+	RR or SMR (95% CI)	Attributable risk (%)
Taiwan [25]	22 707	3454	104.0 (51–212)	93.9
Japan [26]	32 177	496	10.4 (5.0–19.1)	12.7
Japan, Osaka [27]	—	8646	6.6 (4.0–10.2)	10.1[a]
USA, New York [28]	—	6850	9.7 (2.0–28.3)	1.0[b]
England and Wales [29]	—	3934	42.0 (14.0–100.0)	4.0[b]

[a] Using a prevalence rate of HBsAg in the general population of 2.0%
[b] Assuming a prevalence rate of HBsAg in the general population of 0.1%; *RR*, relative risk; *SMR*, standardized mortality ratio

exception of the one from Taiwan. The low RRs observed in the cohort studies of Japan and the USA probably represent underestimates of the true RR due to the passive method of follow-up used. The very high RRs reported in the above-mentioned studies indicate that the association between HBV and HCC is one of the strongest associations so far recorded. That this association is specific as well as strong is suggested by the lack of association of HBV with other cancers [17] and with metastatic liver cancer [30].

Indirect evidence of HBV infection preceding HCC is derived from the analysis of age-specific prevalence curves of HBsAg carriers in high-risk populations for HCC showing a peak in the first decade of life [31]. Since the chances of becoming an HBsAg carrier are higher the earlier the age at infection, HBV perinatal infection could be one of the crucial factors in determining the risk of developing HCC. The relative contribution of the mother and other family members as sources

of HBV perinatal infection may differ in various high-risk populations.

In addition, epidemiological features of HBV infection fit quite well with certain features of the descriptive epidemiology of HCC. The higher prevalence rates of HBsAg carriers among males than among females is in accordance with the fact that males are more prone to develop HCC than females although the range of the sex ratio is wider for the HCC incidence rates than for the prevalence of the HBsAg. The high prevalence of HBsAg carriers in childhood among high-risk populations could explain the relatively common occurrence of HCC in the younger age-groups in these populations and the fact that migrants from these high-risk populations retain their high risk when they settle in low-risk countries.

3.1.2 Laboratory studies

Two types of laboratory investigation have provided valuable information on the possible mechanisms by which HBV may lead to HCC.

Molecular biology studies. Hybridization experiments using cloned purified HBV-DNA have shown that HBV-DNA is integrated into the genomes of liver cell lines derived from HCC [32], the genomes of malignant liver cells from patients with HCC [33], and the genomes of liver cells of long-term asymptomatic HBsAg carriers [33]. The occurrence of integration in patients without HCC indicates that integration itself is not sufficient for the development of HCC.

Investigations in animal models. Viruses which closely resemble human HBV in three species—woodchuck hepatitis virus (WHV), ground squirrel hepatitis virus (GSHV), and Chinese domestic duck virus (DHBV) [34]. WHV produces a chronic persistent infection in woodchucks, which eventually progresses to chronic active hepatitis and HCC. Moreover, integration of WHV-DNA has been demonstrated in the genomes of liver cells of woodchucks with HCC [34], providing a remarkable parallel between HBV and HCC. The oncogenic potential of GSHV and DHBV remains to be established.

In conclusion, the strength, specificity, and consistency of the association between HBV and HCC in several human populations, the clear evidence that HBV infection precedes the development of HCC, and the biological plausibility as derived from laboratory investigations indicate that the association between HBV and HCC is causal. Ultimate proof of the causality will be provided by the demonstration that elimination of HBV infection by vaccination prevents HCC.

3.2 Aflatoxins

Aflatoxins are mycotoxins elaborated by *Aspergillus flavus* fungi. There are four major members of this group—aflatoxins B1, B2, G1, and G2. There is strong evidence of carcinogenic effects of aflatoxin in animals, AFB1 being the most potent. The evidence is less strong in humans.

3.2.1 Laboratory studies

Aflatoxins are powerful liver carcinogens for many animal species, including fish (rainbow trout and salmon), rodents (rats and mice), lower primates (tree shrews and marmosets), and primates (rhesus, cynomolgus, and African green monkeys). Liver tumors have also been induced in ducklings and ferrets [36]. Susceptibility to tumor induction varies greatly between species and between strains of the same species [35]. Dose-response relationships have been docu-

Table 1.8. Correlation studies on human exposure to aflatoxin B1 and HCC incidence

Country	Incidence rate of HCC in males over 15 years (per 100 000/year)	Aflatoxin B1 (ng/kg body wt/day)
Kenya [41]		
High altitude	3.11	4.88
Middle altitude	10.80	7.84
Low altitude	12.92	14.81
Swaziland I [42]		
Highveld	7.02	8.34
Middleveld	14.79	14.43
Lubombo	18.65	19.89
Lowveld	26.65	53.34
Swaziland II [43]		
Highveld	4.39	14.3
Middleveld	10.62	40.0
Lubombo	11.07	32.9
Lowveld	23.02	127.1
Transkei [12]	9.1	16.5
Mozambique [12]		
Massinga	9.3	38.6
Manhica-Magude	12.1	20.3
Inharrime	17.8	86.9
Inhambane	21.8	77.7
Zavala	28.8	183.7
Morrumbene	29.1	87.7
Homoine-Maxixe	47.9	131.4
Panda	60.7	
Thailand [44]		
Ratburi	6.0	31.48
Songkhla	2.0	5.6

mented in trout [36, 37] and rats [38]. Sex differences in response to aflatoxin have also been noted; latent periods were significantly shorter in male than in female Fisher rats, though the final tumor incidence was similar for both sexes [39].

Although the primary target organ for orally administered aflatoxin is usually the liver, a significant occurrence of tumors at other sites such as the kidney, colon, and skin has been observed, depending on the species, sex, age, strain of animals, route and dose of aflatoxin used [35]. In addition to the carcinogenic effects, aflatoxin has been shown to produce acute liver toxicity in several animal species and humans [35].

3.2.2 Epidemiological studies

Epidemiological studies on the role of aflatoxin in the development of HCC have been hampered by a lack of appropriate methods to assess chronic aflatoxin exposure at the individual level. The development of tests for measuring recent exposure at the individual level through the detection of aflatoxin metabolites or DNA adducts in biological fluids could be the first step in this direction [40]. Two types of epidemiological study have been conducted on the association of aflatoxin and HCC.

Correlation studies. Table 1.8 summarizes the most relevant of these studies [12, 41–44]. The methods used to obtain estimates of aflatoxin exposure vary from study to study, as does the completeness of cancer registration. Comparisons on absolute values between these studies are thus difficult to interpret. It should be kept in mind that estimates of aflatoxin exposure in these studies indicate aflatoxin contamination at the time each survey was performed. However, each of them indicates that HCC rates tend to increase with increasing levels of aflatoxin in the diet.

Case-control studies. Two case-control studies have been reported. In the Philippines, assessment of aflatoxin exposure was attempted using a dietary recall questionnaire and a table which provided measurements of aflatoxins in the local foodstuffs. In cases of HCC, there was exposure to a higher aflatoxin load per day than in matched controls. The differences in risk were higher among heavy alcohol consumers [45].

A second study in Hong Kong did not show any effect of aflatoxin. However, the assessment of aflatoxin exposure by means of a food frequency questionnaire was not reliable [19].

3.3 Joint effect of HBV and aflatoxin

The impossibility of assessing chronic exposure to aflatoxin at the individual level is, again, the major obstacle in the evaluation of the joint effect of HBV and aflatoxin. Attempts to assess this joint effect have been made in high-risk populations in Africa through correlation studies. Van Rensburg et al. [12], in a study involving nine areas in Mozambique and Transkei, observed that the prevalence of HBsAg carriers was low to intermediate in regions where the rate of HCC was extremely high. They also noted that gold miners, whose diet changed after moving to South Africa for work, experienced a reduction in HCC risk within a year. These findings led them to conclude that the HBsAg carrier state was an indicator of initiation, and that aflatoxin was reponsible for late-stage or promoting effects. In Swaziland, a joint International

Agency for Research on Cancer (IARC)/Food and Agriculture Organization (FAO)/United Nations Environment Programme (UNEP) project was set up in 1982 to measure aflatoxin exposure and the prevalence of HBsAg carriers throughout the country [43]. As in a previous survey [42], a positive correlation was found between the estimates of aflatoxin exposure from diets and crop samples and the HCC minimal incidence rates in males. A positive correlation was also found with the prevalence of HBsAg carriers. Multivariate analysis was used to assess the joint effects of aflatoxin and HBsAg on HCC rates. Aflatoxin was implicated as the most important determinant of the geographical variation of HCC incidence in Swaziland [43].

3.4 Tobacco smoking

A moderate excess for liver cancer has been observed in some of the major cohort studies on smoking and cancer [46–47]. However, the results should be interpreted with caution because these studies are based on death certificates, which are known to be unreliable as diagnostic sources of primary liver cancer. In addition, the confounding with other risk factors cannot be ruled out in these cohort studies. A case-control study within a cohort was made in one of the cohort studies of HBsAg carriers in Japan and an RR of 5.8 [95% confidence interval (CI), 1.0–34.2] was found for heavy smokers (more than 30 cigarettes/day). The increased risk persisted after adjusting for drinking but a dose-response relationship could not be detected [27].

Two case-control studies have reported an increased risk for HCC among smokers negative for HBsAg. One was conducted in Greece (which has an intermediate incidence of HCC) and the other in Hong Kong (a high-risk population for HCC). In the Greek study [48], which has been recently expanded, a statistically significant dose-dependent association was found with tobacco smoking among HCC patients negative for HBsAg after controlling, through logistic regression, for the potential confounding effects of age, sex, and alcohol consumption [22]. The adjusted RR for smokers of 20–30 cigarettes/day was 2.4 and 7.3 for those who smoked more than 30 cigarettes/day. In the Hong Kong study, only 19 of 107 HCC cases were HBsAg negative. The RR of developing HBsAg-negative HCC for smokers of 20 or more cigarettes/day was 3.3 compared with light smokers and nonsmokers, but the 95% confidence limits were 1.0 and 13.4. However, the association was stronger and statistically significant for cases over 50 years of age—RR = 8.2 (95% CI, 1.5–91.9) [19].

A further case-control study from the USA reported an excess risk associated with cigarette smoking, but no information was available on the HBsAg status of cases and controls [49]. The significant effect of cigarette smoking remained after adjusting for other risk factors. On the other hand, three case-control studies have shown negative results: One from Sweden [50] and another from the USA [52] showed a small positive association between HCC and smoking which disappeared after controlling for alcohol consumption; the third study, from the USA, did not show any association [51]. The age-adjusted risk for male smokers was 0.73 (95% CI, 0.48 –1.11) and that for females was 0.99 (95% CI, 0.56–1.69) [52]. In conclusion, only in Greece and Hong Kong has a convincing association between tobacco smoking and HBsAg-negative HCC been demonstrated.

3.5 Alcohol consumption

The proportion of alcoholics who develop chronic liver disease is unknown, but it is probably low. Usually, chronic liver disease occurs in those who have been drinking excessively for years. Alcohol is probably the most important factor in the causation of chronic liver disease in most European countries, the Americas, and Australia. The most significant lesion is chronic alcohol hepatitis, characterized by a neutrophil polymorph inflammatory reaction, especially around liver cells containing Mallory's hyaline, fibrosis for the portal tracts and centrilobular areas, and fatty changes [53]. Alcoholic hepatitis usually terminates in cirrhosis, especially when drinking continues.

Although there is no experimental evidence indicating that alcohol per se is carcinogenic, there are some epidemiological studies which suggest that alcohol consumption is associated with an increased risk for HCC. A case-control study conducted in Los Angeles, USA, reported an RR of 4.2 (95% CI, 1.3–13.8) for those who drank 80 g or more ethanol/day as compared with those who drank less than 10 g/day, and this increased risk persisted after adjustment was made for the other risk factors; no information on the HBsAg status of cases and controls was, however, available [49]. A significant dose-response relationship was found for both males and females in another case-control study in New Jersey, USA, but no risk estimates were significantly different from 1.0 [51]. In a case-control

study in Sweden, a fourfold increase in the risk for HCC (95% CI, 1.8–10.8) was found for heavy drinkers (more than 370 ml spirits/week) and a threefold increase (95% CI, 1.0–8.7) for regular drinkers (more than 370 ml spirits/month but less than 370 ml/week) [50]. In the case-control study within a cohort in Japan, a strong positive association with alcohol and a dose-response relationship were demonstrated: For heavy drinkers (more than 80 ml alcohol/day), an RR of 8.0 (95% CI, 1.3–49.5) was found and this increased risk persisted after adjusting for smoking [27]. In four cohort studies in Norway, Finland, Denmark, and Japan, an increased risk for HCC has been observed among groups identified as having an excessive consumption of alcohol [54]. On the other hand, no association with alcohol consumption was observed in two case-control studies in Greece and Hong Kong [19, 22], and in some cohort studies among alcoholics an increased risk for HCC has not been demonstrated [55].

3.6 Cirrhosis and HCC

An association between cirrhosis and HCC has long been recognized but not clearly understood. No correlation has been observed between the mortality from cirrhosis and the mortality from HCC in different geographical areas. The highest death rates for cirrhosis are observed in Chile, Mexico, Portugal, France, Puerto Rico, Italy, Ireland, and Austria, which have low rates for HCC; lower death rates for cirrhosis are reported in Thailand, Hong Kong, and Greece, which have relatively high rates for HCC. This information is derived from material available at the WHO Data Bank [7]. Cirrhosis is a dynamic condition of varied etiologies with different malignant potentials, which may explain why no agreement has been reached concerning a morphological classification and why no correlation has been observed between death rates for cirrhosis as a whole and HCC. The simple morphological classification of macronodular and micronodular is useful in explaining the association of cirrhosis with liver cancer. The macronodular type is more frequent in Africa and Southeast Asia, high-incidence areas for HCC, and the micronodular type is prevalent in the low-risk areas of Europe and the USA. The macronodular type appears to be more often associated with HBV and it tends to be subclinical; in most cases, the first signs of illness appear with the HCC. On the other hand, the micronodular type is prevalent in the low-risk areas for HCC, i.e., Europe and the USA, and is often of alcoholic etiology; HCC in these areas is usually a late development in cirrhosis of several years' duration.

There is no agreement on the oncogenic potential of the different types of cirrhosis. The essential point to determine is whether the etiological agents of the cirrhosis also cause the HCC, the regenerative process associated with any cirrhosis leads by itself to HCC, or both mechanisms are involved. The available evidence indicates that HBV causes both cirrhosis and HCC but that the development of cirrhosis is not a necessary event in the chain leading to HCC. In Senegal, it was estimated that 62% of cases of HCC that were positive for HBsAg arose in non-cirrhotic livers and that the strength of the association with HBV was similar for HCC with and without cirrhosis [17]. However, in a recent study in Greece it was shown that the association between HBV and HCC is stronger among patients with cirrhosis (RR, 31) than among patients without cirrhosis (RR, 7) [22]. In addition, a cohort study of 115 subjects with cirrhosis in Japan has shown a fourfold increase in the risk for HCC among those with HBsAg-positive cirrhosis as compared with those with HBsAg-negative cirrhosis [56]. Another cohort study of 590 patients with cirrhosis in the UK did not yield similar results, but the statistical analysis of their data is questionable [57].

The above data suggest that HBV can cause HCC by initiating the carcinogenic process or by acting both as an initiator and as a late-stage carcinogen through the liver cell regeneration associated with cirrhosis. With respect to alcohol and other cirrhogenic agents, there is no evidence of a direct carcinogenic effect; therefore, if they are accepted as causes of HCC they may act through cirrhosis-related liver regeneration, although an increased risk for HCC in alcoholics in the absence of cirrhosis has been reported [58]. It has been suggested that HBV could be the ultimate cause of HCC in patients with alcoholic liver disease without HBsAg in the serum but with HBV-DNA integrated in the liver cells [59]. However, other studies have shown that HBV-DNA integration is common only in HCC patients with HBsAg in the serum [60].

3.7 Other risk factors

Sex hormones. The increased risk for liver cell adenomas among women using oral contraceptives is well known [61], but an association between the contraceptive pill and HCC has not

been established. The occurrence of HCC in patients with aplastic anemia after long-term treatment with androgenic-anabolic steroids has been reported [62]; however, prolonged survival and even regression have been observed in some patients after discontinuation of the steroid therapy.

Parasites. An association between schistosomiasis and HCC has been suggested, based on reports of the simultaneous occurrence of the two lesions [63] and an inconclusive case-control study [64].

Thorotrast. A few cases of HCC have been reported to occur many years after the administration of Thorotrast. Most of the liver tumors associated with this radioactive element have been classified as hemangiosarcomas and cholangiocarcinomas [65].

Genetic factors. An increased risk for HCC has been suggested in patients with α-antitrypsin deficiency, but this suggestion has not been confirmed [66]. The association with hemochromatosis, a rare inherited metabolic abnormality, is present only in patients who live long enough to develop cirrhosis [66].

4 Perspectives for prevention

Although the future of treatment of liver cancer cannot be considered promising, there may be very real prospects for the primary prevention of this cancer, which affects so many in large, heavily populated countries of the Far East and Africa. It is felt that the emphasis should fall on primary prevention rather than on early detection, as screening would have to be at very frequent intervals in very large populations [67] (Li HK and co-workers, personal communication, 1985). These estimates are based on the extremely rapid growth of the tumor. Studies in China and South Africa indicate that screening would be required at least every 6 months, but it is unlikely that screening would be effective in reducing HCC mortality.

From the previous section it can be concluded that in the high-risk areas of Africa and Southeast Asia, HBV and aflatoxin account for most cases of HCC. The proportion of the risk attributable to HBV in these areas ranges from 50% to 90%; the proportion attributable to aflatoxin cannot be quantified at present. In the low-risk populations, the proportion of the risk attributable to HBV ranges from 5% to 15%, and aflatoxin probably plays a minimal role, if any, in the development of HCC. The proportion of HCC attributable to heavy smoking among HBsAg-negative subjects both in high- and low-risk populations ranges from 27% to 40% and that attributable to heavy alcohol drinking, especially in the low-risk populations, is between 15% and 50%. Consequently, the prevention measures which will have a great impact in the high-risk populations for HCC are those aiming at the elimination of the HBsAg carrier state and the reduction of aflatoxin exposure.

The importance of reducing the contamination of food by mycotoxins such as aflatoxin is obvious, as apart from their potential as carcinogens they are also acute toxic hazards. Such contamination is primarily a problem for developing countries where agriculture is based mainly on small subsistence farms. The measures that will reduce contamination of foodstuffs by aflatoxins—improved methods of harvesting and storage—will also reduce food losses from insect and rodent damage and, therefore, it is generally advantageous for these methods to be adopted by agricultural administrations. However, it is difficult to assess the success of such interventions on liver cancer, as this requires experimental conditions and a long observation period.

It has been suggested that the prevention of hepatitis B could be the most successful form of primary prevention of HCC. Several safe and effective HBV vaccines have been and are being used in large-scale trials [68–71]. Vaccination strategies should take into consideration geographical patterns in the prevalence rates of HBsAg. Mass vaccination of all infants has been recommended for countries with high or intermediate prevalence rates and vaccination of only high-risk groups for populations with low HBsAg prevalence rates [72]. Table 1.9 summarizes the estimated reduction in the incidence of HCC expected after mass vaccination programs aimed at all infants from high-risk populations, where various degrees of vaccination coverage are achieved, assuming that 80% of cases of HCC under 50 years of age are attributable to HBV. It can be seen, then, that under scheme I, in which 85% of the eligible children present themselves for at least one injection of the HBV vaccine, 80% for at least two injections, and 75% for all three injections, a reduction of 58% in the HCC incidence could be expected. This estimate has been calculated taking into consideration that: (1) After only one shot, 20% of the children

Table 1.9. Effect of different degrees of HBV vaccination coverage on the incidence of HCC

	Scheme I	Scheme II	Scheme III
Coverage achieved (%)			
Fully vaccinated (3 shots)	75	50	25
Partially vaccinated (2 shots)	5	10	15
Partially vaccinated (1 shot)	5	10	15
Unvaccinated	15	30	45
Expected proportion of reduction of HCC incidence (%)	58	44	29

respond with the production of anti-HBs, after two shots 80%, and after three injections 95% (2) 10% of the HBsAg carriers are infected perinatally and only 50% of them are protected by vaccination. Scheme I is the anticipated result in a large-scale intervention study which the IARC is just initiating in Gambia [71]. Under scheme III, in which only 25% of the children receive the three injections and 45% remain unvaccinated, a reduction of only one-third in the HCC incidence could be expected.

In summary, in the high-risk populations for HCC, the prospects are bright for the prevention of HBV infection through a safe and efficient HBV vaccine. This may ultimately affect not only the incidence of acute HBV infection and the pool of chronic carriers but may also reduce the morbidity and mortality from chronic active hepatitis, cirrhosis, and HCC. In the low-risk populations for HCC, elimination of heavy smoking and alcohol consumption would probably have a greater impact on HCC incidence than HBV vaccination of high-risk groups. Tobacco smoking and alcohol consumption are worldwide problems, control of which is the subject of much effort in many countries; their important sequelae are undoubtedly heart disease, cancers of the lung, larynx, esophagus, oral cavity, and bladder, chronic lung diseases, and cirrhosis, but their control could also reduce HCC mortality.

References

1. Parkin DM, Stjernswärd J, Muir CS (1984) Estimates of the worldwide frequency of twelve major cancers. Bull Wld Hlth Org 62: 163–182
2. Parkin DM (ed) (1986) Cancer occurrence in developing countries. International Agency for Re-

search on Cancer, Lyon (IARC Scientific Publications no. 75)

3. Doll R, Payne P, Waterhouse J (eds) (1966) Cancer incidence in five continents. A technical report. Springer, Berlin Heidelberg New York

4. Doll R, Muir C, Waterhouse J (eds) (1970) Cancer incidence in five continents, vol. II. Springer, Berlin Heidelberg New York

5. Waterhouse JAH, Muir CS, Correa P, Powell J (eds) (1976) Cancer incidence in five continents, vol. III. International Agency for Research on Cancer, Lyon (IARC Scientific Publications no. 15)

6. Waterhouse JAH, Muir C, Shanmugaratnam K, Powell J (eds) (1982) Cancer incidence in five continents, vol. IV. International Agency for Research on Cancer, Lyon (IARC Scientific Publications no. 42)

7. World Health Organization (1982) World health statistics annual, 1978–1982. Vital statistics and causes of death. WHO, Gereva

8. Chinese Academy of Medical Sciences (1981) Atlas of cancer mortality in the People's Republic of China. China Map Press, Beijing

9. Robertson MA, Harington JS, Bradshaw E (1971) The cancer pattern in Africans at Baragwanath Hospital, Johannesburg. Br J Cancer 25: 377–384

10. Harington JS, McGlashan ND, Bradshaw E, Geddes EW, Purves LR (1975) A spatial and temporal analysis of four cancers in African gold miners from Southern Africa. Br J Cancer 31: 665–678

11. Bradshaw E, McGlashand ND, Fitzgerald D, Harington JS (1982) Analyses of cancer incidence in black gold miners from Southern Africa (1964–79). Br J Cancer 46: 737–748

12. Van Rensburg SJ, Cook-Mozaffari P, van Schalkwyk DJ, van der Watt JJ, Vincent TJ, Purchase IF (1985) Hepatocellular carcinoma and dietary aflatoxin in Mozambique and Transkei. Br J Cancer 51: 713–726

13. Shanmugaratnam K, Lee HP, Day NE (eds) (1983) Cancer incidence in Singapore 1968–1977 (IARC Scientific Publications no. 47). International Agency for Research on Cancer, Lyon

14. Szmuness W (1978) Hepatocellular carcinoma and the hepatitis B virus: evidence for a causal association. Prog Med Virol 24: 40–69

15. Muñoz N, Linsell A (1982) Epidemiology of primary liver cancer. In: Correa P, Haenszel W (eds) Epidemiology of cancer of the digestive tract. Nijhoff, The Hague, pp 161–195

16. Melbye M, Skinhøj P, Højgaard Nielsen N, Vestergaard BF, Ebbesen P, Hart Hansen JP, Biggar RJ (1984) Virus-associated cancers in Greenland: frequent hepatitis B virus infection but low primary hepatocellular carcinoma incidence. J Natl Cancer Inst 73: 1267–1272

17. Prince AM, Szmuness W, Michon J, Desmaille J, Diebolt G, Linhard J, Quenum C, Sankale M (1975) A case-control study of the association between primary liver cancer and hepatitis B infection in Senegal. Int J Cancer 16: 376–383

18. Kew MC, Desmyter J, Bradburne AF, Macnab GM (1979) Hepatitis B virus infection in southern African blacks with hepatocellular cancer. J Natl Cancer Inst 62: 517–520

19. Lam KC, Yu MC, Leung JWC, Henderson BE (1982) Hepatitis B virus and cigarette smoking: risk factors for hepatocellular carcinoma in Hong Kong. Cancer Res 42: 5246–5248

20. Yeh FS, Mo CC, Luo S, Henderson BE, Tong MJ, Yu MC (1985) A serological case-control study of primary hepatocellular carcinoma in Guangxi, China. Cancer Res 45: 872–873

21. Lingao AL, Domingo EO, Nishioka K (1981) Hepatitis B virus profile of hepatocellular carcinoma in the Philippines. Cancer 48: 1590–1595

22. Trichopoulos D, Day N, Kaklamani E, Tzonou A, Muñoz N, Zavitsanos X, Koumantaki Y, Trichopoulou A (1987) Tobacco smoking, hepatitis B virus and ethanol consumption in the etiology of hepatocellular carcinoma. Int J Cancer (in press)

23. Yarrish RL, Werner BG, Blumberg BS (1980) Association of hepatitis B virus infection with hepatocellular carcinoma in American patients. Int J Cancer, 26: 711–715

24. Austin H, Delzell E, Grufferman S, Levine R, Morrison AS, Stolley PD, Cole P (1985) A case-control study of hepatocellular carcinoma and the hepatitis B virus, cigarette smoking, and alcohol consumption. Cancer Res 46: 962–966

25. Beasley R, Lin C, Hwang LY, Chien CS (1981) Hepatocellular carcinoma and hepatitis B virus. A prospective study of 32 707 men in Taiwan. Lancet ii: 1129–1133

26. Iijima T, Saitoh N, Nobutomo K, Nambu M, Sakuma K (1984) A prospective cohort study of hepatitis B surface antigen carriers in a working population. Gann 75: 571–573

27. Oshima A, Tsukuma H, Hiyama T, Fujimoto I, Yamano H, Tanaka M (1984) Follow-up study of HBs Ag-positive blood donors with special reference to effect of drinking and smoking on development of liver cancer. Int J Cancer 34: 775–779

28. Prince AM, Alcabes P (1982) The risk of development of hepatocellular carcinoma in hepatitis B virus carriers in New York. A preliminary estimate using death-records matching. Hepatol 2: 15S–20S

29. Hall AJ, Winter PD, Wright R (1985) Mortality of hepatitis B positive blood donors in England and Wales. Lancet i: 91–93

30. Trichopoulos D, Tabor E, Gerety RJ, Xirouchaki E, Sparros L, Muñoz N, Linsell CA (1978) Hepatitis B and primary hepatocellular carcinoma in a European population. Lancet ii: 1217–1219

31. Szmuness W, Prince AM, Diebolt G, Leblanc L, Baylet R, Masseyeff R, Linhard J (1973) The epidemiology of hepatitis B infections in Africa: results of a pilot survey in the Republic of Senegal. Am J Epidemiol 98: 104–110

32. Edman JC, Gray P, Valenzuela P, Rall LB, Rutter WJ (1980) Integration of hepatitis B virus sequences and their expression in a human hepa-

toma cell line. Nature 286: 535–538

33. Shafritz DA, Shouval D, Sherman HI, Hadziyannis SJ, Kew MC (1981) Integration of hepatitis B virus DNA into the genome of liver cells in chronic liver disease and hepatocellular carcinoma. Studies in percutaneous liver biopsies and post-mortem tissue specimens. N Engl J Med 305: 1067–1073

34. Summers J (1981) Three recently described animal virus models for human hepatitis B virus. Hepatol 1: 179–183

35. Busby WF, Wogan GN (1984) Aflatoxins. In: Searle CE (ed) Chemical carcinogens, 2nd edn. American Chemical Society, Washington, pp 945–1136

36. Sinnhuber RO, Wales JH, Ayres JL, Engebrecht RH, Amend DL (1968) Dietary factors and hepatoma in rainbow trout (Salmo gairdnesi): I. Aflatoxin in vegetable protein foodstuffs. J Natl Cancer Inst 41: 711–718

37. Halver JE (1969) Aflatoxin. In: Goldblatt LA (ed) Academic Press, New York, pp 265–306

38. Wogan GN (1973) In: Busch H (ed) Methods in Cancer Res vol 7: Academic Press, New York pp 309–344

39. Wogan GN, Newberne PM (1967) Aflatoxin carcinogenesis. Cancer Res 27: 2370–2376

40. Garner C, Ryder R, Montesano R (1985) Monitoring of aflatoxins in human body fluids and application to field studies. Cancer Res 45: 922–928

41. Peers FG, Linsell CA (1973) Dietary aflatoxins and liver cancer. A population based study in Kenya. Br J Cancer 27: 473–484

42. Peers FG, Gilman GA, Linsell CA (1976) Dietary aflatoxins and human liver cancer. A study in Swaziland. Int J Cancer 17: 167–176

43. Peers FG, Bosch FX, Kaldor JM, Linsell CA (1987) Aflatoxin exposure, hepatitis B virus and liver cancer in Swaziland. Int J Cancer (in press)

44. Shank RC, Gordon JE, Wogan GN, Nondasuta A, Subhamani B (1972) Dietary aflatoxins and human liver cancer: III. Field survey of rural Thai families for ingested aflatoxins. Fd Cosmet Toxicol 10: 71–84

45. Bulatao-Jayme J, Almero EM, Castro CA, Jardeleza TR, Salamat LA (1982) A case-control dietary study of primary liver cancer risk from aflatoxin exposure. Int J Epidemiol 11: 112–119

46. Garfinkel L (1980) Cancer mortality in non-smokers. Prospective study by the American Cancer Society. J Natl Cancer Inst 65: 1169–1173

47. Hirayama T (1981) A large-scale cohort study on the relationship between diet and selected cancers of digestive organs. In: Bruce WR, Correa P, Lipkin M, Tannenbaum S, Wilkins T (eds) Gastro-intestinal cancer: Endogenous factors, Banbury Report 7. CSH Press, Cold Spring Harbor, pp 409–426

48. Trichopoulos D, MacMahon B, Sparros L, Merikas G (1980) Smoking and hepatitis B-negative primary hepatocellular carcinoma. J Natl Cancer Inst 65: 111–114

49. Yu MC, Mack T, Hanisch R, Peters RL, Henderson BE, Pike MC (1983) Hepatitis, alcohol consumption, cigarette smoking, and hepatocellular carcinoma in Los Angeles. Cancer Res 43: 6077–6079

50. Hardell L, Bengtsson NO, Jonsson U, Eriksson S, Larsson LG (1984) Aetiological aspects on primary liver cancer with special regard to alcohol, organic solvents and acute intermittent porphyria —an epidemiological investigation. Br J Cancer 50: 389–397

51. Stemhagen A, Slade J, Altman R, Bill J (1983) Occupational risk factors and liver cancer. A retrospective case-control study of primary liver cancer in New Jersey. Am J Epidemiol 117: 443–454

52. Austin H, Delzell E, Grufferman S, Levine R, Morrison AS, Stolley PD, Cole P (1986) A case-control study of hepatocellular carcinoma and the hepatitis B virus, cigarette smoking, and alcohol consumption. Cancer Res 46: 962–966

53. Anthony PP (1976) Pathology of hepatocellular carcinoma. In: Cameron HM, Linsell CA, Warwick GP (eds) Liver cell cancer Elsevier, Amsterdam, pp 93–120

54. Tuyns A (1980) Alcohol. In: Schottenfeld D, Fraumeni JF (eds) Cancer epidemiology and prevention. Saunders, Philadelphia, pp 293–303

55. Rothman KJ (1980) The proportion of cancer attributable to alcohol consumption. Prev Med 9: 174–179

56. Obata H, Hayashi N, Motoike Y, Hisamitsu T, Okuda H, Koibayashi S, Nishioka K (1980) A prospective study on the development of hepatocellular carcinoma from liver cirrhosis with persistent hepatitis B virus infection. Int J Cancer 25: 741–747

57. Zaman SN, Melia WM, Johnson RD, Portmann BC, Johnson PJ, Williams R (1985) Risk factors in development of hepatocellular carcinoma in cirrhosis: prospective study of 613 patients. Lancet ii: 1357–1360

58. Lieber CS, Seitz HK, Garro AJ, Worner TM (1979) Alcohol-related diseases and carcinogenesis. Cancer Res 39: 2863–2866

59. Brechot C, Nalpas B, Courouce AM, Duhamel G, Callard P, Carnot F, Tiollais P, Bethelot P (1982) Evidence that hepatitis B virus has a role in liver-cell carcinoma in alcoholic liver disease. N Engl J Med 306: 1384–1387

60. Hino O, Kitagawa T, Sugano H (1985) Relationship between serum and histochemical markers for hepatitis B virus and rate of viral integration in hepatocellular carcinomas in Japan. Int J Cancer 35: 5–10

61. Jick H, Herman R (1978) Oral contraceptive-induced benign liver tumors. The magnitude of the problem. J Am Med Assoc 240: 828–829

62. Guy JT, Smith RE (1980) Androgens and hepatocellular carcinoma. In: Nieburgs HE (ed) Prevention and detection of cancer, part II: Detection, vol. 2: Cancer detection in specific sites. Marcel Dekker, New York, pp 217–285

63. Nakashima T, Okuda K, Kajino M, Sakamoto K,

Kubo Y, Shimokawa Y (1975) Primary liver cancer coincident with schistosomiasis japonica. Cancer 36: 1483–1489

64. Inaba Y, Maruchi N, Matsuda M, Yoshihara N, Yamamoto SI (1984) A case-control study on liver cancer with special emphasis on the possible aetiological role of schistosomiasis. Int J Epidemiol 13: 408–412

65. Battifora HA (1976) Thorotrast and tumours of the liver. In: Okuda K, Peters RL (eds) Hepatocellular carcinoma. Wiley, New York, pp 83–93

66. Okuda K, Mackay I (eds) (1982) Hepatocellular carcinoma. International Union Against Cancer, Geneva (UICC Technical Report Series vol. 74)

67. Leblanc L, Tuyns AJ, Masseyeff R (1973) Screening for primary liver cancer. Digestion 8: 8–14

68. Maupas P, Chiron JP, Barin F, Coursaget P, Goudeau A, Perrin J, Denis F, Diop Mar I (1981) Efficacy of hepatitis B vaccine in prevention of early HBsAg carrier state in children. Controlled trial in an endemic area (Senegal). Lancet i: 289–292

69. Szmuness W, Stevens CE, Harley EJ, Zang EA, Oleszko WR, William DC, Sadovsky R, Morrison JM, Kellner A (1980) Hepatitis B vaccine. Demonstration of efficacy in a controlled clinical trial in a high-risk population in the United States. N Engl J Med 303: 833–841

70. Beasley RP, Hwang LY, Stevens CE, Lin CC, Hsieh FJ, Wang KY, Sun TS, Szmuness W (1983) Efficacy of hepatitis B immune globulin for prevention of perinatal transmission of the hepatitis B virus carrier state: final report of a randomized double-blind, placebo-controlled trial. Hepatol 3: 135–141

71. IARC (1984) Annual Report. International Agency for Research on Cancer, Lyon, pp 50–51

72. World Health Organization (1983) Prevention of Liver Cancer (Technical Report Series vol. 691). World Health Organization, Geneva

Chapter 2

Hepatitis B Virus Infection and Hepatocellular Carcinoma

HARVEY M. LIEBERMAN[1], RAN TUR-KASPA[1], and DAVID A. SHAFRITZ[2]

1 Introduction

The association between persistent infection with hepatitis B virus (HBV) and the development of hepatocellular carcinoma (HCC) has been strengthened by substantial recent evidence. This evidence consists of both retrospective and prospective epidemiological studies, molecular studies of human tissue and HCC cell lines obtained from human HBV carriers who developed liver cancer, and studies of animal models infected with viruses closely related to HBV. Although the mechanism(s) by which persistent HBV infection and development of HCC are related remain largely unknown, techniques of modern molecular biology offer the means by which such answers may be obtained in the future. In this chapter, evidence supporting the association between persistent infection with HBV and the development of primary liver cancer will be examined in the hope of offering insight into the possible mechanism(s) of carcinogenesis as related to HBV infection.

2 Epidemiology of persistent HBV infection and development of HCC

Several lines of epidemiological evidence support an association between persistent HBV infection and development of HCC [1–3].

2.1 Geographical correlation between persistent viral infection and incidence of HCC

The worldwide prevalence of HBV infection, defined by hepatitis B surface antigen (HBsAg)

Department of Medicine[1] and Department of Cell Biology[2], Marion Bessin Liver Research Center, Albert Einstein College of Medicine, 1300 Morris Park Avenue, Bronx, NY 10461, USA

in serum, varies considerably by location, being lowest in North America and Western Europe (0.1%–1.0% of blood donors), while in other regions, such as Southeast Asia and Africa, the prevalence is at least ten fold higher [1, 2]. Although many of these data are poorly documented and subject to bias, it is clear that while the mean proportions of HCC found on autopsy in the USA and Europe are only 0.39% and 0.45% (range 0.22%–1.65%), respectively, the proportion of HCC found at autopsy in Africa and East Asia, where HBV is common, is 2%–8%, a difference of up to ten fold compared with Western countries. HCC constitutes only 2.5% of total cancers in the USA and Western Europe, whereas in areas of Africa and Southeast Asia, it comprises 20%–40% of all cancers, making it one of the commonest malignancies and the most common fatal malignancy among males in these regions. While death from HCC varies from 3 to 7/100 000 population/year in Western countries, this rate varies between 20 and 100/100 000 population/year in some regions of southern Africa and Southeast Asia, thus demonstrating a general correlation between HBsAg carrier rates in different world regions and death rates from HCC [1].

2.2 Increased prevalence of HBV serum markers in patients with HCC

In Africa, between 45% and 80% of patients with HCC have HBsAg in their sera, while the prevalence of serum HBsAg in individuals without HCC in these areas is between 6% and 14%. Similar patterns are seen in countries with a low prevalence of HBsAg carriers, such as the USA and Europe, where the prevalence of HBsAg by radioimmunoassay (RIA) is less than 2% in control populations and 26%–71% in patients having HCC. Such differences in HBV markers between control populations and those with HCC increase if one includes patients with hepatitis B core antibody (anti-HBc) as a marker of HBV infection [1, 2]. In addition, the levels of HBsAg in the sera of patients with HCC appear to be reduced compared with non-HCC carrier patients in the same geographical region, suggesting that HCC occurs after a prolonged carrier state in which virus replication is less active or has ceased.

2.3 Prospective studies on increased risk of developing HCC among HBV carriers

To demonstrate a specific causal relationship between persistent HBV infection and the development of HCC, a prospective study was carried out showing continued viral infection antecedent to the development of HCC and persistent infection during malignant transformation by Beasley and Hwang, involving 22 707 male subjects in Taiwan [3]. All patients were examined for presence of HBV markers at the time of entry into the study; 15.2% had serum HBsAg. During a mean follow-up period of 7 years, 116 cases of HCC occurred, of which 113 patients were positive for HBsAg, and the three HBsAg-negative patients had either serum anti-HBc or serum anti-HBc and anti-HBs. From this study, the relative risk of developing HCC was determined to be more than 200-fold greater in individuals with evidence of HBV infection than in noninfected individuals. The excess risk of developing HCC after exposure to HBV provides the strongest epidemiological evidence for an etiological role of HBV. This study also indicates that development of HCC is not simply related to HBV infection but also requires persistence of virus infection (i.e., to the chronic HBsAg carrier state).

3 Genetic organization of HBV

The hepatitis DNA (hepadna) virus family currently comprises four members—human [4], woodchuck [5, 6], ground squirrel [5, 7], and duck [5, 8]. All have similar virion structure, genome organization, and mechanism of viral replication. The HBV genome is a small, circular, partially double-stranded DNA molecule with a single-stranded region of variable length (Fig. 2.1). The long (L) or minus (−) strand is complete but nicked and is of fixed length (~3200 nucleotides). The short (S) or plus (+) strand is of variable length, ranging from 1700–2800 bases in different molecules. DNA polymerase activity in the virion repairs the single-stranded

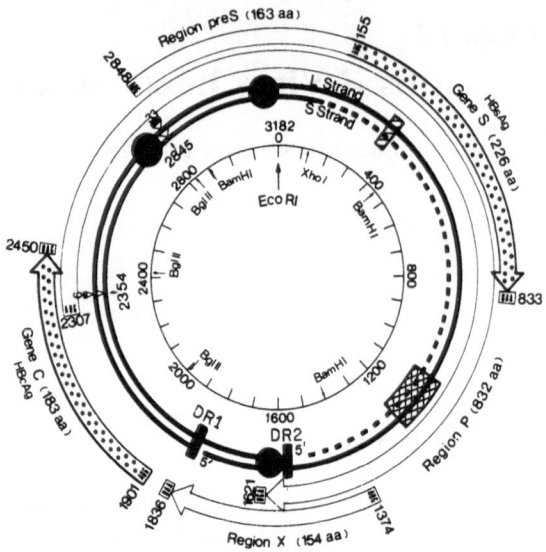

Fig. 2.1. Restriction map of hepatitis B virus genome illustrating the four open reading frames capable of transcribing mRNA for specific viral proteins and regulatory sequences capable of controlling or modulating transcription of specific viral genes. The positions on this map of HBV promoters (●), the known HBV enhancer (▨), and a recently described putative glucocorticoid responsive element (▨) involved in HBV gene expression. After Tiollais et al. [100]

region in viral DNA to make a fully double-stranded molecule. The positions of the 5'-ends of the L (−) and S (+) strands are fixed, while the positions of the 3'-end of the S (+) strand are variable. Maintenance of a circular structure of the genome is assured by base-pairing of the 5'-ends of the two strands. The 5'-ends of the S (+) and L (−) strands were recently mapped to positions 1601 and 1826 from the EcoRl site on viral DNA (Fig. 2.1). At both sides of the cohesive ends, there is an 11-base-pair direct repeat (DR) sequence 5'-TTCACCTCTGC. The two copies of this sequence, which start at nucleotides 1824 and 1590, are termed DR1 and DR2, respectively. If the nicked but repaired DNA were linearized and the overlapping ends filled in, the HBV genome would resemble a retrovirus proviral DNA with a large direct repeat at each end. The structural genes of HBV are also organized in a fashion similar to retroviruses. The complete nucleotide sequences of the cloned DNAs of nine HBV isolates [9] have been reported. There are four open reading frames in the complete L (−) DNA strand (Fig. 2.1) and these have similar locations in each hepadna virus [10]. The C gene codes for the major viral core or nucleocapsid polypeptide. The S gene, including preS1 and preS2 regions, specifies the viral surface antigen polypeptides in the virion envelope and in surface antigen particles, found in the serum and liver of infected individuals. The P gene is thought to code for the DNA polymerase (or reverse transcriptase). The X gene specifies a polypeptide of unknown function. Evidence for X-gene expression in natural HBV infections is limited to the finding of antibodies to synthetic X polypeptides in the serum of some patients [11]. The "e" antigen, a structural protein derived from the C gene, uses the same reading frame as core antigen but a separate ATG initiation site.

3.1 Regulatory sequences

Recent in vitro and in vivo studies [12–14] have revealed that the HBV genome contains at least three RNA polymerase II-dependent promoters— the presurface gene promoter (SPI), the surface gene promoter (SPII), and the core promoter (CP). In addition, an enhancer element has been located at map position 1080–1234, 5' to the core-gene promoter [15]. Gene enhancers are recognized as potent activators of transcription, perhaps by providing an entry site for RNA polymerase II. The regulatory elements, promoters or enhancers, exhibit tissue/host-specific action similar to that reported for a number of viral and cellular genes [16]. For example, the HBV enhancer exhibits a preferred activity in human hepatocytes. In addition, transgenic mice containing integrated HBV DNA express viral proteins, such as HBsAg, in a liver tissue-specific manner [17]. Therefore, it seems that the HBV enhancer requires a transacting factor or factors present in liver cells [18]. This factor is required for HBV enhancer activity. The tissue-specific expression of the HBV enhancer might explain in part the tendency of hepadna viruses to infect or replicate in liver tissue.

We have recently demonstrated that HBV enhancer activity is stimulated by glucocorticoids [19]. This stimulatory effect appears to occur via a glucocorticoid responsive element (GRE) in HBV DNA located 5' to the enhancer on the S gene. Such GRE sequences have been identified in the mouse mammary tumor virus (MMTV) genome and the cellular genes coding for growth hormone and metallothionein IIa, which are known to be regulated by glucocorticoids [20].

3.2 HBV replication

The hepadna virus replication mechanism is different from that of other DNA viruses [21]. The replication cycle involves a reverse transcrip-

tase step using a full-length copy of virion DNA (+) mRNA, transcribed from the L (−) strand of supercoiled virus DNA. This RNA synthesis is initiated at DR1 and is referred to as "pregenome" RNA. It is transported from the nucleus to the cytoplasm, where it binds to viral proteins from core particles. The viral DNA L (−) strand is synthesized within core particles using the presumed viral polymerase. The S (+) strand is then transcribed from the L (−) strand, beginning at DR2. Core particles are assembled into complete virions with HBsAg and a cell membrane lipid-containing envelope. In HBV, virus formation and release from cells can take place at almost any step after intracellular assembly of the core particles, since virions (Dane particles) in blood contain either incompletely partly double-stranded circular DNA molecules or HBV DNA-RNA hybrids [22].

4 Molecular studies of chronic HBV infection

The use of molecular hybridization technology has enabled the study of HBV-related diseases through the detection of specific HBV DNA sequences in serum and human tissues [23–39]. Using cloned HBV DNA probes of high specific activity and Southern blot techniques, HBV DNA has been found in the liver and serum of chronically infected individuals all over the world. HBV DNA in the serum is thought to represent virion DNA and its presence correlates with active viral replication.

Direct analysis of serum by spot hybridization shows a good correlation between serum DNA and other markers of viral replication, such as HBcAg in hepatocyte nuclei and DNA polymerase, but not necessarily with HBeAg/anti-HBe status [25, 31, 37]. During acute viral hepatitis, HBsAg and HBeAg are present in the serum and HBV DNA is detectable. HBeAg-positive chronic carriers are presumed to be infectious and most of these patients have circulating HBV DNA as well as HBcAg in the liver cell nuclei, suggesting that they have active virus replication. Many of these patients have some form of chronic liver disease. In contrast, HBsAg carriers who are anti-HBe positive were previously thought to have passed the stage of active viral replication and were considered to be noninfectious. However, HBsAg-positive/anti-HBeAg-positive patients often have detectable HBV DNA in the serum and also have active chronic liver disease, despite the fact that they are HBeAg negative [38, 39]. Most of these patients are also positive for core antigen in hepatocyte nuclei. In our studies [38], all patients with a normal liver histological condition (i.e., normal except for the presence of "ground-glass" hepatocytes) were serum HBV DNA negative. These findings demonstrated a correlation between continued activity of chronic liver disease, serum HBV DNA, and virus replication in the liver independent of the HBeAg/anti-HBe status. This group of patients with chronic liver disease who are HBeAg negative but serum HBV DNA positive appears to represent a previously unrecognized subgroup. Yokosuka et al. have reported that these patients have a most virulent form of chronic active hepatitis, often progressing rapidly to cirrhosis [40].

HBsAg carriers who have been positive for HBsAg for less than 2 years do not generally have detectable integrated HBV sequences in the liver, as analyzed by restriction enzyme analysis and Southern blot hybridization [24]. HBV DNA is usually found in these patients in a free virion (replicative) form, irrespective of the presence or absence of liver disease. Integrated HBV DNA has been found in longer term chronic HBsAg carriers (more than 2 years), regardless of the histological status of the liver. In some of these latter patients, the HBV DNA is integrated diffusely through the hepatocyte genome, but in others the HBV DNA integration pattern shows unique bands, suggesting its presence in a clonal population of cells.

Thus, chronic infections often progress from a replicating phase, in which virus is secreted into the blood, to a nonreplicating phase, in which no virus is found in the blood and a random integration of viral DNA in the cellular genome is present [41]. Later, it appears that there is a relationship between HBV DNA integration into the host cellular genome, clonal expansion of such cells, and the development of HCC (see sections 5.2 and 8).

5 Molecular studies of HBV-related HCC

Substantial insight into the relationship between persistent HBV infection and HCC has been gained through the use of molecular cloning and DNA sequencing. Through the use of Southern blot analysis, molecular hybridization techniques have been applied to study the relationship of persistent HBV infection to the molecular state of viral DNA and development of HCC. Since most animal tumor viruses (adenovirus, EBV, SV40) integrate into the host cellular genome during the process of viral transformation [42], one would hypothesize that the HBV viral genome should be integrated into the genome of HCC. This has been determined by Southern blot analysis through the finding of specific hybridization bands after restriction enzyme analysis with Hind III, suggesting unique integration of the HBV genome into many liver cells [details, 23, 24]. This finding strongly implies clonal expansion of such cells. Such studies have been conducted with human HCC cell lines, tissues from human HCC, and animal models of closely related DNA viruses.

5.1 Human HCC cell lines

Initial molecular studies demonstrating HBV integration into liver tumor genomes were performed on cell line PLC/PRF/5, established by Alexander and colleagues from a liver tumor of a young male chronic HBV carrier with HCC from Mozambique (43), as shown in Fig. 2.2. This cell line is hepatocytic in origin, secretes liver-specific and oncofetal proteins, and demonstrates a transformed phenotype [44, 45]. Despite copious production of HBsAg [43], other known HBV proteins are not expressed nor are virions produced. Initial Southern blot hybridization analysis of tumor DNA subjected to restriction enzyme digestion has demonstrated HBV DNA to be integrated into eight sites, comprising approximately four total genome equivalents [15, 26, 27, 46]. All of these integrations have been cloned and mapped by restriction enzyme analysis and DNA sequencing, revealing duplication and inversion of viral sequences in one case and deletion in another [47, 48]. Rearrangements of cellular sequences flanking the integrated HBV DNA have also been found [47, 48]. Studies employing DNA sequencing and other techniques have also shown amplification and transposition of integrated viral sequences and cellular flanking sequences in PLC/PRF/5 cells [49–52].

Other, less extensively studied HCC-derived cell lines which express HBsAg [53–57]. Include Hep3B, which has one or two sites of HBV integration. Other HCC cell lines have been shown to have integrated HBV genomes [53, 56, 57], including one cell line derived from an anti-HBs-positive patient [54]. One of the cloned HBV DNA integration sites within cell line HuSP has revealed extensive rearrangement of cellular

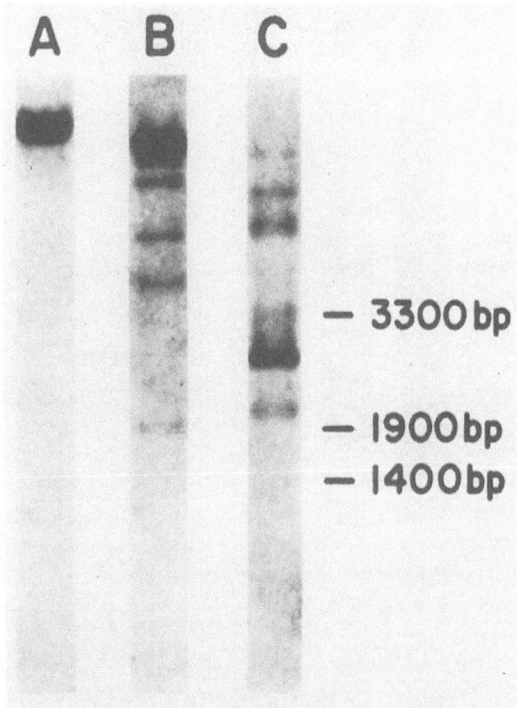

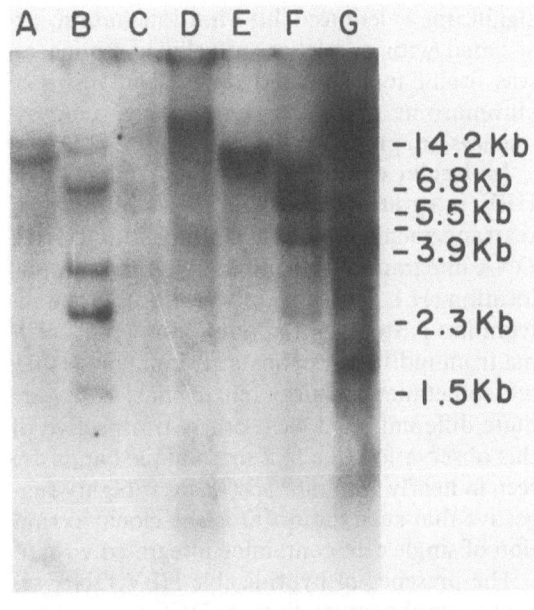

Fig. 2.2. Autoradiogram of HBV DNA sequences in human HCC cell line PLC/PRF/5. *Lane A* shows undigested DNA; *lane B* shows DNA digested with Hind III; *lane C* shows DNA digested with EcoRI. Probe was [^{32}P]-labeled double-purified cloned HBV-DNA insert of 3200 bp. After Shafritz [41], with permission

Fig. 2.3. Autoradiogram of integrated HBV-DNA sequences in DNA extracts of different human HCCs using restriction endonuclease Hind III. [^{32}P]-labeled, purified cloned HBV DNA of 3200 bp (specific activity 4×10^8 cpm/μg DNA) was the hybridization probe. After Shafritz and Kew [23], with permission

flanking sequences adjacent to viral sequences and inverted duplication of both viral and cellular sequences [57].

In summary, work with HCC-derived cell lines has demonstrated integration of HBV viral sequences into cellular DNA, consistent with observations in other tumorigenic viruses. Significant rearrangements of cellular flanking regions and integrated viral sequences have also been observed and are consistent with observations in other viruses known to transform cells [58–60]. However, the interpretation of such observations is difficult because (1) integration of HBV DNA may have occurred in the process of establishing such cell lines, and (2) the derived lines may not represent the major cell type present in the original tumor. Such genetic rearrangements could also represent a nonspecific phenomenon, which often occurs in cell lines undergoing multiple passage [58–60]. Unfortunately, appropriate comparisons of the HBV DNA integration pattern in the initial human tumor with that observed in the derived cell lines have not been performed in most instances.

5.2 Studies with human HCC

Numerous tumors have been analyzed from both serum HBsAg-positive and -negative patients [23, 24, 27, 28, 47]. In the vast majority of cases, HCC has been associated with persistent serum HBsAg, and HBV molecular studies have been performed in which viral DNA has been found to be integrated in tumor genomic DNA. Most of these tumors contained HBV DNA integrated in unique banding patterns (Fig. 2.3). Although restriction patterns have varied with individual tumors, in some instances free HBV DNA has also been noted. This suggests continued viral replication, though these results may also be explained by entrapment of HBV-infected hepatocytes within the tumor specimen. In one integration cloned from a human HCC, cellular flanking sequences at the viral integration site were shown to contain repeated DNA sequences [61]. Several viral integration sites of a second human HCC from a chronic HBV carrier have been cloned. Extensive study of one such integration has revealed that the viral sequences contain only small deletions, while cellular flanking regions contain significant deletions. This viral integration, associated with a deletion of cellular sequences, was found to be located on the short arm of chromosome 11, where known oncogenic sequences are present [62].

Molecular cloning of HCC containing single HBV integrations has also shown substantial rearrangement of cellular DNA adjacent to HBV DNA integration sites and, in some cases, translocation (H.L., personal observation). When integration patterns of tumor and liver parenchyma from individual patients are compared, they are sometimes identical but in most cases are quite different from each other. Irrespective of this observation, the fact that unique bands are seen in nearly all tumor specimens is highly suggestive that such tumors arose by clonal expansion of single cells containing integrated virus.

The presence of hybridizable HBV DNA sequences in the serum, liver, or HCC tissue of patients in whom serum HBsAg was undetected by conventional RIA utilizing polyvalent antibody has recently been noted [24, 32, 63–66]. While some patients were anti-HBs and/or anti-HBc positive, others had no marker of intercurrent or previous HBV infection. The presence of HBV DNA in the tissues of such patients suggests continued presence of the virus despite the absence of viral protein expression or antibody production. Specific HBV integrations have been described in some anti-HBsAg-positive patients with HCC (Fig. 2.4) [24]. A cell line from one such patient has also been established, showing specific viral integration [54]. However, the majority of HBsAg$^-$/anti-HBs$^+$ patients do not have integrated HBV DNA in their tumor genome, nor do they have evidence of continued viral replication.

A series of alcoholic patients with HCC from France without serum HBsAg by conventional RIA has been studied [63, 67]. Each tumor was reported to contain integrated HBV DNA, including specimens from seven of sixteen (44%) patients without any serological marker of HBV infection, past or present. A recent study [67] by the same investigators in collaboration with Wands evaluated patients with chronic liver disease who were serum HBsAg negative by conventional RIA but contained hybridizable HBV DNA sequences in liver tissue. Unfortunately, serum from most patients with HCC in the earlier series was not available for testing with monoclonal anti-HBs. However, an HBV DNA integration from one patient, in whom HBsAg was not detected by conventional RIA, has been

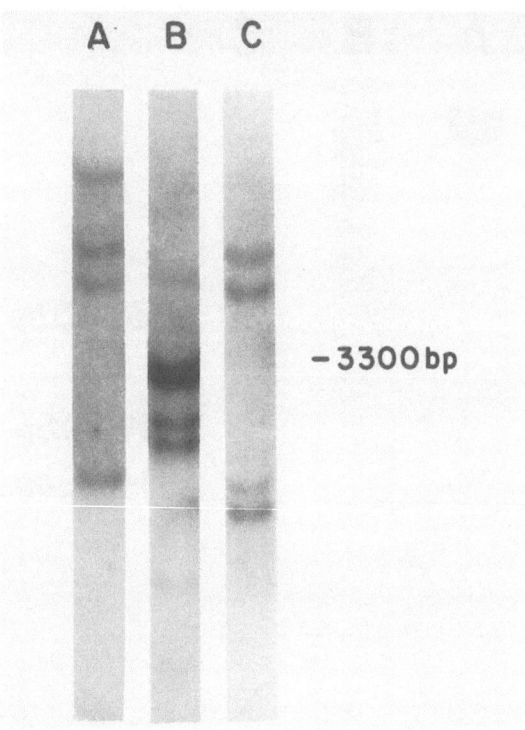

Fig. 2.4. Hybridization pattern of DNA extracts of HCC tissue from three patients negative for HBsAg but anti-HBs positive. Restriction enzyme treatment with EcoRl. HBV probe was used as described in Figs. 2.2 and 2.3. After Shafritz el al. [24], with permission

cloned and characterized by other investigators [68]. A mutation (deletion) was found in the HBsAg coding DNA sequence, which could account for lack of HBsAg expression and/or detection by RIA.

5.3 Studies with HBV-related viruses in animals

Viruses similar to HBV in genome size, organization of viral DNA, virus morphology, and cross-reacting gene products and termed hepatitis associated DNA (hepadna) viruses have been recently discovered in woodchucks (WHV), Beechy ground squirrels (GSHV), and Pekin ducks [5–8]. Amongst these models, chronic liver disease and HCC is commonly found only in the woodchuck [6, 69, 70]. Like human HCC, nearly all woodchuck HCCs in virally infected animals contain integrated WHV DNA sequences [69, 70]. Two of these viral integrations have been cloned and characterized [71], revealing extensive rearrangements of integrated viral sequences, including inversions, duplications, and deletions to produce incomplete viral genomes. Cellular sequences flanking these viral integrations also contain substantial rearrangements. Chronic woodchuck WHV carriers without HCC have also been studied [72–74]. In one case, a WHV integration, undetectable by conventional Southern blot analysis, was cloned in a lambda phage and found to be colinear with the WHV genome except for a minor deletion. In addition, there were no detectable rearrangements of cellular flanking regions in the WHV carrier. This suggests that rearrangement of both viral and cellular flanking regions may be unique to HCC and occurs during the process of transformation after initial viral integration.

Integration of WHV occurs in close proximity to the 5'-end of the virion-plus DNA strand, implicating a possible role for this region in the integration process. This observation is consistent for all WHV and HBV integrations cloned thus far, in which the cohesive end region of the viral genome is often conserved and is located close to the viral cell junction. In both cloned integrations of WHV in HCC, only the X-gene open reading frame was conserved (containing the cohesive end and part of the single-strand region [71], suggesting a possible transforming role for this region of the HBV genome; recent studies also suggest the presence of a specific X-gene product, possibly an early viral gene-transforming protein in the PLC/PRF/5 cell line [75]).

6 HBV as an oncogenic virus

The temporal relationship of HBV DNA integration to persistent viral infection and the finding of integrated viral sequences in tumor genomes of patients with HCC have suggested a role for HBV in oncogenesis. In both DNA and RNA (retrovirus) tumor viruses, integration of viral DNA sequences into the cellular genome is a necessary event for transformation [42, 76]. In SV40, such integration occurs randomly with respect to cellular and viral sites and is commonly associated with significant rearrangements of both viral sequences (oligomers, repeats, partial duplications, deletions, inversions) and flanking cellular sequences. Such findings have been observed for HBV. Also, integration of DNA tumor viruses either precedes or occurs at the time of cell transformation, consistent with results observed in HBV carriers. However, unlike HBV, neoplastic transformation by DNA tumor viruses commonly requires expression of specific

virally coded proteins, such as the transformation or T antigens of papovaviruses [42]. Although such antigens have not been identified to date for HBV, the protein product of the HBV X gene could represent such a function. The X protein appears to be expressed in the liver of HBV carriers and antibodies are present in the serum of some HBV-infected individuals, especially those with HCC [11, 75]. Of 254 serum samples evaluated, antibody to X protein was detected in 5.8% of asymptomatic HBV carriers, 13.4% of patients with HBV-related chronic hepatitis, 15.7% of patients with HBV-related cirrhosis, and 8/11 (72.7%) of patients with HBV-related cirrhosis and HCC, but in no healthy controls [75]. The apparent correlation between development of antibody to X protein and HCC, as well as the role of the X protein, will require further investigation.

HBV also shows similarities with a group of RNA tumor viruses (retroviruses) which are associated with a variety of animal sarcomas, lymphomas, and leukemias and which also have the ability to transform fibroblasts. The life cycle of these single-stranded RNA viruses consists of replication of a DNA-minus (−) strand from the RNA-plus (+) strand (template) by an RNA-dependent DNA polymerase (reverse transcriptase), followed by synthesis of the complementary DNA strand. The double-stranded DNA then integrates into the cellular genome and produces RNA-plus strands which are packaged into viral particles [76]. Adjacent to the retroviral genome on either side are repeated sequences (long terminal repeats), serving not only as the sites of proviral DNA integration but also containing promoter regions for the regulation of viral gene expression [77]. Additional analogies have been made between hepadna viruses, cauliflower mosaic viruses, and retroviruses, since they all replicate by reverse transcription [78]. Miller et al. [79] have compared the sequence of HBV and retroviruses and conclude that the C terminus of the core gene, the middle portion of *pol*, and a large segment of X have considerable homology to retrovirus sequences.

HBV replication occurs in a fashion similar to that in retroviruses, inasmuch as a reverse transcriptase is required and a full-length mRNA intermediate is utilized to copy viral DNA. Despite similar replicative patterns of HBV and retroviruses, however, distinct differences are present. The most striking differences are that HBV is a DNA rather than an RNA virus and that integration into the cellular genome is not a necessary step for replication of HBV. In addition, initiation of replication of retroviruses may depend on specific tRNA molecules, while no such tRNA initiators have been identified in HBV. Finally, the proviral genomes of retroviruses are surrounded by long terminal repeat (LTR) sequences, believed to contain the promoter and initiation sequences for proviral transcription as well as the sequences for integration. Analogous regions of integrated HBV genomes have not been found, although short repeated sequences have been mapped at the junction of several cloned HBV integrations [61]. While the significance of this finding is unknown, some attention has been drawn to the region of the cohesive end of HBV as being analogous to the LTR of retroviruses.

Retroviruses cause malignant transformation by two mechanisms—firstly, by containing specific oncogenes, i.e., DNA sequences found in many vertebrate cells which are also associated with a transformed phenotype in cultured cells [77, 80]. Although such genes have no specific structural function for the virus, many appear to code for proteins with tyrosine phosphorylase activity [81]. Therefore, oncogenic transformation may be related to metabolic changes occurring as a result of increased enzyme activity for tyrosine phosphorylation. A second mechanism of transformation involves integration of a viral promoter or enhancer sequence adjacent to a cellular proto-oncogene [82], resulting in increased expression of the proto-oncogene and subsequent oncogenic transformation. This mechanism has been shown to cause transformation in retroviruses, such as avian leukosis virus, which lack specific oncogenes. However, whereas cells transfected with retroviral oncogenes undergo oncogenic transformation, no transformation has been observed with cells transfected with HBV DNA [83, 84]. Although this may be explained by the selective nature of the cell types used for transfection experiments, HBV DNA does not contain sequences homologous to any currently known oncogene. In regard to the promoter or enhancer insertion mechanism of oncogenesis, it is of interest that several viral promoters have been found in HBV, including one (the core gene promoter) in the "cohesive end" region [12, 13, 15]. However, the presence of a viral promoter adjacent to a cellular oncogene has not been identified to date in any HBV DNA integration studied in HCC tissue or in HCC cell lines.

7 Other factors in development of HCC

Other factors, independent of HBV infection, have been associated with the development of HCC. For example, dietary aflatoxin, alcohol, and a variety of diseases such as hemochromatosis, alpha-l-antitrypsin deficiency, and tyrosinemia have all been associated with the development of HCC in non-HBsAg carriers [85–87]. In most instances (alcoholism, hemochromatosis), hepatic neoplasia occurs only after the development of cirrhosis [88–91]. Although rare instances of HCC have been noted in cases of non-A, non-B hepatitis [92], a number of such patients have been identified as having HBV-related disease when molecular hybridization techniques were applied to the liver, tumor, and/or serum [64, 65, 67], or when HBsAg was detected with high-affinity monoclonal antibodies to HBsAg [64, 67].

The relationship between HCC and cirrhosis in chronic HBV infection is also worth noting. Persistent HBV infection results in cirrhosis in many chronic HBV carriers and the majority of worldwide HCCs also arise in the setting of cirrhosis (usually 80%–90%) [1, 2]. However, 40% of HCC in Africa occurs in the absence of cirrhosis. Prospective studies by Obata et al. [93] also suggest that it is persistent HBV infection, rather than the related cirrhosis, which results in HCC. The overall evidence, therefore, suggests that persistent HBV infection is a common etiological agent which produces two different states, postnecrotic cirrhosis and HCC, which may coexist.

An interaction between HBV and other genetic or environmental factors is suggested by epidemiological studies from South Africa and China. These studies have shown that the incidence of HCC varies with location and urbanization, despite a constant high prevalence of chronic HBV infection in these regions [94]. In China, undefined agents in stagnant water have been shown to be associated with increased incidence of HCC in HBV carriers [95]. The interaction of viral infection with chemical agents in producing a synergistic effects on neoplasia development has been well-documented in both laboratory animals and tissue culture systems [96–99]. From such studies, several carcinogenic mechanisms have been postulated which involve changes or rearrangements of cellular DNA. Chemical carcinogens are known to induce a variety of mutational events involving breaks in

DNA which could serve as integration sites for viral genomes. Rearrangement of cellular DNA may also result in close apposition of cellular transforming genes and viral promoters, resulting in amplification or enhanced activity of those genes. Carcinogens may also directly amplify cellular genes, which, if adjacent to integrated viral sequences, could result in increased promoter and associated oncogene activity, as already demonstrated in non-HBV systems [98].

8 Speculative model of persistent HBV infection and development of HCC

From the above discussion, persistent HBV infection may be viewed as a spectrum with two types of HBV carrier at either end (Fig. 2.5): (1) those who continue to replicate the virus (permissive infection) and demonstrate continued inflammatory liver disease activity; the bulk of viral DNA within the liver is in free replicating forms and integration into unique sites within the host genome is not observed; (2) those who no longer replicate the virus (nonpermissive infection) and show little or no inflammatory liver disease, the liver containing only integrated HBV DNA. In some patients, a mixed type of persistent infection is found in which different regions of the liver contain features of permissive and nonpermissive infection.

Persistence of hepatocytes containing nonreplicating HBV may result from an impaired ability of the host immune system to rid the liver of hepatocytes containing integrated HBV genomes as compared with hepatocytes with active replication. This may result in accumulation of hepatocytes containing integrated viral genomes (stage I). At this stage of persistent HBV infection, the integrated HBV DNA would be randomly distributed over many sites. Under conditions which stimulate hepatocyte division (humoral or hormonal factors, superinfection with other viruses, contact with hepatotoxins or carcinogens), a series of cellular/viral genomic rearrangements may occur leading to altered phenotypic behavior of hepatocytes containing integrated HBV DNA (cellular transformation). These events may occur over many years, during which individual cells may expand into groups or clusters (clonal expansion) with discrete bands of integrated HBV DNA on hybridization analysis (stage II). With further growth of such cells under conditions of stimulation by host or envi-

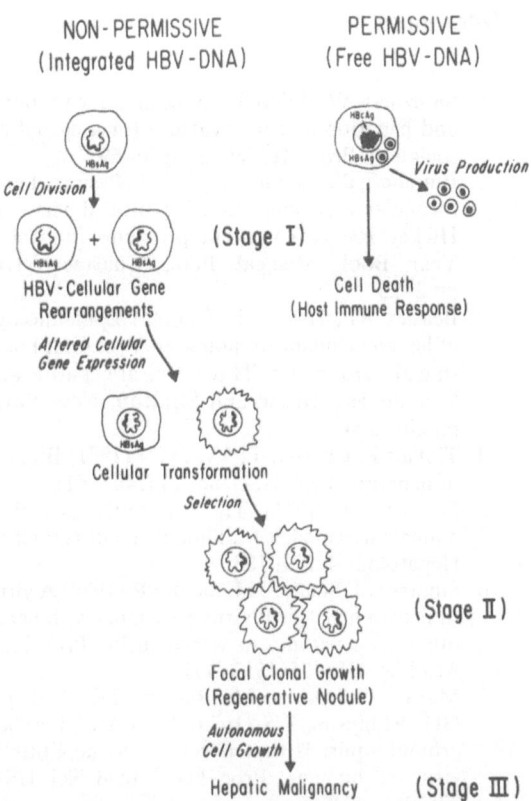

Fig. 2.5. Speculative model showing events following infection with HBV and integration of the viral DNA into liver cell genome, which may lead to development of HCC. See text for details. After Shafritz and Hadziyannis [101], with permission

ronmental factors, some HBV carriers would develop autonomous neoplasia (stage III).

Although this model is entirely speculative, it is consistent with numerous studies noted above. While integration of the HBV genome into cellular DNA is a required initial event for cellular transformation, expression of viral gene products or the ultimate presence of the HBV genome is not required, and a variety of interactions of host and environmental factors are needed to determine which HBV carriers will actually develop HCC. If such a mechanism does initiate celluar transformation, the finding of uniquely integrated HBV DNA in the absence of viral replication in HBsAg-positive carriers in whom active inflammatory liver disease is minimal or absent may possibly identify individuals at increased risk for the development of HCC.

References

1. Smuzness W (1978) Hepatocellular carcinoma and hepatitis B virus: evidence for a casual association. Prog Med Virol 24: 40–69

2. Blumberg BS, London WT (1981) Primary hepatocellular carcinoma and hepatitis B virus. In Hickey RC (ed) Current problems in cancer. Year Book Medical Publ, Chicago VI(I), pp 2–23

3. Beasley RP, Hwang L-Y (1984) Epidemiology of hepatocellular carcinoma. In Vyas GH, Dienstag JL, Hoofnagle JH (eds) Viral hepatitis and liver disease. Grune and Stratton, New York, pp 209–224

4. Tiollais P, Charnay P, Vyas GN (1981) Biology of hepatitis B virus. Science 213: 406–411

5. Summers J (1981) Three recently described animal virus models for human hepatitis B virus. Hepatology 1: 179–183

6. Summers J, Smolec JM, Snyder R (1978) A virus similar to hepatitis B virus associated with hepatitis and hepatoma in woodchucks. Proc Natl Acad Sci USA 75: 4533–4537

7. Marion PL, Oshiro LS, Regnery DC Scullard, GH, Robinson, WS (1980) A virus of Beechey ground squirrels that is related to hepatitis B virus of humans. Proc Natl Acad Sci USA 77: 2941–2945

8. Mason WS, Seal G, Summers J (1980) Virus of Pekin ducks with structural and biological relatedness to human hepatitis B virus. J Virol 36: 829–836

9. Galibert F, Mandart E, Fitoussi F, Tiollais P, Charnay P (1979) Nucleotide sequence of the hepatitis B genome cloned in E. coli. Nature 281: 646–650

10. Mandart E, Kay A, Galibert F (1984) Nucleotide sequence of a cloned duck hepatitis virus genome: Comparison with the human and woodchuck hepatitis B virus sequences. J Virol 49: 782–792

11. Meyers ML, Trepo LV, Nath N, Sninsky JJ (1986) Hepatitis B virus polypeptide X: Expression in E. coli and identification of specific antibodies in sera from hepatitis B virus infected humans. J. Virol 57: 101–109

12. Rall LB, Standring DN, Laub O, Rutter WJ (1983) Transcription of hepatitis B virus by RNA polymerase II. Mol Cell Biol 3: 1766–1773

13. Shaul Y, Rutter WJ, Laub O (1985) A human hepatitis B viral enhancer element. EMBO J 4: 427–430

14. Pourcell C, Louise A, Gervais M, Chenciner N, Dubois MF, Tiollais P (1982) Transcription of the hepatitis B surface antigen gene in mouse cells transformed with cloned viral DNA. J Virol 42: 100–105

15. Chakraborty PR, Ruiz-Opazo N, Shafritz DA (1981) Transcription of human hepatitis B virus core antigen sequences in an in vitro HeLa cellular extract. Virology 111: 647–652

16. Laimonis AL, Khoury G, Gorman C, Howard B, Gruss P (1982) Host-specific activation of transcription by tandem repeats from simian virus 40 and Moloney murine sarcoma virus. Proc Natl Acad Sci USA 79: 6453–6457

17. Chisari FV, Pinkert CA, Milich DR, Filippi P, McLachlan A, Palmiter RD, Brinster RL (1985) A transgenic mouse model of the chronic hepatitis B surface antigen carrier state. Science 230: 1157–1160

18. Jameel S, Siddiqui A (1986) The human hepatitis B virus enhancer requires trans-acting cellular factor(s) for activity. Mol Cell Biol 6: 710–715

19. Tur-Kaspa R, Burk RD, Shaul Y, Shafritz DA (1986) Hepatitis B virus DNA contains a glucocorticoid responsive element. Proc Natl Acad Sci 83: 1627–1631

20. Geisse S, Scheidereit C, Westphal HM, Hynes NE, Groner B, Beato M (1982) Glucocorticoid receptors recognize DNA sequences in and around murine mammary tumor virus DNA. EMBO J 1: 1613–1619

21. Summers J, Mason WS (1982) Replication of the genome of a hepatitis B-like virus by reverse transcription of an RNA intermediate. Cell 29: 403–415

22. Miller RH, Tran C-T, Robinson WS (1984) Hepatitis B virus particles in plasma and liver contain viral DNA-RNA hybrid molecules. Virology 139: 53–63

23. Shafritz DA, Kew MC (1981) Identification of integrated hepatitis B virus DNA sequences in human hepatocellular carcinomas. Hepatology 1: 1–8

24. Shafritz DA Shouval D, Sherman HI, Hadziyannis SJ, Kew MC (1981) Integration of hepatitis B virus DNA into the genome of liver cells in chronic liver disease and hepatocellular carcinoma. N Engl J Med 305: 1067–1073

25. Lieberman HM, LaBrecque DR, Kew MC, Hadziyannis SJ, Shafritz DA (1983) Detection of hepatitis B virus directly in human serum by a simplified molecular hybridization test. Comparison to HBeAg/anti-HBe status in HBsAg carriers. Hepatology 3: 286–291

26. Edman JC, Gray P, Valenzuela P, Rall LB, Rutter WJ (1980) Integration of hepatitis B virus sequences and their expression in a human hepatoma cell. Nature 286: 535–538

27. Brechot C, Pourcel C, Louise A, Rain B, Tiollais P (1980) Presence of integrated hepatitis B virus DNA sequences in cellular DNA of human hepatocellular carcinoma. Nature 286: 533–535

28. Koshy R, Maupas P, Muller R, Hofschneider PH (1981) Detection of hepatitis B virus-specific DNA in the genomes of human hepatocellular carcinoma and liver cirrhosis tissues. J Gen Virol 57: 95–102

29. Brechot C, Hadchouel M, Scotto J, Fonck M, Potet F, Vyas GN, Tiollais P (1981) State of hepatitis B virus DNA in hepatocytes of patients with hepatitis B surface antigen-positive and negative liver disease. Proc Natl Acad Sci USA 78: 3906–3910

30. Brechot C, Poucel C, Hadchouel M, Dejean A,

Louise A, Scotto J, Tiollais P (1982) State of hepatitis B virus DNA in liver diseases. Hepatology 2: 27S–34S

31. Bonino F, Hoyer B, Nelson J, Engle R, Verme G, Gerin J (1981) Hepatitis B virus DNA in the sera of HBs antigen carriers: a marker of active hepatitis B virus replication in the liver. Hepatology 1: 386–391

32. Brechot C, Scotto J, Hadchouel M, Charnay P, Degos F, Trepo C, Tiollais P (1981) Detection of hepatitis B virus DNA in liver and serum: a direct appraisal of the chronic carrier state. Lancet 2: 765–767

33. Berninger M, Hammer M, Hoyer B, Gerin J (1982) An assay for the detection of the DNA genome of hepatitis B virus in serum. J Med Virol 9: 57–68

34. Scotto J, Hadchouel M, Hery C, Yvart J, Tiollais P, Brechot C (1983) Detection of hepatitis B virus DNA in serum by a simple spot hybridization technique: comparison with results for other viral markers. Hepatology 3: 279–284

35. Kam W, Rall LB, Smuckler EA, Schmid R, Rutter WJ (1982) Hepatitis B virus DNA in liver and serum of asymptomatic carriers. Proc Natl Acad Sci USA 79: 7522–7526

36. Weller IVD, Fowler MJF, Monjardino J, Thomas HC (1982) The detection of HBV DNA in serum by molecular hybridization: a more sensitive method for detection of complete HBV particles. J Med Virol 9: 273–280

37. Sherlock S, Thomas HC (1983) Hepatitis B virus infection: the impact of molecular biology. Hepatology 3: 455–456

38. Hadziyannis SJ, Lieberman HM, Karvountzis GG, Shafritz DA (1983) Analysis of liver disease, nuclear HBcAg, viral replication and hepatitis B virus DNA in liver and serum of HBeAg vs. anti-HBe positive carriers of hepatitis B virus. Hepatology 3: 656–662

39. Fattovich G, Rugge M, Brollo L, Portisso P, Noventa F, Guido M, Alberti A, Realdi G (1986) Clinical, virological and histologic outcome following seroconversion from HBeAg to anti-HBe in chronic hepatitis type B. Hepatology 6: 167–172

40. Yokosuka O, Omata M, Imazeki F, Okuda K (1985) Active and inactive replication of hepatitis B virus DNA in chronic liver disease. Gastroenterology 89: 610–616

41. Shafritz DA (1982) Hepatitis B virus DNA molecules in the liver of HBsAg carriers: mechanistic considerations in the pathogenesis of hepatocellular carcinoma. Hepatology 2: 35S–41S

42. Tooze J (1980) DNA tumor viruses. Part 2 of molecular biology of tumor viruses. Cold Spring Harbor Laboratory, New York

43. Macnab GM, Alexander JJ, Lacatsas G, Bey EM, Urbanowitz JM (1976) Hepatitis B surface antigen produced by a human hepatoma cell line. Br J Cancer 34: 504–515

44. Bassendine MF, Arborgh BAM, Shipton U, Monjardino J, Aranguibel F, Thomas HC, Sherlock S (1980) Hepatitis B surface antigen and alphafetoprotein secreting human primary liver cell cancer in athymic mice. Gastroenterology 79: 528–532

45. Desmyter J, Ray MB, Bradburne AF, Alexander JJ (1978) Human HBsAg-positive hepatoma in nude athymic mice. In: Vyas GN, Cohen SN, Schmid R (eds) Viral hepatitis. Proceedings of the Second Symposium on Viral Hepatitis. Franklin Institute, Philadelphia, pp 459–460

46. Marion PL, Salazar FH, Alexander JJ, Robinson WS (1980) State of hepatitis B viral DNA in a human hepatoma cell line. J Virol 33: 795–806

47. Dejean A, Brechot C, Tiollais P, Wain-Hobson S (1983) Characterization of integrated hepatitis B viral DNA cloned from a human hepatoma and the hepatoma derived cell line PLC/PRF/5. Proc Natl Acad Sci USA 80: 2505–2509

48. Koshy R, Koch S, Freytag von Loringhoven A, Kahmann R, Murray K, Hofschneider PH (1983) Integration of hepatitis B virus DNA: evidence for integration in the single-stranded gap. Cell 34: 215–223

49. Ziemer M, Garcia P, Shaul Y, Rutter WJ (1985) Sequence of hepatitis B virus DNA incorporated into the genome of a human hepatoma cell line. J Virol 53: 885–892

50. Koch S, Freytag von Loringhoven A, Hofschneider PH, Koshy R (1984) Amplification and rearrangement in hepatoma cell DNA associated with integrated hepatitis B virus DNA. EMBO J 3: 2185–2189

51. Koch S, Freytag von Loringhoven A, Kahmann R, Hofschneider PH, Koshy R (1984) The genetic organization of integrated hepatitis B virus DNA in the human hepatoma cell line PLC/PRF/5. Nucleic Acid Res 12: 6871–6886

52. Ou J-H, Rutter WJ (1985) Hybrid hepatitis B virus-host transcripts in a human hepatoma cell. Proc Natl Acad Sci USA 82: 83–87

53. Twist EM, Clark HF, Aden DP, Knowles BB, Plotkin SA (1981) Integration pattern of hepatitis B virus DNA sequences in human hepatoma cell lines. J Virol 37: 239–243

54. He L, Shih C, Isselbacher KJ, Goodman HM, Wands JR (1983) Integration of HBV into genome of a new hepatocellular carcinoma cell line (CUSPF). Gastroenterology 84: 1184

55. Das PK, Nayak N, Tsiquaye KN, Zuckerman AJ (1980) Establishment of a human hepatocellular cell line releasing hepatitis B virus surface antigen. Br J Exp Pathol 61: 648–654

56. Koike K, Koyabashi M, Mizusawa H, Yoshida E, Yaginuma K, Taira M (1983) Rearrangement of the surface antigen gene of hepatitis B virus integrated in the human hepatoma cell lines. Nucl Acid Res 11: 5391–5403

57. Mizusawa H, Taira M, Yaginuma K, Kobayashi M, Yoshida E, Koike K (1985) Inversely repeating integrated hepatitis B virus DNA and cellular flanking sequences in the human hepatoma-derived cell line huSP. Proc Natl Acad Sci USA 82: 208–212

58. Geissler E, Theile M (1983) Virus-induced gene mutations of eukaryotic cells. Human Genet

63: 1–12

59. Mounts P, Kelly TJ, Jr. (1984) Rearrangements of host and viral DNA in mouse cells transformed by simian virus 40. J Mol Biol 177: 431–460

60. Matsuo T, Heller M, Petti L, O'Shiro E, Kieff E (1984) Persistence of the entire Epstein-Barr virus genome integrated into human lymphocyte DNA. Science 226: 1322–1324

61. Dejean A, Sonigo P, Wain-Hobson S, Tiollais P (1984) Specific hepatitis B virus integration in hepatocellular carcinoma DNA through a viral 11-base-pair direct repeat. Proc Natl Acad Sci USA 81: 5350–5354

62. Rogler CE, Sherman M, Su CY, Shafritz DA (1985) Deletion in chromosome 11p associated with a hepatitis B integration site in hepatocellular carcinoma. Science 230: 319–322

63. Brechot C, Nalpas B, Courouce AM, Duhamel G, Callard P, Carnot F, Tiollais P, Berthelot P (1982) Evidence that hepatitis B virus has a role in liver cell carcinoma in alcoholic liver disease. New Engl J Med 306: 1384–1387

64. Shafritz DA, Lieberman HM, Isselbacher KJ, Wands JR (1982) Monoclonal radioimmuno-assays for hepatitis B surface antigen. Demonstration of hepatitis B virus DNA or related sequences in serum and viral epitopes in immune conplexes. Proc Natl Acad Sci USA 79: 5675–5679

65. Wands JR, Lieberman HM, Muchmore E, Isselbacher K, Shafritz DA (1982) Detection and transmission in chimpanzees of hepatitis B virus-related agents formerly designated "non-A, non-B" hepatitis. Proc Natl Acad Sci USA 79: 7552–7556

66. Figus A, Blum HE, Vyas GH, De Virgilis S, Cao A, Lippi M, Lai E, Balestrieri A (1984) Hepatitis B viral nucleotide sequences in non-A, non-B or hepatitis B virus-related chronic liver disease. Hepatology 4: 364–368

67. Brechot C, Degos F, Lugassy C, Thiers V, Zafrani S, Franco D, Bismuth H, Trepo C, Benhamou J-P, Wands J, Isselbacher K, Tiollais P, Berthelot P (1985) Hepatitis B virus DNA in patients with chronic liver disease and negative tests for hepatitis B surface antigens. New Engl J Med 312: 270–276

68. Figus A, Fung Y-KT, Blum HE, Vyas GN, Varmus HE (1984) Definition of a deletion mutant of hepatitis B virus DNA that appears to replicate in the chronically infected liver of a Sardinian patient with B°-thalassemia. In: Vyas GN, Dienstag JL, Hoofnagle JH (eds) Viral hepatitis and liver disease. Grune and Stratton, New York, p 632

69. Popper H, Shih JW-K, Gerin JL, Wong DC, Hoyer BH, London WT, Sly DL, Purcell RH (1981) Woodchuck hepatitis virus and hepatocellular carcinoma: correlation of histological and virological observations. Hepatology 1: 91–98

70. Snyder RL, Summers J (1980) Woodchuck hepatitis virus and hepatocellular carcinoma. In: Essex M, Todaro G, ZurHausen M (eds) Viruses

in naturally occurring cancers, vol.7. Proceedings of Cold Spring Harbor Symposium on Cell Proliferation 1979. Cold Spring Harbor Laboratory, New York, pp 446–457

71. Ogston CW, Jonak GJ, Rogler CE, Astrin SM, Summers J (1982) Cloning and structural analysis of integrated woodchuck hepatitis virus sequences from hepatocellular carcinomas of woodchucks. Cell 29: 385–394

72. Rogler CE, Summers J (1984) Cloning and structural analysis of integrated woodchuck hepatitis virus sequences from a chronically infected liver. J Virol 50: 832–837

73. Rogler CE, Summers J (1982) Novel forms of woodchuck hepatitis virus DNA isolated from chronically infected woodchuck liver nuclei. J Virol 44: 852–863

74. Rogler CE, Summers J, Shafritz DA (1984) Molecular characteristics of woodchuck and human hepatitis virus in persistent infections of the liver and associated hepatic neoplasms. In: Gallo RC, Essex M, Gross L (eds) Human T-cell leukemia/lymphoma viruses. Cold Spring Harbor Laboratory, New York, pp 55–67

75. Moriarty AM, Alexander H, Lerner RA, Thornton GB (1985) Antibodies to peptides detect new hepatitis B antigen: serological correlation with hepatocellular carcinoma. Science 227: 429–433

76. Varmus HE (1982) Form and function of retroviral proviruses. Science 216: 812–820

77. Temin HM (1982) Function of the retrovirus large terminal repeat. Cell 28: 3–5

78. Mason WS, Taylor JM, Hull R (1987) Retroid virus genome replication. In: Moramorosch K, Murphy FA, Shortkin AJ (eds) Advances in virus research. Academic Press, New York (in press)

79. Miller RH, Robinson WS (1986) Common evolutionary origin of hepatitis B virus and retroviruses. Proc Natl Acad Sci USA 83: 2531–2535

80. Bishop JM (1981) The enemy within: genesis of retrovirus oncogenes. Cell 23: 5–6

81. Hunter T (1980) Proteins phosphorylated by the RSV transforming function. Cell 22: 647–648

82. Neel BG, Hayward WS, Robinson HL, Fang J, Astrin SM (1981) Avian leukosis virus-induced tumors have common proviral integration sites and synthesize discrete new RNA's: oncogenesis by promoter insertion. Cell 23: 323–334

83. Murray MJ, Shilo B-Z, Shih C, Cowing D, Hsu HW, Weinberg RA (1981) Three different human tumor cell lines contain different oncogenes. Cell 25: 355–361

84. Gough NM, Murray K (1982) Expression of the hepatitis B virus surface, core and e antigen genes by stable rat and mouse cell lines. J Mol Biol 162: 43–67

85. Lieber CS, Seitz HK, Garro AJ, Worner TM (1979) Alcohol-related diseases and carcinogenesis. Cancer Res 39: 2863–2886

86. Bulatao-Jayme J, Alermo E, Castro MC, Jardelezo MT, Salamat L (1982) A case-control dietary study of primary liver cancer risk from afla-

toxin exposure. Int J Epidemiol 11: 112–119
87. Edmondson HA and Peters RL (1982) Neoplasms of the liver. In: Schiff L, Schiff ER (eds) Diseases of the liver, 5th edn. Lippincott, Philadelphia, pp 1101–1157
88. Shikata T (1976) Primary liver carcinoma and liver cirrhosis. In: Okudo K, Peters RL (eds) Hepatocellular carcinoma. Wiley, New York, pp 53–71
89. Falk H (1982) Liver. In: Schrottenfeld D, Franmoni JF (eds) Cancer epidemiology and prevention. Saunders, Philadelphia, pp 668–682
90. Kew MC (1982) Tumors of the liver In: Zakim D, Boyer TD (eds) Hepatology. A textbook of liver diseases Saunders, Philadelphia, pp 1048–1084
91. Eriksson S, Carlson J, Velez R (1986) Risk of cirrhosis and primary liver cancer in alpha-l-antitrypsin deficiency. New Engl J Med 314: 736–739
92. Shibreski K, Soga K, Homma A, Ichida F (1981) Hepatic cancer and non-A non-B type hepatitis. Nippon Rinsko 39: 3251–3256
93. Obata H, Hayashi H, Matoike Y, Hisamitsu T, Okuda H, Kobayashi S, Nishioka K (1980) A prospective study on the development of hepatocullular carcinoma from liver cirrhosis with persistent hepatitis B infection. Int J Cancer 25: 741–747
94. Kew MC, Rossouw E, Hodkinson J, Paterson A, Dusheiko GM, Whitcutt JM (1983) Hepatitis B virus status of South African blacks with hepatocellular carcinoma: Comparison between rural and urban patients. Hepatology 3: 65–68
95. Su DL Drinking water and liver cell cancer: An epidemiological approach to the etiology of this disease in China. Chin Med J 92: 748–756
96. Salaman MH, Rowson KEK, Roe JFC, Ball JK, Harvey JJ, De Benedictis G (1963) The combined action of viruses and other carcinogens. In: Viruses, nucleic acids and cancer. University of Texas MD Anderson Hospital and Tumor Institute, 17th Annual Symposium on Fundamental Cancer Research. Williams and Wilkins, Baltimore, pp 544–558
97. Rous P, Kidel JA (1938) The carcinogenic effect of a papilloma virus on the tarred skin of rabbits: I. Description of the phenomenon. J Exp Med 67: 399–428
98. Casto BC, DiPaulo JA (1973) Viruses, chemicals and cancer. Prog Med Virol 16: 1–47
99. Lavi S (1981) Carcinogen mediated amplification of viral DNA sequences in simian virus 40 transformed Chinese hamster embryo cells. Proc Natl Acad Sci USA 78: 6144–6148
100. Tiollais P, Pourcel C, Dejean A (1985) the hepatitis B virus. Nature 317: 488–496
101. Shafritz DA, Hadziyannis SJ (1984) Hepatitis B virus DNA in liver and serum, viral antigens and antibodies, virus replication and liver disease activity in patients with persistent hepatitis B virus infection. In: Chisari (ed) Advances in hepatitis research. Masson, New York, pp 80–90

Chapter 3
Hepadna Viruses and Hepatocarcinogenesis

Masao Omata, Osamu Yokosuka, Fumio Imazeki, and Kunio Okuda[1]

1 Hepatitis B virus infection and hepatocellular carcinoma

1.1 Epidemiological survey of hepatitis B infection and hepatocellular carcinoma

Since the discovery of Australian antigen, the rate of hepatitis B (HBV) infection among patients with hepatocellular carcinoma (HCC) has been studied in various parts of the world. In 1971, Tong et al. reported that 44 of 55 (88%) patients with HCC in Taiwan were positive for hepatitis B surface antigen (HBsAg) by the agar gel diffusion test [1]. Subsequently, many studies in Africa and Asia showed that the positivity rate for HBsAg varied from 35% to 90% in patients with HCC [2]. When additional serum testings for anti-HBs and anti-HBc (core) were included, HBV infection rates reached 75%–81% in Africa [3], the USA [4], and Japan [5] (Table 3.1). These data indicate that the majority of patients with HCC had a previous infection or current antigenemia.

In 1971, Denison et al. [6] and Ohbayashi et al. [7] reported familial clustering of asymptomatic carriers and patients with HCC. Later, it was shown that the familial clustering of HBV infection was through "vertical transmission" from HBeAg-positive mothers to babies [8]. The importance of HBV infection in hepatocarcinogenesis may be elucidated by following the infected persons, which takes a great deal of time and effort. However, this was done by Beasley [9], who recruited (between December 1975 and June 1978) 22 707 male government employees, of whom 3454 were seropositive and 19 253 negative for HBsAg. After 6.2 years of follow-up, 113 men in the positive group and

Table 3.1. Serum hepatitis B virus markers in patients with HCC in Uganda, the USA, and Japan

	HBsAg alone (%)	HBsAg, anti-HBs, and/or anti-HBc (%)	Reference
Uganda	40	96	3
USA	21	75	4
Japan	46	81	5

only three in the negative group had developed primary liver cancer (mostly HCC), and the relative risk of developing HCC in the seropositive group was 217 [9]. In Japan, Sakuma et al. [10] followed 202 HBsAg-seropositive and 2928 seronegative employees of the Japan National Railways (98% men) for 5 years and observed the development of HCC in four individuals in the former group and in none in the latter (Table 3.2). The relative risk could not be calculated because there was no cancer development in the seronegative group. However, the calculated annual incidence of HCC/100 000 HBsAg-seropositive individuals was 528 in Taiwan [9] and 396 in Japan [10] (Table 3.2). Epidemiological studies indicate that the annual mortality due to HCC/100 000 persons in the general population (male) is 1.4 in the USA (low-incidence area), 4.4 in Switzerland (intermediate-incidence area), and 12.5 in Japan (high-incidence area) [11]. Thus, these prospective data in Taiwan provide strong evidence that HBV is etiologically closely related to HCC in male carriers.

1.2 Molecular biology of HBV infection and HCC

In 1980, four groups demonstrated that HBV DNA was integrated in the genome of HCC [12–15]. There have since been molecular biological studies analyzing the structure and func-

---

[1] First Department of Medicine, Chiba University School of Medicine, Chiba, 280 Japan

Table 3.2. Comparison of two prospective studies of adult male HBsAg carriers and noncarriers for the development of HCC in Japan and Taiwan

	Serum HBsAg	No. of subjects	Follow-up (years)	Development of HCC	HCC/100 000/ year	Relative risk	Reference
Beasley, Taiwan	+	3 454	6.2	113	528	217	9
	−	19 253	6.2	3	2.5		
Sakuma et al.,	+	202	5	4	396		10
Japan	−	2 928	5	0	0		

tion of integrated viral DNA in this carcinoma in order to elucidate the mechanism of cell transformation.

1.2.1 Studies by Southern blot hybridization

A procedure known as Southern transfer [16] is of great utility in recombinant DNA technology, since it allows physical mapping of regions complementary radiolabeled HBV DNA. With this technique applied to clinical material, the frequency of HBV DNA integration into the genome of HCC was studied by many investigators [17–21]. A summary of the results of these studies is given in Table 3.3; the studies showed that HBV DNA integration was almost invariably present in HBsAg-seropositive patients with HCC (49 of 51 cases in five studies). However, the results in HBsAg-seronegative patients have been inconsistent. Brechot et al. [18] first reported a very high frequency of viral integration in HBsAg-seronegative patients. Their subsequent study similarly demonstrated the presence of viral integration in the genome of HCC that had arisen in HBsAg-seronegative patients with alcoholic cirrhosis [22]. They reported that all 20 patients with alcoholic cirrhosis and HCC had HBV DNA integrated into the genome of neoplastic liver cells [22]. How can these data be reconciled with others which show the frequency of integration in HBsAg-seronegative HCC to be in the range of 10%–30% [17, 20, 21]? Imazeki, et al. analyzed 34 patients with HCC and found the integration of viral DNA in all nine HBsAg-seropositive and in 3 of 25 (12%) -seronegative cases by the Southern blot hybridization technique [21] (Fig. 3.1). Although the possibility of technical artifacts was suggested [23], no convincing explanation for this discrepancy has been offered. Epidemiological surveys have demonstrated that more of the patients with HCC were seronegative for HBsAg (Table 3.1). These integration data seem to have great implications in HBsAg-seronegative HCC. The only way to

Table 3.3. Reported frequency of HBV integration in HCC (by Southern blot hybridization technique)

	Serum HBsAg	No. of subjects	Positive integration	Reference
Shafritz et al.	+	12	12(100%)	17
	−	8	3(38%)	
Brechot et al.	+	17	17(100%)	18
	−	16	16(100%)	
Koshy et al.	+	4	3(75%)	19
	−	2	0(0%)	
Hino et al.	+	9	8(89%)	20
	−	15	2(13%)	
Imazeki et al.	+	9	9(100%)	21
	−	25	3(12%)	

resolve the discrepancy may be to clone and sequence the integrated viral DNA found in HBsAg-seronegative cases. Yaginuma et al. [24] analyzed the integrated viral DNA in an HCC cell line derived from an HBsAg-seronegative patient and found a single integrated copy of a 1895-base-pair subgenomic region of HBV DNA, spanning from the middle of the pre-S gene to the end of the gene X. With the accumulation of such data, the structure and frequency of the integration and the impact of HBV infection in hepatocarcinogenesis in HBsAg-seronegative patients will be understood.

1.2.2 Studies by cloning and sequencing of integrated viral DNA

Southern blot hybridization is a useful technique to screen for the presence of HBV DNA integration in a large number of specimens, but detailed information on the structure of integrated viral DNA may be gained only by cloning and sequencing the integrated viral DNA and cellular flanking DNA. The data analyzed so far indicate the following [25–30]: (1) Frequently, multiple copies of viral DNA are integrated in the genome of HCC. In the Alexander cell line (PLC/PRF/5), at least eight different clones have

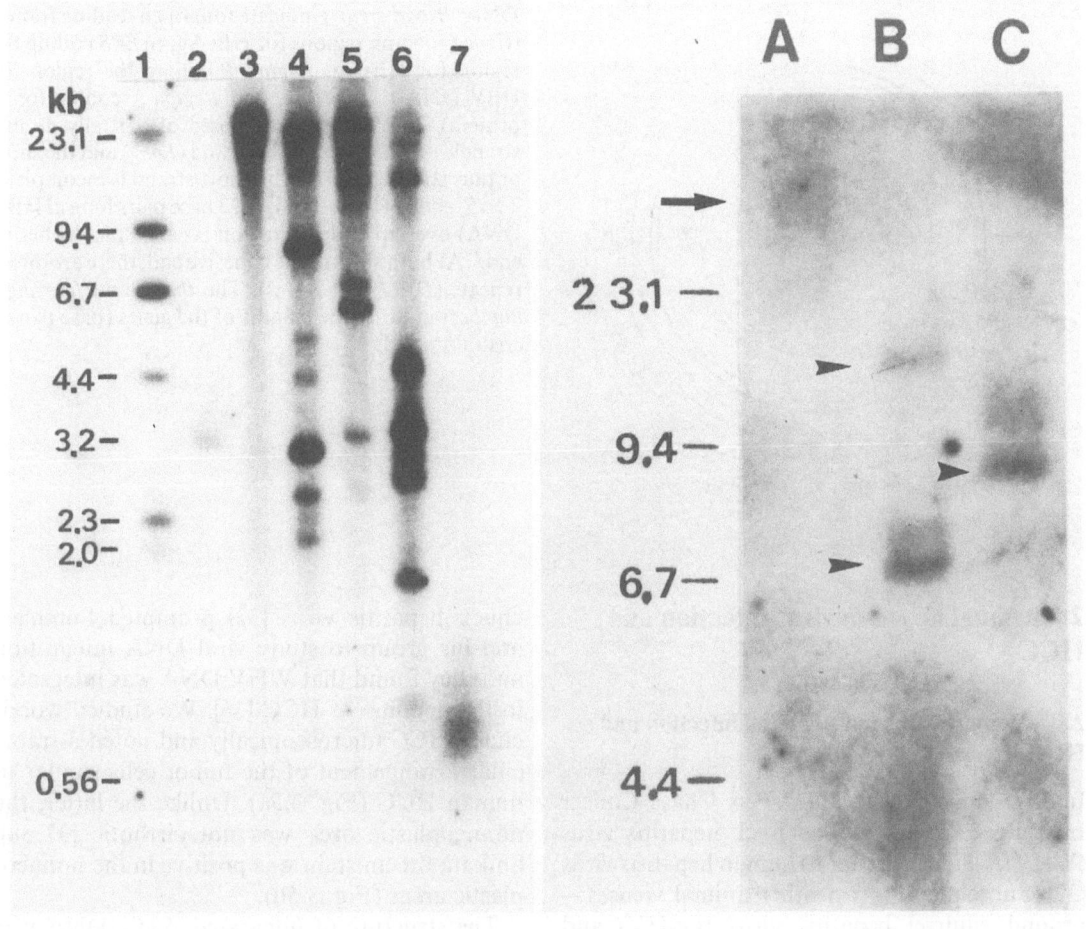

Fig. 3.1a, b. Southern blot hybridization of extracted DNA from HCC in two patients, **a** HBsAg seropositive; a very high molecular radioactive signal (lane *3*) was converted to several discrete bands, some of which were located higher than HBV DNA (lane *2*) after restriction enzyme digestion (lane *4*, Hind III; lane *5*, Eco RI; lane *6*, Bam HI; and lane *7*, Taq I). **b** HBsAg seronegative; the signals were generally weak. The *arrow* indicates very high molecular signals, and the *arrowheads* show bands after enzyme digestion, suggesting integration

been identified [30]. (2) Almost always, the integrated viral DNA found is not full length (3200 base pairs) and is often devoid of a part of the C gene (549-base-pair segment coding for HBcAg) (Fig. 3.2). The S gene (678-base-pair segment coding for HBsAg) is well preserved. In addition to deletion, integrated viral DNA is often rearranged to yield inverted repetition of part of the viral and cellular gene [29]. (3) No specific viral site of integration has been identified. However, a virus-specific site of integration is often within DR 1 or DR 2 (Fig. 3.2). DR 1 and DR 2 (direct repeat) consist of an 11-base-pair repeat sequence (TTCACCTCTGC), which is located at both sides of the "cohesive ends" (Fig. 3.2). This may be analogous to the long terminal

repeat (LTR) seen in retroviruses. (4) No specific structure of the cellular gene has been identified in the integration site.

Most of the time, the integrated viral DNA in HCC is so extensively rearranged that it is difficult to deduce the structure of a virus-cell DNA junction when the virus gene is integrated into the cellular gene. However, most studies suggest that HBV DNA can initially integrate via a specific viral DNA sequence (DR 1 and DR 2) [26, 31]. More information is needed on the integration pattern in the early stage of infection before HCC develops. The role of viral DNA integration in hepatocarcinogenesis will be discussed at the end of this chapter.

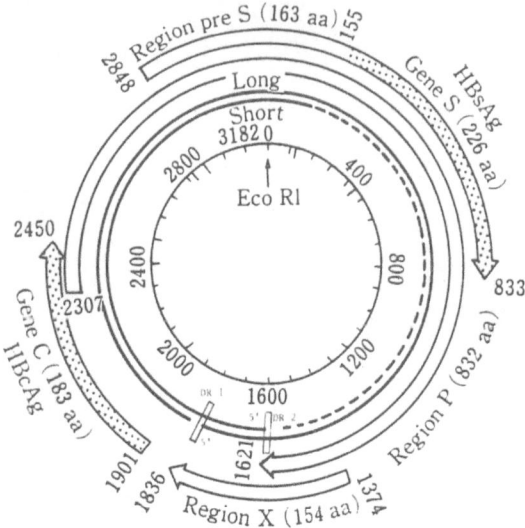

Fig. 3.2. Structure and genetic organization of HBV DNA. *Broad arrows* indicate four open reading frames (*Gene C* coding regions for HBcAg, *Gene S* coding the region for HBsAg, *Region P* coding the region for HBV DNA polymerase, and *Region X* coding for X protein). The DNA is composed of partially double strands—the long or minus strand (*Long*) and the short or plus strand (*Short*). The short strand is incomplete. The 5′-ends of two strands (223 base pairs long in HBV DNA) overlap and this region is called the "cohesive end." At both sides of the cohesive end, there are direct repeats (*DR 1* and *DR 2*). The *three*- and *four-digit numbers* indicate the lengths of the genes (base pairs). *aa* amino acids

2 Animal hepadna virus infection and HCC

2.1 Woodchuck hepatitis virus infection and HCC

In 1978, Summers et al. at Fox Chase Cancer Institute discovered woodchuck hepatitis virus (WHV), which is similar to human hepatitis virus [32]. Subsequently, two other animal viruses—ground squirrel hepatitis virus (GSHV) and duck hepatitis B virus (DHBV)—were described by Marion et al. [33] and Mason et al. [34], respectively. These viruses are termed hepadna viruses, and their characteristics are summarized in Table 3.4. They have partially double-stranded DNA (Fig. 3.2). The structure of DNA is similar among the mammalian viruses (HBV, WHV, and GSHV), but the genetic organization of DHBV DNA is somewhat different from that of the other three: The mammalian viruses have basically four different genes encoding HBsAg (S gene), HBcAg (C gene), DNA polymerase (region P), and an unknown product (region X) (Fig. 3.2), but DHBV lacks region X (Fig. 3.3). The nucleotide homologies between HBV and the three animal hepadna viruses (WHV, GSHV, and DHBV) are around 70%, 55%, and 40%, respectively. The morphology of the virion is similar among the four viruses and shows a Dane particlelike structure with the internal core and the outer surface antigen (Fig. 3.4).

In 1968, Snyder described the frequent occurrence of HCC in woodchucks (9 of 30) at the Philadelphia Zoo [35]. The discovery of wood-chuck hepatitis virus [32] prompted Summers and his group to study viral DNA integration and they found that WHV DNA was integrated in the genome of HCC [36]. We studied woodchuck HCC microscopically and noted a trabecular arrangement of the tumor cells similar to human HCC (Fig. 3.5a). Unlike the latter, the nonneoplastic area was not cirrhotic [37, 38]. Shikata orcein stain was positive in the nonneoplastic areas (Fig. 3.5b).

The structure of integrated WHV DNA was analyzed by Ogston et al. [39]. Analysis of two integrated clones in HCC revealed extensive rearrangement (deletion, duplication, and inverted repetition) and the location of one end of the integrated viral DNA close to the cohesive end (DR 1).

Rogler and Summers [40, 41] studied the structure of viral DNA in a woodchuck with chronic liver disease (without HCC) and found two different types of viral DNA. One was a "novel" form of WHV DNA that was 7–10 kilobase pairs larger than the 3.2-kilobase-pair length of WHV DNA. However, this form was not attached to cellular DNA and, hence, not integrated. The other form was an integrated form which was 2.7 kilobase pairs long. This had a deletion of approximately 500 base pairs in the region between the 1000- and 1500-base position on the viral map (Fig. 3.2), but no internal rearrangement of the viral DNA was recognized. Due to the deletion of 500 base pairs, this form may be incapable of supporting viral replication.

Although there have been a number of studies on the genomic structure of integrated viral

Table 3.4. Characteristics of four hepadna viruses

	Host	Distribution	Prevalence (%)	HCC	Virion size (nm)	Surface particle size (nm)	DNA size (base pairs)	DNA homology with HBV DNA
HBV	Man	Worldwide	0.1–20	Yes	42	20–25	3150	
WHV	*Marmota monax*	Pennsylvania, Maryland	30–35	Yes	40–45	20–25	3200	+ + +
GSHV	*Spermophlus beechey*	California	0–50	Yes	47	18–20	3200	+ + +
DHBV	Domestic duck	China	1–60	Yes	40	35–60	3021	+

HBV Hepatitis B virus, *WHV* woodchuck hepatits virus, *GSHV* ground squirrel hepatitis virus, *DHBV* duck hepatitis B virus

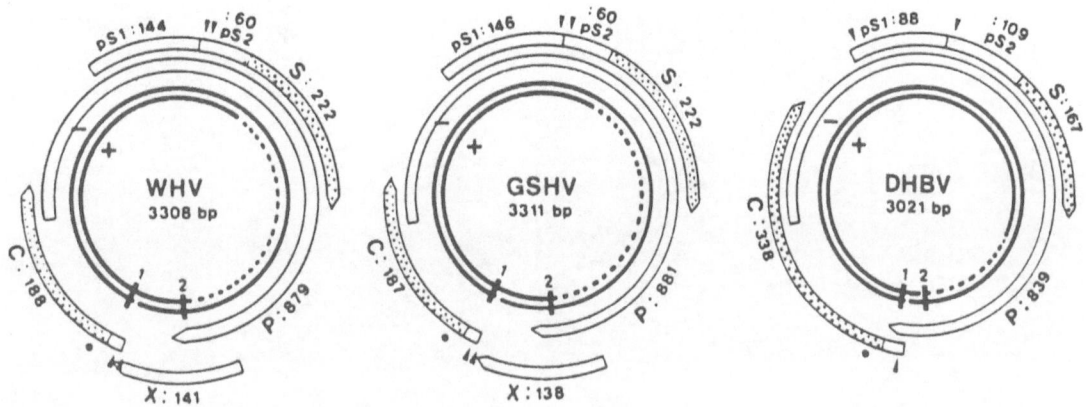

Fig. 3.3. The genetic organization of three hapadna viruses (*WHV, GSHV, DHBV*). DHBV lacks the X region. *C* coding the region for HBcAg; *pS1* coding region for pre-S1 region; *pS2* coding region for pre-S2; *S* coding region for HBsAg; *P* coding region for DNA-polymerase; *X* coding region for X protein. The *two-* and *three-digit numbers* indicate the lengths of the genes (amino acids)

DNA in HCC, data on the structure of the integrated form in nonneoplastic chronic liver disease are limited. The study of WHV infection by Rogler and Summers indicated that integration of viral DNA did occur in nonneoplastic hepatocytes and that the difference in the structure between the integrated form in hepatocytes and in HCC was the absence of extensive internal rearrangement of viral DNA that was often observed in woodchuck [39] and human HCC [25]. However, whether the absence of extensive rearrangement of viral DNA is characteristic of the integration in chronic liver disease has yet to be determined by the analysis of more cases.

The frequent development of HCC has been well documented in woodchucks in zoos. However, to study the pathogenic role of WHV

in HCC, experimental infection of WHV-susceptible woodchucks under controlled laboratory conditions is required. Gerin and colleagues [42] performed a transmission study with WHV and found the development of HCC within 18 months in four of five woodchucks infected at birth but in none of the noninfected woodchucks followed for more than 3 years. These observations have provided experimental support to the view that WHV and, by analogy, HBV may have oncogenic properties.

2.2 DHBV infection and HCC

In 1980, Mason et al. described a virus found in Pekin ducks which was similar to human HBV [34]. It had several properties common to other

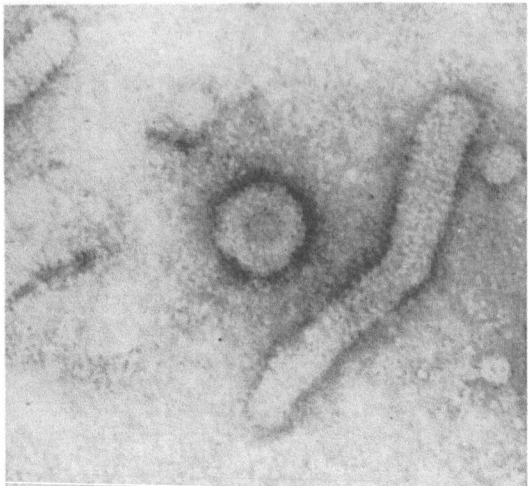

Fig. 3.4. Electron micrograph of WHV particles in serum. Two types are seen—one round virion with an internal core structure, like an HBV Dane particle, and the other tubular

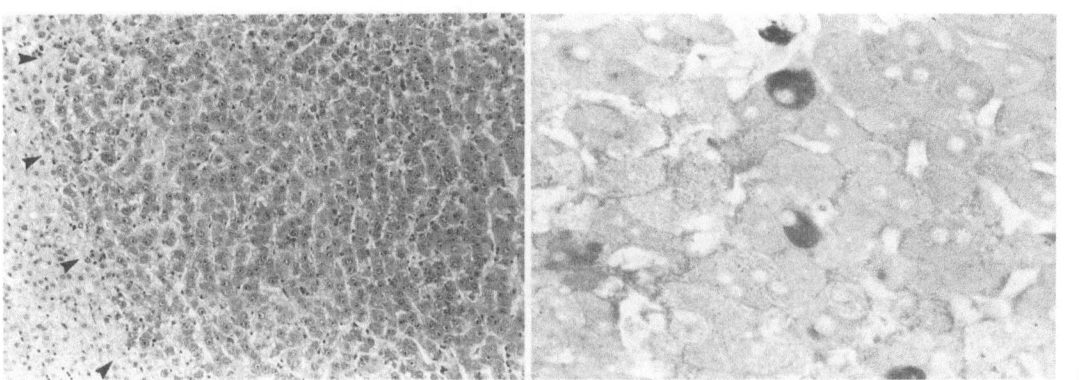

Fig. 3.5. a Photomicrograph of woodchuck HCC. Tumor cells with a trabecular arrangement (*arrow-heads*) are darkly stained and show minimal atypia. H and E, × 80. **b** WHV infected liver. A dark cytoplasmic stain is seen in several cells. Shikata stain, × 400

hepadna viruses (Table 3.4) such as partially double-stranded DNA. Complete analysis of the viral DNA revealed a length of 3021 nucleotides. The nucleic acid homology with other hepadna viruses is rather weak, but four regions located between nucleotides 100 and 200, 300 and 500, 600 and 800 (all these are in gene S), and 1300 and 2100 had about 50% homology with the corresponding regions found in the HBV and WHV. The regions between nucleotides 1300 and 1400 had the highest homology (70%) [43]. One of the characteristic features of DHBV DNA is the absence of an open reading frame for gene X (Fig. 3.3). However, the significance of its absence is not known.

The frequent occurrence of HCC among woodchucks led to the discovery of WHV. Therefore, liver disease in infected ducks was sought in the USA and it was generally reported

that liver disease was infrequent in infected ducks [34, 44]. We first obtained liver tissue of ducks from China and found a high (50%) infection rate among 24 ducks from the Chitung area of China as well as various pathological changes of the liver, which included chronic hepatitis and HCC [45]. However, we were not able to study the molecular state of viral DNA in the liver tissue of these ducks because only formalinfixed tissue was available. It was found further that some livers of noninfected ducks had cirrhotic changes (Fig. 3.6) [45, 46]. We conducted a more extensive study of duck hepatitis and infection by obtaining fresh-frozen livers from 170 ducks in China, 28 ducks in Taiwan, 20 ducks in India, and ten ducks in Indonesia. DHBV infection was observed only in areas along the east coast of China. The specimens obtained from Chitung County, approximately 150 km to the north of

Fig. 3.6. Gross finding of the liver with cirrhotic changes seen in a DHBV-infected duck obtained from China

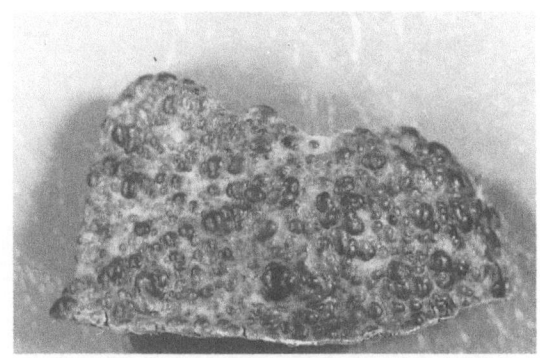

Shanghai, were most heavily infected, and the infection rate turned out to be 70% (16 of 23) when sera and liver specimens were analyzed by DNA hybridization techniques [47]. These infected ducks showed a variety of pathological changes, including advanced chronic liver disease. In contrast, none of the virus-negative ducks had advanced hepatic changes. The livers of two ducks showed neoplastic changes, one being a benign bile duct adenoma and the other a large HCC (Fig. 3.7a, b); no evidence of infection was obtained in the former, whereas integrated viral DNA was found in the latter in the areas of HCC by Southern blot hybridization (Fig. 3.8). Recently, Imazeki cloned the integrated viral DNA of this HCC and analyzed its structure. The results showed extensive rearrangement of viral DNA with inverted repetition (unpublished data).

Although we observed pathological changes in the liver of ducks from China, no significant liver disease was found in infected ducks from the USA [34, 46]. It has been suggested that the difference in duck breed is an important factor in the development of liver disease. Of the ducks we obtained from China, half were "white Pekin" and the other half were colored "Chinese" ducks. The DHBV infection rate was 4% in the former and 64% in the latter. According to the zoological description of the "Chinese" duck, these ducks were reared in China for many years and were kept in fields in very large numbers, where they fed on weeds, waste rice, wild seeds, and water insects [48]. Histological examination revealed that 36% of the infected "Chinese" ducks had chronic active hepatitis, whereas the infection rate for DHBV was low in "white Pekin" ducks, and the two infected white Pekins showed a near normal liver. Our survey of ducks obtained from various areas indicated that the infection rate for DHBV may vary from place to

place and that the difference in duck breed may explain varying results in the development of DHBV infection and liver disease. The ducks with HCC which we found to have integrated viral DNA were colored "Chinese" ducks.

2.3 GSHV infection and HCC

In 1980, Marion et al. [33] reported the presence of another hepatitis virus in Beechey ground squirrels in northern California. A study of the liver pathology in the infected ground squirrels failed to demonstrate significant lesions [49]. WHV and GSHV DNA sequences are very closely related with more than 80% homology. The genetic organization of WHV and GSHV is likewise very similar and is also similar to that of HBV (Fig. 3.3). Despite the similarity of the two viruses, the marked difference in the frequency of HCC development has remained an enigma.

Recently, some of the infected ground squirrels developed HCC after several years in captivity (WS Robinson and PL Marion, personal communication). Whether the difference in hepatocarcinogenesis between the two animal species is explicable only on a molecular biological basis or is somehow related to different host responses to the similar viruses has yet to be determined. One approach to this problem is perhaps to make recombinant WHV and GSHV DNAs and transfect the hybrid DNA to individual hosts in order to evaluate the pathological changes in the liver.

3 Role of viral DNA integration in hepatocarcinogenesis

Viral integration in the genome of HCC has been demonstrated in three of four hepadna viruses [12–15, 25–30, 36, 39, 47]. Detailed analyses of

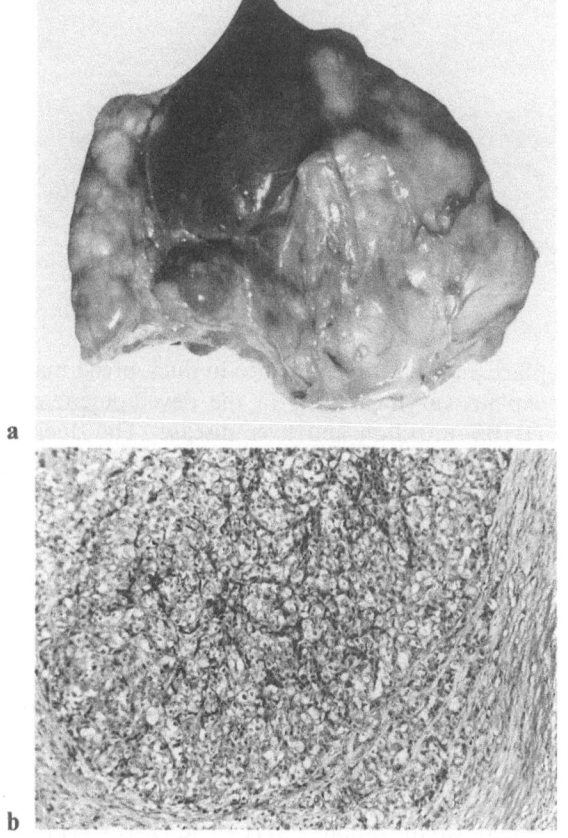

Fig. 3.7. a Massive liver tumor in a "Chinese" duck. **b** Photomicrograph of the tumor. Cancer cells are in a trabecular arrangement and are surrounded by a fibrous capsule. H and E, × 100

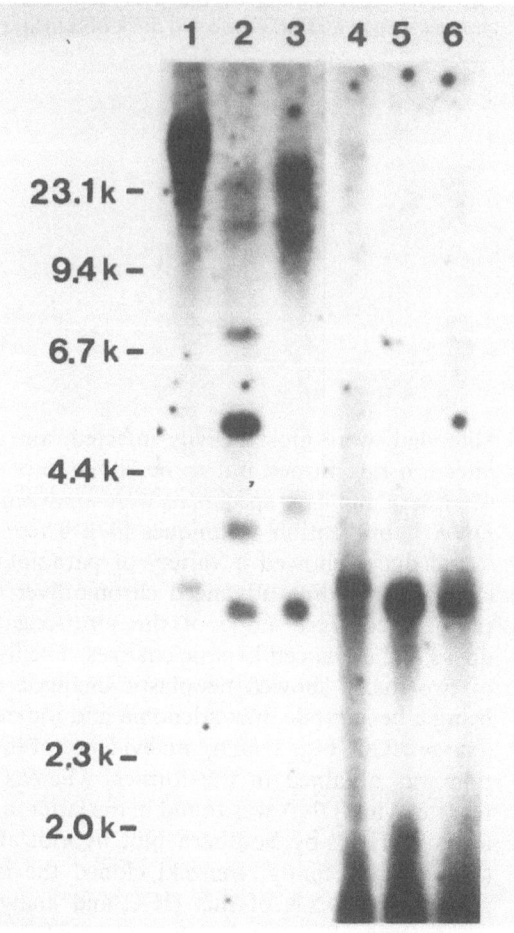

Fig. 3.8. Southern blot hybridization of DNA extracted from the tumor (lanes *1–3*) and adjacent nonneoplastic liver of Fig. 3.9 (lanes *4–6*). Integrated viral DNA was identified in the tumor and episomal DNA was seen in the nonneoplastic tissue. Lanes *1* and *4*, undigested DNA; lanes *2* and *5*, Eco RI; lanes *3* and *6*, Hind III

the integrated viral segment have failed to show any constant site of integration or common viral DNA segments of deletion or duplication. However, studies of integrated viral DNA in humans and animals indicate that at least one end of the integrated viral DNA segment is in the vicinity of the "cohesive end" or one of the direct repeats (DR 1 and DR 2) (Fig. 3.3, 3.9). These direct repeats are composed of an 11-base-pair repeat (TTCACCTCTGC) in HBV, a 10-base-pair repeat (TCACCTGTGC) in WHV, an 11-base-repeat (TTCACCTGTGC) in GSHV, and a 12-base-pair repeat (TACACCCCTCTC) in DHBV. The direct repeats are located at both sides of the "cohesive ends." It is tempting to speculate by analogy with the retroviruses that hepatitis virus DNA is integrated at the direct

repeats (Fig. 3.9). In man, HCC develops after a long incubation period, sometimes as long as 60 to 70 years. Thus, the extensive rearrangement or deletion of viral DNA observed in HCC seems to occur after hepatitis viral DNA was integrated. Initially, viral DNA may integrate at a fixed position, possibly at the direct repeats. It seems necessary here to obtain information on the molecular details of integration in the early phase of infection, namely in chronic hepatitis or in acute hepatitis. An intriguing observation was made by Rogler and Summers [41] in a chronically infected woodchuck. In their study, one of the virus-cell junctions (integrated site) was adjacent to DR 2, and no rearrangement of integrated viral DNA was found. Therefore, there may be a more regular way of integration at the beginning

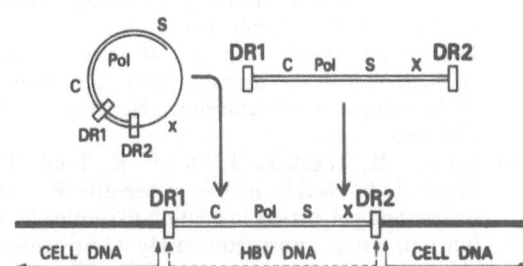

Fig. 3.9. Comparison of Integration models for retro- and hepadna viruses. Retroviral DNA, which has *gag* (this seems to correspond to C gene in HBV DNA), *pol* (region P in HBV), *env* (S gene in HBV DNA), and *x* (region X in HBV DNA) genes from the 5'-end, could be integrated at both long terminal repeats (*LTR*). In HBV infection, the initiation pattern of integration is not known. However, it is conceivable that the viral genome is integrated at both direct repeats (*DR*) and could be rearranged and deleted during the long incubation period of hepatocarcinogenesis

than that extrapolated from the findings in HCC. If this is true, the process could be very similar to that in retroviruses (Fig. 3.9).

How could the virus integration induce transformation of hepatocytes and be related to hepatocarcinogenesis? There are several possibilities.

Transforming gene of virus. The viral DNA itself could contain a transforming gene (oncogene) like some retroviruses. Analysis of the viral DNA structure and studies of the transforming activity of the viral genome have failed to demonstrate a constituent transforming gene or activity. If the virus had an oncogene in its genome, malignancy would develop quite rapidly. Therefore, these results do not explain the long incubation in human HCC.

Promoter insertion model. A cellular oncogene which induces cell transformation and which is inactive under normal conditions could be activated by the integration of viral DNA and its promoter sequence upstream from the cellular oncogene [50, 51]. In this model, the viral DNA would have to be integrated adjacent to a cellular oncogene. A recent study demonstrated that HBV DNA contains an "enhancer" element which is positioned between nucleotides 1080 and 1234 [52]. Thus, an integrated segment of "enhancer" could activate the transcription of the neighboring oncogenes.

Hybrid DNA transcripts. Recent data suggest that hybrid hepatitis B virus-host transcripts may be produced by the integration of viral DNA into the hepatocyte genome [53, 54]. These newly synthesized transcripts and their products

may play a role in HBV-related oncogenesis.

Chromosomal deletion was recently described in an HBV integration site in HCC [55]. Thus, not only the rearrangement, translocation, or duplication of integrated viral DNA, but also the changes of the host chromosome due to integration may be related to hepatocarcinogenesis.

All these mechanisms still remain possibilities. DNA technology and hepadna animal models will probably contribute to the elucidation of the underlying mechanism.

References

1. Tong MJ, Sun S-C, Schaeffer BT, Chang NK, Lo KJ, Peters R (1971) Hepatitis-associated antigen and hepatocellular carcinoma in Taiwan. Ann Int Med 75: 687–691
2. Szmuness W (1978) Hepatocellular carcinoma and the hepatitis B virus: evidence for a causal association. In: Milnick JL (ed) Progress in medical virology, vol. 24. Karger, Basel, pp 40–69
3. Lutwick LI (1979) Relation between aflatoxin and hepatitis B virus and hepatocellular carcinoma. Lancet I: 755
4. Omata M, Aschcavai M, Liew C-T, Peters R (1979) Hepatocellular carcinoma in the U.S.A., etiologic considerations. Localization of hepatitis B antigens. Gastroenterology 76: 279–287
5. Kubo Y, Okuda K, Hashimoto M, Nagasaki Y, Ebata H, Nakajima Y, Musha H, Sakuma K, Ohtake H (1977) Antibody to hepatitis B core core antigen in patients with hepatocellular carcinoma. Gastroenterology 72: 1217–1220
6. Denison EK, Peters RL, Reynolds TB (1971) Familial hepatoma with hepatitis-associated antigen. Ann Int Med 74: 391–394

7. Ohbayashi A, Mayumi M, Okochi K (1971) Australia antigen in familial cirrhosis. Lancet I: 244

8. Okada K, Yamada T, Miyakawa Y, Mayumi M (1975) Hepatitis B surface antigen in the serum of infants after delivery from asymptomatic carriers mothers. J Pediat 87: 360–363

9. Beasley RP (1982) Hepatitis B virus as the etiologic agent in hepatocellular carcinoma-epidemiologic considerations. Hepatology 2: 21S–26S

10. Sakuma K, Takahara T, Okuda K, Tsuda F, Mayumi M (1982) Prognosis of hepatitis B virus surface antigen carriers in relation to routine liver function tests: a prospective study. Gastroenterology 83: 114–117

11. Munoz M, Linsell A (1982) Epidemiology of primary liver cancer. In: Correa P, Haenszel W (eds) Epidemiology of cancer of the digestive tract. Nijhoff, Hague, pp 161–195

12. Marion PL, Salazar FH, Alexander J, Robinson WS (1980) State of hepatitis viral DNA in a human hepatoma cell line. J Virol 33: 795–806

13. Chakraborty PR, Ruiz-Opazo N, Shouval D, Shafritz DA (1980) Identification of integrated hepatitis B virus DNA and expression of viral DNA in an HBsAg-producing human hepatocellular carcinoma cell line. Nature 286: 531–533

14. Brechot C, Pourcel C, Louise A, Rain B, Tiollais P (1980) Presence of integrated hepatitis B virus DNA sequence in cellular DNA of human Hepatocellular carcinoma. Nature 286: 533–535

15. Edman JC, Gray P, Valenzuela P, Rall LB, Rutter WJ (1980) Integration of hepatitis B virus sequences and their expression in a human hepatoma cell. Nature 286: 535–538

16. Southern EM (1975) Detection of specific sequences among DNA fragments separated by gel electrophoresis. J Mol Biol 98: 503–517

17. Shafritz D, Shouval D, Shermann HI, Hadziyannis SJ, Kew MC (1981) Integration of hepatitis B virus DNA into the genome of the liver cells in chronic liver disease and hepatocellular carcinoma. N Engl J Med 305: 1067–1073

18. Brechot C. Pourcell C, Hadchouel M, Dejean A, Lonise A, Scotto J, Tiollais P (1982) State of hepatitis B virus DNA in liver disease. Hepatology 2: 27S–34S

19. Koshy R, Maupas R, Muller R, Hofschneider PH (1981) Detection of hepatitis B virus specific DNA in the genomes of human hepatocellular carcinoma and liver cirrhosis tissues. J Gen Virol 57: 95–102

20. Hino O, Kitagawa T, Koike K, Kobayashi M, Hara M, Mori W, Nakashima T, Hattori N, Sugano H (1984) Detection of hepatitis B virus DNA in hepatocellular carcinoma in Japan. Hepatology 4: 90–96

21. Imazeki F, Omata M, Yokosuka O, Okuda K (1986) Integration of hepatitis B virus DNA in hepatocellular carcinoma: reappraisal after exclusion of possible bacterial contamination. Cancer 58: 1055–1060

22. Brechot C, Nalpas B, Courouce AM, Duhamel G,

Gallard P, Carnot F, Tiollais P, Berthelot P (1982) Evidence that hepatitis virus has a role in liver cell carcinoma in alcoholic liver disease. N Engl J Med 306: 1384–1387

23. Hino O, Kitagawa T, Sugano H (1984) Bacterial contamination of human tumor samples. Nature 225: 670–671

24. Yaginuma K, Kobayashi M, Yoshida E, Koike K (1985) Hepatitis B virus integration in hepatocellular carcinoma DNA: duplication of cellular flanking sequences at the integration site. Proc Natl Acad Sci USA 82: 4458–4462

25. Dejean A, Brechot C, Tiollais P, Wain-Hobson S (1983) Characterization of integrated hepatitis B viral DNA cloned from a human hepatoma and the hepatoma-derived cell line PLC/PRF/5. Proc Natl Acad Sci USA 80: 2505–2509

26. Dejean A, Sonigo P, Wain-Hobson S, Tiollais P (1984) Specific hepatitis B virus integration in hepatocellular carcinoma DNA through a viral 11-base-pair direct repeat. Proc Natl Acad Sci USA 81: 5350–5354

27. Koshy R, Koch S, Freytag von Loringhoven A, Kahmann R, Murray K, Hofschneider PH (1983) Integration of hepatitis B virus DNA: evidence for integration in the single-stranded gap. Cell 34: 215–223

28. Shaul Y, Ziemer M, Garcia PD, Crawford R, Hsu H, Valenzuella P, Ruffer WJ (1984) Cloning and analysis of integrated hepatitis virus sequences from a human hepatoma cell line. J Virol 51: 776–787

29. Mizusawa H, Taira M, Yaginuma K, Kobayashi M, Yoshida E, Koike K (1985) Inversely repeating integrated hepatitis B virus DNA and cellular flanking sequences in the human hepatoma-derived cell line huSP. Proc Natl Acad Sci USA 82: 208–212

30. Ziemer M, Garcia P, Shaul Y, Rutter WJ (1985) Sequence of hepatitis B virus incorporated into the genome of a human hepatoma cell line. J Virol 53: 885–892

31. Tiollais P, Pourcel C, Dejean A (1985) The hepatitis B virus. Nature 317: 489–495

32. Summers J, Smolec J, Snyder RL (1978) A virus similar to human hepatitis B virus associated with hepatitis and hepatoma in woodchuck. Proc Natl Acad Sci USA 75: 4533–4537

33. Marion PL, Oshiro LS, Regnery DC, Scullard GH, Robinson WS (1980) A virus in Beechey ground squirrels that is related to hepatitis B virus of humans. Proc Natl Acad Sci USA 77: 2941–2945

34. Mason WS, Seal G, Summers J (1980) Virus of Pekin ducks with structural and biological relatedness to human hepatitis B virus. J Virol 36: 829–836

35. Snyder RL (1968) Hepatomas of captive woodchucks. Am J Path 52: 32a (abstr)

36. Summers J, Smolec JM, Werner BG, Kelly JJ, Tyler GU, Snyder RL (1980) Hepatitis B and woodchuck hepatitis virus are members of a novel class of DNA viruses. In: Viruses in naturally

occurring cancers. Cold Spring Harbor Conferences on Cell Proliferation 1980, vol. 7, New York, pp 459–470

37. Snyder RL, Summers J (1980) Woodchuck hepatitis virus and hepatocellular carcinoma. In: Viruses in naturally occurring cancers, Cold Spring Harbor Conferences on Cell Proliferation, vol. 7, New York, pp 447–457

38. Popper H, Shih JWK, Gerin JL (1981) Woodchuck hepatitis and hepatocellular carcinoma. Hepatology 1: 91–98

39. Ogston CW, Jonak GJ, Rogler CE, Astrin SM, Summers J (1982) Cloning and structural analysis of integrated woodchuck hepatitis virtus sequences from hepatocellular carcinomas of woodchuck. Cell 29: 385–394

40. Rogler C, Summers J (1982) Novel forms of woodchuck hepatitis virus DNA isolated from chronically infected woodchuck liver nuclei. J Virol 44: 852–863

41. Rogler C, Summers J (1984) Cloning and structural analysis of integrated woodchuck hepatitis virus sequences from a chronically infected liver. J Virol 50: 832–837

42. Gerin J, Tennant B, Popper H, Tyeryar F, Purcell R (1985) Chronic hepatitis and hepatocellular carcinoma in woodchuck following experimental woodchuck hepatitis virus infection. In: H Varmus, J Summers (eds) Molecular biology of hepatitis B viruses. Cold Spring Harbor, New York, p 26 (abstr.)

43. Mandart E, Kay A, Galibert F (1984) Nucleotide sequence of a cloned duck hepatitis B virus genome: comparison with woodchuck and human hepatitis B virus sequences. J Virol 49: 782–792

44. Mason WS, Taylor JM, Seal G, Summers J (1982) An HBV-like virus of domestic ducks. In: Alter H, Maynard J, Szmuness W (eds) Viral hepatitis. Franklin Institute Press, Philadelphia, pp 107–116

45. Omata M, Uchiumi K, Ito Y, Yokosuka O, Mori J, Terao K, Weifa Y, O'Connell AP, London WT, Okuda K (1983) Duck hepatitis B virus and liver disease. Gastroenterology 85: 260–267

46. Marion PL, Knight SS, Ho BK, Guo YY, Robinson WS, Popper H (1984) Liver disease associated with duck hepatitis B virus of domestic ducks. Proc Natl Acad Sci USA 81: 898–902

47. Yokosuka O, Omata M, Zhou Y–Z, Imazeki F, Okuda K (1985) Duck hepatitis B virus DNA in liver and serum of Chinese ducks: integration of viral DNA in a hepatocellular carcinoma. Proc Natl Acad Sci USA 82: 5180–5184

48. Howard H, Weller MW, Humphrey PS, Clark GA (1973) Domestic waterfowl. In: Delacour J (ed) The waterfowl of the world, vol. 4. Country Life, London, pp 154–166

49. Marion PL, Knight SS, Salazar FH, Popper H, Robinson WS (1983) Ground squirrel hepatitis virus infection. Hepatology 3: 519–527

50. Hayward WS, Neel BG, Astrin SM (1981) Activation of a cellular oncogene by promoter insertion in ALV induced lymphoid leukosis. Nature 290: 475–480

51. Neel G, Hayward WS, Robinson HL, Fang J, Astrin SM (1981) Avian leucosis virus-induced tumor have common proviral integration sites and synthesize discrete new RNAs: oncogenes by promoter insertion. Cell 23: 323–334

52. Shaul Y, Rutter J, Laub O (1985) A human hepatitis B viral enhancer element. EMBO J 4: 427–430

53. Ou J, Rutter WJ (1985) Hybrid hepatitis B virus-host transcripts in a human hepatoma cell. Proc Natl Acad Sci USA 82: 83–87

54. Freytag von Loringhoven A, Koch S, Hofschneider PH, Koshy R (1985) Co-transcribed 3' sequences augment expression of integrated hepatitis B virus DNA. EMBO J 4: 249–255

55. Rogler C, Sherman M, Su CY, Shafrits DA, Summers J, Shows TB, Henderson A, Kew M (1985) Deletion in chromosome 11p associated with a hepatitis B integration site in hepatocellular carcinoma. Science 230: 319–322

Chapter 4
Human Hepatoma Cell Lines

JENNIFER J. ALEXANDER[1]

1 Introduction

A major biological component of cancer is that of uncontrolled growth. Viable cells do not maintain stasis with the organ of origin although they may retain some of its specialized metabolic functions. This seemingly unlimited growth potential in vivo should be transplantable to in vitro conditions where repeatable and comparative studies could be carried out on many different cell lines, originating from tumors of the same histological type but from different individuals. However, the establishment of human tumors as permanent cell lines in vitro is a rare event.

Normal hepatocytes in vitro do not readily divide although they can be maintained as monolayer cultures and retain many specialized hepatocyte functions. Many attempts have been made to develop cell lines from human hepatomas, and within the last decade a number of these cell lines have been established. While some of these cultures have been more extensively studied than others, some comparisons between the findings on different hepatoma lines can be made. Human hepatoma cell lines provide material for the following investigations: (1) metabolic similarities or differences among cultures derived from well-differentiated and poorly differentiated tumors, (2) possible etiological agents, and (3) the nature of hepatoma at the molecular level.

In this overview, hepatoma is defined as hepatocellular carcinoma and excludes hepatoblastoma since the two are differentiated pathologically, although metabolically they may have many common features.

2 Established hepatoma cell lines

The methods used to establish hepatoma cell lines vary and no single method has been developed with a reasonable success rate. In general tumor tissue which contains no necrotic areas and which is processed for culture as rapidly as possible is the ideal starting material, even though there is generally less than a 20% chance for successful establishment as a continuously growing cell line outside the original host. Direct inoculation of nude mice with human tumor material is proving a more successful way of maintaining tumor growth than direct explantation in vitro for some malignancies.

During the establishment of any cell line, normal cells within the tumor specimen may grow preferentially and after a long period in vitro become established as a cell line. Cross-contamination with other cell lines may also occur. Thus, any cell line reportedly established from a human hepatoma should demonstrate in vitro features consistent with the cell type from which it originated, and, secondly, the cell line should have malignant properties.

Table 4.1 lists most of the hepatoma cell lines which have been established. A few, such as SK Hep-1 [1] and Chen [2] hepatoma lines, have been omitted because the former was derived from an adenocarcinoma and the latter has no morphological or metabolic features consistent with hepatocytes. Two further cell lines, Hep G-2 [3] and HuH-6 [4], which retain many liver specific functions in vitro, have been omitted as they were derived from hepatoblastomas. All of the cell lines listed in Table 4.1 were derived from tumors which were histologically diagnosed as hepatoma or, synonymously, hepatocellular carcinoma, primary liver cell carcinoma or primary liver cancer.

[1] Department of Microbiology, University of the Witwatersrand, P.O. WITS 2050, Republic of South Africa

Table 4.1. Patient characteristics and hepatoma cell lines

Patient						Cell line		Reference
Age (years)	Sex	Origin	Histological diagnosis	Serology		Morphology	Designation	
				AFP	HBsAg			
NS	F	South Africa	Hepatoma	NS	−	Epithelioid	Mahlavu	5
64	M	Japan	Undifferentiated HCC	+	NS	Epithelial Fibroblast	HLE HLF	6
24	M	Mozambique	Hepatoma	+	+	Epithelial	PLC/PRF/5	7
8	M	USA	HCC	NS	+	Epithelial	Hep 3B	3
53	M	People's Rep. China	PLCC	+	ND	Epithelial	BEL 7402	8
69	M	People's Rep. China	PLCC	+	ND	Epithelial	BEL 7404	
41	F	People's Rep. China	PLCC	+	+	Epithelial	BEL 7405	
50	M	India	HCC	NS	+	Hepatocyte	DELSH-5	9
53	M	Japan	Hepatoma	NS	+	Epithelial	HUH-1	10
51	M	Japan	Hepatoma	NS	+	Epithelial	HUH-4	
57	M	Japan	Well differentiated HCC	+	−	Epithelial	HUH-7	11
63	M	USA	Poorly differentiated HCC	−	−[a]	Epithelioid	FOCUS	12
NS	NS	Thailand	HCC	+	−	Polygonal	HHP-40	13
NS	NS	Thailand	HCC	+	−	and mixed	HHP-85	
NS	NS	Thailand	HCC	+	−	spindle	HHP-89	
NS	NS	Thailand	HCC	+	−	shaped	HHP-56	
53	M	Japan	HCC	+	−[a]	Polygonal	KG55T	14
59	M	USA	HCC	+	+	Epithelial	TONG/PHC	15
NS	F	UK	PLC	+	−[b]	Epithelial	PLC/NUT/1	16
NS	M	Japan	HCC	NS	+	Epithelial	HCC-M	17
56	M	Taiwan	HCC	NS	NS	Polygonal	HA22T/VGH	18
49	M	Taiwan	HCC	NS	NS	Polygonal	HA47T/VGH[d]	
58	M	Japan	HCC	NS	−[c]	NS	HuH-2	19

PLCC primary liver cell carcinoma, *NS* not stated, *ND* not done
[a] HBsAb+
[b] No HBV markers
[c] HBcAb+
[d] Chang, C (1985) personal communication

2.1 Patient characteristics

The reported age range of the hepatoma patients (Table 4.1) was 8–69 years, 12 of these 16 patients being over 50 years of age. Two patients were from Africa, where the majority of cases present between the third and fifth decades of life. Patients from the Far East were generally about 20 years older, and 18 of the cell lines were derived from these patients. The male to female ratio of the hepatoma patients was about 5 : 1, which is in accordance with the world-wide male predominance of hepatoma.

Of the 15 patients tested for alphafetoprotein (AFP), 14 were serologically positive; 8 of the 18 tested had serum hepatitis B surface antigen (HBsAg). Of the ten negative for HBsAg, two were hepatitis B surface antibody (HBsAb) positive and one was hepatitis B core antibody (HBcAb) positive, demonstrating previous exposure to hepatitis B virus (HBV). Thus, the reported total HBV association with hepatoma was 61% (11 of 18); however, this may be an underestimate since most HBsAg-negative patients were not tested for other markers.

2.2 Cell-line characteristics

2.2.1 Markers of liver-associated functions

Twelve of the hepatoma cell lines have been suffi-

Table 4.2. In vitro characteristics of 12 hepatoma cell lines

Cell line	Secretion		Chromosome number	Nude mouse tumors	Reference
	AFP	Plasma proteins			
Mahlavu	−	+[a]	ND	+[b]	
PLC/PRF/5	−	+	56–59	+	7, 20
Hep 3B	+	+	60	+	20
Delsh-5	+	ND	61	ND	
HuH-1	+	+	69	NS	11
HuH-4	+	+	70	NS	11
HuH-7	+	+	ND	+	
Focus	−[c]	+	61–70	+	
Tong/PHC	+	+	63	+	
PLC/NUT/1	+	NS	63	+	
HA22T/VGH	NS	+	ND	+[b]	
HA47T/VGH[a]	−	+	69	+	

ND not done, *NS* not stated
[a] Chang, C (1985) personal communication
[b] Aspinall S (1985) unpublished results
[c] Cells positive by immunofluorescence

ciently characterized to enable a more detailed comparison between some of their similarities and differences. A number of the cell lines have been shown to synthesize AFP and a range of plasma proteins which are secreted into the growth medium. Besides the cell lines listed in Table 4.2, BEL 7402, 7404 and 7405 lines together with the HHP 40, 85, 89 and 56 lines also synthesize and release AFP. The FOCUS line was established from the tumor of a patient whose serum was AFP negative and the absence of AFP secretion by these cells in vitro is consistent with the in vivo findings. PLC/PRF/5 cells express undetectable to low levels of AFP in vitro, but high levels are measurable in the sera of tumor-bearing nude mice [21]. While any cell line theoretically may express any gene in vitro, the demonstration of AFP or plasma protein production by these cells is consistent with the differentiated function of hepatocytes in vivo. AFP-producing cell lines also provide material for a detailed experimental study of the control of oncofetal gene expression and, in particular, whether AFP production precedes or succeeds the commitment to malignancy.

2.2.2 Malignant properties
Criteria used to define the malignancy of cell lines are either growth in soft agar and/or the production of tumors in athymic/nude mice. All eight of the twelve hepatoma cell lines tested (Table 4.2) produce tumors in nude mice. These tumors are histologically similar to the original

hepatomas. Subcutaneous inoculation of 10^7 PLC/PRF/5 cells into either newly weaned or 4-month-old nude mice produces palpable nodules within 2–3 weeks. Within 8 weeks these nodules develop into large subcutaneous tumors with an extensive blood supply. The tumors constitute up to 60% of the total mouse body weight.

The fact that both liver-associated metabolic features and malignant properties are measurable can be used to define many of the cell lines as representative cultures in vitro of human hepatomas in vivo.

2.2.3 Metabolic similarities
A recent study has shown that AFP production in response to combinations of hormones is different among five human hepatoma cell lines tested [22]. The levels of AFP produced under non-stimulated tissue culture conditions also varied among AFP-positive cell lines. This suggests that there are inherent differences in the degree of AFP gene activation in the cell lines. The amount of AFP produced by each particular cell line may reflect the degree of differentiation of the hepatoma in vivo, since poorly differentiated tumors may show closer metabolic similarities to early fetal organ development, while highly differentiated tumors might reflect the metabolic status measurable in later fetal organogenesis. In the former situation a higher level of AFP expression could be expected, reflecting the higher AFP levels expressed during early fetal development, and lower levels may be syn-

thesized in more differentiated tumors, as found in the later stages of fetal development. The levels of AFP which have been determined by different investigators have not supported this hypothesis, however. HuH-7 cells, established from a highly differentiated hepatocellular carcinoma (HCC), secrete approximately 80 ng AFP/10^4 cells/day [22], whereas no AFP was detected in the growth medium from FOCUS cells which were derived from a poorly differentiated HCC, although the cells were positive for AFP by immunofluorescence staining [12]. The histological diagnoses of other hepatomas from which cell lines were established were not specific as to the degree of differentiation. Future correlations between the detailed histology of the original hepatomas and the levels of AFP expression in vitro by cell lines established from these tumors may confirm or reject the above hypothesis.

In comparative studies among a limited number of hepatoma cell lines the activity of a number of liver-specific enzymes was measured as well as the presence of liver cell surface receptors [23]. PLC/PRF/5 cells also displayed many characteristics in vitro similar to HCC in vivo when analysed by immune and histochemical techniques [24].

2.2.4 Chromosome studies

All of the cell lines analysed have human karyotypes and are heteroploid (Table 4.2), and most have marker chromosomes. The PLC/PRF/5 cell line was examined at passages 17–28 [25] and, with banding techniques, at passages 60–90 [26] and 110 [27]. The modal chromosome number remained stable at 56–59. In these studies a high degree of concordance was found in two laboratories between the banded karyotypes, and a number of similarities were detected between the marker chromosomes of Hep 3B and PLC/PRF/5 cells. In another study [28], however, the karyotype of PLC/PRF/5 cells was shown to alter significantly when HBsAg-producing cells, morphologically different from the parental cells, were isolated from pancreas and muscle tissue of nude mice bearing PLC/PRF/5 tumors. These cells were metastatic in nude mice and contained an average of 99 human chromosomes. The authors could detect cells with the same morphology in standard PLC/PRF/5 tissue cultures.

Since it has proved impossible to obtain metaphase spreads from liver biopsies, direct comparisons between the karyotypes of hepatomas and the cell lines cannot be done. Selective pressure, reflected by rearrangements or alterations of certain chromosomes, may occur during the establishment of cells to in vitro growth before chromosomal studies are possible. Only detailed comparative analyses on a large number of hepatoma cell lines will determine whether or not common chromosomal abnormalities occur.

3 Hepatoma cell lines and HBV

3.1 HBsAg production

A number of cell lines produce HBsAg (Table 4.3) and the amounts detected in the growth medium range from about 0.1 μg to 1 μg/10^6 cells 24 h. Cell line-derived HBsAg consists only of small 20-nm-diameter spheres and tubular forms [32, 33] and has the same biophysical and biochemical characteristics and HBsAg derived from human serum [33, 34]. Antigen is rapidly released from the cells after synthesis and no 20-nm particles have been detected in PLC/PRF/5 cells by electron microscopy [35]. The largest polypeptide of HBsAg is glycosylated and cells grown in the presence of Tunicamycin, an inhibitor of glycosylation, continue to synthesize and export non-glycosylated but antigencially active HBsAg [36].

PLC/PRF/5, HuH-1, HuH-4, Tong/PHC and DELSH-5 cells produce HBsAg continuously

Table 4.3. Hepatoma cell lines and HBV

Cell line	HBsAg synthesis	Integrated HBV DNA	Reference
Mahlavu	−	−	29
PLC/PRF/5	+	+	30
Hep 3B	+	+	
Bel 7402	−	−	29
7404	−	−	29
7405	−	−	29
Delsh-5	+	ND	
HuH-1	+	+	31
HuH-4	+	ND	
HuH-7	−	ND	
Focus	−	+	
KG 55T	−	+	31
TONG/PHC	+	+	
PLC/NUT/1	+	+	
HCC-M	−	ND	
HA22T/VGH	−	+[a]	
HA47T/VGH	−	+	
HuH-2	−	+	19, 31

ND not done

[a] Chang, C (1985) personal communication

although it is only measurable in concentrated media taken from DELSH-5 cultures. In contrast, Hep 3B cells synthesize detectable HBsAg only as the cultures become confluent. The mode of antigen production by PLC/PRF/5 cells was examined in synchronized cultures [36]. The cells did not synthesize HBsAg during the S phase, but thereafter continuous production was measured, indicating that in this cell line antigen synthesis was not confined to a single phase of the growth cycle. Both PLC/PRF/5 and Hep 3B cells have been cloned [37–39], and all clones produce HBsAg, suggesting that the original tumors were derived from one or more HBV-positive liver cells.

3.1.1 Interferon and immunotherapy
HBsAg expression in infected patients has been inhibited following interferon (IFN) treatment [40]. PLC/PRF/5 cells did not produce endogenous IFN when stimulated with poly I poly C but did respond to exogenously added IFN as the treated cells induced 2'5'-oligo (A) synthetase [41, 42] and inhibited sindbis, vesicular stomatitis, and encephalomyocarditis virus replication. Low doses of IFN which induced the antiviral state, however, did not inhibit HBsAg production. High IFN doses caused a cytostatic effect and, indirectly, a decrease in HBsAg synthesis. IFN treatment of nude mice inoculated with PLC/PRF/5 cells did not affect tumor growth [41].

PLC/PRF/5 cells in vitro were not inhibited in the presence of polyclonal HBsAb with or without complement [43]. However, more detailed studies have shown that monoclonal HBsAb together with complement were cytotoxic to these cells [44], and the production of PLC/PRF/5 tumors was inhibited in nude mice treated with specific monoclonal HBsAb [45].

3.1.2 Antiviral chemotherapy
The effects of antiviral compounds such as adenine arabinoside, ribavirin [46], 3'-deoxyadenosine and 6-azauridine [47] have shown that a decrease in HBsAg production is concomitant with a decrease in cell viability or protein synthesis. Similar effects were found when cells were treated with Hygromicin B [47], an inhibitor of translation, and the antifungal agents ketoconazole and amphotericin B [48].

Dexamethasone, betametasone, cortisone [49] and sodium butyrate [50] enhanced HBsAg production by 40% to 200% in PLC/PRF/5 cells. Dexamethasone, however, induced a ten-fold increase of HBsAg in HuH-1 cells, but antigen production was only slightly increased in HuH-4 cells [10]. Differences in response to glucocorticoid treatment may be due to differences in expression of steroid membrane receptors in different cell lines.

No 42-nm complete infectious HBV particles have been induced in any HBsAg-positive cell line. Neither the spent growth medium nor the cells were infectious when inoculated into chimpanzees [51, 52].

The inherent differences between the amounts of HBsAg produced by each hepatoma cell line may be due to: (1) different numbers of HBV S-gene copies; (2) differences in the activation mechanisms of S-gene transcription in individual cell lines, such as the presence or absence of viral enhancer or promoter elements or host cell factors [53]; (3) differences in the sites of viral DNA integration in host chromosomes.

3.2 Other HBV gene products
Four coding regions have been identified in HBV DNA: (1) S region, which codes for HBsAg; (2) C region, which codes for hepatitis B core antibody (HBcAg) and hepatitis Be antigen (HBeAg), the latter being a breakdown product of HBcAg; (3) P region, coding for viral DNA polymerase; (4) X region—the product or function of this gene has not been determined. Apart from the S gene no human hepatoma cell line has been shown consistently to express C, P or X gene products.

Miller and Robinson [54] have shown that the C-gene region of HBV DNA in PLC/PRF/5 cells is highly methylated while the S gene is not. Treatment of these cells with an inhibitor of methylation, 5-azacytidine, has given conflicting results. Aspinall and Alexander [55] detected neither HBcAg nor HBeAg following prolonged growth in the presence of this inhibitor; Yoakum et al. [56] found HBcAg in these cells after 3–6 days of 5-azacytidine treatment.

Extracts from tumors produced in nude mice by PLC/PRF/5 cells have been reported to contain C gene-like products with a density of 1.3 g/ml in CsCl gradients, similar to that measured for viral core particles [57]. Earlier studies from the same laboratory described two HBV-specific particles in PLC/PRF/5 cells grown in tissue culture— particles with a buoyant density of 1.2 g/ml which contained HBsAg and particles with a density of 1.3 g/ml which had HBV DNA-specific sequences [58]. Aspinall (personal communication, 1985) has detected non-specific HBeAg reactivity in extracts from tumors induced in nude mice following inoculation of different human hepatoma cell lines. Non-specific reactivity was also found in concentrated extracts from normal human and mouse livers.

Antisera raised against synthetic peptides representing different regions of the HBV DNA X gene were reacted with extracts from PLC/PRF/ 5 cells and the HBV-negative hepatoblastoma cell line Hep G2. A 28-kilodalton protein from the HBV-positive cell line reacted positively while Hep G2 cell extracts did not react. Antibodies to the synthetic X protein were detected in sera from four hepatoma patients positive for HBV markers [59].

Wen et al. [60] detected a nuclear antigen by anticomplement immunofluorescence in PLC/ PRF/5 and Hep 3B cells; the antigen was not present in Mahlavu or Hep G2 cells. Antibody to this nuclear antigen was present in a low percentage of sera from HBsAg-positive hepatoma patients, but not in sera from HBsAg-negative hepatoma patients. The authors postulate that this nuclear antigen may represent expression of either (1) the X gene region of HBV DNA, (2) another as yet unidentified HBV gene, or (3) enhanced expression of a transformation-associated cellular gene.

All observations on the synthesis of HBV gene products other than HBsAg need further confirmation and comparative analyses among a variety of HBV-associated hepatoma cell lines.

3.3 HBV DNA and hepatoma cell lines

The association between HBV DNA and HCC is discussed in detail in Chapters 2 and 3. The following are brief comments which refer more specifically to studies on hepatoma cell lines. Viral DNA when present in hepatoma cell lines is integrated into host chromosomal DNA. Since integrated HBV DNA has been found in normal non-tumorous liver cell DNA, a preferred site or sites of integration may be necessary for transformation in vivo.

3.3.1 Chromosomal localization

In two studies the chromosomal site of HBV DNA integration was investigated in Hep 3B [61] and PLC/PRF/5 cells [62]. A single integration site was detected in chromosome 12 in a clone derived from the parental Hep 3B cell line. The viral DNA was located at 12q13-q14, which contains a known fragile site but does not correlate with any known oncogene location. In situ hybridization of radiolabelled HBV DNA to metaphase spreads of PLC/PRF/5 cells identified three chromosomal integration regions—15q22-q23, 11q22 and 18q12. The hybridization signal at 15q22-q23 was the most intense. In this connection, Rogler et al. [63] reported that one of three HBV DNA integration sites in a HCC was accompanied by a deletion of cellular sequences in chromosome 11 at the 11p13-11p14 location. These results, though limited, have not identified a common chromosomal site.

3.3.2 Molecular studies

A number of cell lines (Table 4.3) contain HBV DNA sequences but do not express HBsAg. This may be due to total or partial S-gene deletions. Both HuH2 and KG-55T cells have S-gene sequences although they may be incomplete genes. Different HBV DNA inserts cloned from PLC/ PRF/5 cells produce different amounts of HBsAg following transfection [64].

The number of identifiable HBV DNA sequences integrated into the DNA of different hepatoma cell lines varies from one [39] to seven [53], and different researchers have found different numbers of integrated viral DNA sequences in the same cell line. Hind III restriction analyses of PLC/PRF/5 cell DNA have yielded three [30], five [65] and six [66] high-molecular-weight HBV DNA-containing fragments. HuH-2 cells digested with Hind III had one major HBV DNA band at 5.2 kb [31], while a clone, HuH 2-2, contained a single band at 9.8 kb [39]. DNA extracted from hepatoma cell lines HuH-1 and KG 55T [31] contained, respectively, three and two high-molecular-weight bands of viral DNA. Twist et al. [39] analysed HBV DNA in three hepatoma cell lines cloned from Hep 3B. The patterns of integration differed significantly among the clones.

These results suggest that integrated HBV sequences in many hepatoma call lines are probably unstable. Instability may also result in inversions, duplications and deletions of viral and host DNA sequences, which might have occurred in vitro after a presumed molecular event had taken place which precipitated the onset of malignancy in vivo.

4 Hepatoma cell lines without HBV

A number of cell lines have been established which by virtue of their in vitro properties appear to be representative hepatoma cell lines. They include the Bel series, HuH-7, HCC-M and Mahlavu. The patients from whom the BEL 7405 and the HCC-M lines were established were serologically postive for HBsAg. Mahlavu and HuH-7 donors had no HBsAg, but other serological HBV markers were not tested. None of these cell lines secrete HBsAg and the BEL lines and Mahlavu had no detectable HBV DNA sequences. The four Thailand hepatoma cell lines, all derived from HBsAg-negative patients, synthesized no HBsAg although three of the lines were only tested by the relatively insensitive counter-immuno-electrophoresis test. Tests for the presence of HBV DNA sequences have not been reported for the Thailand, HCC-M or HuH-7 cells lines.

5 Discussion

Hepatoma is a common malignancy in certain parts of the world, and concomitant environmental factors, showing an equally highly regionalized distribution, may be causally related to the development of this tumor. One of these factors is HBV infection. A number of hepatoma cell lines have been established providing unlimited amounts of material for investigating the biochemical features which may be specific to hepatoma and the nature of the virus-cell association in many of these cell lines.

The establishment of a permanently growing cell line from any human tumor is more the result of serendipity than of science. No single laboratory has been able to compare the characteristics of all the cell lines reportedly established from human hepatomas; some published results are not always independently verifiable and therefore must remain anecdotal. Thus, in this overview of human hepatoma cell lines emphasis has been placed, as far as possible, on results which have been corroborated by independent investigators. Most of the cell lines which have been discussed fulfill the requirements of both malignancy and liver-specific metabolic features in vitro. Large amounts of tumor can be grown in nude mice and histologically these tumors are indistinguishable from human hepatoma, providing controlled systems for testing a wide range of pharmacological and immunostimulatory agents.

Epidemiological and prospective studies have shown a striking association between HBV infection and hepatoma. Molecular studies on hepatoma cell lines have not yet provided any explanation of a common mechanism whereby the virus may induce the tumor, and HBV contains no known oncogene. HBV is liver-tropic, replicates via an RNA intermediate and is able to integrate into chromosomal DNA. This combination alone may be sufficient to destabilise any persistently infected hepatocyte by more than one mechanism over a period of years and may manifest as one of a number of functional instabilities such as cell death, dedifferentiation or transformation. Transformation may arise following viral DNA integration at any of a number of host DNA sites.

Comparisons between cell lines and even between the same cell line in different laboratories suggest that HBV DNA integration, when present, may not be stable in vitro.

The correlation between serological markers of HBV in cell-line donor patients with hepatoma (Table 4.1) is 61%. The number of hepatoma cell lines having an HBV association (Table 4.3) is 66%. Such close agreement may be fortuitous as not all serological markers were tested in the patients, a number of cell lines negative for HBsAg have not been examined for HBV DNA, and not all of the cell lines listed in Table 4.1 have been included in Table 4.3.

Three of the cell lines which do not produce HBsAg but have integrated HBV DNA sequences were taken from patients who were not HBsAg carriers but were serologically positive for antibodies to HBV.

All persistently infected cell lines which constitutively synthesize any viral antigen produce only HBsAg, suggesting that the mechanisms of viral DNA integration may be similar in all HBV-associated hepatomas.

A significantly high proportion of hepatoma cell lines contain integrated HBV DNA sequences; the S gene, but no other viral gene, is expressed in over 50% of these cell lines.

References

1. Fogh J, Trempe G (1975) New human tumor cell lines. In: Fogh J (ed) Human tumor cells in vitro. Plenum, London, pp 115–159
2. Chen J, Tang S, Chu T, Shen T (1962) Preliminary report on the establishment of a strain of human liver cancer cells in vitro. In: VIII International Cancer Congress Abstracts. Moscow, p 136
3. Aden D, Fogel A, Plotkin S, Damjanov I, Knowles B (1979) Controlled synthesis of HBsAg in a differentiated human liver carcinoma-derived cell line. Nature 282: 615–616
4. Doi I (1976) Establishment of a cell line and its clonal sublines from a patient with hepatoblastoma. Gann 67: 1–10
5. Prozesky O, Brits C, Grabow W (1973) In vitro culture of cell lines from Australia Antigen posi-

tive and negative hepatoma patients. In: Saunders S, Terblanche J (eds) Liver. Pitman, London, pp 358–360

6. Doi I, Namba M, Sato J (1975) Establishment and some biological characteristics of human hepatoma cell lines. Gann 66: 385–392

7. Alexander J, Bey E, Geddes E, Lecatsas G (1976) Establishment of a continuously growing cell line from primary carcinoma of the liver. S Afr Med J 50: 2124–2128

8. Chen R, Zhu D, Ye X, Shen D, Lu R (1980) Establishment of three human liver carcinoma cell lines and some of their biological characteristics in vitro. Scientia Sinica 23: 236–247

9. Das P, Nayak N, Tsiquaye K, Zuckerman A (1980) Establishment of a human hepatocellular carcinoma cell line releasing hepatitis B virus surface antigen. Br J Exp Pathol 61: 648–654

10. Huh N, Utakoji T (1981) Production of HBs-antigen by two new hepatoma cell lines and its enhancement by dexamethasone. Gann 72: 178–179

11. Nakabayashi H, Taketa K, Miyano K, Yamane T, Sato J (1982) Growth of human hepatoma cell lines with differentiated functions in chemically defined medium. Cancer Res 42: 3858–3863

12. He L, Isselbacher K, Wands J, Goodman H, Shih C, Quaroni A (1984) Establishment and characterization of a new human hepatocellular carcinoma cell line. In Vitro 29: 493–504

13. Laohathai K, Bhamarapravati N (1985) Culturing of human hepatocellular carcinoma: A simple and reproducible method. A J P 118: 203–208

14. Matsuura H (1983) Primary cultured cells and an established cell line of human hepatocellular carcinomas. Acta Med Okayama 37: 341–352

15. Lin J-H, Tong M, Stevenson D (1984) A new human hepatocellular carcinoma cell line secreting hepatitis B surface antigen and alpha-fetoprotein. In: Vyas G, Deinstag J, Hoofnagle J (eds) Viral hepatitis and liver disease. Grune and Stratton, Orlando, p 673

16. Bassendine M, Curtin N, Ince P, Gaunt K, Fowler M, James O (1984) Establishment of a cell line (PLC/NUT/1) containing integrated hepatitis B virus (HBV) DNA from a hormone associated human primary liver cell cancer. In: Vyas G, Deinstag J, Hoofnagle J, (eds) Viral hepatitis and liver disease. Grune and Stratton, Orlando, p 625

17. Watanabe T, Morizane T, Tsuchimoto K, Inagaki Y, Munakata Y, Nakamura T, Kumagai N, Tsuchiaja M (1983) Establishment of a cell line (HCC-M) from a human hepatocellular carcinoma. Int J Cancer 32: 141–146

18. Chang C, Lin Y, O'Lee T-W, Chow C-K, Lee T-S, Liu T-S, P'Eng F-K, Chen T-Y, Hu C-P (1983) Induction of plasma protein secretion in a newly established human hepatoma cell line. Mol Cell Biol 3: 1133–1137

19. Yaginuma K, Kobayashi M, Yoshida E, Koike K (1985) Hepatitis B virus integration in hepatocellular carcinoma DNA: Duplication of cellular flanking sequences at the integration site. Proc Natl Acad Sci USA 82: 4458–4462

20. Knowles B, Howe C, Aden D (1980) Human hepatocellular carcinoma cell lines secrete the major plasma proteins of hepatitis B surface antigen. Science 209: 497–499

21. Bassendine M, Arborgh B, Shipton N, Monjardino J, Aranguibel F, Thomas H, Sherlock S (1980) Hepatitis B surface antigen and alphafetoprotein secreting human primary liver cancer in athymic mice. Gastroenterology 79: 528–532

22. Nakabayashi H, Taketa K, Yamane T, Oda M, Sato J (1985) Hormonal control of α-fetoprotein secretion in human hepatoma cell lines proliferating in chemically defined medium. Cancer Res 45: 6379–6383

23. Knowles B, Searls D, Aden D (1984) Human hepatoma derived cell lines. In: Chisari F (ed) Advances in hepatitis research. Masson, New York, pp 196–202

24. Gerber M, Garfinkel E, Hirschman S, Thung S, Panagiotatos T (1981) Immune and enzyme histochemical studies of a human hepatocellular carcinoma cell line producing hepatitis B surface antigen. J Immunol 126: 1085–1089

25. Robinson K, Bey E, Alexander J, Gear J (1976) Chromosome analyses of two recently established human tumor cell lines derived from a carcinoma of the oesophagus and a primary liver tumor. S Afr J Med Sci 41: 285–295

26. Simon D, Aden D, Knowles B (1982) Chromosomes of human carcinoma cell lines. Int J Cancer 30: 27–33

27. Pinto M, Bey E, Bernstein R (1985) The PLC/PRF/5 human hepatoma cell line: 1. Re-evaluation of karyotype. Cancer Genetics Cytogenetics 18: 11–18

28. Marquardt O, Freytag von Loringhoven A, Miller K, Desmyter J (1984) Two types of cells are present in in vitro and in vivo cultures of PLC/PRF/5 cells. In: Vyas G, Deinstag J, Hoofnagle J (eds) Viral hepatitis and liver disease. Grune and Stratton, Orlando, p 669

29. Koshy R, Maupas Ph, Muller R, Hofschneider PH (1981) Detection of hepatitis B virus-specific DNA in genomes of human hepatocellular carcinoma and liver cirrhosis tissue. J Gen Virol 57: 95–102

30. Marion P, Salazar F, Alexander J, Robinson W (1980) State of hepatitis B viral DNA in a human hepatoma cell line. J Virol 33: 795–806

31. Koike K, Kobayashi M, Mizusawa H, Yoshida E, Yaginuma K, Taira M (1983) Rearrangement of the surface antigen gene of hepatitis B virus integrated in the human hepatoma cell lines. Nuc Acid Res 11: 5391–5402

32. Stannard L, Alexander J (1977) Electron microscopy of HBsAg from human hepatoma cell line. Lancet 2: 713–714

33. Alexander J, Macnab G, Saunders R (1978) Studies on in vitro production of hepatitis B surface antigen by a human hepatoma cell line. In: Pollard M (ed) Perspectives in virology, vol. 10. Raven, New York, pp 103–120

34. Marion P, Salazar F, Alexander J, Robinson W (1979) Polypeptides of hepatitis B virus surface antigen produced by a hepatoma cell line. J Virol 32: 796–802

35. Aoki N, Thung S, Gerber M (1982) Ultrastructural analysis of hepatitis B surface antigen production in vitro. Lab Invest 47: 465–470

36. Alexander J, van der Merwe C, Saunders R, McElligott S, Desmyter J (1982) A comparison between in vitro experiments with a hepatoma cell line and in vivo studies. Hepatology 2: 92S–96S

37. Saunders R, Alexander J (1977) HBsAg production by parental and cloned cell cultures. Lancet 2: 714

38. Wen Y, Copeland J, Mann G, Howard C, Zuckerman A (1981) Detection of HBsAg in a clone derived from the PLC/PRF/5 human hepatoma cell line. Arch Virol 68: 157–163

39. Twist E, Clark H, Aden D, Knowles B, Plotkin S (1981) Integration pattern of hepatitis B virus DNA sequences in human hepatoma cell lines. J Virol 37: 239–243

40. Desmyter J, De Groote G, Bradburne A, Desmet V, Edy V, Billiau A, De Somer P, Mortelans J (1976) Administration of human fibroblast interferon in chronic hepatitis B infection. Lancet 2: 645–647

41. Desmyter J, De Groote G, Ray M, Bradburne A, Desmet V, De Somer P, Alexander J (1981) Tumorigenicity and interferon properties of PLC/PRF/5 human hepatoma cell line. Prog Med Virol 27: 103–108

42. Nakajima Y, Kuwata T, Tomita Y, Okuda K (1982) Effect of interferon on the production of HBsAg and induction of an antiviral state in human hepatoma cell line PLC/PRF/5. Microbiol Immunol 26: 705–712

43. Alexander J, McElligott S, Saunders R (1978) Antibody to hepatitis B surface antigen is not cytotoxic to antigen-secreting hepatocytes. S Afr Med J 54: 973–974

44. Shouval D, Wands J, Zurawski V, Isselbacher K, Shafritz D (1982) Selecting binding and complement-mediated lysis of human hepatoma cells (PLC/PRF/5) in culture by monoclonal antibodies to hepatitis B surface antigen. Proc Natl Acad Sci USA 79: 650–654

45. Shouval D, Shafritz D, Zurawski V, Isselbacher K, Wands J (1982) Immunotherapy in nude mice of human hepatoma using monoclonal antibodies against hepatitis B virus. Nature 298: 567–569

46. Lemon S, Bancroft W (1979) Lack of specific effect of adenine arabinoside, human interferon and ribavirin on in vitro production of hepatitis B surface antigen. J Infect Dis 140: 798–801

47. Clementi M, Bagnarella P, Pauri P, Calegari L (1984) Modulation of production of hepatitis B surface antigen by a human hepatoma cell line. J Med Virol 13: 117–123

48. Pottage J, Kessler H (1985) Inhibition of in vitro HBsAg production by amphotericin B and ketoconazole. J Med Virol 16: 275–281

49. Marshall J, Coulepsis A, Pringle R, Dimitrakakis M, Gust I (1983) The effect of glucocorticoid hormones on release of HBsAg from PLC/PRF/5 (Alexander) hepatoma cells. Acta Virol 27: 429–433

50. Barin F, Goudeau A, Brechot C, Romet-Lemonne J, Sureau C, Lesage G (1983) Further studies on production and characterization of HBsAg derived from a human hepatoma cell line (PLC/PRF/5). Develop Biol Standard 54: 81–92

51. Daemer R, Feinstone S, Alexander J, Tully J, Tully W, London W, Wong W, Purcell R (1980) PLC/PRF/5 (Alexander) Hepatoma cell line. Studies on infectivity and synthesis of hepatitis B virus antigens. Infect Immun 30: 607–611

52. Tabor E, Copeland J, Mann G, Howard C, Skelly J, Snoy P, Zuckerman A, Gerety J (1981) Nondetection of infectious hepatitis B virus in a human hepatoma cell line producing hepatitis B surface antigen. Intervirol 15: 82–86

53. Rutter W, Zeimer M, Ou J, Shaul Y, Laub O, Garcia P, Standring D (1984) Transcription units of hepatitis B virus genes and structure and expression of integrated viral sequences. In: Vyas G, Deinstag J, Hoofnagle J (ed) Viral hepatitis and liver disease. Grune and Stratton, Orlando, pp 67–86

54. Miller R, Robinson W (1983) Integrated hepatitis B virus DNA sequences specifying the major viral core polypeptide are methylated in PLC/PRF/5 cells. Proc Natl Acad Sci USA 80: 2534–2538

55. Aspinall S, Alexander J (1985) Hepatitis B virus gene expression in two cell lines, one derived from a natural human infection, the other experimentally infected in vitro. S Afr Med J 68: 751–754

56. Yoakum G, Korba B, Lechner J, Tokiwa T, Gazdar A, Seeley T, Siegel M, Leeman L, Autrup H, Harris C (1983) High frequency transfection and cytopathology of the hepatitis B virus core antigen gene in human cells. Science 222: 385–389

57. Marquardt O, Freytag von Loringhoven A, Frosner G (1984) PLC/PRF/5 cells grown as nude mouse tumor express HBV core antigen genes. In: Vyas G, Deinstag J, Hoofnagle J (eds) Viral hepatitis and liver disease. Grune and Stratton, Orlando, p 669

58. Zaslavsky V, Marquardt O, Wong T-K, Hofschneider PH (1980) Hepatitis B virus (HBV)-specific structures found in cytoplasmic extracts of cells producing HBV surface antigen (HBsAg) in vitro. J Gen Virol 51: 341–349

59. Moriarty A, Alexander H, Lerner R, Thornton G (1985) Antibodies to peptides detect new hepatitis B antigen: serological correlation with hepatocellular carcinoma. Science 227: 429–433

60. Wen Y-M, Mitamura K, Merchant B, Tang Z, Purcell R (1983) Nuclear antigen detected in hepatoma cell lines containing integrated hepatitis B virus DNA. Infec Immun 39: 1361–1367

61. Simon D, Searls D, Cao Y, Sun K, Knowles B (1985) Chromosomal site of hepatitis B virus (HBV) integration in a human hepatocellular carcinoma-derived cell line. Cytogenet Cell Genet 39: 116–120

62. Bowcock A, Pinto M, Bey E, Kuyl J, Dusheiko G, Bernstein R (1985) The PLC/PRF/5 hepatoma cell line: II. Chromosomal assignment of hepatitis B virus integration sites. Cancer Genetics Cytogenet 18: 19–26

63. Rogler C, Sherman M, Su C, Shafritz D, Summers J, Shows T, Henderson A, Kew M (1985) Deletion in chromosome 11p associated with a hepatitis B integration site in hepatocellular carcinoma. Science 230: 319–322

64. Freytag von Loringhoven A, Koch S, Hofsch-neider PH, Koshy R (1985) Co-transcribed 3′ host sequences augment expression of integrated hepatitis B virus DNA. EMBO J 4: 249–255

65. Brechot C, Pourcel C, Louise A, Rain B, Tiollais P (1980) Presence of integrated hepatitis B virus DNA sequences in cellular DNA of human hepatocellular carcinoma. Nature 286: 533–535

66. Edman J, Gray P, Valenzuela P, Rall L, Rutter W (1980) Integration of hepatitis B virus sequences and their expression in a human hepatoma cell. Nature 286: 535–538

Chapter 5

Analysis of Proto-oncogene Expression During Liver Regeneration and Hepatocarcinogenesis

NELSON FAUSTO[1] and PETER R. SHANK[2]

1 Introduction

The discovery and characterization of viral oncogenes and the cellular genes from which they originated (cellular or proto-oncogenes) represents one of the most dramatic advances in the field of cancer research in recent years. Elucidation of the role of these genes in the process of oncogenesis and the role of the proto-oncogenes in the control of normal cellular growth and/or differentiation has united the fields of cancer research and cell biology. Despite the vast amount of information which has become available recently on the molecular nature of the alterations which lead to the "activation" of proto-oncogenes, the precise role of these genes in the development of natural tumors remains to be established. Some investigators have gone so far as to state that "there is as yet no convincing evidence that activated proto-oncogenes are even necessary, much less sufficient for carcinogenesis" [1]. Although this rather extreme view is a minority opinion, it is important to remember that in the complex process encompassing the development of a tumor, the oncogene may be but one player with several others remaining to be elucidated. Given this still unsettled picture, it is particularly important to define the role which various proto-oncogenes play in normal cells and tissues.

The vast majority of studies designed to examine the role of proto-oncogenes have used cell culture systems to examine expression of these genes during replication or differentiation [2–7]. The regenerating liver remains one of the few systems in which the relationship between proto-oncogene expression and cell replication

can be examined during a physiological growth response in vivo [8]. Studies of the regenerating liver have revealed a precise regulation of proto-oncogene expression in the whole organ and have paved the way for a detailed analysis of the stages which precede hepatocyte DNA replication during liver regeneration [9].

In this report, we will first briefly describe the proto-oncogenes which have been studied in liver regeneration and hepatocarcinogenesis. For a more detailed and comprehensive review of oncogenes, several excellent review articles have recently been published [10, 11]. We will then examine the expression of proto-oncogenes in the regenerative response of rat liver and propose a working hypothesis which links the sequential expression of proto-oncogenes during liver regeneration with circulating and autocrine growth factors. In the last section, we will examine the role of proto-oncogenes in the development of hepatic cell carcinoma.

2 Proto-oncogenes

Most of the proto-oncogenes studied in liver regeneration and hepatocarcinogenesis (src, mos, abl, Ha-ras, Ki-ras, and myc) were first characterized as part of the genome of acute transforming retroviruses and were subsequently shown to have homologues in uninfected cell DNA [10, 11]. In addition to these genes, we have also studied the expression of p53 in rat liver, a gene whose product was first described as a cellular protein complexed with the large T antigen of simian virus (SV) 40 [12].

Oncogenes have been isolated through four basic routes: (1) The majority of known oncogenes have been transduced from the cell into the genome of acutely transforming retroviruses and have been isolated from these genomes; (2) several oncogenes, from primary tumors and cell

Department of Pathology and Laboratory Medicine[1] and Section of Molecular, Cell and Developmental Biology[2], Division of Biology and Medicine, Brown University, Providence RI 02912, USA

lines, have been isolated by the ability of their DNA to transform NIH-3T3 cells or other indicator cells in culture; (3) some oncogenes have been detected by characteristic chromosomal anomalies associated with certain neoplastic diseases; and (4) a set of oncogenes which, unlike those in the first three classes appear to have no counterpart in normal cell DNA, have been found within the genome of DNA tumor viruses.

Although the structures and functions of the 40 or so described oncogenes seemed initially quite disparate, recent experiments indicate that they may fall into a small number of classes. Members of each class might transform cells by a common route. Transformation of a "normal" cell could then require the cooperation of two types of oncogenes, one acting at the cell membrane and one acting in the nucleus. Evidence for this hypothesis came first from the observation that neither *myc* nor Ha-*ras* acting alone could transform normal rat cells, yet acting in concert they were able to transform such cells [13]. Extensions of these initial observations have shown that p53, N-*myc*, SV40, polyoma large T antigen, or adenovirus E la are capable of cooperating with an "activated" *ras* gene to transform normal cells. Implicit in these studies is the view that NIH-3T3 cells are not "normal" but have undergone changes, perhaps associated with their immortalization, similar to those mediated by the nuclear oncogenes. It should be pointed out that there are exceptions to this model in that under certain conditions the *ras* gene alone is sufficient to transform early passage rodent fibroblasts [14, 15].

Weinberg points out [10] that as a general rule those proto-oncogenes which act in the cytoplasm become "activated" by a qualitative change in the coding region of the gene while those proto-oncogenes which act in the nucleus usually become "activated" by quantitative changes in the expression of an unaltered gene product. The most extensively characterized "activated" cytoplasmic oncogene is the *ras* gene product p21. Mutations in the *ras* protein at residues 12, 13, or 61 can lead to "activation." Alternatively, the cytoplasmic *myc* protein can be "activated" by insertion of a viral promoter/enhancer near the gene [16], translocation to proximity to the immunoglobulin heavy chain enhancer [17], or chromosomal amplification [18]. All these *myc* alterations lead to a deregulation of the *normal* gene and enhanced expression of the gene product. A similar but distinct mechanism of enhanced expression of a nuclear oncogene is the stabilization of p53 achieved by association with

the large T antigen in SV40-infected cells [12].

Some of the oncogenes are members of a related family of genes. This is true of the *ras* family, which is composed of two members initially isolated from acute transforming retroviruses, Ha-*ras* and Ki-*ras* [19], and one member, N-*ras*, isolated from a human neuroblastoma by transfection of NIH-3T3 cells [20]. Similarly, the *myc* gene was originally isolated from an acute leukemia virus, MC29 [21], and a distantly related gene, N-*myc*, was isolated from human neuroblastomas [22]. An even more distant relationship exists between the nuclear oncogenes *myc*, E la, and *myb*, the oncogene of avian myeloblastosis virus [23].

The role of the proto-oncogenes in normal cell growth has perhaps been most extensively explored for the *ras* genes, which have been shown to be cytoplasmic guanosine nucleotide-binding proteins. Progress in the analysis of the function of the *ras* genes has been aided by detection of homologous sequences in yeast cells which allow very powerful genetic analysis essentially unavailable in other eukaryotic organisms. These studies have shown that yeast requires one functional copy of the *ras* gene for viability and that the mammalian *ras* can complement defects in the yeast *ras* genes. The current hypothesis is that the yeast *ras* genes are positive regulators of adenylate cyclase analogous to "G" proteins in mammals [24]. However, this observation is not directly applicable to mammalian systems [25]. It has been reported that mammalian *ras* genes induce meiosis in xenopus oocytes without any effect on the levels of cyclic AMP [26].

Although the nuclear oncogenes may function as "trans" activators of transcription, their precise role in the normal cell is unclear. The c-*myc* gene may function as a "competence" factor in the cell cycle [27, 28]; however, other reports indicate that the level of c-*myc* mRNA or protein is essentially invariant in the cell cycle [29, 30]. Given the ambiguity which still remains regarding the function of proto-oncogenes in normal cells, it seems more appropriate than ever to examine the role of these genes in physiological growth responses in vivo.

3 Proto-oncogene expression during liver regeneration

3.1 RNA populations in normal and regenerating liver

Polysomes of normal rat liver contain 20 000–25 000 different polyadenylated mRNAs [31].

These species can be roughly divided into three abundance classes: (1) the most abundant group comprises about 20 mRNAs which are present at more than 5000 copies/cell; (2) the moderate frequency group contains approximately 700 species, with a cellular distribution of 100–200 copies/cell; (3) the rare group comprises the bulk of cytoplasmic mRNAs (about 20 000 species) present at one to five copies/cell [31–34].

Only a subset of polyadenylated RNAs which are transcribed in liver nuclei reaches the cytoplasm. The range of sequence abundance for nuclear RNAs is much narrower than that of cytoplasmic RNAs, varying from 1 (or less) to about 30 copies/cell. This implies that post-transcriptional mechanisms might play an important role in determining the distribution of mRNAs in liver cytoplasm [31, 35–37].

Given this very complex picture, it is easy to understand why detailed analyses of mRNA populations had to be undertaken to determine whether or not changes occur in these populations when liver cells are stimulated to replicate after partial hepatectomy (PH). The major experimental findings from these studies may be summarized as follows:.

a) The rate of synthesis of hepatic poly(A)$^+$ mRNA changes very rapidly after PH [38, 39]. The total amount of polysomal poly(A)$^+$ mRNA increases by 2.5-fold during the first 12 h after PH, but nuclear poly(A)$^+$ RNA amounts are unchanged during the first 2 days after the operation [40].

b) Only 6%–7% of the single-copy haploid genome is transcribed into RNA in normal rat liver. The percentage of genes transcribed does not change during liver regeneration [41–44].

c) Polysomal poly(A)$^+$ mRNA populations in the normal liver are almost entirely homologous to the corresponding regenerating liver RNA populations. However, the abundance of normal liver mRNAs may change (increase or decrease) during liver regeneration [31, 32, 43, 45].

d) Screening of 6000 individual clones from a cDNA library constructed from poly(A)$^+$ mRNA from 18-h regenerating liver failed to identify clones unique to the regenerating liver. Three clones appeared to be more abundant (by at least twofold) in partially hepatectomized than in sham-operated rat liver [46].

e) The analysis of 800 cytosol and 800 membrane proteins by 2-D gel electrophoresis revealed many quantitative changes but only three qualitative changes in comparisons between normal and 18-h regenerating liver proteins. A subset of these quantitative changes was also detected in proteins extracted from the livers of sham-operated rats [46].

3.2 Proto-oncogene expression

The extensive homology existing between mRNAs and proteins of normal and regenerating rat liver made clear that key changes in mRNA populations associated with the entry of hepatocytes into the cell cycle were likely to be confined to changes in the abundance of rare mRNAs. Although it was not immediately obvious which among the 20 000 or more mRNA species that constitute the low-abundance class of liver RNA should be selected for study, the discovery that the *src* gene of Rous sarcoma virus had a counterpart in DNA of higher organisms (and indeed itself had originated by transduction of the cellular sequence) suggested a class of mRNAs which might be important in the regenerative response [47]. Initially, an analysis of c-*src* expression was undertaken in normal and regenerating livers. Subsequently, the expression of several other newly discovered proto-oncogenes was also examined. These studies, discussed below and illustrated in Fig. 5.1, showed that the expression of the proto-oncogenes c-*fos*, c-*myc*, p53, c-Ha-*ras*, and c-Ki-*ras* increases transiently and at relatively defined points after PH in rats. In contrast, the abundance of c-*src* and c-*abl* transcripts does not change during liver regeneration while c-*mos* mRNA is not detected in normal or regenerating livers [8, 9, 48, 49].

3.2.1 c-*myc* and c-*fos* expression

Transcripts of c-*fos* are already elevated 15 min after PH in rats, the earliest time investigated. They reach a maximum during the next hour and decline by 2 h after the operation [9]. Transcripts from c-*myc* are unchanged at 15 min, increase between 30 min and 2 h, and decline to normal by 4 h [9, 50]. From these results, it appears that while elevation of mRNAs encoded by both of these genes is quite rapid, c-*fos* changes precede those of c-*myc*. Similar sequential expression of c-*fos* and c-*myc* has been reported in fibroblasts stimulated by growth factors [4]. However, it is equally possible that the activation of the two genes occurs simultaneously, but a positive balance between synthesis and degradation rates is reached first by c-*fos* mRNA, resulting in an earlier rise in its steady state levels. Such a possibility must be entertained because c-*myc* mRNA (and probably also c-*fos* mRNA) has a very short half-life, at least in some culture cell systems [51].

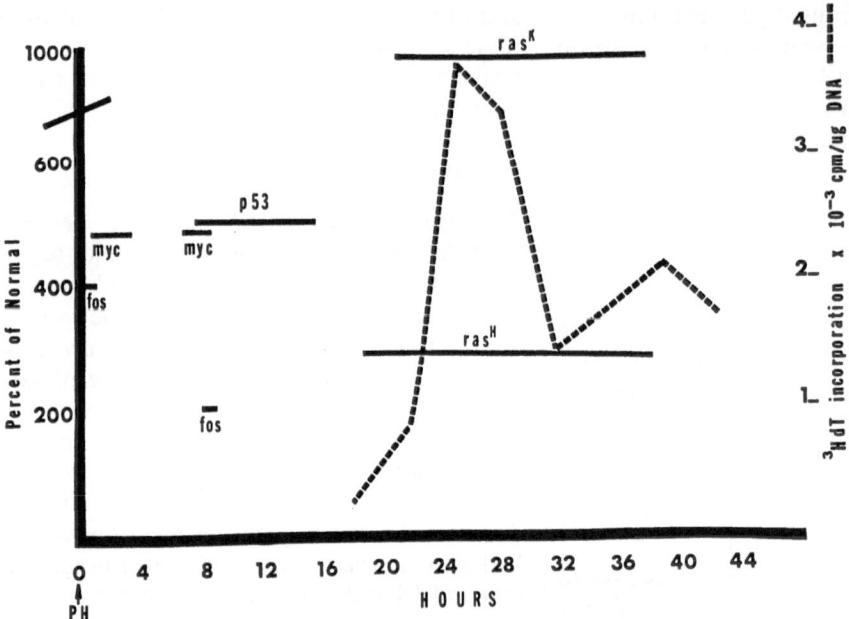

Fig. 5.1. Proto-oncogene expression during liver regeneration after partial hepatectomy in rats. The *abscissa* shows the times after partial hepatectomy. The *left ordinate* shows the level of expression of various proto-oncogenes in relation to the expression of the corresponding genes in normal rat liver. The *horizontal bars* represent the times during liver regeneration at which expression of each oncogene is elevated; the level of expression indicated corresponds to peak values, which generally occur at the middle of the time period represented by the *bars*. Expression of *mos, src,* and *abl* proto-oncogenes is either undetectable in rat liver (*mos*) or does not change during liver regeneration (*src, abl*). The *right ordinate* shows the amount of ³HdT incorporation into DNA at various times after partial hepatectomy as indicated by the *dashed line* [9]

c-*myc* and c-*fos* have different sensitivities to actinomycin D (Act D) during the first 2 h after PH, as measured by the respective abundance of their mRNAs [9]. Act D injected at the time of PH entirely suppresses the increase of c-*myc* at 2 h; the same dose of the inhibitor given at the time of the operation or 45 min before it has little if any effect on c-*fos* mRNA levels at 2 h or 30 min, respectively, after PH [9].

Although results from in vitro nuclear transcription are not yet available for the regenerating rat liver, the differential sensitivity to Act D suggests that post-transcriptional events may play an important role in the activation of c-*fos* shortly after PH, while transcription seems to be the predominant regulatory mechanism for c-*myc*.

It has also been shown that cycloheximide causes an increase in liver c-*myc* transcripts both in intact and in partially hepatectomized rats [50]. A similar effect of cycloheximide on c-*myc* mRNA levels in lymphocytes has been interpreted as evidence for the existence of a labile repressor protein for c-*myc* [52]. Alternatively, transcript stabilization could explain the cycloheximide effect. If the mechanisms by which

cycloheximide and the PH growth stimulus act are similar, it might be suggested that such a hypothetical repressor protein stops being synthesized or is more rapidly degraded almost immediately after PH. To explain the sensitivity of c-*myc* levels to Act D at the start of liver regeneration, one would have to assume that the repressor protein directly or indirectly modifies the rate of c-*myc* transcription. In any event, changes in the levels of this protein are likely to be transient and not to persist beyond 4 h after the operation.

An unusual feature of c-*myc* and c-*fos* expression during liver regeneration is that it occurs with a biphasic pattern. In addition to the early phase discussed above, transcripts of these two proto-oncogenes increase again at around 8 h after PH and decline very quickly thereafter [9]. For c-*fos*, the early and later peaks of expression correspond to a four- and two fold elevation over normal, respectively; for c-*myc*, both early and late peaks represent a fivefold increase over normal. Injections of Act D at 6 h after PH do not alter c-*fos* mRNA levels at 8 h, while c-*myc* mRNA shows ca. 30% inhibition. Thus, c-*fos* mRNA levels are not changed by the inhibitor at either the early or late phase, while c-*myc* RNA decreases drastically in response to Act D at the early phase but only slightly at the late stage [9].

The biological significance of the biphasic increase in c-*fos* and c-*myc* transcripts in the initial stages of liver regeneration is at present unknown. In the absence of in situ hybridization data, it is not possible to establish whether the first and second phases of expression of these genes occur in the same cells or even in the same cell types. It appears unlikely, on the basis of the timing and pattern of the second phase of expression, that the late phase reflects the entry into the cell cycle for endothelial, Kupffer or ductular cells which replicate 1–3 days after hepatocytes during liver regeneration [53, 54]. It is also not likely that c-*fos* expression during liver regeneration is a reflection of macrophage infiltration in the liver because the experimental data show that macrophage infiltration does not occur during the 1st day after PH [55]. It remains to be determined whether the transient expression of c-*fos* and c-*myc* at 8 h after PH corresponds to late entry of a subset of hepatocytes into the cell cycle or reflects some specific signal at the G_1/S transition in hepatocytes which entered the cell cycle immediately after PH. Although c-*myc* mRNA levels increase rapidly after the application of growth stimuli to quiescent fibroblasts and lymphocytes, these levels remain elevated for may hours and may fluctuate during the growth response [4, 6, 52], while in continuously dividing cells c-*myc* mRNA levels are elevated throughout the cell cycle [29, 56].

Corral et al. [57] reported that c-*fos* transcripts are elevated at 30 h after PH. Given that 15%–20% of hepatocytes participate in a second wave of DNA synthesis (which is maximal at 44 h but far less synchronous than the first wave), the elevation of c-*fos* mRNA at this late time is probably related to the second hepatocyte replicative cycle.

3.2.2 p53 Expression
p53 is a cellular protein (or a family of related proteins) which does not have a counterpart in oncogenic viruses but has been associated with cellular transformation and normal cell replication [12, 58, 59]. Microinjection of monoclonal antibodies to p53 protein into the nuclei of quiescent cells prevents the growth response of these cells upon serum stimulation [60]. p53 is considered a "competence" factor in the cell cycle, that is, a factor which although not a complete stimulator of DNA synthesis by itself may make the cell responsive to factors which induce progression of the cell into DNA synthesis [61].

In contrast to c-*fos* and c-*myc*, there is only one phase of p53 expression during the prereplicative phase of liver regeneration. The increase in mRNA levels begins at about 4 h, reaches a maximum between 8 and 12 h (fivefold greater than normal), and the levels decline to normal by 24 h. Act D injection at 6 h after PH decreased p53 mRNA levels at 8 h by approximately 70% [9].

The amounts of p53 protein in rat liver extracts which are precipitable by a monoclonal antibody to mouse p53 have been measured during liver regeneration. The protein levels are similar to those of sham-operated rats at 8 h after PH, increase by about fourfold at 12–15 h, and return to basal levels at 18 h after PH. Thus, there seems to be a reasonable correlation between p53 mRNA changes and the levels of the corresponding protein during liver regeneration [9].

3.2.3 *ras* Expression
Expression of both c-Ha-*ras* and c-Ki-*ras* genes is a late event in regeneration and takes place more or less in parallel with the first wave of DNA synthesis and mitosis of hepatocytes between 24 and 48 h after PH [48, 49]. The magnitude of the change in c-Ki-*ras* mRNA abundance (about 10- to 20-fold greater than normal) is greater than that for c-Ha-*ras* mRNA (three- to fivefold), but the timing of the changes for both genes is similar. In the regeneration of the liver after CCl_4 injury, the peaks of c-Ha-*ras* and c-Ki-*ras* expression again coincide with DNA synthesis, which in this regenerative process occurs 48 h after the administration of the chemical [48, 49].

The levels of p21 proteins in rat liver are very low but the proteins can be demonstrated by immunoprecipitation with either monoclonal antibodies against rat p21 or with rabbit polyclonal anti-p21 antibodies. With both methods, the amount of p21 protein in regenerating livers was found to increase by two- to threefold at 48 and 72 h after PH. The rat monoclonals precipitate two bands which are likely to correspond to precursor and product forms of the p21 protein [62]. Only the faster migrating band was increased after PH. It is unlikely that these two bands represent different phosphorylation states in p21 proteins because endogenous p21 proteins do not appear to be phosphorylated in normal cells [63].

3.3 Working hypothesis for the regulatory events of liver regeneration

To what extent does the sequential expression of proto-oncogenes after PH described above help

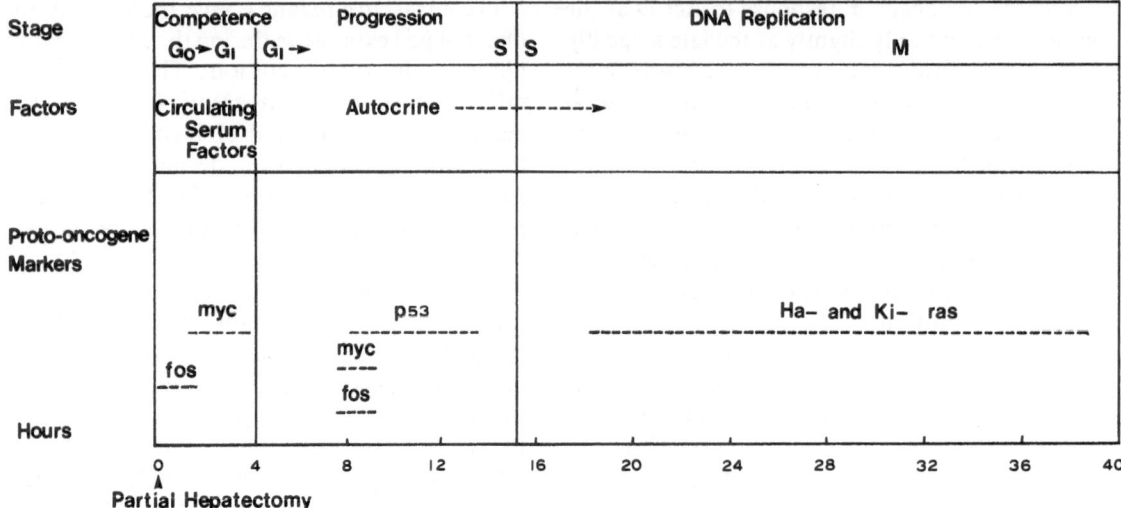

Fig. 5.2. Growth stages and proto-oncogene expression in regenerating rat liver

us elucidate the mechanisms which regulate the regenerative response? As Thompson et al. [7] have aptly stated: "A gene that exhibits a transient increase in expression during the cell cycle could, therefore, either be a regulator of a restriction point, or be responding to a cell-cycle-specific regulatory signal." Viewed in this light, the expression of proto-oncogenes during liver regeneration permits the recognition of stages in the prereplicative phase of the process and at the same time provides some clues as to the nature of the regulatory signals which might operate at each of these stages. The early responses of c-*fos* and c-*myc* are very quick and not present in sham-operated animals [9]. The timing of the response suggests that this is a primary event, probably triggered by factors which are already present in the blood. It is conceivable that the decrease in organ mass brought about by the operation has the effect of raising the concentration of amino acids [64] and hormones such as vasopressin and norepinephrine to which liver cells are exposed [65–67]. Some of these hormones, under appropriate conditions, can stimulate DNA synthesis in hepatocyte cultures [68–70], but it is not known whether these hormones can induce hepatocyte "competence" [71] in vitro, signaled by an incease in c-*fos* and c-*myc* mRNAs.

An alternative way to explain some of the early changes in proto-oncogene expression after PH is that hormones or the metabolic adaptive changes imposed upon the liver remnant immediately after PH do not lead to a direct stimu-latory effect on gene transcription but to a decrease in the steady state levels of hypothetical c-*myc* "repressor protein," which would also result in increases in c-*myc* mRNA levels. Similar mechanisms might also regulate c-*fos* expression, but it is well to remember that the Act D experiments suggest that post-transcriptional events may play a prominent role in the regulation of c-*fos* mRNA levels in the regenerating liver [9].

The expression of p53, which follows that of c-*fos* and c-*myc* by several hours, likely represents the progression of committed hepatocytes through the cell cycle (Fig. 5.2). Hepatocytes at this stage of the prereplicative phase might be able to produce and respond to their own growth factors by an autocrine stimulatory loop. Alternatively, hepatocytes progressing through the cell cycle may, by exhibiting the appropriate receptors [72, 73], acquire the capability to respond to growth factors which normally circulate in the serum or are made in the liver by other cell types. Preliminary experiments from our laboratory suggest that liver nonparenchymal epithelial cells may produce insulin-like growth factor (IGFII), a growth factor synthesized by the fetal liver [74, 75]. Another growth factor, transforming growth factor (TGFβ), may function as a negative effector for hepatocyte replication [76, 77]. This balance between positive and negative effectors [78, 79] and the interplay between hepatocytes and nonparenchymal cells as producer/responder cells may provide clues as to why liver regeneration is a self-limited process which never becomes autonomous and ceases at a point where liver mass is restored [54].

Most of the postulates predicted by this hypothesis can be tested experimentally in vivo and in hepatocyte cultures.

4 Oncogenes and liver carcinogenesis

Work in this area has not yet progressed sufficiently so that a summary of the existing data can give a coherent picture of the role various oncogenes may play in hepatocarcinogenesis. We will first summarize studies of proto-oncogene expression during carcinogenesis and in animal or human tumors. The second part of this section will review work which makes use of transfection assays to detect activated proto-oncogenes in liver tumors.

4.1 Proto-oncogene expression during liver carcinogenesis

It is not yet possible to determine whether the increased expression of some proto-oncogenes, which takes place during chemically induced hepatocarcinogenesis, is directly related to transformation or reflects changes in the proliferative state of the involved cells. The expression of c-*myc*, c-Ha-, and c-Ki-*ras* increases in the liver of rats fed a choline-deficient diet containing ethionine [80] or a diet containing 3′-methyl-4-dimethylaminoazobenzene [81, 82]. In rats receiving diethylinitrosamine (DENA) after PH, the expression of c-*fos*, c-Ha-, c-Ki, and N-*ras* is elevated [57, 83]. In animals fed 3-Me-DAB, c-Ha-*ras* expression increases progressively with feeding, while c-*myc* expression reaches maximal values (two- to threefold above normal) 2–3 months after the start of the feeding and does not increase further despite continuous feeding of the carcinogen [81, 82]. In these animals, both tumors and the nontumorous parts of the liver have higher levels of c-Ha-*ras* mRNA than the livers of normal rats, while c-*myc* mRNA increases appear to be confined to the tumorous parts [82]. Similarly, in livers of rats which received DENA, c-Ha-, c-Ki-, and N-*ras* expression is elevated both in tumors and in the surrounding cells [83]. The significance of these observations is not clear as yet, but it seems safe to conclude that the expression of these various proto-oncogenes is neither specific to nor unusually high in tumor cells. However, it is not known whether the cells of the nontumorous parts of the liver included in these assays are quiescent, proliferating, or if they have been altered by the development of tumors in adjacent portions of the liver. The ambiguities inherent in these studies point out the difficulties in interpreting measurements of proto-oncogene expression in animal or human tumors [84] in the absence of a detailed histological examination of the cellular composition of the tumors and surrounding tissues.

Jagirdar et al. [85] have recently analyzed the expression of the *ras* p21 protein in human liver biopsies and postmortem specimens using the *ras* monoclonal antibody RAP-5 developed by Thor et al. [86] and the avidin-biotin peroxidase method. Intense p21 staining was detected in neoplastic and non-neoplastic cells containing hepatitis B surface antigen. "Dysplastic" cells and focal areas of differentiated hepatocellular carcinomas also displayed high levels of expression, but no staining was present in undifferentiated tumors. Thus, elevation of p21 *ras* proteins appears to be an early event in liver tumorigenesis, but no obvious correlation between the abundance of these proteins and progression to malignancy could be established. Similarly, elevation of c-*ras* gene expression has been detected in premalignant lesions of the gastrointestinal tract in humans [87] and in mouse skin papillomas [88], suggesting that elevated expression of these genes also occurs relatively early in these systems. However, augmented *ras* expression alone is not sufficient to produce malignancy. In contrast to the findings with *ras* genes, studies of N-*myc* expression and amplification in human neuroblastomas [89] indicate that elevated N-*myc* expression correlates with the progression of malignancy and is associated with tumors of advanced clinical stages (stages III and IV).

In HepG2 cells, a human hepatoma cell line, c-*myc* expression was elevated relative to levels of normal adult rat liver in all clones examined and in the tumors but not in the cells in culture. C-Ha-*ras* transcripts were not changed in the cells or the tumors [90]. C-*myc* mRNA elevation in this cell line or in the tumors could not be explained by gene amplification or hepatitis B virus integration [90]. In four different Morris hepatomas analyzed by Cote et al. [82], c-*myc* and c-Ha-*ras* mRNAs were increased two- to threefold above normal liver levels. There seems to be, however, no direct correlation between the expression of these genes and the differentiation state or growth properties of the tumors.

In rats fed a choline-deficient diet containing 0.1% ethionine there is also an increase in the expression of c-*myc*, c-Ha-*ras*, and c-Ki-*ras* [80]. However, in the liver of these animals, proto-oncogenes are differentially expressed in different cell populations during carcinogenesis. The abundance of c-Ki-*ras*, c-Ha-*ras*, and c-*myc* in polysomal poly(A)$^+$ RNA from whole livers increase 2 weeks after the start of the carcinogenic diet, whereas c-Ki-*ras* and c-*myc* expression remained elevated during the 35 weeks the rats were kept on this diet; c-Ha-*ras* increased only transiently during the first 4 weeks of feeding [80]. The tumors which developed in these animals had high levels of c-Ki-*ras* and c-*myc* transcripts but near normal levels of c-Ha-*ras* mRNAs. Oval cells isolated from livers of rats fed the carcinogenic diet [80] contain high levels of c-Ki-*ras* and c-*myc* transcripts, which increase progressively throughout carcinogenesis. At 16 weeks on the diet, oval cells have approximately 6- and 25-fold higher levels of c-*myc* and c-Ki-*ras* mRNA, respectively, than normal hepatocytes. In contrast, hepatocytes isolated from rats fed the diet for 2–4 weeks contain high levels of c-Ha-*ras* transcripts [80].

Although such studies have established the pattern of expression of some proto-oncogenes in different cell populations during hepatocarcinogenesis induced by feeding rats a carcinogenic diet, the results obtained do not directly address the question of the relationships which may exist between the pattern of proto-oncogene expression in different cell types and tumor development. To explore this question, oval cells isolated by centrifugal elutriation [91, 92] from livers of rats fed the carcinogenic diet for 2 or 6 weeks were placed in culture and two cell lines were derived from these isolates (LE/2 and LE/6 lines, respectively). These two liver epithelial cell lines are similar in phenotypic properties, do not grow in soft agar, and are not tumorigenic when inoculated into nude mice. However, with passage in culture, LE/6 cells become sensitive to epidermal growth factor (EGF) and in the presence of this growth factor acquire the capacity to grow in soft agar. In these cell lines (even in late-passage LE/6 cells, which can be induced to grow in soft agar by EGF), the expression of c-Ki-*ras*, c-Ha-*ras*, c-*myc*, and p53 is regulated in relation to the cell cycle, that is, quiescent cells have low levels of mRNAs encoded by these genes, but the abundance of the transcripts is increased as cells are stimulated to grow. From these studies, one concludes that the changes in the expression of proto-oncogenes detected in oval cells in vivo during hepatocarcinogenesis

induced by the choline-deficient/ethionine diet reflect primarily the proliferative state of these cells rather than their progression to a transformed state. It remains to be determined whether the acquired sensitivity of EGF displayed by late-passage cells in culture correlates with alterations in proto-oncogene expression or with the expression of genes encoding growth factors or growth factor receptors.

Beer et al. [93] have analyzed the expression of c-Ha-*ras* and c-*myc* proto-oncogenes in γ-glutamyl transpeptidase-positive and -negative hepatocytes isolated from livers and tumors of rats which were given DENA after PH and maintained on a diet containing 0.05% phenobarbital. These authors observed no differences in the expression of proto-oncogenes between these two cell populations and also found that in the tumors the levels of expression of c-Ha-*ras* and c-*myc* were highly variable. Beer et al. [93] also point out that differences in proto-oncogene expression in various primary tumors may reflect the heterogeneity in the cellular composition of these tumors and emphasize that in situ hybridization using tissue sections of livers and tumors might clarify questions regarding the specificity of proto-oncogene expression and progression to malignancy.

4.2 Detection of activated proto-oncogenes in liver tumors by transfection assays

Transforming proto-oncogenes have been found in a significant proportion of chemically induced tumors in animals [94–98]. So far, however, there have been few definitive reports of activated proto-oncogenes in chemically induced liver tumors. A survey for activated oncogenes in such tumors yielded negative results [99]. In contrast to these results, Reynolds et al. [100] detected activated oncogenes in spontaneously occurring benign and malignant hepatocellular tumors in B6C3F1 mice. However, DNAs from 29 spontaneous tumors which developed in various tissues of Fischer 344/N rats were all negative in transfection assays. In male B6C3F1 mice, which have a high natural incidence of liver adenomas and carcinomas, 3/10 liver adenomas and 10/13 hepatocellular carcinomas were positive in transfection assays. The DNA of NIH-3T3 cells transfected with 13 tumor DNA samples, which were positive in transfection assays, were analyzed by Southern blot hybridization using c-Ha-, c-Ki-, and N-*ras* as probes. Although no changes were found in bands corresponding to c-Ki- and N-*ras*, 11 of the 13 DNAs from the transfected cells showed amplification of c-Ha-*ras*. In three of these, there were also extra bands corresponding to c-Ha-*ras*. The activated oncogene contained in two DNA samples (which show no abnormalities in c-Ha-*ras* bands) has not been identified so far [100].

There are preliminary reports that the *raf* gene might be activated in some primary rat hepatocellular carcinomas [101] and that hepatocarcinogenesis induced by certain alkylating agents might also be associated with transforming oncogenes (M. Goyette, in preparation). N-*ras* is reported to be activated in HepG2 cells and a solid liver tumor [94], while an activated c-Ha-*ras* gene apparently interacts with genes from other families in rat hepatocellular carcinomas induced by 2-amino-3-methyl-imidazo-quinoline [102]. In studies with human primary hepatocellular carcinomas [103], no genes were detected in these tumors capable of transforming rodent cells in culture. In addition, oncogene amplification, deletion, or translocation was not found in the tumors analyzed [103]. In a survey of human epithelial tumors from other sites, deletion of c-Ha-*ras* and c-*myc* was detected in 17% and 9% of samples while amplification of c-*myc* and c-Ki-*ras* was found in 11% and 1% of tumors sampled, respectively [104].

4.3 Activation of proto-oncogenes as an optional path in hepatocarcinogenesis

Increased expression of proto-oncogenes occurs in rat liver tumors induced by chemicals, but the specificity of these changes in relation to the development of malignancy has not been established. At the same time, no activated oncogenes have been found so far in primary human hepatocellular carcinomas and there are only preliminary reports on the detection of activated oncogenes in chemically induced hepatic tumors, despite the fact that such tumors are easy to produce and constitute one of the best-studied models of experimental carcinogenesis. It is also to be noted that in the B6C3F1 mouse, activated c-Ha-*ras* was detected in both benign (adenomas) and malignant (hepatocellular carcinomas) spontaneous tumors and that no activated proto-oncogenes have been detected in rat tumors which develop spontaneously in various tissues [100]. One interpretation for these findings is that activation of proto-oncogenes is not an obligatory component of the process of hepatocarcinogenesis. The augmented expression of one or more proto-oncogenes during liver carcinogenesis might reflect either the enhanced proliferative state of certain cell populations or be a marker for losses in normal cellular regulatory controls. As exemplified by the experiments with oval cells in culture, such changes are probably reversible and not in themselves sufficient to transform cells fully [92]. Further changes are required for transformation but such steps may or may not involve proto-oncogene activation, that is, mutation or deregulation of these genes. It appears, so far, that such activation is present in only a small minority of liver tumors. Thus, if this view is correct, the presence of activated proto-oncogenes in spontaneously or chemically induced rat tumors reflects a particular path which normal or partially transformed cells may utilize as they progress into a transformed state. Under other circumstances, the same cell might progress to malignancy by an entirely different series of steps, which may not involve proto-oncogene activation. Such a hypothesis gains support from the results of Garte et al. [105], who demonstrated that tumors which develop in rats and mice exposed to three direct-acting alkylating agents which bind to DNA and induce tumors with similar histological characteristics in the rat nasal cavity exhibit variable activity in transfection assays. The presence of transforming genes in these tumors, detected in NIH-3T3 transfection assays, appears to be mainly a function of the carcinogen used. Thus, 8/8 DNAs obtained from methylmethane sulfonate (MMS)-induced tumors scored positive, while none of the DNAs obtained from dimethylcarbamyl chloride (DMCC)-induced tumors were positive (0/10) and 2/5 DNAs extracted from β-propiolactone (BPL)-induced tumors were positive in the transfection assays. Although the specificity of the carcinogen effect might be explained by the different pattern of adduct formation elicited by each agent (DMCC produces O^6 guanine and O^4 thymine adducts; BPL and MMS lead to adduct formation on guanine and adenine endocyclic nitrogens), it should be remembered that a very high proportion of mammary tumors induced by methylnitrosourea (a direct alkylating agent which produces O^6 guanine adducts) are positive in transfection assays [94, 95]. Garte et al. [105] conclude that carcinogen specificity determines to a large extent whether or not activation of proto-oncogenes occurs, but that other factors related to the cellular and tissue alterations caused by specific agents may also be of importance.

Alternatively, the difficulties in detecting activated proto-oncogenes in hepatocarcinogenesis may be a consequence of the inadequacy of methods to detect such genes. It is known that the usual NIH-3T3 transfection assay primarily detects activation of the *ras* gene family, but such genes may perhaps not be very important in liver carcinogenesis. Proto-oncogene activation (including *ras*-gene activation) in liver tumors might be much more readily detected if liver cells (hepatocytes, normal liver epithelial cells, or oval cells) were used as recipients in transfection assays. The development of reliable methods to introduce foreign genes into primary hepatocytes in culture [106] might permit the analysis of proto-oncogene activation during hepatocarcinogenesis under much more physiological conditions. With such methods, it may be possible to demonstrate the presence of activated proto-oncogenes in a larger proportion of liver tumors in humans and animals.

Acknowlegment. We thank Anna-Louise Baxter and Christine Levesque for their help in preparing the manuscript, Nancy L. Thompson for her suggestions and ideas, and Dr. Henry C. Pitot for making available unpublished data from his laboratory. The authors' research discussed in this chapter is supported by grants CA-23226 and CA-35249 from the National Cancer Insitute (USA).

References

1. Duesberg PH (1985) Activated proto-oncogenes: sufficient or necessary for cancer? Science 228: 669–677
2. Campisi J, Gray HE, Pardee AB, Dean M, Sonenshein GE (1984) Cell-cycle control of c-*myc* but not c-*ras* expression is lost following chemical transformation. Cell 36: 241–247
3. Greenberg ME, Ziff EB (1984) Stimulation of 3T3 cells induces transcription of the c-*fos* proto-oncogene. Nature 311: 433–438
4. Muller R, Bravo R, Burckhardt J, Curran T (1984) Induction of c-*fos* gene and protein by growth factors precedes activation of c-*myc*. Nature 321: 716–720
5. Reed JC, Nowell PC, Hoover RG (1985) Regulation of c-*myc* mRNA levels in normal human lymphocytes by modulators of cell proliferation. Proc Natl Acad Sci USA 82: 4221–4224
6. Kaczmarek L, Calabretta B, Baserga R (1985) Expression of cell cycle-dependent genes in phytohemagglutinin-stimulated human lymphocytes. Proc Natl Acad Sci USA 82: 5375–5379
7. Thompson CB, Challoner PB, Neiman PE, Groudine M (1986) Expression of the c-*myb* proto-oncogene during cellular proliferation. Nature 319: 374–380
8. Fausto N, Shank PR (1983) Oncogene expression in liver regeneration and hepatocarcinogenesis. Hepatology 3: 1016–1023
9. Thompson NL, Mead JE, Braun L, Goyette M, Shank PR, Fausto N (1986) Sequential proto-oncogene expression during liver regeneration. Cancer Res 46: 3111–3117
10. Weinberg RA (1985) The action of oncogenes in the cytoplasm and nucleus. Science 230: 770–776
11. Bishop JM (1983) Cellular oncogenes and retroviruses. Ann Rev Biochem 52: 301–354
12. Oren M (1985) The p53 cellular tumor antigen: gene structure, expression and protein properties. Biochem Biophys Acta 823: 67–78
13. Land H, Parada LF, Weinberg RA (1983) Cellular oncogenes and multistep carcinogenesis. Science 222: 771–778
14. Spandidos DA, Wilkie NM (1984) Malignant transformation of early passage rodent cells by a single mutated human oncogene. Nature 310: 469–475
15. Muschel RJ, Williams JE, Lowy DR, Liotta LA (1985) Harvey *ras* induction of metastatic potential depends upon oncogene activation and the type of recipient cell. Am J Pathol 121: 1–8
16. Hayward SW, Neel BG, Astrin SM (1981) Activation of a cellular *onc* gene by promoter insertion in ALV-induced lymphoid leukosis. Nature (London) 290: 475–480
17. Leder P, Battey J, Lenoir G, Moulding C, Murphy W, Potter H, Stewart T, Taub R (1983) Translocations among antibody genes in human cancer. Science 222: 765–771
18. Collins S, Groudine M (1982) Amplification of endogenous *myc*-related DNA sequences in a human myeloid leukemia cell line. Nature 298: 679–681
19. Scolnick EM (1981) Transformation by rat-derived oncogenic retroviruses. Microbiol Revs 45: 1–8
20. Shimizu K, Goldfarb M, Perucho M, Wigler M (1983) Isolation and preliminary characterization of the transforming gene of a human neuroblastoma cell line. Proc Natl Acad Sci USA 80: 383–387
21. Roussel M, Saule S, Langrou C, Rommens C, Beug H, Graff T, Stehelin D (1979) Three new types of viral oncogene of cellular origin specific for haematopoietic cell transformation. Nature 281: 452–455
22. Schwab M, Alitalo K, Klempnauer K-H, Varmus HE, Bishop JM, Gilbert F, Brodeur G, Goldstein M, Trent J (1983) Amplified DNA with limited homology to *myc* is shared by human neuroblastoma cell lines and a neuroblastoma tumor. Nature (London) 305: 245–248
23. Ralston R, Bishop JM (1983) The protein products of the *myc* and *myb* oncogenes and adenovirus *Ela* are structurally related. Nature 306: 803–806
24. Toda T, Uno I, Ishikawa T, Powers S, Kataoka T, Broek D, Cameron S, Broach J, Matsumoto K, Wigler M (1985) In yeast, *ras* proteins are controlling elements of adenylate cyclase. Cell 40: 27–36
25. Beckner SK, Hattori S, Shih TY (1985) The *ras*

oncogene product p21 is not a regulatory component of adenylate cyclase. Nature 317: 71–72

26. Birchmeier C, Broek D, Wigler M (1985) *ras* proteins can induce meiosis in xenopus oocytes. Cell 43: 615–621

27. Armelin HA, Armelin MCS, Kelly K, Stewart T, Leder P, Cochran BH, Stiles CD (1984) Functional role for c-*myc* in mitogenic response to platelet-derived growth factor. Nature. 310: 655–660

28. Kaczmarek L, Hyland JK, Watt R, Rosenberg M, Baserga R (1985) Microinjected c-*myc* as a competence factor. Science 228: 1313–1315

29. Thompson CB, Challoner PB, Neiman PE, Groudine M (1985) Levels of c-*myc* oncogene mRNA are invariant throughout the cell cycle. Nature. 314: 363–366

30. Hann SR, Thompson CB, Eisenman RN (1985) c-*myc* oncogene protein synthesis is independent of the cell cycle in human and avian cells. Nature. 314: 366–369

31. Fausto N (1984) Messenger RNA in regenerating liver: implications for the understanding of regulated growth. Mol Cell Biochem 59: 131–147

32. Scholla CA, Tedeschi MV, Fausto N (1980) Gene expression and the diversity of polysomal messenger RNA sequences in regenerating liver. J Biol Chem 255: 2855–2860

33. Fausto N, Schultz-Ellison G, Atryzek V, Goyette M (1982) Distribution and specificity of sequences in polyadenylated nuclear RNA of normal, regenerating and neoplastic liver. J Biol Chem 257: 2200–2206

34. Savage MJ, Sala-Trepat JM, Bonner J (1978) Measurement of the complexity and diversity of poly (adenylic acid) containing messenger RNA from rat liver. Biochemistry 17: 462–467

35. Sippel AE, Hynes N, Groner B, Schutz G (1977) Frequency distribution of messenger sequences within polysomal mRNA and nuclear RNA from rat liver. Eur J Biochem 77: 141–151

36. Jacobs H, Birnie GD (1980) Post-transcriptional regulation of messenger abundance in rat liver and hepatoma. Nucleic Acids Res 14: 3087–3103

37. Powell DJ, Friedman JM, Oulette AJ, Krauter KS, Darnell JE Jr (1984) Transcriptional and post-transcriptional control of specific messenger RNAs in adult and embryonic liver. J Mol Biol 179: 21–35

38. Glazer RI (1977) The action of N-hydroxy-2-acetylamino-fluorene on the synthesis of ribosomal and poly(A)-RNA in normal and regenerating liver. Biochem Biophys Acta 475: 492–500

39. Walker PR, Whitfield JF (1981) Regulation of the prereplicative changes in the synthesis and transport of messenger and ribosomal RNA in regenerating livers of normal and hypocalcemic rats. J Cell Physiol 108: 427–437

40. Atryzek V, Fausto N (1979) Accumulation of polyadenylated mRNA during liver regeneration. Biochemistry 18: 1281–1287

41. Tedeschi MV, Colbert DA, Fausto N (1978) Transcription of the non-repetitive genome in liver hypertrophy and the homology between nuclear RNA of normal and 12h-regenerating liver. Biochem Biophys Acta 521: 641–649

42. Fausto N, Colbert DA, Greene RF, Tedeschi M (1976) Transcriptional activity and gene expression during liver regeneration. In: Fishman WH, Sell S (eds) Onco-developmental gene expression. Academic Press, New York, pp 35–45

43. Wilkes PR, Birnie GD, Paul J (1979) Changes in nuclear and polysomal polyadenylated RNA sequences during rat liver regeneration. Nucleic Acids Res 6: 2193–2208

44. Grady LJ, Campbell WP, North AB (1979) Non-repetitive DNA transcription in normal and regenerating rat liver. Nucleic Acids Res 7: 259–269

45. Grady LJ, Campbell WP, North AB (1981) Sequence diversity of nuclear and polysomal polyadenylated and non-polyadenylated RNA in normal and regenerating rat liver. Eur J Biochem 115: 241–245

46. Huber BE, Heilman CA, Wirth PJ, Miller MJ, Thorgeirsson SS (1986) Studies in gene transcription and translation in regenerating rat liver. Hepatology. 6: 209–219

47. Spector DH, Varmus HE, Bishop JM (1978) Nucleotide sequences related to the transforming gene of avian sarcoma virus are present in DNA of uninfected vertebrates. Proc Natl Acad Sci USA 75: 4102–4106

48. Goyette M, Petropoulos CJ, Shank PR, Fausto N (1983) Expression of a cellular oncogene during liver regeneration. Science 219: 510–512

49. Goyette M, Petropoulos CJ, Shank PR, Fausto N (1984) Regulated transcription of c-Ki-*ras* and c-*myc* during compensatory growth of rat liver. Mol Cell Biol 4: 1493–1498

50. Makino R, Hayashi K, Sugimura T (1984) C-*myc* transcript is induced in rat liver at very early stage of regeneration or by cycloheximide treatment. Nature 310: 697–698

51. Dani CH, Blanchard JM, Piechaczyk MS, El Sabouty S, Marty L, Janteur PH (1984) Extreme instability of myc mRNA in normal and transformed human cells. Proc Natl Acad Sci USA 81: 7046–7050

52. Kelly K, Cochran BH, Stiles CD, Leder P (1983) Cell-specific regulation of the c-*myc* gene by lymphocyte mitogens and platelet-derived growth factor. Cell 35: 603–610

53. Grisham J (1962) Morphologic study of deoxyribonucleic acid synthesis and cell proliferation in regenerating rat liver: autoradiography with thymidine H³. Cancer Res 22: 842–849

54. Bucher NLR, Malt RA (1971) Regeneration of liver and kidney. Little Brown, Boston, pp 1–176

55. Bouwens L, Baekeland M, Wisse E (1984) Importance of local proliferation in the expanding Kupffer cell population of rat liver after zymosan stimulation and partial hepatectomy. Hepatology 4: 213–219

56. Rabbits PH, Watson JV, Lamond A, Forster A, Stinson MA, Evan G, Fischer W, Atherton E, Sheppard R, Rabbits TH (1985) Metabolism of

c-*myc* gene products: c-*myc* mRNA and protein expression in the cell cycle. EMBO J 4: 2009–2015

57. Corral M, Tichonicky L, Guguen-Guillouzo C, Corcos D, Raymondjean M, Paris B, Kruh J, Defer N (1985) Expression of c-*fos* oncogene during hepatocarcinogenesis, liver regeneration and in synchronized HTC cells. Exptl Cell Res 160: 427–434

58. Reich NC, Levine AJ (1984) Growth regulation of a cellular tumor antigen, p53, in nontransformed cells. Nature 308: 199–201

59. Mercer WE, Baserga R (1985) Expression of the p53 protein during the cell cycle of human peripheral blood lymphocytes. Exptl Cell Res 160: 31–46

60. Mercer WE, Nelson D, DeLeo L, Old LJ, Baserga R (1982) Microinjection of monoclonal antibody to protein p53 inhibits serum-induced DNA synthesis in 3T3 cells. Proc Natl Acad Sci USA 79: 6309–6312

61. Kaczmarek L, Oren M, Baserga R (1986) Cooperation between the p53 protein tumor antigen and platelet-poor plasma in the induction of cellular DNA synthesis. Exptl Cell Res 161: 268–272

62. Tabin CJ, Bradley SM, Bargmann CI, Weinberg RA, Papageorge AG, Scolnick EM, Dhar R, Lowy DR, Chang EH (1982) Mechanisms of activation of a human oncogene. Nature 300: 143–149

63. Furth ME, Davis LJ, Fleurdelys B, Scolnick EM (1982) Monoclonal antibodies to the p21 products of the transforming gene of Harvey murine sarcoma virus and of the cellular *ras* gene family. J Virol 43: 294–304

64. McGowan JA, Atryzek V, Fausto N (1979) Effects of protein-deprivation on the regeneration of rat after partial hepatectomy. Biochem J 180: 25–35

65. Russell WE, Bucher NLR (1983) Vasopressin modulates liver regeneration in the Brattleboro rat. Am J Physiol 245: 321–324

66. Cruise JL, Houck K, Michalopoulos GK (1985) Induction of DNA synthesis in cultured rat hepatocytes through stimulation of α' adrenoreceptor by norepinephrine. Science 277: 749–751

67. Bucher NLR, Patel U, Cohen S (1978) Hormonal factors concerned with liver regeneration. In: Hepatotrophic factors. Ciba Foundation Symp 55. Elsevier, Amsterdam, pp 95–107

68. Richman RA, Clause TH, Pilkis SJ, Friedman DL (1976) Hormonal stimulation of DNA synthesis in primary cultures of rat hepatocytes. Proc Natl Acad Sci USA 73: 3589–3593

69. Leffert HL, Koch KS (1978) Proliferation of hepatocytes. In: Hepatotrophic factors. Ciba Foundation Symp 55. Elsevier, Amsterdam, pp 61–82

70. McGowan JA, Strain AJ, Bucher NRL (1981) DNA synthesis in primary cultures of adult rat hepatocytes in a defined medium: effects of epidermal growth factor, insulin, glucagon and cyclic AMP. J Cell Physiol 108: 353–363

71. Pledger WJ, Stiles CD, Antoniades HN, Sher CD (1977) Induction of DNA synthesis in BALB/c3T3 cells by serum components: reevaluation of the commitment process. Proc Natl Acad Sci USA 74: 4481–4485

72. Earp HS, O'Keefe EJ (1981) Epidermal growth factor receptor number decreases during rat liver regeneration. J Clin Invest 67: 1580–1583

73. Francavilla A, Ove P, Polimeno L, Sciascia C, Coetzee ML, Starzl TE (1986) Epidermal growth factor and proliferation in rat hepatocytes in primary culture isolated at different times after partial hcpatectomy. Cancer Res 46: 1318–1323

74. Soares MB, Ishii DN, Efstratiadis A (1985) Developmental and tissue-specific expression of a family of transcripts related to rat insulin-like growth factor II mRNA. Nucleic Acids Res 13: 1119–1134

75. Rechler MM, Eisen HJ, Higa OZ, Nissley SP, Moses AC, Schilling EE, Fenoy I, Bruni CB, Phillips LS, Baird KL (1979) Characterization of a somatomedin (insulin-like growth factor) synthesized by fetal rat liver organ cultures. J Biol Chem 254: 7942–7950

76. Nakamura T, Tomita Y, Hirai R, Yamaoka K, Kaji K, Ichihara A (1985) Inhibitory effect of transforming growth factor β on DNA synthesis of adult rat hepatocytes in primary culture. Biochem Biophys Res Commun 133: 1042–1050

77. McMahon JB, Richards WL, del Campo AA, Song MKH, Thorgeirsson SS (1986) Differential effects of transforming growth factor β on proliferation of normal and malignant rat liver epithelial cells in culture. Cancer Res 46: 4665–4671

78. Sporn MB, Roberts AB (1985) Autocrine growth factors and cancer. Nature 313: 745–747

79. Goustin AS, Leof EB, Shipley GD, Moses HL (1986) Growth factors and cancer. Cancer Res 46: 1015–1029

80. Yaswen P, Goyette M, Shank PR, Fausto N (1985) Expression of c-Ki-*ras*, c-Ha-*ras* and c-*myc* in specific cell types during hepatocarcinogenesis. Mol Cell Biol 5: 780–786

81. Makino R, Hayashi K, Sato S, Sugimura T (1984) Expression of the c-Ha-*ras* and c-*myc* genes in rat liver tumors. Biochem Biophys Res Commun 119: 1096–1102

82. Cote GJ, Lastra BA, Cook JR, Huang DP, Chiu JF (1985) Oncogene expression in rat hepatomas and during hepatocarcinogenesis. Cancer Lett 26: 121–127

83. Corcos D, Defer N, Raymondjean M, Paris B, Corral M, Tichonicky L, Kruh J (1984) Correlated increase of the expression of the c-*ras* genes in chemically induced hepatocarcinomas. Biochem Biophys Res Commun 122: 259–264

84. Slamon DJ, deKernion JB, Verma IM, Cline MJ (1984) Expression of cellular oncogenes in human malignancies. Science 224: 256–262

85. Jagirdar J. Nonomura A, Patil J, Paronetto F (1985) Activated *ras* oncogene p21 expression in hepatocellular carcinoma (HCC) and HBsAg-positive liver cells. Hepatology 5: 1055 (Abst.)

86. Thor A, Horand Hand P, Wunderlich D, Caruso A, Muraro R, Schlom J (1985) Monoclonal anti-

bodies define differential *ras* gene expression in malignant and benign colonic diseases. Nature 311: 562–565

87. Spandidos DA, Kerr IB (1984) Elevated expression of the human *ras* oncogene family in premalignant and malignant tumors of the colorectum. Br J Cancer 49: 681–688

88. Balmain A, Ramsden M, Bowden GT, Smith J (1984) Activation of the mouse cellular Harvey-*ras* gene in chemically induced benign skin papillomas. Nature 307: 658–660

89. Schwab M, Ellison J, Busch M, Rosenau W, Varmus HE, Bishop JM (1984) Enhanced expression of the human gene N-*myc* consequent to amplification of DNA may contribute to malignant progression of neuroblastoma. Proc Natl Acad Sci USA 81: 4940–4944

90. Huber BE, Dearfield KL, Williams JR, Heilman CA, Thorgeirsson SS (1985) Tumorigenicity and transcriptional modulation of c-*myc* and N-*ras* oncogenes in a human hepatoma cell line. Cancer Res 45: 4322–4329

91. Yaswen P, Hayner NT, Fausto N (1984) Isolation of oval cells by centrifugal elutriation and comparison with other cell types purified from normal and preneoplastic livers. Cancer Res 44: 324–331

92. Braun L, Goyette M, Yaswen P, Thompson NL, Fausto N (1987) Liver epithelial cells from carcinogen treated rats: Growth in culture and tumorigenicity after transfection with the *ras* oncogene. Cancer Res (in press)

93. Beer DG, Schwarz M, Swada N, Pitot HC (1986) Expression of H-*ras* and c-*myc* proto-oncogenes in isolated γ-glutamyl transpeptidase-positive rat hepatocytes and in hepatocellular carcinomas induced by diethylnitrosamine. Cancer Res 46: 2435–2441

94. Notario V, Sukumar S, Santos E, Barbacid M (1984) A common mechanism for the malignant activation of *ras* oncogenes in human neoplasia and in chemically induced animal tumors. In: Vande Woude GF, Levine AJ, Topp WC, Watson JD (eds) Cancer Cells: II. Oncogenes and viral genes. Cold Spring Harbor Laboratory, Cold Spring Harbor, NY, pp 425–432

95. Sukumar S, Notario V, Martin-Zanca D, Barbacid M (1983) Induction of mammary carcinomas in rats by nitroso-methyl-urea involves the malignant activation of the H-*ras*-1 locus by single point mutations. Nature 306: 658–661

96. Eva A, Aaronson SA (1983) Frequent activation of c-Kis as a transforming gene in fibrosarcomas induced by methylcholanthrene. Science 220: 955–956

97. Balmain A, Pragnell IB (1983) Mouse skin carcinomas induced in vivo by chemical carcinogens have a transforming Harvey-*ras* oncogene. Nature 303: 72–74

98. Guerrero I, Villasante A, Mayer, A, Pellicer A (1984) Carcinogen and radiation-induced mouse lymphomas contain an activated c-*ras* oncogene. In: Vande Woude GF, Levine AJ, Topp WC, Watson JD (eds) Cancer cells: II. Oncogenes and viral genes. Cold Spring Harbor Laboratory, Cold Spring Harbor, NY, pp 455–461

99. Farber E (1984) Cellular biochemistry of the stepwise development of cancer with chemicals. Cancer Res 44: 5463–5474

100. Reynolds SH, Stowers SJ, Maronpot RR, Anderson MW, Aaronson SA (1986) Detection and identification of activated oncogenes in spontaneously occurring benign and malignant hepatocellular tumors of the B6C3F1 mouse. Proc Natl Acad Sci USA 83: 33–37

101. Zurlo J, Yager J (1985) Oncogene expression during pancreatic regeneration and in chemically induced pancreatic and liver carcinomas in the rat. Fed Proc 44: 1493 (Abst).

102. Ishikawa F, Takaku F, Nagao M, Ochiai M, Hayashi K, Takayama S and Sugimura T (1985) Activated oncogenes in a rat hepatocellular carcinoma induced by 2-amino-3-methyl-imidazo [4, 5-f] quinoline. Jpn J Can Res (Gann) 76: 425–428

103. Varmus HE (1984) Do hepatitis B viruses make a genetic contribution to primary hepatocellular carcinoma? In: Vyas GN, Dienstag JL, Hoofnagle JH (eds) Viral hepatitis and liver disease. Grune and Stratton, Orlando, pp 411–414

104. Yokota J, Tsunetsugu-Yokota Y, Battifora H, LeFevre C, Cline MJ (1986) Alterations of *myc*, *myb* and *Ras* Ha proto-oncogenes in cancers are frequent and show clinical correlation. Science 231: 261–264

105. Garte SJ, Hood AT, Hochwalt AE, D'Eustachio P, Snyder CA, Segal A, Albert RE (1985) Carcinogen specificity in the activation of transforming genes by direct-acting alkylating agents. Carcinogenesis 6: 1709–1712

106. Tur-Kaspa R, Teicher L, Levine BJ, Skoultchi AI, Shafritz DA (1986) Use of electroporation to introduce biologically active foreign genes into primary rat hepatocytes. Mol Cell Biol 6: 716–718

Note added in proof. Since the writing of this chapter (references up to March 1986), several new reports on oncogene activity in hepatocarcinogenesis have been published. Ishikawa et al. (1986, Proc Natl Acad Sci USA 83: 3209–3219) showed that the c-*raf* activation originally reported to occur in rat liver hepatocellular carcinomas induced by 2-amino-3-methylimidazo [4, 5-f] quinoline actually took place during the transfection experiments and might not be present in the tumors. McMahon et al. (1986, Proc Natl Acad Sci USA 83: 9418–9422) showed that 11 of 13 rat DNA samples from aflatoxin-induced hepatocellular carcinomas has transforming DNA sequences, but a highly amplified c-Ki-*ras* oncogene was detected in only two of eight individual tumors. Ochiya et al. (1986, Proc Natl Acad Sci USA 83: 4993–4997) reported the isolation of a new oncogene (*lca* gene) from human hepatocellular carcinomas. In contrast with findings in human and rat hepatic tumors, *ras*-gene activation seems to be a common event in chemically induced hepatocellular tumors in B6C3F1 mice (Wiseman et al. 1986, Proc Natl Acad Sci USA 83: 5825–5829). Finally, Braun et al. (Cancer Res, in press) showed that the transfection of oval cells in vitro with an activated c-Ha-*ras* oncogene (EJ gene) produced differentiated hepatocellular carcinomas after innoculation of the cells into nude mice.

Chapter 6

Hepatitis B Virus Infection, Its Sequelae, and Prevention in Taiwan

DING-SHINN CHEN[1]

1 Introduction

Viral hepatitis, liver cirrhosis, and hepatocellular carcinoma (HCC) are common in Taiwan [1–3]. In 1984, malignant neoplasms ranked first in the causes of death with an annual rate of 81.95/ 100 000 population, and cirrhosis was sixth at a rate of 16.65/100 000 [4]. Among the cancer deaths, 21% were attributed to HCC, which was the leading cause of cancer mortality for men and the third for women [4]. These statistics reflect the prevalence and importance of chronic liver diseases and HCC in Taiwan.

The discovery of Australia antigen two decades ago [5] and the subsequent solid link of the antigen to the hepatitis B virus (HBV) [6, 7] prompted active research in Taiwan, and chronic HBV infection was soon found to be extremely common. The high prevalence of chronic HBV infection and liver diseases in Taiwan provide an unusual opportunity to study the relationship between these disorders. The progress of research has been dramatic and culminated in a nationwide immunoprophylaxis program in Taiwan in 1984.

The purpose of this chapter is to review and discuss the epidemiology of HBV infection, the sequelae of chronic infection, and its prevention in Taiwan.

2 Epidemiology of HBV infection in Taiwan

2.1 The prevalence of HBsAg carriers in the general population

A very high hepatitis B surface antigen (HBsAg) carrier rate in the Chinese on Taiwan was found

[1] Department of Internal Medicine and Graduate Institute of Clinical Medicine, National Taiwan University College of Medicine, Taipei, Taiwan, Republic of China

shortly after the relatively insensitive first generation test for HBsAg was introduced in the early 1970s. By micro-Ouchterlony immunodiffusion, the carrier rate in the general population was found to range from 2% to 17% with an average of 8% [8]. Subsequent studies with sensitive methods revealed that 80%–90% of adults were infected, with 15%–20% carrying HBsAg [9–12]. The infection is contracted at an early age and continues to occur as is indicated by the steadily increasing prevalence of antibody to hepatitis B core antigen (anti-HBc) in Fig. 6.1. The prevalence of HBsAg reaches its peak in the first decade of life and then decreases gradually. The decrease may be due to: (1) decrease of HBsAg titers to undetectable levels with increasing age of chronic HBsAg carriers [11], (2) mortality due to HBV-related liver diseases, or (3) seroconversion to antibody to HBsAg (anti-HBs) in chronic carriers. Cross-sectional seroepidemiological studies suggest that HBV infection contracted at a younger age more frequently results in the carrier state, while infection in older age-groups does not. A study of 1200 healthy children in Taipei revealed that HBV infections contracted after the age of 3 years contribute minimally to the HBsAg carrier rate [13]. Prospective studies in Taiwan have shown that the younger the age at which HBV infection is contracted, the higher the HBsAg carrier rate [14–16].

In every age-group, the carrier rate is 1%–6% lower in females and females are better anti-HBs responders [11]. Chronic HBV infections occur less frequently in people who originally came from northern mainland China (11.2%) than in those who came from the south (17.7%) [17].

Based on these seroepidemiological data, it is estimated that there are currently 3 million HBsAg carriers among the 19 million population in Taiwan. They act as reservoirs of HBV and transmit the virus to others. Additionally, the

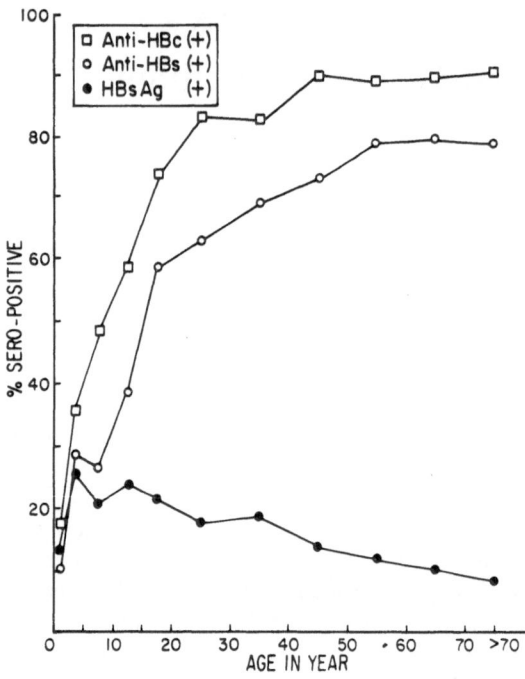

Fig. 6.1. Prevalence of hepatitis B virus markers by age in 2003 healthy subjects in Taiwan. The viral markers in the serum were studied by radioimmunoassay

carriers have a higher risk of developing chronic liver diseases and HCC, as will be described below.

2.2 The important role of perinatal transmission

Prospective [14] and retrospective [18] studies have indicated the key role of perinatal transmission in producing chronic carriage of HBsAg. This mechanism alone accounts for 40% of the HBsAg carriers in Taiwan [14]. Most of the infections develop in infants of hepatitis B e antigen (HBeAg)-positive-carrier mothers. As high as 86%–96% of these babies become chronic HBsAg carriers, in contrast to 6%–21% of babies born to anti-HBe-positive carrier mothers [19, 20]. The infection is essentially asymptomatic and occurs despite the presence of high titers of anti-HBc passively transferred from the mothers. The anti-HBc IgM response is often short-lived and of low titer and so may escape serological detection [21].

Although the exact mechanism of perinatal transmission is unclear, maternal HBeAg [19] and HBsAg titers [14, 20] are good predictors of the infection. Approximately 3% of the cord blood samples from the newborn of HBsAg-carrier mothers contain high-titer HBsAg; these

are probably instances of intrauterine infection. However, preliminary studies with molecular hybridization of liver specimens from five stillbirths of HBsAg-carrier mothers failed to reveal any intrahepatic HBV DNA (Chen DS et al. 1985, unpublished data).

The annual incidence of horizontal HBV infection is 5% in preschool children [15], 1.2% in adolescents [22], and 1.5% in young adults [16]. Despite the fact that HBsAg is frequently present in the various body fluids of the carrier [23], the major mode of horizontal transmission is unclear. Although inadequately sterilized syringes and needles have been suspected to play some role in Taiwan [15], it is insufficient to explain the high frequency of HBV infections.

2.3 Subtypes of HBsAg and family clustering of HBsAg

The main subtypes of HBsAg in Taiwan are adw and adr [24]; the y subtype is rare but is found in some tribes of the island's indigenous population [9]. The subtype does not correlate with the types of liver disease, since in each group of patients adw always predominates [24]. A geographical difference is evident, however; adw is dominant in people coming from southern mainland China (76%) and in Taiwanese (91%), whereas adr is present in 78% of the HBsAg carriers who originated from northern mainland China, the Yangtze River being the boundary. It is interesting to note that in those whose families originated in northern China, the adr subtype still dominates in the younger generations who were born and have lived exclusively in Taiwan, where adw is the main subtype. This observation strongly emphasizes the importance of intrafamilial transmission [24].

Familial clustering of HBsAg is common [18, 25], and the subtype in members of a given family is usually identical, particularly when the mother is a carrier of HBsAg [18, 25, 26]. However, there are some families with clusters of carriers of different HBsAg subtypes [27]. This has been observed only in families with an adr-carrier father and adw-carrier children. Horizontal infection of children by the locally dominant adw subtype accounts for this occasional discordance of subtypes between carrier fathers and their children.

Studies on the heterotypic anti-HBs in HBsAg carriers have also been revealing. Most of the anti-HBs-positive HBsAg sera are with HBsAg/ adr and anti-HBs of the w-subtype. HBsAg/adw with anit-HBs/adr is rare [28]. This observation is in keeping with HBV/adw as the main subtype in Taiwan.

3 The sequelae of chronic hepatitis B virus infection

3.1 The carrier state of HBsAg

A chronic carrier of HBsAg is an individual with the antigen detectable in the serum for 6 months or longer [29]. Our knowledge of the natural history of chronic HBsAg carriers is incomplete. The spectrum of hepatic derangement ranges widely from a normal liver to well-established cirrhosis, or even asymptomatic HCC. Despite the lack of symptomatology, the liver in young HBsAg carriers almost always shows some histological abnormalities, albeit mild.

A histopathological study in 18 perinatally infected HBsAg-carrier children revealed no abnormalities in only one instance (5.6%); four carriers (22.2%) had minimal histological changes, two (11.1%) had mild lobular hepatitis, and 11 (61.1%) had chronic persistent hepatitis (CPH) [30]. In 44 asymptomatic young military recruits with HBsAg, three (6.8%) had normal histology, 22 (50%) nonspecific abnormalities, nine (20.5%) lobular hepatitis, nine (20.5%) CPH, and one (2.3%) chronic active hepatitis (CAH) [31]. In another study of 82 asymptomatic carriers (university students), only 12 (14.6%) had normal histology, 43 (52.4%) had nonspecific reactive hepatitis, 24 (29.3%) acute viral hepatitis, and three (3.7%) CAH [32]. A study from National Taiwan University Hospital (Yang PM et al. 1985, unpublished data) in 44 asymptomatic carriers over 40 years of age suggests that the frequency of both cirrhosis and minimal histological changes increase with age. Cirrhosis was found in eight (18.2%), CPH in 18 (40.9%), lobular hepatitis in one (2.3%), and minimal histological changes in 17 (38.6%).

The majority of young asymptomatic HBsAg carriers have a good prognosis histologically over a period of 1.5–2 years [33]. Apparently, the long-term consequences of chronic HBsAg carriage remain to be determined.

Although serum HBsAg titers tend to decrease after prolonged carrier status [11], detectable antigenemia persists refractorily. HBsAg becomes undetectable in only about 1% of chronic carriers/year in our experience, and seroconversion to anti-HBs is even rarer.

The serum levels of HBsAg in chronic carriers range from 0.01 to 325 μg/ml. Serum HBeAg and HBV DNA correlate well with the HBsAg levels, with a mean level 15 times higher in the HBeAg- or HBV DNA-positive HBsAg carriers [34].

The prevalence of HBeAg varies with the age of the HBsAg carriers [13, 35–37]. In those younger than 20 years, HBeAg is positive in 70%–100% and decreases steadily with age. By contrast, anti-HBe increases in a reversed tendency with >90% of carriers older than 60 years positive for anti-HBe [12]. The prolonged interval in HBeAg/anti-HBe seroconversion and the age-dependent declining prevalence of HBeAg, accompanied by a reciprocal increase in anti-HBe, suggest HBeAg/anti-HBe as chronological indicators in chronic HBV infection in Taiwan [38].

Because of the close association of the infectivity and the presence of HBeAg in HBsAg carriers [19, 34, 39], the detection of HBeAg in asymptomatic HBsAg carriers identifies these individuals as a reservoir of HBV infection. In a large-scale screening of 82 084 pregnant women in Taiwan, 48% of 15 867 who were HBsAg positive were also positive for HBeAg [40]. In the absence of intervention, these women will transmit HBV perinatally to their offspring, as described above.

In summary, chronic HBV infection can be divided into two phases—an early replicative phase followed by a nonreplicative phase. The early phase is characterized by higher serum HBsAg levels and the presence of HBeAg and HBV DNA, and the later phase by the opposite findings. Although described as "early," the replicative phase may last for decades.

3.2 Chronic hepatitis

Probably because of the frequency of persistent HBV infections, chronic hepatitis is common in Taiwan [1–3, 32], and the HBsAg prevalence in chronic hepatitis is surprisingly high. By radioimmunoassay, HBsAg is present in 91% of patients with CAH, 82% with CPH, and 60% with chronic lobular hepatitis (CLH) (Table 6.1). Although in one study from Taiwan [41] it was stated that CLH accounts for 31% of 259 patients with chronic hepatitis, other studies have not borne out this finding (Table 6.1; Tsai YT 1985, personal communication). The reason may be due to a difference in patient populations [41] or different criteria for the histological diagnosis of CLH.

The male to female ratio in chronic hepatitis is 4–7 : 1 and the peak age is 20–30 years [42,

Table 6.1. Prevalence of hepatitis B virus markers in patients with chronic liver diseases and hepatocellular carcinoma in Taiwan

Diagnosis	No. tested	HBsAg(+)		Anti-HBs(+)		Anti-HBc(+)		HBeAg(+)[a]		Anti-HBe(+)[a]	
		No.	Percent	No.	Percent	No.	Percent	No.	Percent	No.	Percent
Chronic hepatitis											
Chronic active hepatitis	231	209	90.5	51	22.1	229	99.1	145	69.4	50	23.9
Chronic persistent hepatitis	106	87	82.1	28	26.4	103	97.1	66	75.9	18	20.7
Chronic lobular hepatitis	10	6	60.0	4	40.0	10	100.0	5	83.3	1	16.7
Cirrhosis	112	90	80.4	25	22.3	109	97.3	29	32.2	57	63.3
Hepatocellular carcinoma	273	241	88.3	51	18.7	269	98.5	45	18.7	187	77.6
Healthy adults	1454	213	14.6	1036	71.3	1293	88.9	68	31.9	126	59.2

Hepatitis markers detected by radioimmunoassay
[a] Only HBsAg-positive patients were tested

43]. HBeAg is positive in most patients (Table 6.1), reflecting the association of HBV replication with active hepatitis. Seroconversion from HBeAg to anti-HBe occurs at an annual rate of 12%–18% in CAH [44, 45], and exacerbations of the hepatitis, manifested by lobular inflammation and elevated serum aminotransferases, are observed frequently, sometimes before the HBe seroconversion [44]. Transient mild elevation of serum α-fetoprotein (AFP) is observed in 15%–51% of patients with chronic hepatitis, particularly in HBsAg-positive patients [46]. Elevation of serum AFP in chronic hepatitis B may precede the clearance of HBeAg [47]. Although seroconversion to anti-HBe is generally associated with a markedly reduced activity of hepatitis, it does not always indicate a favorable prognosis. Observations from Italy [48] and Taiwan [38] have independently indicated a higher frequency of cirrhosis in anti-HBe-positive patients with HBsAg-positive CAH. That anti-HBe does not necessarily indicate a favorable prognosis is further supported by a very high prevalence of anti-HBe in patients with inactive cirrhosis and HCC [37, 38, 49, 50] (Table 6.1).

In about 10% of HBeAg-negative patients with CAH in Taiwan, active hepatitis still persists with repeated exacerbations despite seroconversion to anti-HBe. Serum HBV DNA was present in all of 11 such patients studied and the levels increased during the exacerbations. Furthermore, the free forms of HBV DNA were also present in the liver tissue [51], indicating the important role of viral replication in causing active hepatitis in CAH.

It has been claimed that the prognosis of HBsAg-positive CAH is very poor in Taiwan [52]. Sixty-five patients with HBsAg-positive CAH were evaluated in National Taiwan University Hospital by follow-up liver biopsy at least 1 year after initial biopsy (median, 3.9 years; range, 1–15 years; Chen DS et al. 1985, unpublished data). Among 49 patients with an initial histological diagnosis of severe CAH, follow-up biopsies showed cirrhosis in 21(43%), portal fibrosis or posthepatitic scarring in 9(18%), and minimal histological change or normal histology in seven (14%). The prognosis in 16 patients with mild to moderate CAH seemed better than in severe CAH. Among the 24 cirrhotic patients in this study, two or 8% eventually developed HCC (Fig. 6.2). Thus, approximately 40% of HBsAg-positive patients with CAH in Taiwan will develop cirrhosis and another 40% will regress at some stage of the disease process, with liver histological findings showing only portal fibrosis, post-hepatitic scarring, or even minimal histological changes. This longitudinal study revealed that when HBe seroconversion had occured, liver histology was the most important determinant of the prognosis in CAH. If there is no cirrhotic change at the time of seroconversion, then the CAH will generally regress to an inactive state with a well-preserved liver architecture. By contrast, if cirrhosis is already present at the time of seroconversion, then the disease will progress, though slowly and asymptomatically. A significant number of such patients may eventually develop HCC.

Until now, δ agent, a defective RNA virus

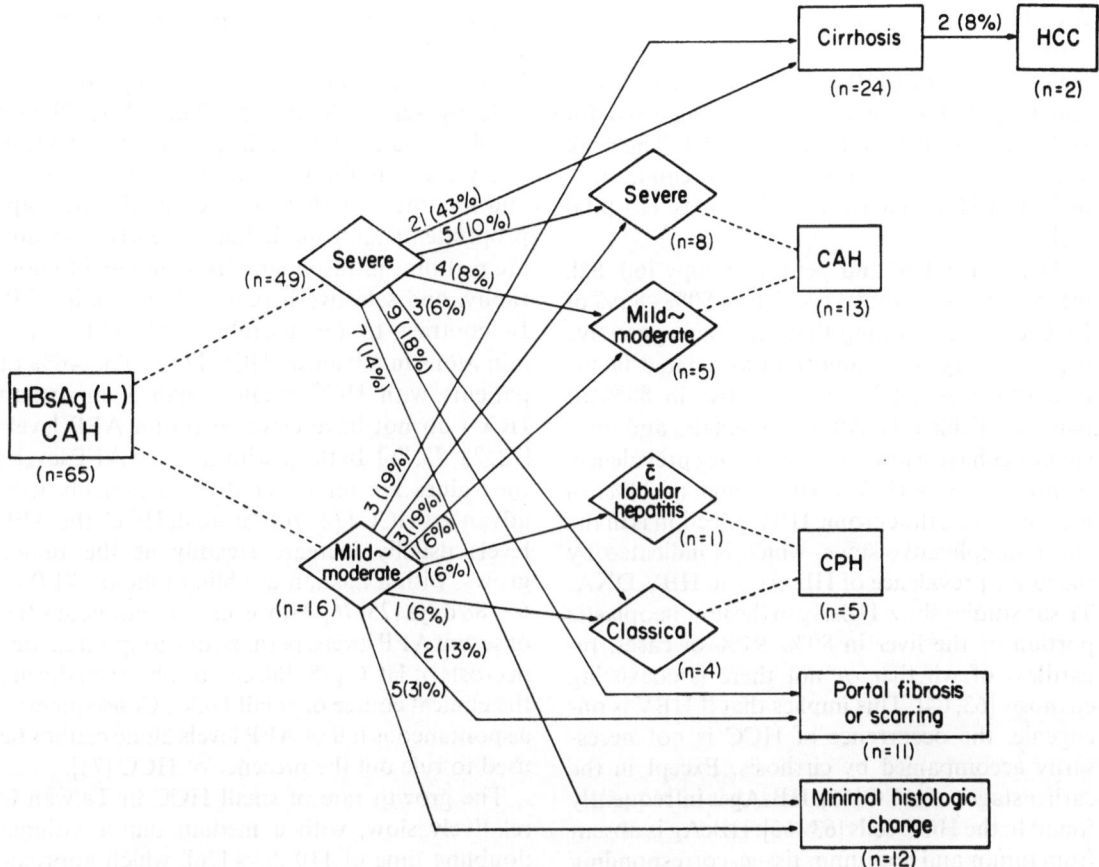

Fig. 6.2. Results of follow-up liver biopsies in 65 patients with HBsAg-positive chronic active hepatitis. Follow-up biopsies were performed at least 1 year after the initial biopsy (median, 3.9 years; range, 1–15 years). *CAH* chronic active hepatitis, *CPH* chronic persistent hepatitis, *HCC* hepatocellular carcinoma

requiring the "helper" function of HBV [53], seems to have played little or no role in the sequelae of chronic HBV infection in Taiwan [54, 55]. However, HBsAg carriers who are intravenous drug abusers in Taiwan have a prevalence of anti-δ of 67%–79% [55, 56], indicating that δ agent could potentially have a disastrous impact among the many HBsAg carriers in Taiwan, if appropriate routes of transmission should develop.

3.3 Cirrhosis

Alcoholic liver disease and other causes of cirrhosis are relatively uncommon in Taiwan. The peak age of patients with cirrhosis is 50–60 years and the male to female ratio is 3–4 : 1. A past history of hepatitis is seen in only about

10%–20% of cases, indicating the subclinical nature of the preceding disease process in most patients. The prevalence of HBsAg is high (Table 6.1), which indicates again the strong association of cirrhosis with persistent HBV infection in Taiwan. This is not unexpected, because cirrhosis is a sequela to chronic aggressive liver disorder which is mainly caused by HBV in Taiwan. The prolonged period of HBV infection is indicated by the predominance of anti-HBe (Table 6.1).

Because the peak age of CAH is 20–30 years and that of decompensated cirrhosis is 50–60 years, the cirrhosis is likely to have progressed asymptomatically for several decades before it is manifested by decompensation in its terminal stage. Initially, the cirrhosis is micronodular but it later becomes macronodular in type. As is shown in Fig. 6.2, a significant proportion of the cirrhotics in Taiwan will develop HCC.

3.4 Hepatocellular carcinoma

This malignancy is common in Taiwan with an incidence of 25/100 000 males and 10/100 000 females [57]. HBsAg carriers are at high risk for HCC, as described in Chaps. 1 and 3. The peak age is 50–60 years with a male to female ratio of 7 : 1 in National Taiwan University Hospital [58].

At autopsy [59] and peritoneoscopy [60–62], macronodular cirrhosis coexists in 80%–85% of HCC cases, suggesting that previous aggressive hepatic injury is an important associated factor in pathogenesis. HBsAg is positive in 88% of patients (Table 6.1). Although females and non-cirrhotics have a lower serum HBsAg prevalence, its prevalence in HCC is still as high as 70%. In most patients, the chronic HBV infection is in the late nonreplicative stage, which is indicated by the lower prevalence of HBeAg and HBV DNA. Tissue studies show HBsAg in the non-neoplastic portion of the liver in 80%–91% of cases, regardless of whether or not there is coexisting cirrhosis [63, 64]. This implies that if HBV is oncogenic, the occurrence of HCC is not necessarily accompanied by cirrhosis. Except in the earlier stages of HCC [65], HBsAg is infrequently found in the HCC cells [63–65]. HBcAg is absent from tumor and nontumor tissue, corresponding to the nonreplicative stage of the HBV infection.

At the molecular level, HBV DNA is found to be integrated to host chromosomal DNA in most patients with HCC in Taiwan [66–68]. The integration occurs at multiple sites and there seems to be no unique site of integration. The number of HBV genomes integrated varies widely from <0.01 to several hundred per cell [66, 67], and stoichiometric analysis may yield evidence suggesting a monoclonal origin of HCC [67]. Similarly, integration of HBV genomes is also present in the non-neoplastic portion of the liver with HCC. The patterns of integration are different in neoplastic and non-neoplastic tissues from individual patients. The presence of integrated HBV DNA in the non-neoplastic portions suggests that the integration precedes the development of HCC. The molecular viral oncogenesis of hepadna viruses is discussed in Chaps. 3 and 4.

The prevalent chronic HBV infection in Taiwanese patients with HCC is most likely of maternal origin. In a retrospective study, eight of eleven mothers of HBsAg-positive HCC patients were also positive for HBsAg, invariably with an identical subtype [26]. Occasionally, HCC is seen in perinatally infected carrier children [69, 70] as young as 5 years of age.

The high incidence of HCC in Taiwan provides a special opportunity to study this cancer. Early detection in asymptomatic high-risk subjects by serum AFP surveillance [71, 72] and regular hepatic sonography [72] has been fruitful and yielded useful information on the diagnosis and treatment of HCC. Currently, the most appropriate imaging modalities for early detection are real-time ultrasonography, computed tomography, and selective hepatic arteriography [73]. In contrast to the usefulness of AFP determinations in advanced HCC [74], 25%–46% of patients with HCC smaller than 3 cm (small HCC) do not have elevated serum AFP levels [72, 73, 75, 76]. In those with elevated AFP levels, the values are far lower than in patients with advanced HCC [72–76]. In small HCC, the AFP levels usually increase steadily as the tumor grows, with a median doubling time of AFP of 60–88 days [75, 76]. However, a spontaneous fall of serum AFP levels, perhaps due to spontaneous necrosis of HCC [65, 76], can be observed during the clinical course of small HCC. Consequently, a spontaneous fall of AFP levels alone cannot be used to rule out the presence of HCC [75].

The growth rate of small HCC in Taiwan is relatively slow, with a median tumor volume doubling time of 110 days [76], which approximates the experience in Japan [77]. The median detectable subclinical period of HCC in Taiwan is calculated to be 3.2 years (range, 0.8–10.9 years). Therefore, the perception of HCC in the past as a rapidly progressing fatal malignancy is probably erroneous, being the result of late diagnosis [76].

In a prospective study [78], cirrhotics and middle-aged HBsAg-positive family members of HCC patients were shown to be at increased risk of HCC. The annual incidence of HCC in 193 cirrhotics followed for 338 person-years is 5.6% (7.7%/year in the HBsAg positives and 5.1%/year in the HBsAg negatives, $P > 0.05$). The annual incidence for 117 middle-aged asymptomatic HBsAg carriers (138 person-years) is 0.7%. It is interesting to note that in 120 patients with chronic hepatitis alone, none has developed HCC during the follow-up period of 205 person-years.

Liver function tests in patients with small HCC show only mild abnormalities or reflect the underlying cirrhosis, with increased BSP retention as the most common abnormal finding [73]. The familiar pattern of increased serum alkaline phosphatase [79] or a disproportionate increase of the GOT/GPT ratio [80] in advanced HCC is not encountered. When the non-neoplastic portion of the liver is studied by peritoneoscopy, the coexisting cirrhosis in small HCC seems less severe than that of advanced HCC [81], indicating that the cirrhosis progresses along with the growth of HCC.

When HCC is detected in the symptomatic patient with advanced HCC, the prognosis is extremely poor [82]. In National Taiwan University Hospital, observations on more than 300 patients with advanced HCC (1971–1978) revealed a resectability rate of 8.5%; 40% of the patients had a recurrence in the 1st year after surgery. In recent years, early detection of asymptomatic small HCC has had a substantial impact on this situation. With the aid of intraoperative ultrasonography [83], the resectability has increased to more than 80% [73]. However, the recurrence rate after surgery is still as high as 10% per year [84]. This fact strongly calls for measures not only to prevent chronic HBV infection, but also to prevent carcinogenesis in chronically infected persons in Taiwan.

4 The national strategy for hepatitis B immunoprophylaxis

Because hepatitis B is so important in Taiwan, a hepatitis B control program was established in 1981 in an attempt to interrupt transmission of HBV and to decrease the prevalent chronic HBsAg carriage.

Studies in Taiwan have shown that in the newborns of HBeAg-positive mothers, combination of hepatitis B immune globulin (HBIG) and hepatitis B vaccine is highly effective in preventing chronic HBsAg carriage [85, 86]. Thus, a 10-year nationwide hepatitis B vaccination program was started in July 1984, with newborn infants of HBsAg-carrier mothers as the top priority for vaccination [87, 88]. These infants receive 5 μg hepatitis B vaccine (HEVAC, Institut Pasteur Production, France) at 1 week, 5 weeks, 9 weeks, and 12 months of age. If the mother's HBeAg is positive or if her serum HBsAg titer by reversed passive hemagglutination is $\geqslant 1:2560$, then the newborn receives an additional dose of 0.5 ml HBIG immediately after birth. The vaccines and HBIG and HBsAg testing reagents are all provided by the government free of charge. To combat horizontal infections, the program will be extended to all newborns in 1986, and in a stepwise fashion all persons susceptible to HBV infection will be vaccinated within 10 years [87].

The program in the 1st year has been successful. Up to June 1985, a total of 107 071 doses of vaccines has been given to infants of HBsAg-carrier mothers with an estimated coverage of 70% (Department of Health, Republic of China, 1986, unpublished data).

All data from carrier mothers and vaccinees are stored in a data center through an efficient registration system. This will be extremely helpful in providing information on whether or not hepatitis B immunoprophylaxis will reduce the prevalence of chronic liver diseases and HCC in future years. If prevention of chronic HBV infection actually decreases the occurrence of HCC, then the solid proof will very possibly come from observations in Taiwan. That chronic HBV infection can induce HCC will then be firmly established at this stage on the basis of these observations.

References

1. Yeh S (1966) Some geographic aspects of common disease in Taiwan. Internatl Path 7: 24–28
2. Cooper WC, Gershon RK, Sun SC, Fresh JW (1966) Anicteric viral hepatitis. A clinicopathological follow-up study in Taiwan. N Engl J Med 274: 585–595
3. Yu JY, Hsieh SC, Tai TY, Wang TH, Chen JS, Shih PL, Chen TS (1970) Endemic anicteric infectious hepatitis in the dormitories of National Taiwan University. J Formosan Med Assoc 69: 353–361
4. Department of Health, Executive Yuan (1985) Health statistics: Vital statistics of Republic of China. 1984(2): 33, 44–45, 100–101
5. Blumberg BS, Alter HJ, Visnich S (1965) A "new" antigen in leukemia sera. JAMA 191: 541–546
6. Okochi K, Murakami S (1968) Observations on Australia antigen in Japanese. Vox Sang 15: 374–385
7. Prince AM (1968) An antigen detected in the blood during the incubation period of serum hepatitis. Proc Natl Acad Sci USA 60: 814–821
8. Shih PL, Chang CK, Sung JL (1971) Hepatitis-associated antigen and antibody in Taiwan. J Formosan Med Assoc 70: 697–706
9. Beasley RP, Stevens CE (1974) Epidemiology of hepatitis B infection in Taiwan. In: Sung JL, Yu, JY, Wang TH (eds) Proceedings of the International Symposium on Hepatitis, The Gastroenterological Society of the Republic of China, Taipei, pp 1–10
10. Sung JL, Chen DS (1976) Hepatitis B surface antigen and antibody in liver disease in Taiwan. In: Lee SK, Sinniah R, Tan LKA, Phua KB, Chow KW (eds) Proceedings of the 5th Asian-Pacific Congress of Gastroenterology. Gastro-

enterological Society of Singapore, Singapore, pp 265–269

11. Chen DS, Sung JL, Lai MY (1978) A seroepidemiologic study of hepatitis B virus infection in Taiwan. J Formosan Med Assoc 77: 908–918

12. Sung JL, Chen DS, Lai MY, Yu JY, Wang TH, Wang CY, Lee CY, Chen SH, Ko TM (1984) Epidemiological study on hepatitis B infection in Taiwan. Chinese J Gastroenterol 1: 1–9

13. Hsu HY, Chang MH, Chen DS, Lee CY, Sung JL (1986) Baseline seroepidemiology of hepatitis B virus infection in children in Taipei, 1984—A study just before mass hepatitis B vaccination program in Taiwan. J Med Virol 18: 301–307

14. Stevens CE, Beasley RP, Tsui J, Lee WC (1975) Vertical transmission of hepatitis B antigen in Taiwan. N Engl J Med 292: 771–774

15. Beasley RP, Hwang LY, Lin CC, Leu ML, Stevens CE, Szmuness W, Chen KP (1982) Incidence of hepatitis B virus infection in preschool children in Taiwan. J Infect Dis 146: 198–204

16. Beasley RP, Hwang LY, Lin CC, Ko YC, Twu SJ (1983) Incidence of hepatitis among students at a university. Am J Epidemiol 117: 213–222

17. Beasley RP, Lin CC, Chien CS, Chen CJ, Hwang LY (1982) Geographic distribution of HBsAg carriers in China. Hepatology 2: 553–556

18. Chen DS, Sung JL (1978) Studies on the subtypes of hepatitis B surface antigen in Taiwan—Demonstration of vertical and intrafamilial transmission of hepatitis B virus. J Formosan Med Assoc 77: 263–271

19. Stevens CE, Neurath RA, Beasley RP, Szmuness W (1979) HBeAg and anti-HBe detection by radioimmunoassay: Correlation with vertical transmission of hepatitis B virus in Taiwan. J Med Virol 3: 237–241

20. Ko TM, Lin KS, Ho MM, Hwang WF, Hwang KC, Hsieh FJ, Yang CL, Chen DS (1986) Perinatal transmission of hepatitis B in the Taoyuan area. J Formosan Med Assoc 85: 341–351

21. Chen DS, Sung JL, Lai MY, Sheu JC, Yang PM, Lee SC, Chen SH, Chang MH, Ko TM, Lee TY (1985) Inadequacy of immunoglobulin M hepatitis B core antibody in detecting acute hepatitis B virus infection in infants of HBsAg carrier mothers. J Med Virol 16: 309–314

22. Chen DS, Twu SJ, Lin JT, Lai MY, Sheu JC, Wang CY, Wang TH, Yu JY, Sung JL (1983) Annual incidence of hepatitis A and hepatitis B virus infection in junior college students in northern Taiwan. Abstracts of papers presented at 13th Annual Meeting of the Gastroenterological Society of the Republic of China, 19–20 March 1983, Taipei, pp 56–57

23. Sung JL, Chen DS (1983) Hepatitis B surface antigen in saliva, urine and ascites. Hepato-Gastroenterology 30: 59

24. Sung JL, Chen DS (1977) Geographical distribution of the subtypes of hepatitis B surface antigen in Chinese. Gastroenterol Jpn 12: 58–63

25. Beasley RP, Tsui J, Stevens CE (1974) Hepatitis B antigen occurrence in families in Taiwan. In: Sung JL, Yu JY, Wang TH (eds) Proceedings of the International Symposium on Hepatitis, The Gastroenterological Society of the Republic of China, Taipei, pp 27–33

26. Sung JL, Chen DS (1980) Maternal transmission of hepatitis B surface antigen in patients with hepatocellular carcinoma in Taiwan. Scand J Gastroenterol 15: 321–324

27. Sung JL, Chen DS (1978) Clustering of different subtypes of hepatitis B surface antigen in families of patients with chronic liver diseases. Am J Gastroenterol 69: 559–564

28. Chen DS, Lai MY, Sung JL (1982) Anti-HBs reactivity in hepatitis B surface antigen positive serum samples—with special emphasis on heterotypic antibody. J Formosan Med Assoc 81: 1357–1364

29. Sampliner RE (1985) Follow-up and management of hepatitis B carriers. In: Gerety RJ (ed) Hepatitis B. Academic Press, Orlando, pp 155–172

30. Chang MH, Beasley RP, Hsu HC, Hwang LY, Lee CY (1984) A clinical and liver histology study in the perinatally transmitted HBV carrier children. Chinese J Gastroenterol 1: 86

31. Anderson KE, Sun SC, Berg HS, Chang NK (1974) Liver function and histology in asymptomatic Chinese military personnel with hepatitis B antigenemia. Am J Dig Dis 19: 693–703

32. Sung JL, Shih PL, Liaw YF, Lin WSJ, Tai TY, Hsieh SC, Wang CY, Chang CK, Wang TH, Yu JY, Chen JS (1979) A survey and follow-up study of anicteric hepatitis, other asymptomatic liver diseases and hepatitis B surface antigen carriers. J Formosan Med Assoc 78: 452–459

33. Sun SC, Beasley RP, Anderson KE, Berg HS, Hsu CP, Lee WC (1976) Serial liver biopsy observations in hepatitis B antigen carriers by light and electron microscopy. Am J Dig Dis 21: 366–369

34. Chen DS, Lai MY, Lee SC, Yang PM, Sheu JC, Sung JL (1986) Serum HBsAg, HBeAg, anti-HBe, and hepatitis B viral DNA in asymptomatic carriers in Taiwan. J Med Virol 19: 87–94

35. Chen DS, Sung JL, Lai MY (1981) HBeAg and anti-HBe in chronic hepatitis B virus infection. Gastroenterology 80: 880–881

36. Sung JL, Chen DS, Lai MY, Wang TH, Wang CY, Yu JY, Lee CY (1982) Hepatitis B e antigen and antibody in asymptomatic Chinese with hepatitis B surface antigenemia in Taiwan. Gastroenterol Jpn 17: 341–346

37. Liaw YF, Chu CM, Lin DY, Sheen IS, Yang CY, Huang MJ (1984) Age-specific prevalence and significance of hepatitis B e antigen and antibody in chronic hepatitis B virus infection in Taiwan: A comparison among asymptomatic carriers, chronic hepatitis, liver cirrhosis and hepatocellular carcinoma. J Med Virol 13: 385–391

38. Chen DS, Sung JL, Lai MY (1981) Hepatitis B e antigen and antibody in chronic liver diseases and hepatocellular carcinoma. Hepato-Gastroenterology 28: 288–291

39. Shikata T, Karasawa T, Abe K, Uzawa T, Suzuki H, Oda T, Imai M, Mayumi M, Moritsugu Y

(1977) Hepatitis B e antigen and infectivity of hepatitis B virus. J Infect Dis 136: 571–576

40. Lin CC, Hsu LC, Liu JY, Lee TC (1984) Prevalence rate of HBsAg and HBeAg in pregnant women in Taiwan, August 1982–December 1983. In: Vyas GN, Dienstag JL, Hoofnagle JH (eds) Viral hepatitis and liver disease. Grune and Stratton, Orlando, pp 637–638

41. Liaw YF, Chu CM, Chen TJ, Huang MJ, Lin DY, Chang-Chien CS, Chen PJ, Wu CS (1981) Chronic hepatitis in Taiwan: I. A histological and etiological study. J Formosan Med Assoc 80: 952–960

42. Liaw YF, Chu CM, Chen TJ, Lin DY, Chang-Chien CS, Wu CS (1982) Chronic lobular hepatitis: A clinicopathological and prognostic study. Hepatology 2: 258–262

43. Liaw YF, Chen DS, Wang TH, Sung JL (1974) The study on chronic aggressive hepatitis. In: Sung JL, Yu JY, Wang TH (eds) Proceedings of the International Symposium on Hepatitis. Gastroenterological Society of the Republic of China, Taipei, pp 133–138

44. Liaw YF, Chu CM, Su IJ, Huang MJ, Lin DY, Chang-Chien CS (1983) Clinical and histological events preceding hepatitis B e antigen seroconversion in chronic type B hepatitis. Gastroenterology 84: 216–219

45. Sung JL, Chen DS, Lai MY, Sheu JC, Yang PM, Lin JT, Yu JY (1984) Studies on HBeAg/anti-HBe—with special reference to its persistence and seroconversion. Abstracts papers presented at 14th Annual Meeting of the Gastroenterological Society of the Republic of China, 17–18 March 1984, Taipei, pp 76–77

46. Chen DS, Sung JL (1979) Relationship of hepatitis B surface antigen and serum α-fetoprotein in nonmalignant diseases of the liver. Cancer 44: 984–992

47. Liaw YF, Chu CM, Huang MJ, Sheen IS, Yang CY, Lin DY (1984) Determinants for hepatitis B e antigen clearance in chronic type B hepatitis. Liver 4: 301–306

48. Realdi G, Alberti A, Rugge M, Bortolotti F, Rigoli AM, Tremolada F, Ruol A (1980) Seroconversion from hepatitis B e antigen to anti-HBe in chronic hepatitis B virus infection. Gastroenterology 79: 195–199

49. Eleftheriou N, Thomas HC, Heathcote J, Sherlock S (1975) Incidence and clinical significance of e antigen and antibody in acute and chronic liver disease. Lancet 2: 1171–1173

50. Werner BG, Murphy BL, Maynard JE, Larouzé B (1976) Anti-e in primary hepatic carcinoma. Lancet 1: 696

51. Lai MY, Chen DS, Lee SC, Yang PM, Su IJ, Hsu HC, Sung JL (1985) Serum HBV DNA in anti-HBe-positive patients with chronic active hepatitis B: Evidence of HBV replications during acute exacerbations. Abstracts of papers presented at International Symposium on Chronic Hepatitis, 28–29 November 1985, Taipei, p 35

52. Lo KJ, Tong MJ, Chien MC, Tsai YT, Liaw YF,

Yang KC, Chian H, Liu HC, Lee SD (1982) The natural course of hepatitis B surface antigen-positive chronic active hepatitis in Taiwan. J Infect Dis 146: 205–210

53. Rizzetto M, Canese MG, Gerin JL, London WT, Sly DL, Purcell RH (1980) Transmission of the hepatitis B virus-associated delta antigen to chimpanzees. J Infect Dis 141: 590–602

54. Chen DS, Lai MY, Sung JL (1984) δ Agent infection in chronic liver diseases and hepatocellular carcinoma—An infrequent finding in Taiwan. Hepatology 4: 502–503

55. Chen DS, Su IJ, Lai MY, Hsu HC' Yang PM, Sheu JC, Sung JL (1987) Delta agent infection in Taiwan. J Gastroenterol Hepatol (in press)

56. Lee SD, Wang JY, Wu JC, Chiang YT, Tsai YT, Lo KJ (1986) Hepatitis B and D virus infection among drug abusers in Taiwan. J Med Virol 20: 247–252

57. Lin TM, Chang LC, Chen KP (1977) A statistical analysis on mortality of malignant neoplasms in Taiwan. J Formosan Med Assoc 76: 656–668

58. The Staff of Cancer Registry (1984) Cancer in NTUH. In: Department of Medical Records, National Taiwan University Hospital (ed) National Taiwan University Hospital Cancer Registry Annual Report 1983. National Taiwan University Hospital, Taipei, p 16

59. Lin WSJ (1980) Hepatoma in Taiwan. A pathologic study. Trans Gastroenterol Soc ROC 9: 3–5

60. Chen DS, Wang TH, Lai MY, Sung JL (1978) Peritoneoscopic diagnosis in hepatoma. J Formosan Med Assoc 77: 764–765

61. Liu JD (1982) Peritoneoscopic diagnosis of hepatocellular carcinoma. Gastroenterol Endosc 24: 3–12

62. Lin DY, Liaw YF, Chu CM, Chang-Chien CS, Wu CS, Chen PC, Sheen IS (1984) Hepatocellular carcinoma in non-cirrhotic patients. Cancer 54: 1466–1468

63. Chen DS, Sung JL (1978) Cellular localization of hepatitis B surface antigen in the non-cirrhotic liver with hepatocellular carcinoma. Ital J Gastroenterol 10: 81–84

64. Hsu HC, Lin WSJ, Tsai MJ (1983) Hepatitis B surface antigen and hepatocellular carcinoma in Taiwan. Cancer 52: 1825–1832

65. Hsu HC, Sheu JC, Lin YH, Chen DS, Lee CS, Hwang LY, Beasley RP (1985) Prognostic histologic features of resected small hepatocellular carcinoma (HCC) in Taiwan. A comparison with resected large HCC. Cancer 56: 672–680

66. Chen DS, Hoyer BH, Nelson J, Purcell RH, Gerin JL (1982) Detection and properties of hepatitis B viral DNA in liver tissue from patients with hepatocellular carcinoma. Hepatology 2: 42s–46s

67. Miller RH, Lee SC, Liaw YF, Robinson WS (1985) Hepatitis B viral DNA in infected human liver and in hepatocellular carcinoma. J Infect Dis 151: 1081–1092

68. Chen CY, Harrison TJ, Lee CS, Chen DS, Zuckerman AJ (1986) Detection of hepatitis B virus DNA in hepatocellular carcinoma. Br J Exp Path

67: 279–288

69. Beasley RP, Shiao IS, Wu ZC, Hwang LY (1982) Hepatoma in an HBsAg carrier: Seven years after perinatal infection. J Pediatr 101: 83–84

70. Chang MH, Hsu HC, Lee CY, Chen DS, Lee CH, Lin KS (1984) Fraternal hepatocellular carcinoma in young children in two families. Cancer 53: 1807–1810

71. Beasley RP, Hwang LY (1984) Epidemiology of hepatocellular carcinoma. In: Vyas GN, Dienstag JL, Hoofnagle JH (eds) Viral hepatitis and liver disease. Grune and Stratton, Orlando, pp 209–224

72. Sheu JC, Sung JL, Chen DS, Lai MY, Wang TH, Yu JY, Yang PM, Chuang CN, Yang PC, Lee CS, Hsu HC, How SW (1985) Early detection of hepatocellular carcinoma by real-time ultrasonography. A prospective study. Cancer 56: 660–666

73. Chen DS, Sheu JC, Sung JL, Lai MY, Lee CS, Su CT, Tsang YM, How SW, Wang TH, Yu JY, Yang TH, Wang CY, Hsu CY (1982) Small hepatocellular carcinoma—A clinicopathological study in thirteen patients. Gastroenterology 83: 1109–1119

74. Chen DS, Sung JL (1977) Serum α-fetoprotein in hepatocellular carcinoma. Cancer 40: 779–783

75. Chen DS, Sung JL, Sheu JC, Lai MY, How SW, Hsu HC, Lee CS, Wei TC (1984) Serum α-fetoprotein in the early stage of human hepatocellular carcinoma. Gastroenterology 86: 1404–1409

76. Sheu JC, Sung JL, Chen DS, Yang PM, Lai MY, Lee CS, Hsu HC, Chuang CN, Yang PC, Wang TH, Lin JT, Lee CZ (1985) Growth rate of asymptomatic hepatocellular carcinoma and its clinical implications. Gastroenterology 89: 259–266

77. Yoshino M (1983) Growth kinetics of hepatocellular carcinoma. Jpn J Clin Oncol 13: 45–52

78. Chen DS, Sheu JC, Sung JL (1985) A prospective study on the occurrence of hepatocellular carcinoma in patients with cirrhosis, chronic hepatitis and asymptomatic HBsAg carriers. Abstracts of papers presented at Symposium on Epidemiology and Clinical Trials, 10–12 June 1985, Taipei, pp 75–76

79. Sung JL, Wang TH, Yu JY (1967) Clinical study on primary carcinoma of the liver in Taiwan. Am J Dig Dis 12: 1036–1049

80. Shimokawa Y, Okuda K, Kubo Y, Kaneko A, Arishima T, Nagata E, Hashimoto M, Sawa Y, Nagasaki Y, Kojiro M, Sakamoto K, Nakashima T (1977) Serum glutamic oxalacetic transaminase/glutamic pyruvic transaminase ratios in hepatocellular carcinoma. Cancer 40: 319–324

81. Lai MY, Chen DS, Sheu JC, Wang TH, Sung JL, How SW, Hsu HC (1982) Peritoneoscopic observations of non-tumorous portion of the liver with small hepatocellular carcinoma. Abstracts of papers presented at the 12th Annual Meeting of the Gastroenterological Society of the Republic of China. 13–14 March 1982, Taipei, p 101

82. Yang PM, Chuang JN, Chen DS, Lai MY, Sheu JC, Wang CY, Wang TH, Yu JY, Sung JL (1983) Systemic chemotherapy of hepatocellular carcinoma with Adriamycin alone and with the FAM regimen. In: Ogawa M, Okamura J, Nagasue N (eds) Proceedings of the 2nd International Workshop for Chemotherapy of Hepatic Tumors. Excerpta Medica, Amsterdam, pp 41–47

83. Sheu JC, Lee CS, Sung JL, Chen DS, Yang PM, Lin TY (1985) Intraoperative hepatic ultrasonography—An indispensable procedure in resection of small hepatocellular carcinomas. Surgery 97: 97–103

84. Lee CS, Sung JL, Hwang LY, Sheu JC, Chen DS, Lin TY, Beasley RP (1986) Surgical treatment of 109 patients with symptomatic and asymptomatic hepatocellular carcinoma. Surgery 99: 481–490

85. Beasley RP, Hwang LY, Lee GCY, Lan CC, Roan CH, Huang FY, Chen CL (1983) Prevention of perinatally transmitted hepatitis B virus infections with hepatitis B immune globulin and hepatitis B vaccine. Lancet 2: 1099–1102

86. Lo KJ, Tsai YT, Lee SD, Yeh CL, Wang JY, Chiang BN, Wu TC, Yeh PSH, Goudeau A, Coursaget P, Tong MJ (1985) Combined passive and active immunization for interruption of perinatal transmission of hepatitis B virus in Taiwan. Hepato-Gastroenterology 32: 65–68

87. Chen DS (1984) National strategy of hepatitis B vaccination in Taiwan, Republic of China. Abstracts of papers presented at the International Symposium on Immunization against HBV in the Developing World, 22–23 October 1984, Seoul, p 30

88. The Hepatitis B Control Committee and the Epidemiology Division, Bureau of Disease Control, Department of Health, Executive Yuan (1985) Hepatitis B control in Taiwan. Epidemiol Bull ROC 1: 17–19

Chapter 7
Pathology of Hepatocellular Carcinoma

Masamichi Kojiro and Toshiro Nakashima[1]

1 Introduction

Primary liver cancer is divided into two major types—hepatocellular carcinoma (HCC) derived from the hapatocytes and cholangiocarcinoma from the intrahepatic bile ducts. The less common malignant epithelial tumors primary to the liver include combined hepatocellular and cholangiocarcinoma and a few others types. The description of liver cancer by Galen and Aretaeus, physicians in ancient Greece, in the second century after Christ has been cited as the oldest record of liver cancer [1]. Virchow [2] gave a detailed account of the difference between primary and metastatic liver cancer. Von Hanseman [3], who reviewed a total of 258 cases of malignant hepatic tumors at the Berlin Pathological Institute, found that the incidence of primary liver cancer was far less common than that of metastatic liver cancer in Europe. The first gross classification of primary liver cancer was proposed in 1888 by Hanot and Gilbert [4] and then by Eggel [5] in 1901. In 1911, Yamagiwa [6] and Goldzieher and Bokay [7] classified primary liver cancer histologically. Yamagiwa [6] histologically differentiated "hepatoma" arising from the hepatocyte from "cholangioma" arising from the bile duct epithelium, and his histological classification was commonly used throughout the world until quite recently. The outstanding studies in this field by Berman [1] and Edmondson and Steiner [8] form the basis for current investigations into primary liver cancer.

After a long hopeless period in the management of HCC, the diagnosis and treatment of HCC have made remarkable progress in the past decade. In particular, significant advances have been made in diagnostic imaging techniques, such as angiography, computed tomography, and ultrasonography in addition to the measurement of serum alpha-fetoprotein, which have made early diagnosis of HCC easier. Much attention has ben paid recently to the histopathology of HCC because of the increased availability of surgically resected cases. The etiological factors of HCC have also been extensively investigated, and a close correlation between HCC and hepatitis B virus infection is currently being studied at the molecular level [9–13].

2 Gross pathology

The gross anatomical classification of HCC proposed by Eggel [5] in 1901 has been widely used up to the present time. He classified HCC into three types on the basis of the gross appearance and size of the mass—nodular, massive, and diffuse forms. The nodular form occurs as a solitary nodule or multiple nodules, which vary in size and are sharply demarcated. This type accounted for 64.4% of Eggel's cases, which were collected mainly from the literature. Tumors involving the entire right or left lobe, or which are as large as a single lobe, are designated as the massive form. This type is not clearly demarcated and is frequently accompanied by small intrahepatic metastatic nodules. It accounted for 23% of Eggel's cases. The diffuse form consists of numerous small foci (about the size of pseudolobules of cirrhosis) scattered throughout the liver, and each focus is encircled by connective tissue. Grossly, it is often difficult to distinguish this form from the pseudolobules of a cirrhotic liver. This type accounted for 12.4% of Eggel's cases.

According to Steiner [14], who compared HCC in Africa (known for its high incidence of HCC) with that in the United States, the macroscopic and histological features of HCC in Africa were basically similar irrespective of race and region, except that the affected livers among

[1] The First Department of Pathology, Kurume University School of Medicine, Kurume, 830 Japan

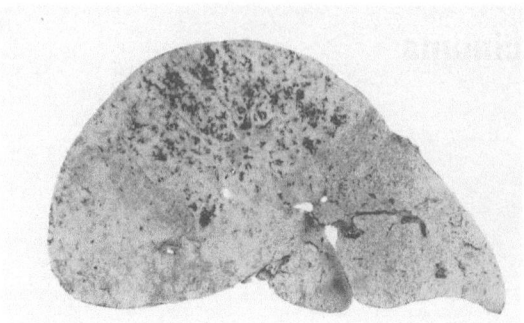

Fig. 7.1. Infiltrative type of HCC. Tumor-nontumor boundary is indistinct. There is no associated liver cirrhosis.

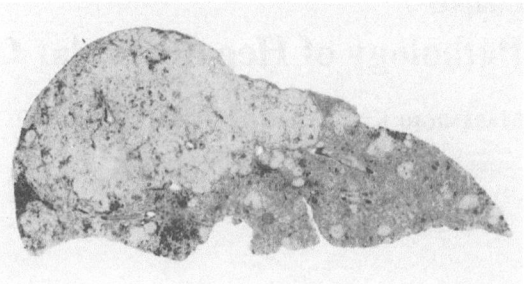

Fig. 7.2. Infiltrative type of HCC, massive. Confluent tumor is proliferating in a cirrhotic liver

African Blacks weighed between 3045 and 3891 g and were heavier (by about 800 g) than those of the Whites. Recent active cultural exchanges between Japan and foreign countries have provided us with increasing information about HCC from Western as well as African countries. As a result, it has become increasingly evident that HCC varies strikingly in its gross features in different parts of the world. According to Okuda et al. [15], who compared the gross features of HCC in the United States, South Africa, and Japan in 1984, the most striking difference among these three countries was the high incidence of encapsulated HCC in Japan in contrast to the other two countries.

2.1 Gross classification of HCC

Okuda et al. [15] proposed a new gross anatomical classification in 1984 based more on what appears to be the mode of tumor growth in relation to the nontumorous parenchyma, with consideration of the growth pattern within the main tumor mass. In their classification, they roughly divided HCC into two basic types—expanding and spreading types. In the expanding type, in which the boundary between the tumor and parenchyma is discrete, the tumor expands, compresses, and distorts the surrounding parenchyma. This type is further subdivided into cirrhotomimetic, pseudoadenomatous, and sclerosing patterns. According to Okuda et al. [15] only 17% of the HCCs from the United States were of this type, whereas 38% and 36% from Japan and South Africa, respectively, were of the expanding type. The term "spreading" was used to indicate poorly defined tumor margins and was subdivided into cirrhotomimetic and infiltrative types. Okuda et al. [15] also recognized a multifocal type (composed of several small tumors of simi-

lar size found at multiple sites in the liver), an indeterminate type (for cases in which classification was not possible because of the extensive growth, hemorrhage, or necrosis), and others which presented a combination of patterns precluding classification into one group.

2.2 Gross classification by the present authors

Our classification is based on the difference in growth pattern with consideration of the following three factors—capsule, liver cirrhosis, and tumor thrombus in the portal vein.

2.2.1 Infiltrative type

This type is virtually the same as the spreading type of the Okuda-Peters-Simson classification [15]. A typical morphological feature of this type is seen in HCC without liver cirrhosis, in which the tumor-nontumor boundary is irregular and indistinct (Fig. 7.1). In cases associated with cirrhosis, the neoplastic foci are not clearly demarcated even if all liver slices have been examined and foci of varying sizes have fused to form larger foci. Such findings suggest that HCC of this type spreads in the liver mainly through tumor thrombi in the portal venous system. At the tumor-nontumor boundary, the tumor extends as if it were replacing the cirrhotic pseudolobules. In the infiltrative type of HCC involving the entire or most of the right or left hepatic lobe, the modifier "massive," is added (Fig. 7.2). The infiltrative type of HCC accounted for approximately 33% of our 439 cases.

2.2.2 Expansive type

This type of HCC extends as if it were pushing intact tissues aside. The mass is sharply demarcated and usually nodular. Most HCCs of this type which are associated with liver cirrhosis have a fibrous capsule. In the early stages of the

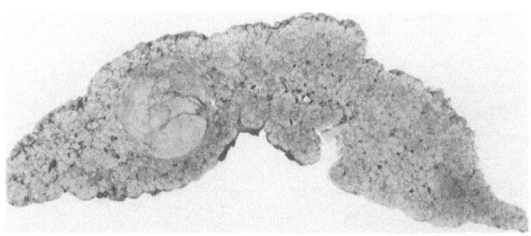

Fig. 7.3. Expansive type of HCC, single nodular (so-called encapsulated HCC). Well-encapsulated tumor in a liver with mixed macro- and micronodular cirrhosis.

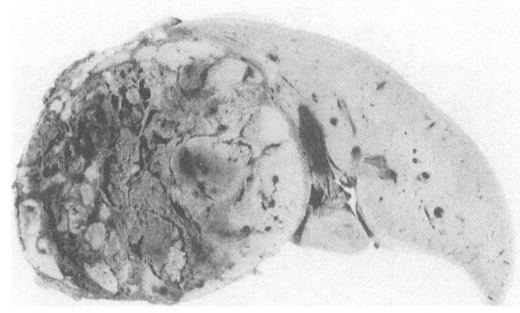

Fig. 7.4. Expansive type of HCC, single nodular, massive. A huge expansive tumor with necrosis occupies the entire right lobe of a noncirrhotic liver

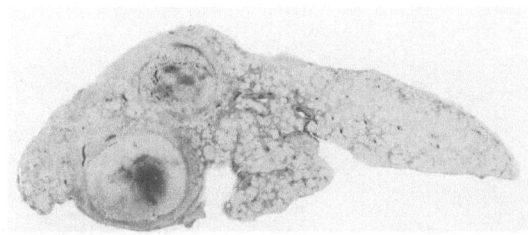

Fig. 7.5. Expansive type of HCC, multinodular. Two well-encapsulated tumors are located in the right lobe of the liver with mixed macro- and micronodular cirrhosis

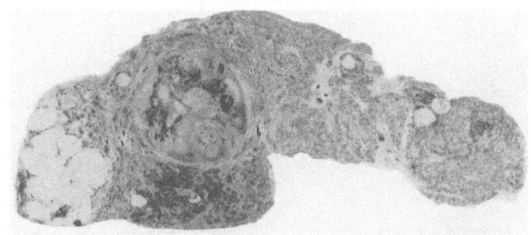

Fig. 7.6. Mixed infiltrative and expansive type of HCC, single nodular. A solitary encapsulated tumor, a possible primary focus, is seen together with tumors showing infiltrative growth and intrahepatic metastases

expansive type of HCC, tumor infiltration across the capsule and portal vein tumor thrombi are usually absent or minimal. Therefore, the earlier the diagnosis is made the greater the chance of complete cure by surgery. This type is subclassified into the single nodular and multinodular types according to the number of tumor nodules. It accounted for 18% of HCCs in our series.

Single nodular type. This type of HCC is quite clearly demarcated. In particular, HCCs of this type associated with liver cirrhosis have a distinct fibrous capsule; they are also termed encapsulated HCCs (Fig. 7.3). The capsule, however, is often indistinct in livers with no associated liver cirrhosis. "Satellite" nodules, which also grow in an expansive fashion, form around the main tumor, and the tumor grows expansively by merging with daughter nodules; the portal vein system is occasionally involved. In an HCC of this type occupying the entire right or left hepatic lobe, the modifier "massive" is added (Fig. 7.4).

Multinodular type. This type involves no fewer than two nodules of the expansive type, regardless of intrahepatic metastasis or multicentric origin. The foci are uniform in size and greater than 2 cm in diameter, with or wihtout liver cirrhosis (Fig. 7.5).

2.2.3 Mixed infiltrative and expansive type

The primary foci of the expansive type can be identified in association with infiltrative foci outside the capsule and/or intrahepatic metastases. This type is further divided into two subtypes according to the number of the expansive tumors. The mixed type accounted for 33% of HCCs in our series.

Mixed type, single nodular. In this type, a solitary encapsulated HCC with a distinct fibrous capsule, a possible primary focus, is seen together with tumor infiltration beyond the capsule and/or apparent intrahepatic metastases (Fig. 7.6).

Mixed type, multinodular. Here, no fewer than two encapsulated HCCs are seen in association with tumor infiltration beyond the capsule and/or prominent intrahepatic metastases (Fig. 7.7).

2.2.4 Diffuse type

This type of HCC occurs as numerous small nodules, 0.5–1.0 cm in diameter, scattered throughout the liver which do not fuse with each other and are always associated with liver cir-

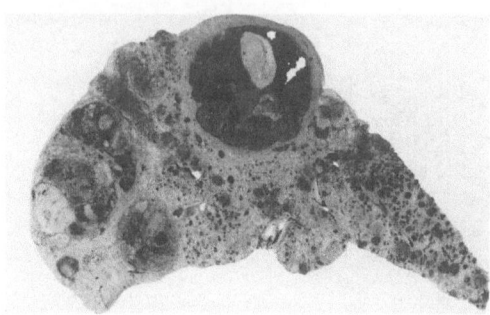

Fig. 7.7. Mixed infiltrative and expansive type of HCC, multinodular. Three encapsulated tumors are seen in association with infiltrative tumors and numerous small intrahepatic metastases

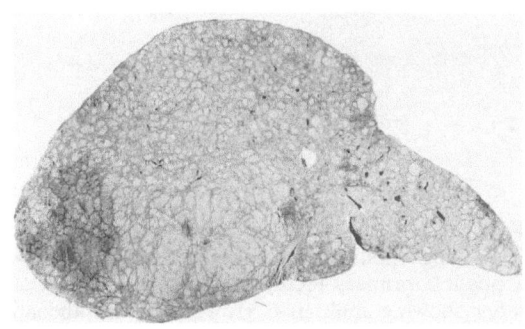

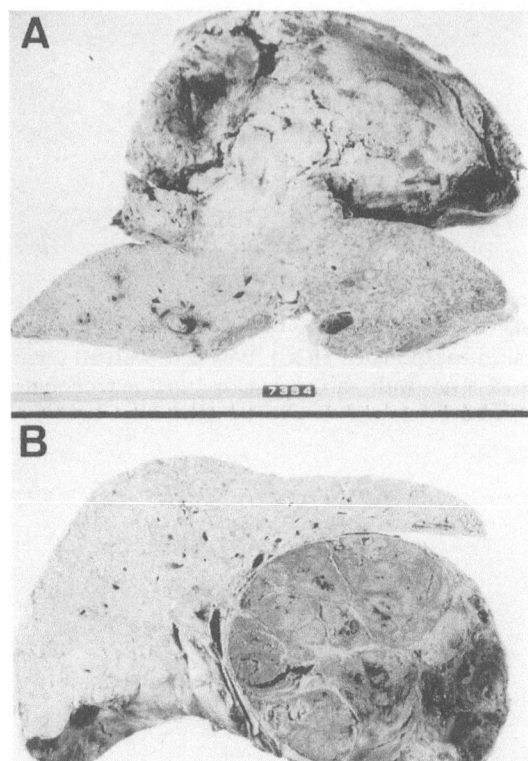

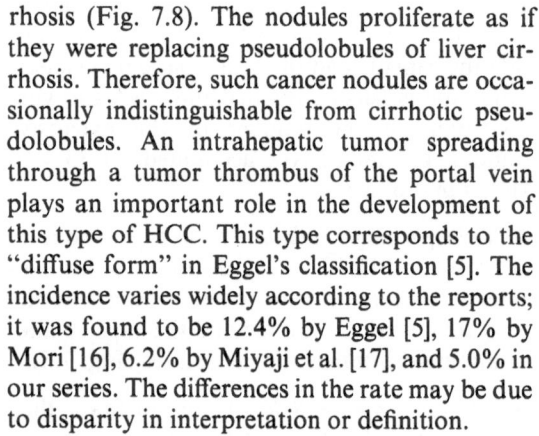

Fig. 7.8. Diffuse type of HCC. Numerous small tumor nodules are scattered throughout the liver

Fig. 7.9A, B. Pedunculated HCC. **A** Pedunculated HCC with little cancerous invasion in the liver. **B** Pedunculated HCC, possibly occurring in an accessory lobe

rhosis (Fig. 7.8). The nodules proliferate as if they were replacing pseudolobules of liver cirrhosis. Therefore, such cancer nodules are occasionally indistinguishable from cirrhotic pseudolobules. An intrahepatic tumor spreading through a tumor thrombus of the portal vein plays an important role in the development of this type of HCC. This type corresponds to the "diffuse form" in Eggel's classification [5]. The incidence varies widely according to the reports; it was found to be 12.4% by Eggel [5], 17% by Mori [16], 6.2% by Miyaji et al. [17], and 5.0% in our series. The differences in the rate may be due to disparity in interpretation or definition.

2.2.5 Specific type
In addition to these four basic gross type of HCC there are two other specific types—pedunculated HCC and HCC characterized by prominent tumor thrombosis of the portal vein without a recognizable tumor mass.

Pedunculated HCC. A massive tumor proliferat-

ing extrahepatically with little cancerous invasion into the liver is occasionally seen. In Japan, since Kato et al. [18] first described one case of pedunculated HCC, a numer of similar cases, including our cases, have been reported [19–22]. In most pedunculated HCCs, a tumor arising in the subcapsular area of the liver grows extrahepatically with or without a pedicle (Fig. 7.9A). There are rare cases of a tumor arising in an accessory or ectopic hepatic lobe (Fig. 7.9B). Although a diagnosis of pedunculated HCC was difficult in the past, the current imaging techniques have made the diagnosis easy. We have encountered 11 cases (2.5%) of pedunculated HCC among our 439 autopsy cases and one HCC which was thought to have arisen from an accessory hepatic lobe.

HCC characterized by prominent tumor thrombus of portal vein with no recognizable main tumor mass. We have experienced only two cases of this type in our series (Fig. 7.10).

Fig. 7.10. HCC characterized only by prominent tumor thrombosis of the portal vein system with no recognizable tumor in the liver. The massive tumor thrombus in the portal vein has invaded the bifurcation of the hepatic duct (*arrow*)

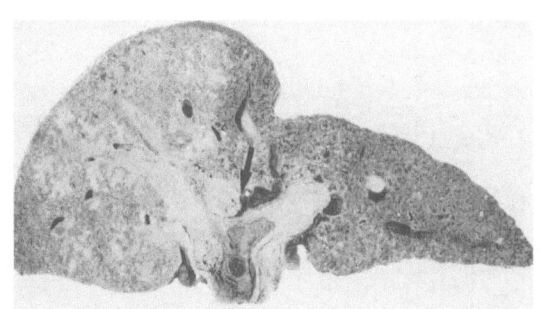

3 Histopathology

The histological structure of HCC resembles that of the normal liver. The tumor parenchyma comprises a liver cell cordlike structure (trabecular pattern) and the stroma consists of sinusoidlike spaces, which contain blood and are lined by a single layer of endothelial cells. The histopathology of HCC varies depending on combinations of the following features: (1) the structural pattern (trabecular, pseudoglandular, solid, or sclerosing); (2) differences in the degree of cell differentiation (well, moderately, or poorly differentiated), and (3) cytological variants (bile production, clear cells, fatty change, cytoplasmic hyalin, pleomorphism, etc).

Edmondson and Steiner [8] classified HCC into four types on the basis of the degree of differentiation of the tumor cells. Their classification has been widely employed in Japan since the early 1970s when studies of the relationship between alpha-fetoprotein and histological differentiation of HCC began. In 1978, the WHO classification [23] was proposed and it has gained worldwide recognition.

3.1 Edmondson and Steiner's classification of HCC

Grade I. This type is the most differentiated and consists of tumor cells with a thin trabecular pattern.

Grade II. Although the tumor cells show a resemblance to normal liver cells, their nuclei are larger and more hyperchromatic and their cytoplasm is abundant and acidophilic. Acinar or glandular structures are frequently associated with the trabecular pattern, which is the basic structure.

Grade III. In this type the nuclei are usually larger and more hyperchromatic than those of grade II. Giant tumor cells are very numerous in this type.

Grade IV. Here, the cancer cells are least differentiated. The nuclei are intensely hyperchromatic and occupy a greater part of the cell. The cytoplasm is often scanty. The growth in the liver is more medullary, the trabecular pattern is uncommon, and tumor cells often lack cohesiveness.

3.2 WHO classification

3.2.1 Trabecular type (sinusoidal)

The tumor cells grow in cords of variable thickness separated by prominent sinusoids (blood spaces) lined by flat endothelial cells (Figs. 7.11, 7.12). The endothelial cells, usually inconspicuous, may sharply define the trabeculae. Fibrous connective tissue is absent between the tumor cords and cells, but a few collagen fibers may sometimes be detected in the sinusoidal walls. When, as in some cases, there is wide and regular dilatation of the blood spaces, the tumor cells may be grouped around the vascular spaces in rosette arrangements, which at first glance resemble glands.

3.2.2 Pseudoglandular type (acinar)

A variety of glandlike structures may be seen in this type (Fig. 7.13). Canaliculi, with or without bile, are often recognizable and may be dilated into glandlike spaces. Larger cystic spaces, lined by a layer of cells, are apparently formed by central degeneration and breakdown in otherwise solid trabeculae. The contents may be periodic acid-Schiff (PAS)-positive but should not be mistaken for mucin. The basic trabecular pattern, with intervening blood spaces, often remains detectable.

3.2.3 Compact type

This is basically a trabecular pattern, but the tumor cells grow in apparently solid masses and the blood spaces are rendered inconspicuous by compression (Fig. 7.14).

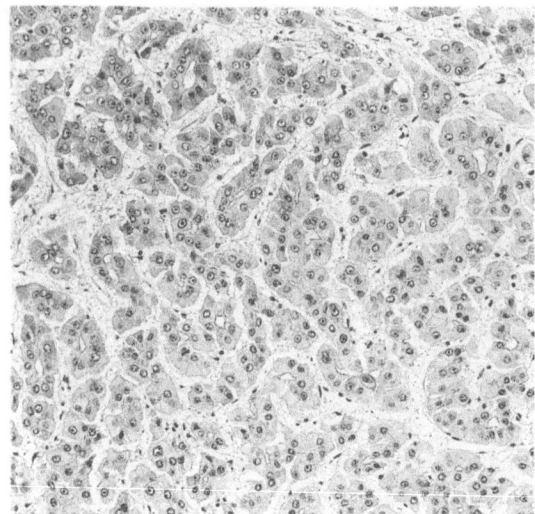

Fig. 7.11. Well-differentiated thin trabecular HCC corresponding to Edmondson and Steiner grade I carcinoma. H and E, × 200

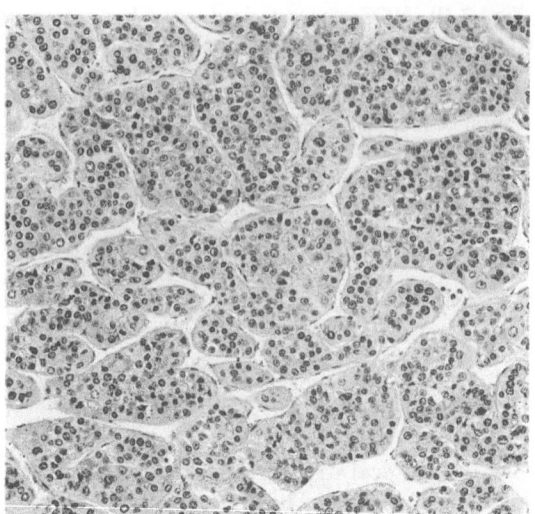

Fig. 7.12. Moderately differentiated trabecular HCC. Tumor cells are arranged in cords of variable thickness separated by blood spaces lined by flat endothelial cells. H and E, × 200

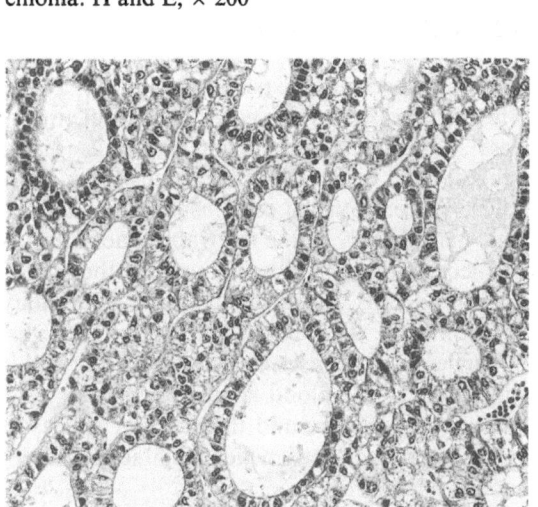
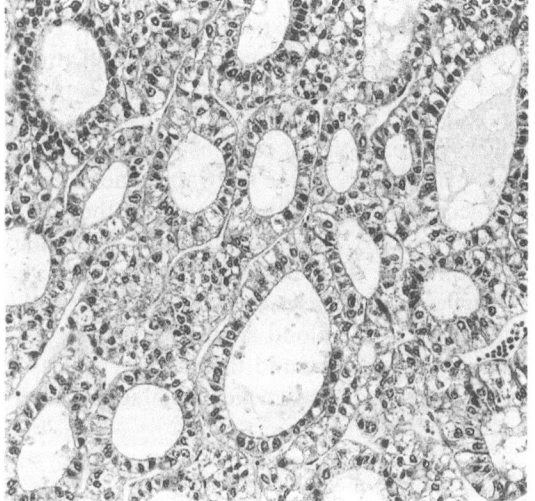

Fig. 7.13. Pseudoglandular (acinar) type HCC. A variety of glandlike structures is evident. H and E, × 200

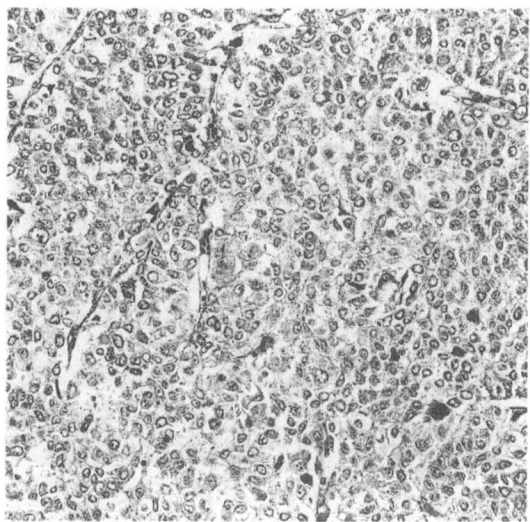

Fig. 7.14. Compact (solid) type HCC. Tumor cells are growing in a solid pattern. H and E, × 200

3.2.4 Scirrhous type

Areas with abundant fibrous stroma separating cords of tumor cells are most often seen following radiation exposure, chemotherapy or infarction. This appearance should be distinguished from those of cholangiocarcinoma and metastatic tumors (Fig. 7.15).

3.2.5 Cytological and other variants

The following cytological and other variants are also listed: pleomorphism, clear cells, tumor cells with little cytoplasm, spindle-shaped tumor cells, bile production, glycogen, fat, and cytoplasmic inclusions.

Clear cells. Occasionally, clear cells almost indistinguishable from clear-cell adenocarcinoma of the kidney and adrenal glands are seen (Fig. 7.16). Buchanan and Huvos [24] reported that clear cells constituted 30%–100% of tumor cells in 13 of their 150 cases. A favorable prognosis of the clear-cell type of HCC was observed by Wu et al. [25]. In HCC of the clear-cell type, the clear

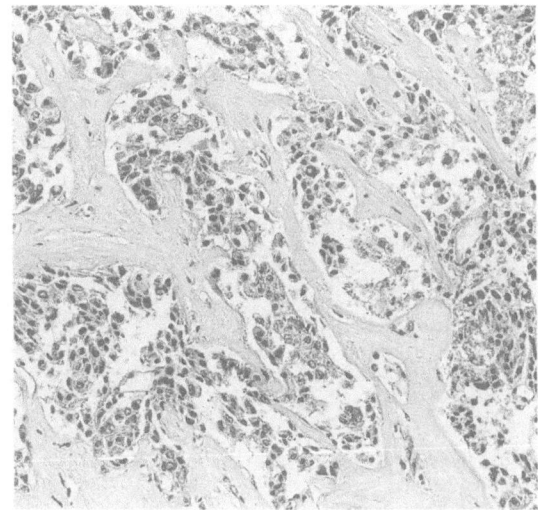

Fig. 7.15. Scirrhous (sclerosing) type of HCC. Tumor nests are separated by a thick fibrous stroma. H and E, × 200

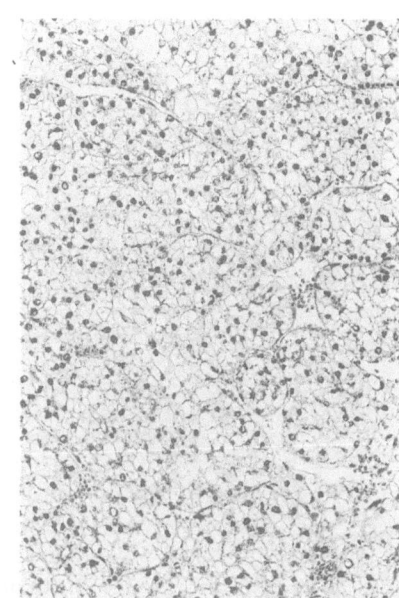

Fig. 7.16. HCC of clear-cell type. H and E, × 100

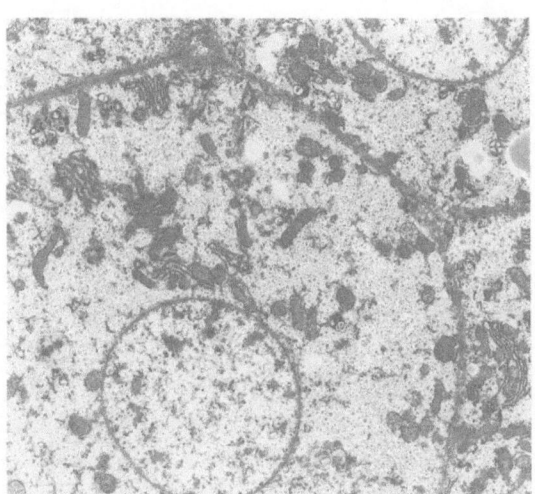

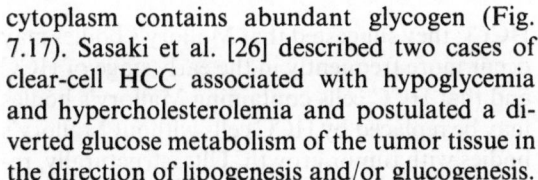

Fig. 7.17. Electron micrograph of HCC of the clear-cell type. Tumor cells contain numerous glycogen granules in the cytoplasm. × 4700

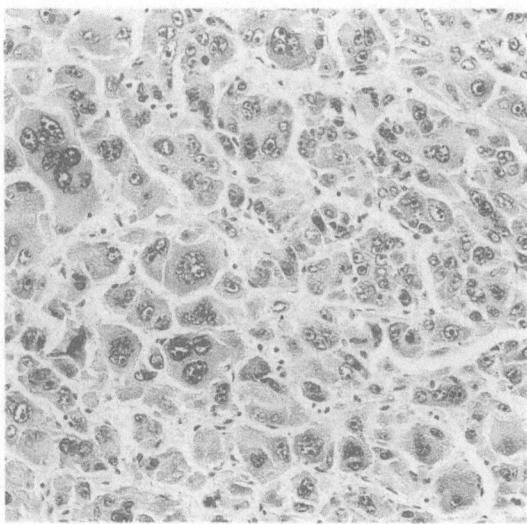

Fig. 7.18. HCC of the giant-cell type. Bizarre multinucleated giant cells are prominent, and the cancer cells lack mutual contact. H and E, × 200

cytoplasm contains abundant glycogen (Fig. 7.17). Sasaki et al. [26] described two cases of clear-cell HCC associated with hypoglycemia and hypercholesterolemia and postulated a diverted glucose metabolism of the tumor tissue in the direction of lipogenesis and/or glucogenesis.

Giant cells. Mutlti- or single-nucleated giant cells are frequently observed in HCC. Peters [27] observed that 14% of HCCs had some giant-cell change. We found varying numbers and degrees of giant cells in 25% of HCCs. Although the basic trabecular structure is retained in most giant-cell HCCs, pleomorphic giant cells have poor mutual contact (Fig. 7.18). HCC with giant cells is considered relatively less differentiated and is classed as grade III carcinoma in the classification of Edmondson and Steiner [8].

Cytoplasmic hyaline inclusions. It is not uncommon to encounter HCC cells containing intracytoplasmic hyalin. Intracytoplasmic hyalin may be in the form of PAS-positive or -negative globules, irregular-shaped (reticular) hyalin, or

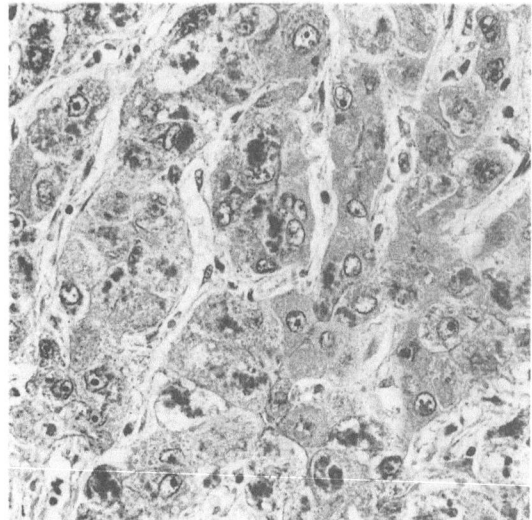

Fig. 7.19. Reticular hyaline inclusions (Mallory's bodies). H and E, × 400

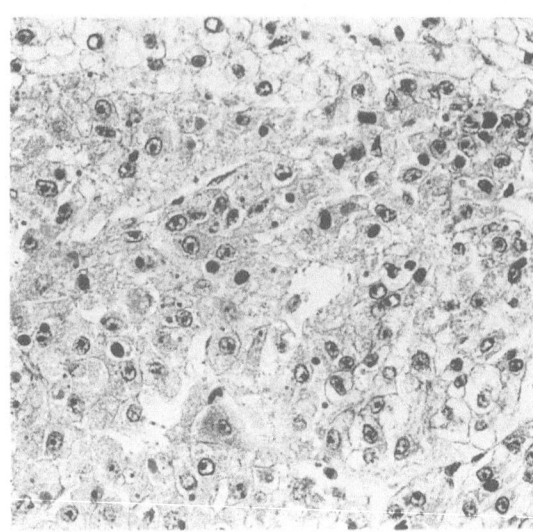

Fig. 7.20. PAS-negative globular hyaline inclusions (darkly stained). H and E, × 200

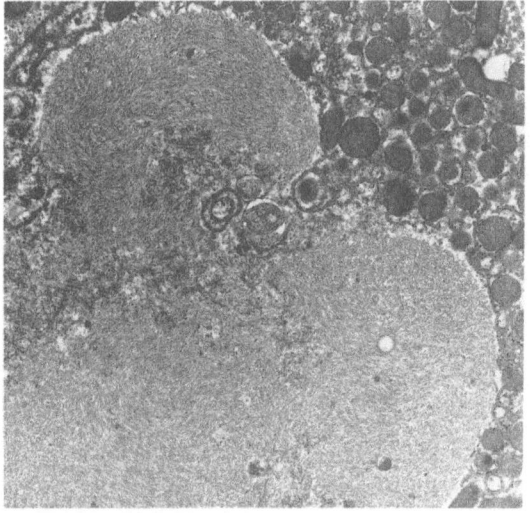

Fig. 7.21. Ultrastructurally, the PAS-negative globular hyaline inclusions consist of a fibrillar substance and are indistinguishable from Mallory's bodies in alcoholic liver disease

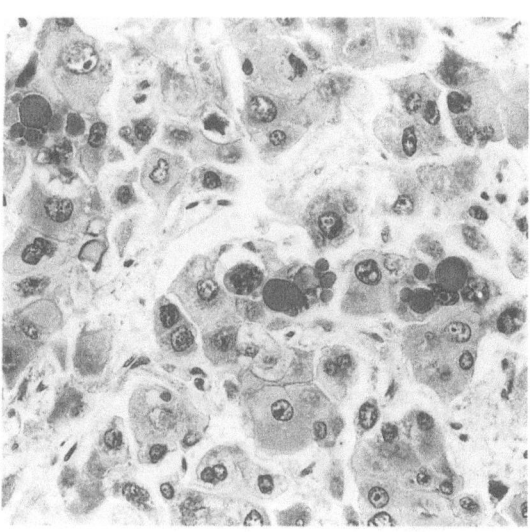

Fig. 7.22. PAS-positive globular hyaline inclusions. H and E, × 400

ground-glass inclusions.

The reticular hyalins (Fig. 7.19) and most of the PAS-negative globular hyalins (Fig. 7.20) are histochemically and ultrastructurally similar to Mallory's alcoholic hyalin. We have found reticular hyalin and PAS-negative globular hyalin in 15.7% and 9.5%, respectively, of 146 consecutive autopsy cases of HCC, and both types coexisted in four cases. Nakanuma and Ohta [28] found Mallory's bodies in 43.5% of minute HCCs but only in 12.6% of advanced

HCCs; they suggested that Mallory's bodies may occur more frequently in the early stage of HCC and that HCC cells containing Mallory's bodies may be replaced by HCC cells without Mallory's bodies with tumor growth. Ultrastructurally, reticular hyalins and PAS-negative globular hyalins are seen as fibrillar deposits without a limiting membrane and are indistinguishable from classic Mallory's bodies (Fig. 7.21). The light-microscopic difference between reticular hyalin and PAS-negative globular hyalin is due

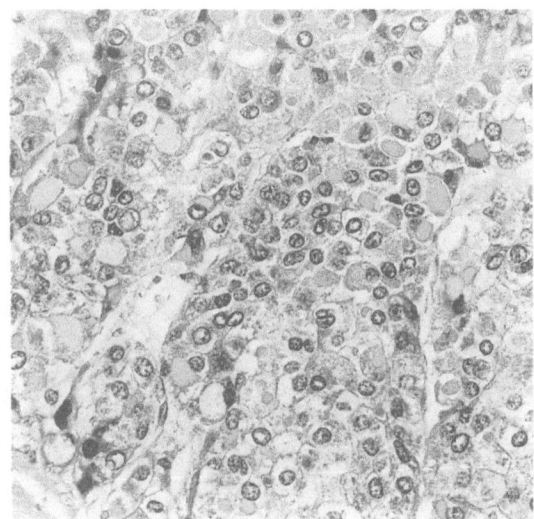

Fig. 7.23. Ground-glass inclusions. H and E, × 200

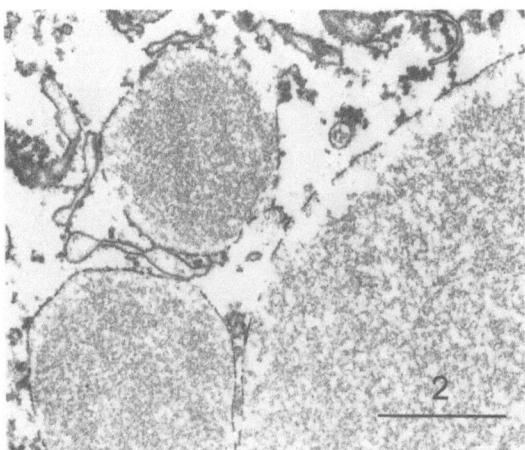

Fig. 7.24. Electron micrograph of ground-glass inclusions. They consist of a membrane-bound fibrillar material. Formalin-fixed section (*scale*, 2 μm)

to an ultrastructural difference of the margin of fibrillar deposits, being regular in the former and irregular in the latter [29].

Diastase-resistant PAS-positive globular hyaline inclusions were seen in 6 (4.1%) of the 146 consecutive autopsy cases of HCC. The inclusions are brightly stained with eosin and are round to oval in shape; they measure 3–30 μm in diameter and are usually seen in groups (Fig. 7.22). All of them are negative for alpha$_1$-antitrypsin.

Stromeyer et al. [30] described ten cases of HCC with the ground-glass appearance that corresponded to the presence of nonmembrane-bound amorphous or fibrillar inclusions, and the ground-glass materials reacted with antifibrinogen. We have found similar inclusions in 3 (2.0%) of 147 consecutive autopsy cases of HCC. All of them reacted with antifibrinogen (Fig. 7.23) and ultrastructurally were composed of membrane-bound fibrillar material. In all three cases of ground-glass inclusions, the endoplasmic reticulum exhibited varying degrees of dilatation and contained fibrillar material similar to that seen in inclusions (Fig. 7.24). Thus, we conclude that the ground-glass inclusion is the result of accumulation of synthesized proteins, mainly fibrinogen, in the endoplasmic reticulum (showing cystic dilatation) due to deranged secretory function of HCC cells.

3.3 Hepatitis B surface antigen-positive cells in HCC

There are several reports of the presence of hepatitis B surface antigen (HBsAg)-positive cells in

HCC tissue. The reported positivity rates are 4.3% by Tanaka et al. [31], 16.7% by Ilardi et al. [32], and 8% by Nayak et al. [33]. In our study [34], the majority of HBsAg-positive cells were thought to be hepatocytes containing HBsAg that were retained in the HCC tissue; HBsAg-positive HCC cells were found in only one case of encapsulated HCC. If HBsAg-positive cells are seen in HCC tissue at the reported incidence, a similar incidence should also be expected in tumor thrombi and/or extrahepatic metastases. However, we never found HBsAg-positive cells in tumor thrombi and pulmonary metastases. Although we do not deny the existence of HBsAg-positive cancer cells in HCC tissue, the incidence must be much lower than that reported.

3.4 Sarcomatous change of HCC

Among a variety of histological features of HCC, the coexistence of sarcomatous-appearing cells has been sporadically reported [8, 35–38]. In many such cases, it is difficult to determine whether the appearance is caused by the sarcomatous change of part of the HCC or by the coexistence of HCC and sarcoma. We found 14 HCC cases (3.9%) which exhibited a sarcomatous appearance among 355 consecutive autopsy cases. Clinically, HCCs with a sarcomatous appearance were characterized by negative or low serum alpha-fetoprotein levels and frequent extrahepatic metastases. Histologically, the tumor consisted mainly of spindle-shaped cells but also contained bizarre multinucleated cells (Fig. 7.25); transitions between trabecular HCC and

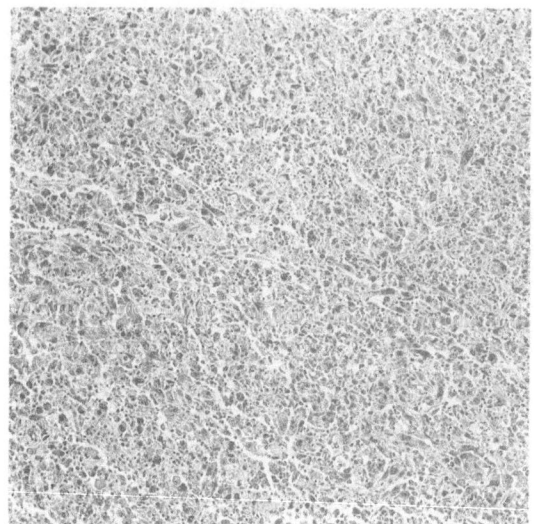 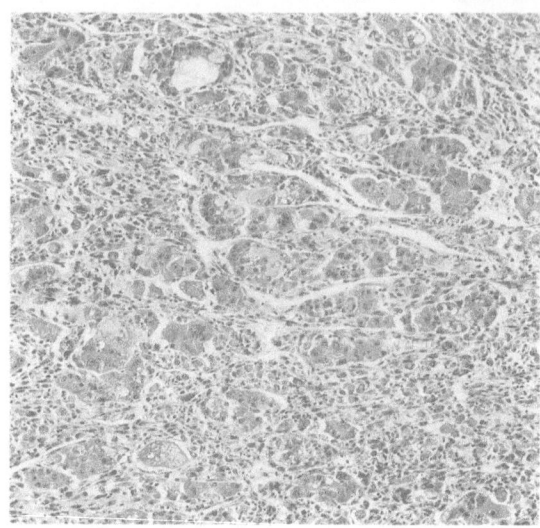

Fig. 7.25. HCC of the sarcomatous type. The tumor consists of spindle-shaped cells and bizarre giant cells. H and E, × 100

Fig. 7.26. Transition between trabecular HCC and sarcomatous carcinoma. H and E, × 100

the sarcomatous areas were occasionally observed (Fig. 7.26). Immunohistochemically, the "sarcomatous" tumor cells were frequently positive for keratin, albumin, alpha-fetoprotein, and/or fibrinogen. These results strongly suggest that the sarcomatous appearance seen in HCC is not due to the coexistence of HCC and sarcoma. Regarding the development of sarcomatous changes in HCC, it is possible that HCC undergoes morphological or phenotypic changes as a result of chemotherapy or some other unknown factor.

3.5 Sarcoidlike reaction in HCC

A sarcoidlike reaction within malignant tumors or in the regional lymph nodes that drain an area involved by malignant tumors has long been recognized; however, it is believed to be rare in HCC. Although Neville et al. [39] reported one case of HCC with granulomas among 138 patients with liver granulomas, the histological details were not published. We encountered only two cases of HCC with a granulomatous reaction in the cancerous tissue among the 439 autopsy cases. The granulomas were characterized by epithelioid cells, Langhans' type giant cells, and varying numbers of lymphocytes (Fig. 7.27); there were a few granulomas in tumor thrombi of the portal vein branches but none in the noncancerous area and extrahepatic metastasis. No evidence of tuberculosis or systemic sarcoidosis was found in any case. Pathogenetic processes proposed for the granulomatous reaction, none

of which are widely accepted, include: (1) a tissue response against the malignant tumor, including an immunological mechanism and (2) nonspecific, fortuitous phenomena. We favor the notion that development of granulomas in HCC is a nonspecific reaction to metabolic or disintegration products of HCC.

3.6 Extramedullary hematopoiesis in HCC

Although it should not be surprising to find extramedullary hematopoiesis in HCC tissue, since the liver is one of the hematopoietic organs, we found foci of extramedullary hematopoieses in cancerous areas in only 4 (3.4%) of 116 consecutive autopsy cases of HCC. The hematopoietic cells were mostly nucleated red blood cells (Fig. 7.28).

3.7 Histological growth pattern of HCC

The growth patterns at the tumor-nontumor boundary can be histologically divided into two basic patterns—sinusoidal and replacing [40].

3.7.1 Sinusoidal growth pattern
In the sinusoidal growth pattern, tumor cells grow in the sinusoids at the boundary in an infiltrative fashion and compress the liver cell cords (Fig. 7.29A). Some eventually contain atrophied liver cell cords and hepatocytes. By silver impregnation, reticulin fibers can be seen to be condensed in the areas where liver cells had disap-

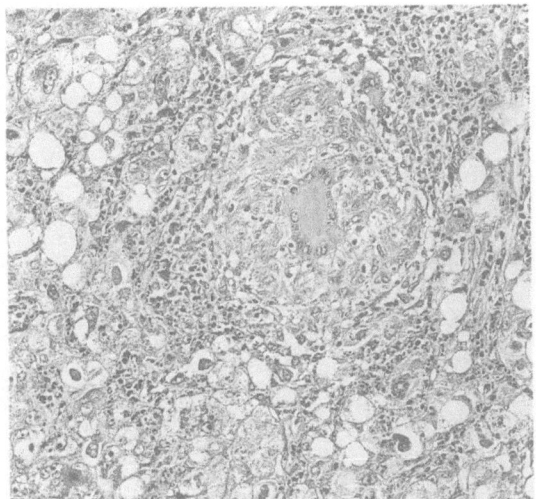

Fig. 7.27. Sarcoidlike reaction in HCC tissue. Epithelioid granuloma with Langhans' type giant cells in evident. H and E, × 200

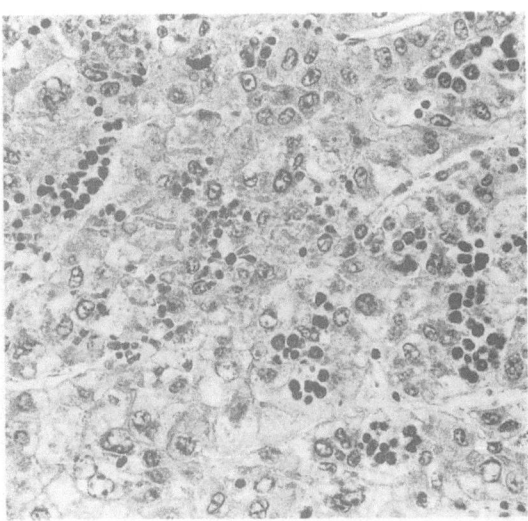

Fig. 7.28. Foci of extramedullary hematopoiesis in HCC consist mostly of nucleated erythrocytes. H and E, × 200

peared, with irregular destruction of the reticulin framework (Fig. 7.29B).

3.7.2 Replacing growth pattern

In this pattern, tumor cells replace hepatocytes within the liver cell cords; this is considered to be the basic growth pattern in HCC (Fig. 7.30A). In Disse's space immediately beneath the sinusoidal lining cells, there is some increase of collagen fibers, but the basic reticulin framework is well preserved (Fig. 7.30B). Thus, in the area where HCC cells are arranged along the liver cell cords with the replacing growth pattern, the sinusoids communicate with the blood spaces of the cancerous tissue.

3.7.3 Pseudocapsular growth pattern

Although it is primarily of the replacing type, this tumor frequently compresses nontumorous tissue in an expansive fashion. A pseudocapsule of reticulin fibers (condensed along the boundary) is formed; such tumors are designated the pseudocapsular growth type and are distinguished from the other two growth patterns (Fig. 7.31). HCC for which surgical resection is indicated is mostly of the encapsulated type. Among 97 surgical cases in our hospital, 87 (89%) were of the encapsulated type. Although they were encapsulated, extracapsular tumor growth was found in 42 (43%) of the resected cases, and all the extracapsular tumors were growing in a replacing fashion (Fig. 7.32).

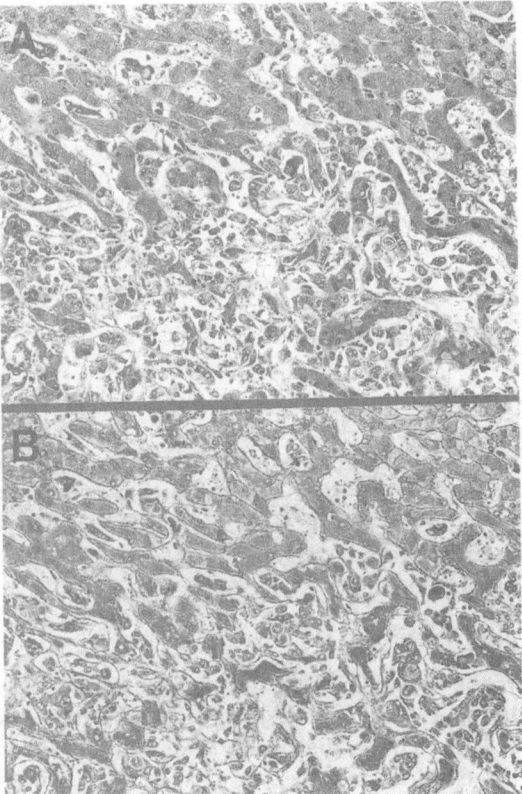

Fig. 7.29A, B. Sinusoidal growth pattern. **A** Tumor cells are growing in the sinusoids at the tumor-nontumor boundary in an infiltrative fashion. H and E, × 100. **B** Reticulin framework is condensed at the boundary. Reticulin, × 100

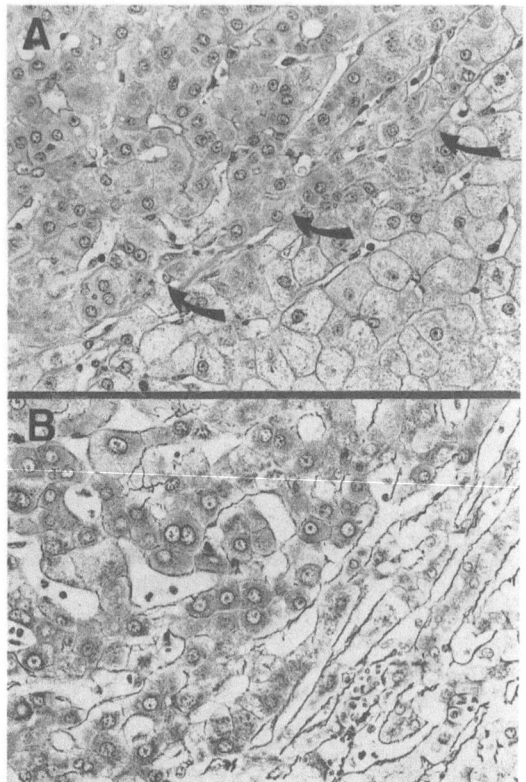

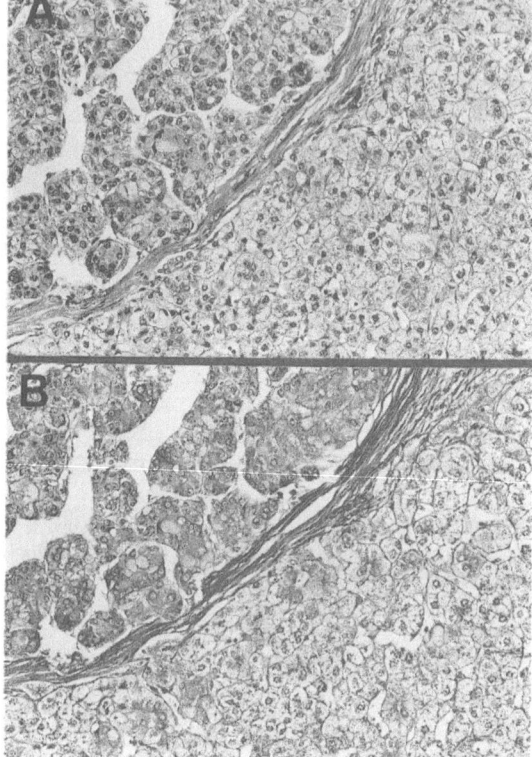

Fig. 7.30A, B. Replacing growth pattern. **A** Tumor cells are seen replacing hepatocytes within the liver cell cords and the tumor-nontumor boundary is ill defined (*arrows*). H and E, × 200. **B** The basic reticulin framework of the liver cell cords is preserved. Reticulin, × 200

Fig. 7.31A, B. Pseudocapsular growth pattern. **A** Thin fibrous capsule forms at the tumor-nontumor boundary. H and E, × 100. **B** Fibrous capsule is thought to be formed by the condensation of reticulin fibers at the boundary. Reticulin, × 100

4 Ultrastructure of HCC

The ultrastructural features of HCC vary with the degree of differentiation. In well- to moderately differentiated HCC, the ultrastructure of the tumor cells is similar to that of normal hepatocytes. When HCC is less differentiated, the nuclei are larger and nuclear irregularity is more evident.

4.1 Trabecular HCC

In the normal liver, the hepatocytes are arranged in one-cell-thick plates, which radiate from the central vein to the portal triad, while two- to three-cell-thick plates are seen in the cirrhotic liver. In trabecular HCC, a structure reminiscent of normal liver cell cords is seen, but the plates form trabeculae of varying thickness, from thin to thick. The relationship between the blood spaces and trabecular tumor nests is similar to that between the sinusoids and liver cell cords in

the normal liver (Fig. 7.33). Isomura [41], however, distinguished the blood space from the normal sinusoid based on the sparsity of pores in the endothelial cells and the existence of a basement membrane-like substance in HCC (which corresponds to capillarization of sinusoids in chronic liver disease, including liver cirrhosis). Microvilli on the free surface in the subendothelial space of HCC are prominent when the tumor is well differentiated. Sugihara et al. [42] demonstrated that the sinusoids in the noncancerous areas are continuous with the blood spaces of the cancerous tissue in HCC of the replacing growth type and that the tumor cells grow along the liver cell cords.

4.2 Pseudoglandular HCC

In this type, the tumor forms tubular structures in varying degrees. The tubules, with microvilli on the free surface of the lumen, are similar to the normal bile canaliculi. In addition, they oc-

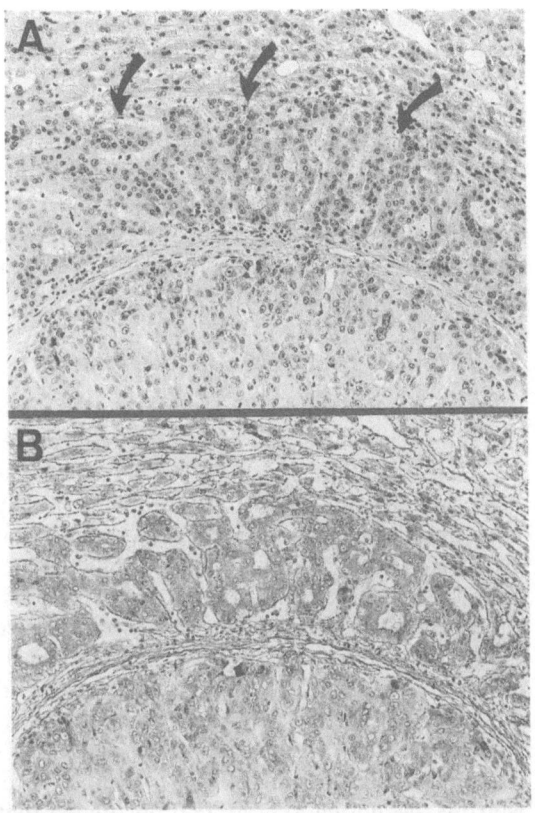

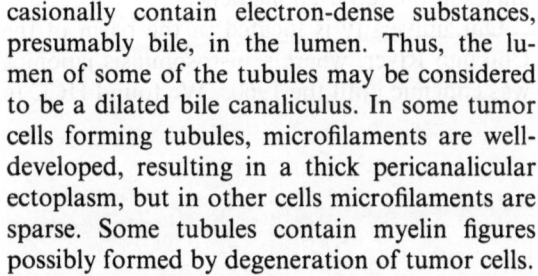

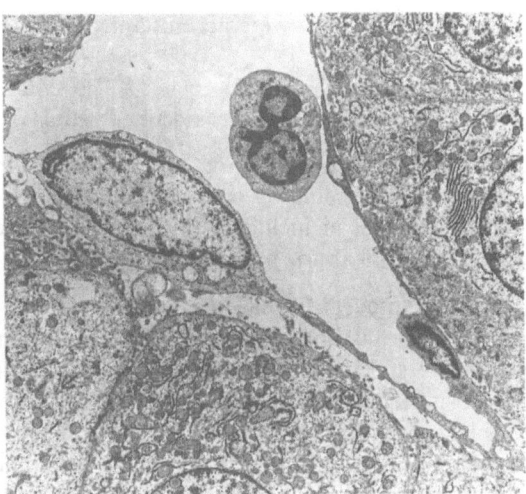

Fig. 7.33. Ultrastructural feature of moderately differentiated trabecular HCC. Tumor cell cords are covered by a single layer of endothelial cells that forms blood spaces (sinusoids). Tumor cells have well-developed cytoplasmic organelles and show tight mutual contact. Microvilli are observed on the free surface in the subendothelial space (*scale*, 6 μm).

Fig. 7.32A, B. Extracapsular tumor growth. A The tumor growing beyond the pseudocapsule shows a replacing growth pattern (*arrows*). H and E, × 100. B Reticulin, × 100

casionally contain electron-dense substances, presumably bile, in the lumen. Thus, the lumen of some of the tubules may be considered to be a dilated bile canaliculus. In some tumor cells forming tubules, microfilaments are well-developed, resulting in a thick pericanalicular ectoplasm, but in other cells microfilaments are sparse. Some tubules contain myelin figures possibly formed by degeneration of tumor cells.

4.3 Solid HCC

In this type, the nuclear/cytoplasmic ratio is large, development of cytoplasmic organelles is poor, mutual contact of tumor cells is poor, and bile canaliculi are scanty. All these ultrastructural findings suggest that the solid HCC is poorly differentiated.

5 HCC and liver cirrhosis

HCC is usually associated with some form of liver cirrhosis. This association, however, varies in frequency with the investigator and geographical location. The incidence ranges from 60% to 90% but is mostly around 80%. Shikata [43] questioned the accuracy of the reports of a low incidence of cirrhosis with HCC and suggested that figures of only 65%–75% may have been based on material that did not convincingly exclude cholangiocarcinoma. Peters [27] further suggested that in regions with a low incidence of HCC, cholangiocarcinoma may make up a larger percentage of the cases of primary liver cancer. Thus, since cholangiocarcinoma is less frequently superimposed on cirrhosis, grouping cholangiocarcinoma and HCC together would cause a significant error in the frequency of associated cirrhosis. However, it is known that the incidence of associated cirrhosis is low among certain African Blacks who have a high incidence of HCC. Geddes and Falkson [44] reported that 60% of 189 autopsy cases of liver cancer, including two cases of cholangiocarcinoma, were associated with liver cirrhosis. In our 439 autopsy cases of HCC, 80% were accompanied by liver cirrhosis.

5.1 Types of liver cirrhosis associated with HCC

The association of HCC and cirrhosis varies in frequency depending on the etiology of the cirrhosis, which can include viral hepatitis, toxic injury, alcohol abuse, and malnutrition.

5.1.1 Cryptogenic cirrhosis
Cryptogenic cirrhosis, in which the causal factor cannot be specified, is the most common type of cirrhosis associated with HCC. Among the various histopathological types of cirrhosis, macronodular and mixed macro- and micronodular cirrhoses are most frequently associated with HCC (Figs. 7.3, 7.5). About 65% of our 439 HCC cases had such types of cirrhosis (serum HBsAg was positive in only 36.5% of them).

5.1.2 Alcoholic cirrhosis
This may follow hepatic injury resulting from alcohol abuse. Liver cirrhosis and HCC in the Tokyo area were compared with those in Cincinnati (USA) by Mori [45]. In Tokyo, HCC was found in 23% of livers with cirrhosis, while this frequency was as low as 7% in Cincinnati. Despite such remarkable differences, the association of liver cirrhosis occurred in 70% and 60% of HCC cases in Tokyo and Cincinnati, respectively. The proportion of alcoholic cirrhosis in the United States was much higher than that in Japan, and HCC seldom occured in association with alcoholic cirrhosis. Lee [46] reported that patients with alcoholic cirrhosis in London who gave up drinking had a higher incidence of coarsely nodular (macronodular) cirrhosis and HCC than those who continued to drink.

Kage in our department found 25 cases (15.0%) of HCC associated with alcoholic cirrhosis among 166 consecutive autopsy cases of HCC, and the serum HBsAg was positive in 5 (20%) of the 25 cases (unpublished data). He suggests that hepatitis B virus infection may be superimposed on alcoholic cirrhosis in a certain proportion of patients with HCC.

5.2 Parasitic cirrhosis due to schistosomiasis

A high prevalence of HCC in patients with schistosomiasis japonica and mansoni has been reported from the endemic areas [47–49], and it has been suggested that schistosomal infection may have an etiological role in the development of HCC. However, there have been conflicting accounts on the relationship between the two diseases. Edington [50] reported that the incidence of HCC was low in Egypt where schistosomiasis mansoni is endemic. According to Cheever and Andrade [51], HCC was more common in uninfected cases than in those suffering from schistosomaisis mansoni in Brazil. Furthermore, Martinez-Maldonado et al. [52] postulated that *Schistosoma mansoni* played no role in the etiology of HCC in Puerto Rico. Thus, the suggested close relationship between HCC and schistosomiasis based only on statistical analyses must be viewed with caution because of discrepancies in the reported incidence.

Our university is located in the basin of the Chikugo River, where schistosomiasis japonica was endemic until the 1960s. We found HCC in

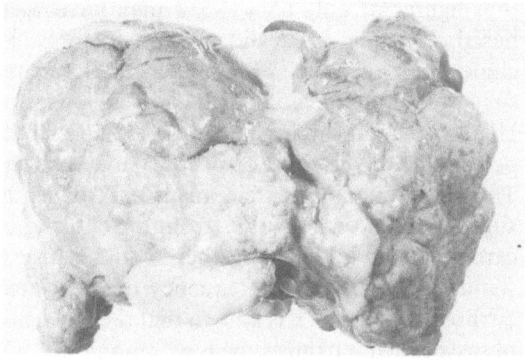

Fig. 7.34. Association of HCC and liver cirrhosis due to *Schistosoma japonicum*. Various-sized tumor nodules on the surface show a coarse nodular pattern (tortoise-shell appearance) characteristic of schistosomal cirrhosis

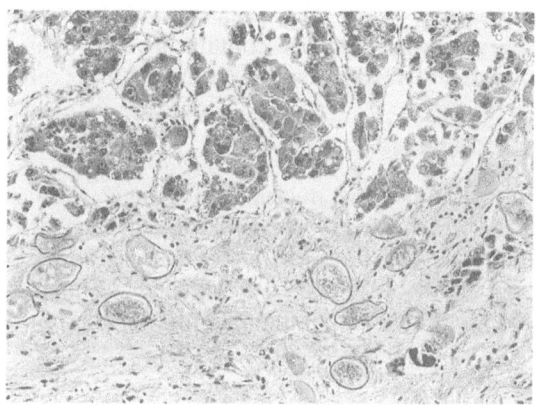

Fig. 7.35. Calcified schistosomal eggs near an HCC. H and E, × 200

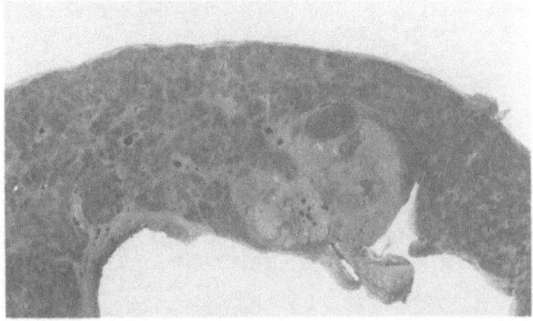

Fig. 7.36. HCC in a liver with marked fibrosis due to Thorotrast deposition

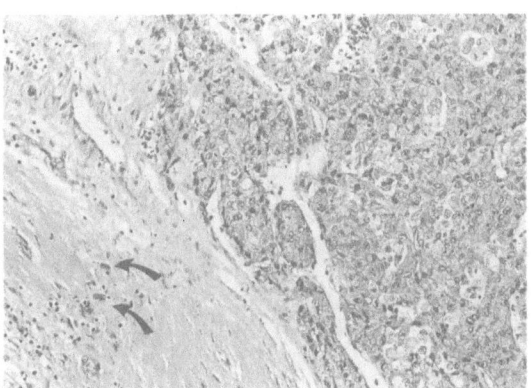

Fig. 7.37. Thorotrast deposits near HCC tissue (*arrows*). H and E, × 200

59 (25.7%) of 229 autopsy cases of chronic schistosomiasis japonica (Figs. 7.34, 7.35). Thus, the incidence of HCC associated with schistosomiasis japonica was significantly higher than the 8.5% in other autopsy cases. However, HBsAg was positive in 28% of these HCC cases associated with schistosomiasis, and anti-HBs and/or anti-HBc was positive in 62.1% of the HBsAg-negative cases. Thus, most of the HCC cases associated with schistosomiasis japonica had had a previous hepatitis B virus infection. Furthermore, morphological examination revealed varying degrees of nonschistosomal hepatic changes, including macronodular or mixed macro- and micronodular cirrhosis superimposed on schistosomal fibrosis, in about two-thirds of the cases. Thus, it is suggested that the additional nonschistosomal factors, particularly hepatitis B virus infection, might play a synergistic role in hepatocarcinogenesis.

5.3 HCC and Thorotrast

Thorotrast, a stabilized 25% colloidal solution of thorium dioxide, was used in many countries in the 1930s and 1940s as a contrast medium for various roentgenographic examinations. Despite the warning that Thorotrast would have a carcinogenic effect, particularly in the liver, it was increasingly used because it lacked acute toxicity and was an excellent radiological contrast medium. Since MacMahon et al. [53] first described Thorotrast-related hepatic angiosarcoma in 1947, many cases of Thorotrast-related malignancies have been reported worldwide. Among 143 autopsy cases with previous Thorotrast injection collected from all over Japan, hepatic malignancies were found in 93 cases. Of these 93 cases, 40 were cholangiocarcinoma, 37

were angiosarcoma, 13 were HCC (Figs. 7.36, 7.37), and three were double cancers. HCC was relatively infrequent among Thorotrast-induced hepatic malignancies. In the 13 HCC cases, although hepatic fibrosis due to Thorotrast deposits was observed, there was an associated cirrhosis in only one case. Thus, it is suggested that the rare association of cirrhosis with Thorotrast may be one of the reasons for such a low frequency of HCC. Furthermore, the suggestion has been made that thorium dioxide itself may not affect hepatocytes as much as it does the bile duct epithelium and endothelial cells.

6 Preneoplastic conditions

According to Peters [27], it is sometimes difficult to distinguish an adenomatous regenerative nodule from an extremely well-differentiated trabecular carcinoma. As discussed in the chapter on small liver cancer (chap. 16), we believe that an adenomatous regenerative focus (Fig. 7.38) in a cirrhotic liver is one of the most likely preneoplastic conditions. Among 14 resected HCCs that presented a variety of cellular differentiation within one tumor mass, it was uncommon to find a highly differentiated Edmondson and Steiner grade I carcinoma in tumors larger than 5 cm, but highly differentiated HCC was frequent (8 of 14 cases, 57%) in tumors smaller than 5 cm. Furthermore, most of the resected minute (smaller than 2 cm) HCCs consisted of extremely well-differentiated cells, which were often difficult to distinguish from those of adenomatous regenerative nodules (Fig. 7.39). The proportion of well-differentiated HCCs tended to diminish in area and the area of less-differentiated HCCs tended to increase with in-

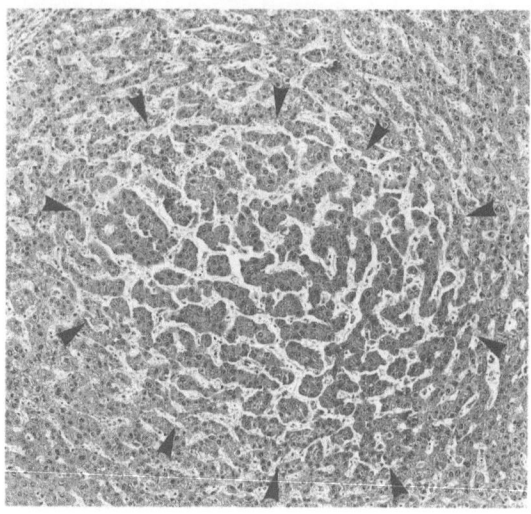

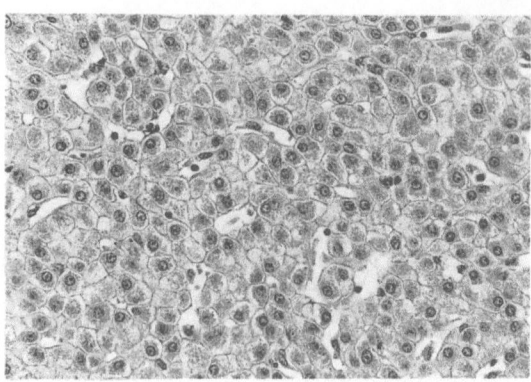

Fig. 7.39. An extremely well-differentiated HCC in a surgically resected minute tumor. H and E, × 200

Fig. 7.38. An adenomatous regenerative focus (*arrowheads*) in a macronodular cirrhosis. H and E, × 100

creasing tumor size. We studied the relationship between the size of HCC and grade of differentiation. The majority of the tumors that were histologically monomorphic and smaller than 2 cm were well-differentiated, but the frequency of moderately to poorly differentiated HCCs increased as the tumors increased in size. In addition, poorly differentiated HCCs grew infiltratively or expansively in the boundary of well-differentiated HCCs. Based on these observations, we conclude that most HCCs may begin as extremely well-differentiated HCC; they transform into less-differentiated HCCs with cell proliferation and growth, and such a conversion may be responsible for the proliferation and growth of the tumor.

7 Paraneoplastic changes

Various histological alterations are encountered in a liver bearing HCC. Peters [27] described histological changes which he called "paraplastic changes." Paraplastic changes become more prominent with the development of carcinoma and are not a prerequisite to the development of carcinoma. They may be found, usually in a less striking fashion, in cirrhotic livers not bearing HCC.

7.1 Liver cell dysplasia

Liver cell dysplasia (LCD) was defined by An-thony [54] in 1973 as the occurrence of nuclear and cytoplasmic enlargement, nuclear pleomorphism, and occasional mitoses in groups of liver cells or in whole cirrhotic nodules. Ever since he described LCD as a premalignant condition, its significance has been disputed [55–57] and no agreement has as yet been reached.

The reported incidence of LCD ranges from 25% to 65.7% [58–59], but it is prevalent in cirrhotic livers bearing HCC in all reports. Furthermore, its close relationship to HBsAg has also been suggested. In our 221 consecutive autopsy cases of HCC, LCD was found in 67 or 30.3%, and there was liver cirrhosis in all cases. Serum HBsAg was found to be positive in 15 (42.8%) of 35 cases with LCD and in 19 (22.1%) of 86 cases without LCD. LCD is multifocal in the noncancerous areas; some of the dysplastic foci may be compressed by adjacent hyperplastic foci (Fig. 7.40A). Because of the unequivocally high incidence of LCD in cases of HCC, it is likely that LCD is closely related to HCC (Fig. 7.40B). Okita et al. [58] suggested that LCD is a premalignant condition because the affected cells show a positive reaction to alpha-fetoprotein. We consider LCD to a paraplastic alteration, not a premalignant condition, because many minute HCCs are highly differentiated and display little cellular atypia and because LCD is very uncommon in livers without HCC. Henmi et al. [59] also denied the possibility of LCD being premalignant on the basis of a karyometric analysis of LCD.

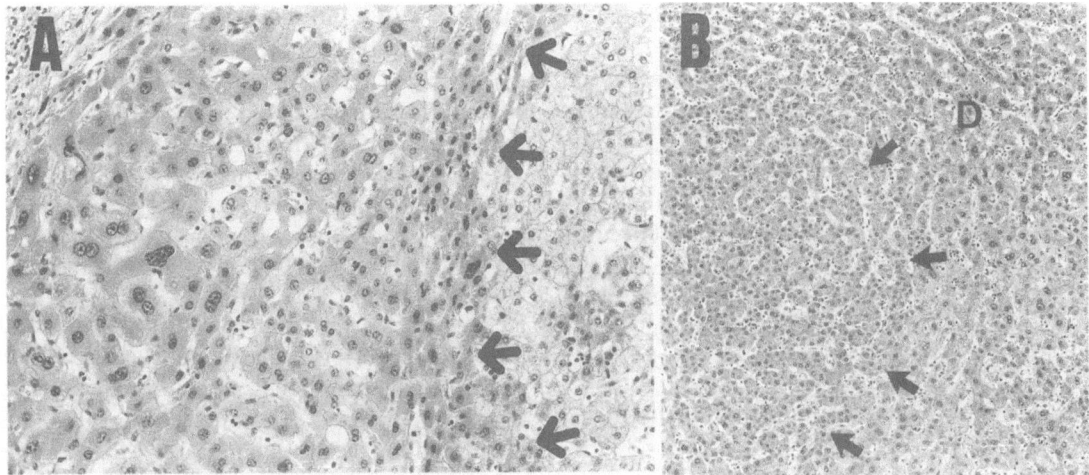

Fig. 7.40. A Liver cell dysplasia in an area compressed by hydropic hepatocytes. H and E, × 200. **B** Moderate dysplastic changes (*D*) of the hepatocytes adjacent to an adenomatous hyperplastic focus. *Arrows* in **A** and **B** show the hyperplastic focus. H and E, × 100

8 Angioarchitecture of HCC

A comparative study of the angiograms made ante and post mortem provides valuable information on the blood vessel structure of HCC. When seen in postmortem angiograms and transparent preparations, the angioarchitecture is complex because vessel structures of the primary focus, tumor thrombus, and intrahepatic metastasis are combined *en bloc* in the angiogram.

The angioarchitecture of HCC varies a great deal depending on the presence or absence of liver cirrhosis and of a capsule [60]. By contrast, a cancer nodule comprises exclusively arterial tumor vessels (Fig. 7.41). The vessels branch off, forming a treelike pattern within the tumor nodule. The degree of ramification of the vessels varies in different areas; the vessels show fine branches at the site of active proliferation of cancer cells but sparse branching where there is an abundant fibrous stroma or necrosis. In encapsulated HCC, the portal vein branches over the capsule are collapsed and flattened; they never penetrate the capsule to supply the nodule.

In nonencapsulated HCC with a replacing or sinusoidal growth pattern, although the tumor vasculature is exclusively arterial, the neoplastic tissue around the boundary receives portal blood through the sinusoids communicating with its blood spaces.

In the capsule, large arterial branches which have been replaced and dislocated are dilated, and numerous regenerating arterial branches

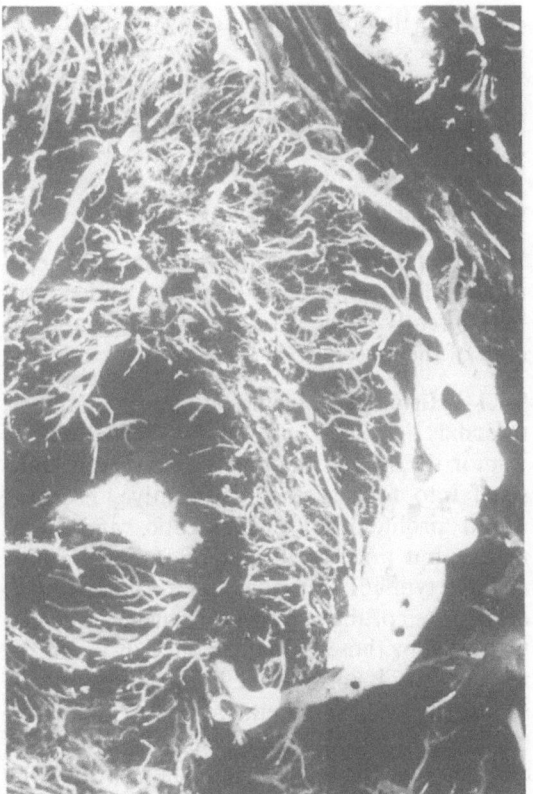

Fig. 7.41. The vasculature of the tumor consists solely of the arterial tumor vessels branching from dilated interlobular arteries around the nodule

form irregular clusters. The portal vein branches are also markedly pushed and flattened. There is, however, no evidence indicating penetration of such capsular blood vessels into the tumor nodule.

The angioarchitecture of daughter nodules is independent of that of the primary nodule, because the vessels arise from arteries that are different from those entering the primary nodule. Thus, not only does a fibrous capsule intervene between the primary and daughter nodules, but the pattern of their angioarchitecture is different.

8.1 Angioarchitecture of tumor thrombus of portal vein

Besides tumor nodules, tumor thrombus of the portal vein contributes greatly to the formation of a complicated vasculature in HCC. Dilatation with increased branching is seen in the arterial branches around the portal vein containing a tumor thrombus. Tumor vessels extend from such arterial branches into the tumor thrombus, indicating that the thrombus is also nourished by arterial vessels.

9 Tumor Thrombus of portal and hepatic veins

9.1 Tumor thrombus of portal vein

HCC frequnetly invades the portal and/or hepatic veins, causing tumor thrombi, and contributes greatly to the variety in the gross appearance of the mass.

9.1.1 Histological findings of portal vein tumor thrombus

Tumor thrombi of the portal vein may be classified into four types—proliferative, necrotic, mixed proliferative and necrotic, and organized—but none of the tumor thrombi are of a single type [61]. In many cases, the histological features of the peripheral branches vary distinctly from those of the portal vein trunk. In medium-sized portal vein branches (fifth and sixth order), the proliferative type is dominant (64.7%), followed by the mixed proliferative and necrotic type (28%) and the necrotic type (18.7%). With the recent improvement in the survival time of patients wtih HCC, the number of cases that manifest organization of tumor thrombi in the portal vein seems to be increasing.

9.1.2 Tumor thrombus of portal vein and intrahepatic metastasis

Although distant metastasis is relatively infrequent in HCC, intrahepatic metastasis through tumor thrombi of the portal vein occurs at an early stage, resulting in intrahepatic tumor spread. Intrahepatic metastases form around the branches of the portal vein (Fig. 7.42). The vascular architecture in an isolated intrahepatic metastasis is solely arterial.

9.1.3 Shunt formation between hepatic artery and portal vein

Retrograde portal circulation through a shunt between the artery and the portal vein (A-P shunt) results from HCC much more frequently than from cirrhosis. The affected portal vein is delineated by celiac angiography (during the arterial phase) because of A-P communication through the tumor thrombus of the portal vein. A large tumor thrombus that has grown within the portal vein has a predisposition to form a shunt between the artery and the portal vein because virtually the entire vascular framework consists of arterial tumor vessels.

The A-P shunts can be divided into three types according to the developmental process: (1) Blood flows from the periportal arterial branches into the arterial vessels of the tumor thrombus and then into its blood spaces, which drain its arterial blood into the portal lumen; (2) dilated periportal arterial branches are directly destroyed by the rapidly expanding tumor thrombus, and arterial blood from the interlobular artery drains directly into the portal vein; (3) tumor invasion extending to the periportal collateral circulation to involve the interlobular arteries destroys the arterial branches, with resultant communication between the hepatic artery and the portal vein.

9.2 Tumor thrombus of hepatic vein

In contradistinction to tumor thrombus of the portal vein, identification of a tumor thrombus in the hepatic vein is difficult because the peripheral branches of the hepatic vein are destroyed earlier by the tumor. Since only tumor thrombi in the relatively large branches of the hepatic vein can be identified, the reported incidence is perhaps much lower than the actual one.

10 Unusual tumor growth in HCC

10.1 Intra-atrial tumor growth

Tumor growth in the right atrium occurs occasionally in malignant neoplasms, including

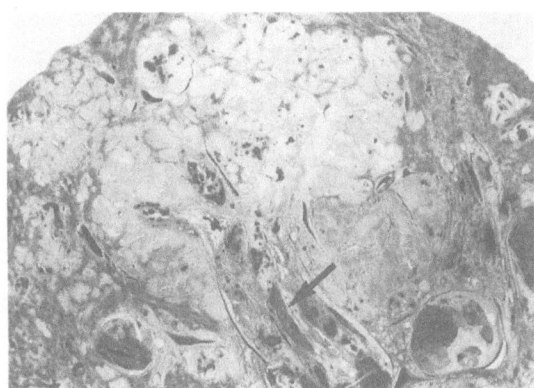

Fig. 7.42. Widespread intrahepatic metastasis via a massive tumor thrombus of the portal vein. The *arrow* shows the massive tumor thrombus

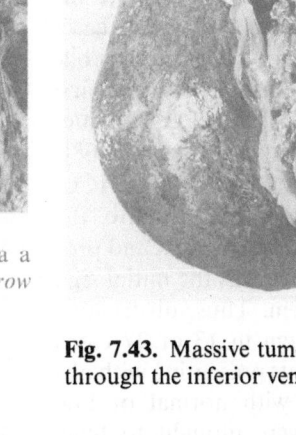

Fig. 7.43. Massive tumor growth in the right atrium through the inferior vena cava and the hepatic vein

HCC, renal cell carcinoma, pulmonary carcinoma, and pancreatic carcinoma. Although tumor growth into blood vessels, particularly the portal vein, is one of the characteristic features of HCC, tumor extension into the right atrium has been considered to be relatively rare. With recent prolongation of survival of patients with HCC, the number of patients who develop intra-atrial tumor growth seems to be increasing [62].

Edmondson and Steiner [8] observed tumor extension into the right atrium in only 1 of 100 cases of primary liver cancer. In the series of MacDonald [63], a tumor thrombus extended into the right atrium in 3 of 108 cases of HCC. As the incidence of HCC in Japan is about ten times that in Western countries, such tumor extension is encountered more frequently. In our 439 HCC cases, tumor thrombi were seen in the hepatic vein in 72 (16.4%) cases, in the inferior vena cava in 48 (10.9%) cases, and in the right atrium in 18 (4.8%) cases (Fig. 7.43). A tumor bolus crossed the tricuspid valves and entered the ventricle in 5 of 18 cases with intra-atrial tumor growth. Of these 18 cases, 17 were grossly of the infiltrative type. A continuous tumor thrombus involved the right atrium, inferior vena cava, and the hepatic vein in 15 cases; the tumor thrombi in all cases were loosely adherent to the vascular endothelium or endocardium. Direct tumor invasion into the myocardium was observed in two cases.

Clinically, hematemesis occurred early in the course of the disease in one patient. Diuretic-resistant marked edema of the lower extremities was seen in 14 cases (77.7%), and marked venous dilatation of the abdominal wall in five cases

(27.7%). The frequency of these symptoms was significantly higher than in the control cases. Continuous tachycardia that ranged from 90 to 110 beats/min was seen in three cases. In five patients, tumor growth into the right atrium through the inferior vena cava was detected by angiography and/or ultrasonography 3–4 months before death. However, in none of these cases symptoms suggestive of obstruction of the inferior vena cava and the right atrium were noted prior to death.

Only one of our patients with intra-atrial tumor growth died of sudden cardiac arrest. However, cases of sudden cardiac arrest or severe dyspnea due to a tumor thrombus in the right atrium have been reported [64, 65]. In these patients, a ball-shaped tumor thrombus was found in the right atrium. It is known that intermittent tricuspid obstruction by a ball-shaped thrombus in the right atrium causes the so-called ball-valve thrombus syndrome [66]. The symptoms are dyspnea of an oxygen-hunger type, enlargement of the liver with or without pulsation, feeble or absent pulse during the attack, a changing heart murmur, and relief produced by changing the position. In our series, however, the tumor thrombi were adherent to the endocardium of the right atrium and the ventricle, which may explain why so few serious cardiac complications developed.

10.2 Intrabile duct tumor growth

Intrabile duct tumor growth presents a variety of clinical and pathological features. Tumor invasion into the hepatic duct and/or common bile duct is frequently detected at autopsy in patients who had developed obstructive jaundice during life. Lin [67] classified such cases as "icteric hepatoma" and stated that they presented difficult problems in differential diagnosis. Despite the recent progress in imaging diagnosis such cases are often, and still incorrectly, diagnosed as bile duct carcinoma or cholelithiasis. In 1982, we first described the clinicopathological characteristics of HCCs with intrabile duct tumor growth [68].

In 27 (6.1%) of our 439 autopsy cases of HCC, we found prominent tumor growth into the hepatic ducts and/or common bile duct and progressive obstructive jaundice was the initial sign or a major clinical problem. Thus, obstructive jaundice was the initial sign in 13 of 27 cases (48.1%). Among the patients presenting with obstructive jaundice, those with normal or low alpha-fetoprotein levels were thought to have biliary carcinoma or stones. Intraductal tumor growth is mostly caused by direct invasion from the primary tumor and occasionally from an adjacent massive tumor thrombus in the portal vein. Only when intraductal tumor growth occurs in a large hepatic duct and/or common bile duct does obstructive jaundice become a clinical problem. Massive hemorrhage in the bile duct (hemobilia) due to intraductal tumor growth is occasionally observed (Fig. 7.44). Of our 27 cases with intrabile duct growth, the HCC was grossly of the infiltrative type in 25 and of the expansive type in two. Thus, the incidence of intraductal tumor growth varies significantly depending on the gross type of HCC, as is the case with intra-atrial tumor growth, suggesting that the tumor growth in the biliary tract is not merely a terminal event. In one of the surgically resected cases, a minute HCC of the infiltrative type, which had arisen in the porta hepatis close to the common bile duct, had invaded the common bile duct; this patient was operated on because he was thought to have a stone in the common bile duct. Patients with HCC growing into the bile duct have a significantly shorter survival after diagnosis than do other HCC patients.

11 Extrahepatic metastases

In general, HCC metastasizes outside the liver in its late stages, although widespread intrahepatic metastases through the portal vein occur relatively early. In our 439 HCC cases, extrahepatic metastases were evident in 63.3%. In the series of

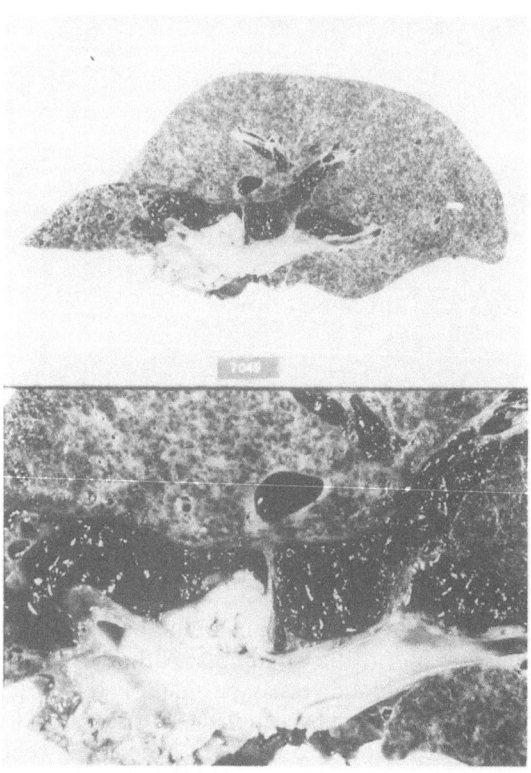

Fig. 7.44. Intrabile duct tumor growth with massive hemorrhage. The tumor has invaded the bifurcation of the hepatic duct and the dilated hepatic ducts are filled with blood clots (the bifurcation is enlarged in the lower picture)

Mori [69] of metastases in Japanese patients with HCC, 52.8% were hematogenous (and commonly involved the lungs and bone) and 29.8% were lymphatic (and involved the lymph nodes of the hepatic hilum, retroperitoneum, mediastinum, and the periaortic area). Peters [27] reported that metastases were more frequent in HCC without cirrhosis than in HCC with cirrhosis, the incidence for the former being 67.0% and for the latter 46.2%. Our results in 439 HCC cases are similar to those reported by Peters [27] with the corresponding figures of 76.1% and 60.1% respectively.

11.1 Hematogenous metastases

In our series, 48.7% of metastases were hematogenous. The lung was the most common site (94.3%) of hematogenous metastases. The adrenal gland, gastrointestinal tract, bone, spleen, heart, and kidney were also involved (in order of decreasing frequency).

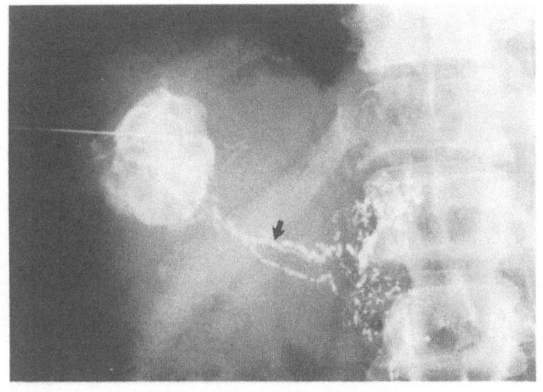

Fig. 7.45. Lymphatic channels (arrow) connecting an HCC tumor nodule and abdominal lymph nodes

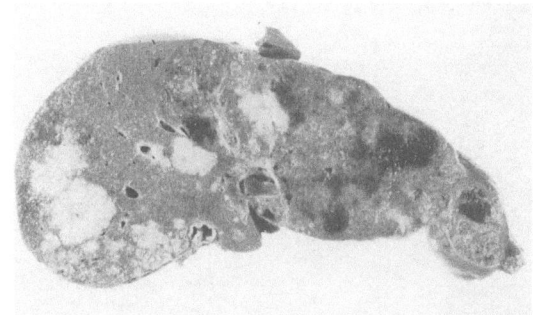

Fig. 7.46. Combined hepatocellular and cholangiocarcinoma. Part of the HCC is dark and part of the cholangiocarcinoma is white. It is relatively easy to identify both components

11.2 Lymphatic metastases

Lymphatic metastases in HCC have not been well documented in the literature, perhaps because the majority of extrahepatic metastases are hematogenous. In our 439 cases, peripancreatic lymph nodes had metastases in 15.2%, this being the highest rate among lymphatic metastases at various sites. Lymph node metastases were found in the hepatic hilum in 14.3% of cases, the second highest frequency. Of the 439 cases of HCC, 32 had massive lymph node metastases which were so large as to lead to an erroneous diagnosis of malignant lymphoma. Kawabata [70] found that free-cell-type HCC was frequent in such massive lymph node metastases. Saitsu et al. [71] demonstrated the lymphatics connecting tumor nodules within the liver and the abdominal lymph nodes by the percutaneous injection of contrast medium (Lipiodol) into the tumor (Fig. 7.45).

12 Combined hepatocellular and cholangiocarcinoma

Combined hepatocellular and cholangiocarcinoma (combined HCC–CCC) is a relatively rare tumor in which both HCC and cholangiocarcinoma are present in the same liver. Allen and Lisa [72] described five of their own cases and 11 cases from the literature and classified these tumors into three types: (1) tumors in which the elements of HCC and cholangiocarcinoma are present separately; (2) tumors in which HCC exists adjacent to a cholangiocarcinoma and the two elements are mixed together as one mass; (3) tumors in which HCC and cholangiocarcino-

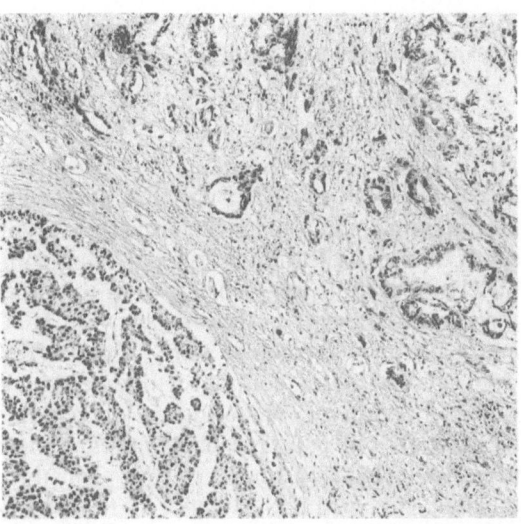

Fig. 7.47. HCC showing a trabecular pattern (*lower left*) and cholangiocarcinoma are clearly separated. H and E, × 50

ma are intimately mixed. Goodman et al. [73] studied 24 cases of combined HCC-CCC and classified them histologically into three types— collision, transitional, and fibrolamellar tumors.

In 393 consecutive autopsy cases of primary liver cancer in our institute, ten cases (2.5%) were combined HCC–CCC. The average age, sex ratio, clinical symptoms, and biochemical data were not much different from those of HCC. However, alpha-fetoprotein levels were relatively low (all within 10 000 ng/ml) with a positivity rate of 60%. Carcinoembyonic antigen (CEA) was positive in 88% of cases, with a mean value of 7.5 ng/ml.

Grossly, eight cases were of the infiltrative type and none was encapsulated, as is common in

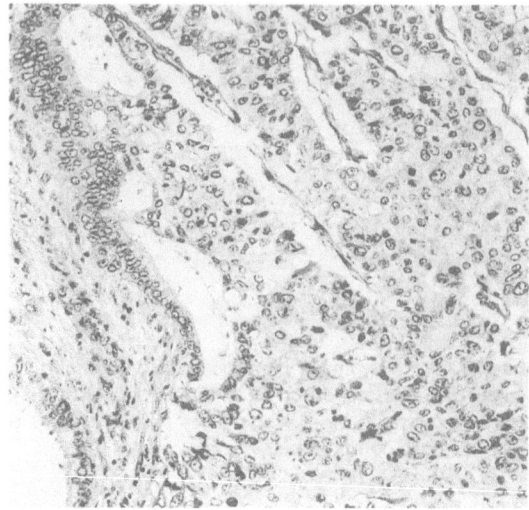

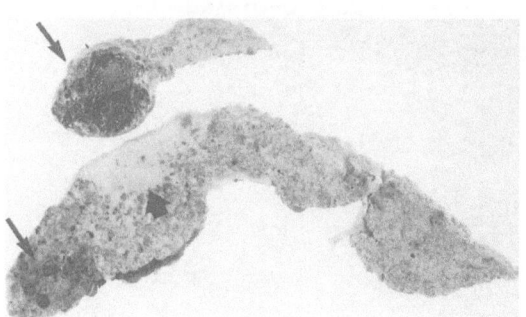

Fig. 7.49. Double cancer. HCC (*thin arrows*) and cholangiocarcinoma (*thick arrow*) are located independently

Fig. 7.48. A transitional feature between HCC and cholangiocarcinoma. H and E, × 200

HCC. Liver cirrhosis was found in five of the cases. The area of HCC and that of cholangiocarcinoma could be distinguished grossly in seven of the cases, the two tumors being completely separate (Figs. 7.46, 7.47). In the other three cases, transitional features between HCC and cholangiocarcinoma were found (Fig. 7.48). One case was confirmed to have double cancer because of the evidence of separate localization of HCC and cholangiocarcinoma (Fig. 7.49). Hematogenous metastases, mostly in the lung, consisted exclusively of an HCC component, while lymphatic metastases were mainly cholangiocarcinoma; metastases of both components in the same lymph node were seen in one case.

As to the histogenesis of combined HCC–CCC, the following three concepts are possible: (1) double cancer; (2) the cancer first arises either from the hepatocyte or bile duct epithelium and part of it differentiates to the other component; (3) the cancer arises in an intermediate (transitional) cell that differentiates in both directions, i.e., HCC and cholangiocarcinoma. The evidence for the transitional feature between HCC and cholangiocarcinoma in a certain proportion of combined HCC–CCC supports the second and third concepts.

Recently, we established a new cell line (KYN-1) from a resected HCC that exhibited a typical trabecular growth pattern with alpha-fetoprotein production [74]. Morphologically, however, KYN-1 cells show mucin production and hetero-

transplanted tumors in nude mice consist exclusively of a solid growth of mucin-containing tumor cells, with occasional tubular structures. These findings may support the second concept of the histogenesis of combined HCC–CCC.

References

1. Berman C (1951) Primary carcinoma of the liver. Lewis, London
2. Virchow R (1862) Krankheiten Geschwulste. Hirschwald, Berlin
3. Von Hansemann D (1890) Über den primare Krebs der Leber. Ber Klin Wchnschr 27: 353–356
4. Hanot V, Gilbert A (1888) Études sur les maladies du foie. Asselin and Houzeau, Paris
5. Eggel H (1901) Über das primare Carcinom der Leber. Beitr path Anat u z allg Path 30: 506–604
6. Yamagiwa K (1911) Primäre Leber Krebs (Hepatom). Gann 5: 226–282
7. Goldzieher M, Bokay Z (1911) Der primäre Leber Krebs. Virchows Arch A (Pathol Anat) 203: 75–131
8. Edmondson HA, Steiner, PE (1954) Primary carcinoma of the liver. A study of 100 cases among 48 900 necropsies. Cancer 7: 462–503
9. Szmuness W (1978) Hepatocellular carcinoma and the hepatitis B virus: evidence for a causal association. Prog Med Virol 24: 40–69
10. Beasley RP (1982) Hepatitis B virus as the etiologic agent in hepatocellular carcinoma—epidemiologic considerations. Hepatology 2: 21S–26S
11. Brechot C, Hadchouel M, Scotto J (1981) State of hepatitis B virus DNA in hepatocytes of patients with hepatitis B surface antigen-positive and

-negative liver diseases. Proc Natl Acad Sci USA 78: 3906–3910

12. Shafrits D, Shouval D, Sherman HI, Hadziyannis SJ, Kew MC (1981) Integration of hepatitis B virus DNA into the genome of liver cells in chronic liver disease and hepatocellular carcinoma. N Engl J Med 305: 1067–1073

13. Chen DS, Hoyer BH, Nelson J, Purcell RH, Gerin SL (1982) Detection and properties of hepatitis B viral DNA in liver tissues from patients with hepatocellular carcinoma. Hepatology 2: 42S–46S

14. Steiner PE (1960) Cancer of the liver and cirrhosis in Transaharan Africa and the United States of America. Cancer 13: 1085–1166

15. Okuda K, Peters RL, Simson IW (1984) Gross anatomic features of hepatocellular carcinoma from three disparate geographic areas. Proposal of new classification. Cancer 54: 2165–2173

16. Mori W (1956) Study on metastasis in hepatoma. Its relationship with liver cirrhosis. Tr Soc Pathol Jpn 45: 224–236

17. Miyaji T, Yu K, Oda T, Nagatomo T, Sawada K (1960) Pathomorphological study on primary liver cancer in recent 10 years in Japan. Acta Hepatol Jpn 1: 17–36

18. Kato M, Minamisuhara T, Kiwaki M, Daima M (1957) An interesting case of hepatocellular carcinoma. J Jpn Soc Intern Med 46: 1218 (Abst)

19. Arakawa M, Kage M, Isomura T, Motoyama F, Nakashima T, Kubo Y, Nakayama T (1982) Pathomorphological studies on hepatocellular carcinoma (HCC)—Seven cases of HCC with an extrahepatic tumor growth, so-called "pedunculated hepatoma". Acta Hepatol Jpn 23: 942–948

20. Horie Y, Katoh S, Yoshida H, Omaoka T, Suou T, Hirayama C (1983) Pedunculated hepatocellular carcinoma. Report of three cases and review of literature. Cancer 51: 746–751

21. Miyoshi M, Iwata N, Fujii H, Katake K (1977) A case of pedunculated hepatoma with spontaneous rupture. Acta Hepatol Jpn 18: 765–771

22. Gyotoku Y, Sugihara H, Amagasaki T, Mori I, Konoshita I (1980) An autopsy case of pedunculated liver cell carcinoma and its review. Jap J Cancer Clin 26: 92–96

23. Gibson JB (1978) Histological typing of tumors of the livers, biliary tract and pancreas. International Histological Classification of Tumors. No. 20, WHO, Geneva

24. Buchanan TF, Huvas AG (1974) Clear cell carcinoma of the liver. Am J Clin Pathol 61: 529–539

25. Wu PC, Lai CL, Lam KC, Lam KC, Lok ASF, Lin HJ (1983) Clear cell carcinoma of the liver. An ultrastructural study. Cancer 52: 504–507

26. Sasaki K, Okuda K, Takahashi M (1981) Hepatic clear cell carcinoma associated with hypoglycemia and hypercholesterolemia. Cancer 47: 820–822

27. Peters RL (1976) Pathology of hepatocellular carcinoma. In: Okuda K, Peters RL (eds) Hepatocellular carcinoma. Wiley, New York, pp 107–168

28. Nakanuma Y, Ohta G (1985) Is Mallory body formation a preneoplastic change? A study of 181 cases of liver bearing hepatocellular carcinoma and 82 cases of cirrhosis. Cancer 55: 2400–2404

29. Tomimatsu H (1983) Ultrastructural study of Mallory body in hepatocellular carcinoma. Acta Hepatol Jpn 24: 513–520

30. Stromeyer FW, Ishak KG, Gerber MA, Mathew T (1980) Ground-glass cells in hepatocellular carcinoma. Am J Clin Pathol 74: 254–258

31. Tanaka K, Toyokawa H, Uchida T, Uzawa T, Karasawa T, Shikata T, Kitano M (1977) Hepatitis B related antigens in hepatoma cells. Acta Hepatol Jpn 18: 689

32. Ilardi CF, Ying YY, Ackerman LV, Elias JM (1980) Hepatitis B surface antigen and hepatocellular carcinoma in the People's Republic of China. Cancer 46: 1612–1616

33. Nayak NC, Dhar A, Sachdeva R, Mittal A, Seth HN, Sudarsanam D, Reddy B, Wagholikar UL, Reddy CRRM (1977) Association of human hepatocellular carcinoma and cirrhosis with hepatitis B virus surface antigens in the liver. Int J Cancer 20: 643–654

34. Kawano Y (1983) Localization of hepatitis B surface antigen in hepatocellular carcinoma. Acta Pathol Jpn 33: 1087–1093

35. Jaffe RH (1924) Sarcoma and carcinoma of the liver following cirrhosis. Arch Int Med 33: 330–342

36. William WL, Agha FP, Morgan WS (1983) Primary sarcoma of the liver in adult. Cancer 51: 1510–1517

37. Shin P, Ohmi S, Sakurai M (1981) Hepatocellular carcinoma combined with hepatic sarcoma. Acta Pathol Jpn 31: 815–824

38. Nagamine Y, Sasaki M, Kaku K, Takahashi M (1978) Hepatic sarcoma associated with hepatoma. Acta Pathol Jpn 28: 645–651

39. Neville E, Piyasena KHG, James DG (1975) Granulomas of the liver. Postgrad Med J 51: 361–365

40. Nakashima T, Kojiro M, Kawano Y, Shirai F, Takemoto N, Tomimatsu H, Kawasaki H, Okuda K (1982) Histologic growth pattern of hepatocellular carcinoma. Relationship to orcein (hepatitis B surface-antigen)-positive cells in cancer tissue. Hum Pathol 13: 563–568

41. Isomura T (1979) Pathological study of primary liver cancer. Ultrastructural study of hepatocellular carcinoma—structure of blood space (tumor vessel). Acta Hepatol Jpn 20: 164–174

42. Sugihara S, Kojiro M, Nakashima T (1985) Ultrastructural study of hepatocellular carcinoma with replacing growth pattern. Acta Pathol Jpn 35: 549–559

43. Shikata T (1959) Studies on the relationship between hepatic cancer and liver cirrhosis. Acta Pathol Jpn 9: 267–331

44. Geddes FW, Falkson G (1970) Malignant hepatoma in the Bantu. Cancer 25: 1271–1278

45. Mori W (1967) Cirrhosis and primary cancer of the liver. Comparative study in Tokyo and Cincinnati. Cancer 20: 627–631

46. Lee FI (1966) Cirrhosis and hepatoma in alcoholics. Gut 7: 77–95

47. Nakashima T, Okuda K, Kojiro M, Sakamoto K, Kubo Y, Shimokawa Y (1975) Primary liver cancer coincident with schistosomiasis japonica. A study of 24 necropsies. Cancer 36: 1483–1489

48. Iuchi M, Hayakawa M, Kitani K, Yamada H, Iio M, Sasaki Y, Kameda H (1973) Hepatocellular carcinoma and chronic schistosomiasis japonica: II. Acta Hepatol Jpn 11: 249–252

49. Kamo E, Ebato T (1982) A clinical analysis of primary carcinoma of the liver in relation with schistosomiasis japonica. J Yamanashi Med Assoc 9: 23–37

50. Edington GM (1979) Schistosomiasis and primary liver cancer. Tran R Soc Trop Med Hyg 73: 351–352

51. Cheever AW, Andrade ZA (1967) Pathological lesions associated with Schistosoma mansoni infection in man. Tran R Soc Trop Med Hyg 61: 629–639

52. Martinez-Maldonado M, Girod CE, Arellano GR, Ramirez EA (1965) Liver cell carcinoma (hepatoma) in Puerto Rico. A study of 26 cases. Am J Dig Dis 10: 522–529

53. MacMahon E, Murphy AS, Bates MI (1947) Endothelial cell sarcoma of the liver following Thorotrast injection. Am J Pathol 23: 585–613

54. Anthony PP (1973) Primary carcinoma of the liver. A study of 282 cases in Ugandan Africans. J Pathol 110: 37–48

55. Sakurai M (1978) Liver cell dysplasia and hepatitis B surface and core antigens in cirrhosis and hepatocellular carcinoma of autopsy cases. Acta Pathol Jpn 28: 705–719

56. Omata M, Mori J, Yokosuka O, Ito Y, Okuda K (1982) Hepatitis B virus antigens in liver tissue in hepatocellular carcinoma and advanced chronic liver disease—relationship to liver cell dysplasia. Liver 2: 125–132

57. Cohen C, Berson SD, Geddes FW (1979) Liver cell dysplasia. Association with hepatocellular carcinoma, cirrhosis and hepatitis B antigen carrier status. Cancer 44: 1671–1676

58. Okita K, Kodama T, Harada T, Takemoto T (1977) Early lesions and development of primary hepatocellular carcinoma in man—association with hepatitis B viral infection. Gastroenterologia Jpn 12: 51–57

59. Henmi A, Uchida T, Shikata T, (1985) Karyometric analysis of liver cell dysplasia and hepatocellular carcinoma. Cancer 55: 2594–2599

60. Nakashima T, Kojiro M (1986) Hepatocellular Carcinoma: An Atlas of Its Pathology. Springer-Verlag, Tokyo

61. Jimi A (1983) Pathomorphological study on hepatocellular carcinoma—a study of tumor thrombus of the portal vein. Acta Hepatol Jpn 24: 641–647

62. Kojiro M, Nakahara H, Sugihara S, Murakami T, Nakashima T, Kawasaki H (1984) Hepatocellular carcinoma with intra-atrial tumor growth. A clinicopathologic study of 18 autopsy cases. Arch Pathol Lab Med 108: 989–992

63. MacDonald RA (1957) Primary carcinoma of the liver: A clinicopathologic study of 108 cases. Arch Intern Med 99: 266–279

64. Kitagawa T, Sugiura G, Takazawa Y, Ohya K (1963) An autopsy case of hepatic cirrhosis associated with acute Budd-Chiari syndrome due to complicating hepatoma. Naika 12: 1178–1182 (in Japanese)

65. Kato Y, Kurosaki Y, Kobayashi K, Sugimoto T, Takada A, Tsuda I (1971) A case of hepatocellular carcinoma with large ball-shaped tumor thrombus in the right atrium. Naika 28: 349–353 (in Japanese)

66. Hahne OH, Climie ARH (1962) Right atrial thrombus with ball-valve action. Am J Med 32: 942–949

67. Lin TY (1976) Primary malignant tumors. In: Bockus HL (ed) Gastroenterology, Saunders, Philadelphia, pp. 522–533

68. Kojiro M, Kawabata K, Kawano Y, Shirai F, Takemoto N, Nakashima T (1982) Hepatocellular carcinoma presenting as intrabile duct tumor growth. A clinicopathologic study of 24 cases. Cancer 49: 2144–2147

69. Mori W (1956) Study of metastasis in hepatoma: its relation to liver cirrhosis. Tr Soc Pathol Jpn 45: 224–236

70. Kawabata K (1980) Pathomorphological studies on hepatocellular carcinoma. A study of the lymph node with marked metastasis of hepatocellular carcinoma. Acta Hepatol Jpn 21: 203–215

71. Saitsu H, Yoshida K, Nakayama T, Okuda K, Sato M, Koga M, Sugihara S, Kojiro M (1986) Demonstration of lymphatics between tumor nodules and the regional lymph nodes in hepatocellular carcinoma. Acta Hepatol Jpn 27: 1296–1302

72. Allen RA, Lisa JR (1949) Combined liver cell and bile duct carcinoma. Am J Pathol 25: 647–655

73. Goodman ZD, Ishak KG, Langloss JM, Sesterhenn IA, Rabin L (1985) Combined hepatocellular-cholangiocellular carcinoma. A histological and immunohistological study. Cancer 55: 124–135

74. Yano H, Kojiro M, Nakashima T (1986) A new human HCC cell line (KYN-1) with a transformation to adenocarcinoma. In Vitro 22: 637–646

Chapter 8
Benign Tumors of the Liver*

Zachary D. Goodman[1]

Benign tumors of the liver are all uncommon or relatively rare entities. Some are true neoplasms, others are tumorlike masses, while still others are of uncertain pathogenesis. They have diverse clinical manifestations that parallel their pathological features. The classification of benign hepatic tumors (Table 8.1), based on their principal histological features, is adapted from several previously published reviews [1–4].

1 Nodular regenerative hyperplasia

Nodular regenerative hyperplasia (NRH) has been described by many authors under many names. Synonyms include nodular transformation of the liver, partial nodular transformation, miliary hepatocellular adenomatosis, hepatocellular adenomatosis, liver adenomatosis, nodular noncirrhotic liver, noncirrhotic nodulation of the liver, adenomatous hyperplasia of the liver, and diffuse nodular hyperplasia of liver [5–12]. The livers described by these names are all very similar morphologically. They have a preserved architectural framework in which are scattered multiple hepatocellular nodules with intervening areas of hepatic atrophy. However, some differences exist between cases, perhaps indicating multiple pathogenetic mechanisms.

1.1 Clinical features

NRH has been reported in patients of all ages (8 months to 82 years) with an approximately equal sex distribution. Of great interest is the association of this condition with a variety of nonhepa-

tic chronic diseases [5, 13–19]. These include especially myeloproliferative disorders (polycythemia vera, chronic myelogenous leukemia, myeloid metaplasia), lymphoproliferative disorders (Hodgkin's and non-Hodgkin's lymphomas, chronic lymphocytic leukemia, plasma cell dyscrasias), and collagen-vascular disorders (rheumatoid arthritis, Felty's syndrome, polyarteritis nodosa, scleroderma, CRST syndrome, lupus erythematosus). The true incidence of NRH is not known. In one series, 500 consecutive autopsies at a medical examiner's office were

Table 8.1. Histological classification of benign neoplasms and tumorlike lesions of the liver

Hepatocellular
    Nodular regenerative hyperplasia
    Hepatocellular adenoma
    Focal nodular hyperplasia
Cholangiocellular
    Bile duct adenoma
    Biliary microhamartoma (von Meyenberg complex)
    Biliary cystadenoma
    Biliary papillomatosis
Vascular
    Hemangioma
    Infantile hemangioendothelioma
    Hereditary hemorrhagic telangectasia
    Lymphangiomatosis
Mesenchymal (nonvascular)
    Leiomyoma
    Lipoma
    Myelolipoma
    Angiomyolipoma
    Pseudolipoma
    Fibrous mesothelioma
Mixed mesenchymal-epithelial
    Mesenchymal hamartoma
    Benign teratoma
Miscellaneous
    Adrenal rest tumor
    Pancreatic heterotopia
    Inflammatory pseudotumor
    Focal fatty change

---

*The opinions and assertions contained herein are the private views of the author and are not to be construed as official or as reflecting the views of the Department of the Army or the Department of Defense.
[1] Department of Hepatic Pathology, Armed Forces Institute of Pathology, Washongton, DC 20306, USA

reviewed and three cases of NRH were found, an incidence of 0.6% [15]. However, among patients who die in hospitals, the incidence is undoubtedly much higher, due to the associations noted above. Indeed, in one recent study it was found that nearly 30% of bone marrow transplant patients had NRH [20].

Three presentations are seen in patients with NRH.

1.1.1 Incidental finding
Patients without symptoms or signs of liver disease are sometimes found to have NRH at autopsy or at laparotomy for an unrelated condition (e.g., at staging laparotomy for lymphoma). Often the surgeon will note that the liver appeared "cirrhotic," prompting the biopsy.

1.1.2 Portal hypertension
NRH is probably a major cause of noncirrhotic portal hypertension in the Western world. The exact mechanism of increased portal pressure is not known but has been postulated to be due to obstruction of portal venous inflow, either by the hyperplastic nodules themselves [5, 6, 14] or by a primary portal venopathy [15]. Up to 60% of reported patients had esophageal varices and/or ascites [5], and many have died as a result of this.

1.1.3 Rupture of liver and hemorrhage
In a few patients, a nodule may become large enough to rupture, causing hemoperitoneum, similar to what occurs with hepatocellular adenoma [5].

1.2 Pathology

The hallmark of NRH is a diffuse nodularity of the liver. The liver may be small, normal-sized, or large. The capsular surface and cut surface show numerous cirrhosislike nodules that usually range from 0.1 to 1.0 cm (Fig. 8.1), but occasional cases may have adenomalike nodules up to 10 cm or larger. The nodules are usually paler than the intervening hepatic parenchyma, which may be dark and congested, but not fibrotic.

Microscopically, the nodules are formed by hyperplasia of hepatocytes, usually distorting but not obliterating the lobular landmarks. The nodules may be apparent on routine H and E stain, but they usually are best appreciated with a reticulin stain showing expanding masses of hepatocytes in cell plates two or more cells thick (Figs. 8.2, 8.3). The hepatocytes composing the nodules are usually somewhat large but otherwise normal. In some cases, however, the cytoplasm of the cells is pale due to an increased

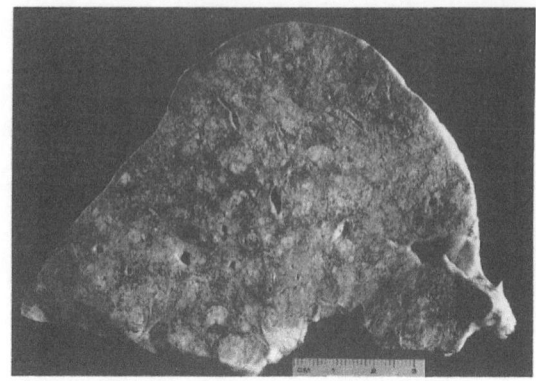

Fig. 8.1. Nodular regenerative hyperplasia. Portion of fixed liver tissue with numerous small, pale nodules, measuring up to 1 cm in diameter. AFIP neg 78-6566

content of fat and/or glycogen. A few cases show liver cell dysplasia. The smallest nodules occupy less than an entire hepatic acinus and tend to occupy the periportal region. In some cases, all of the nodules are this size and may not be grossly visible. Larger nodules may incorporate or push aside vascular structures and portal tracts. Some large nodules appear to form by confluence of small nodules. The hepatic parenchyma between the nodules is atrophic with small hepatocytes and thin, compressed liver cell plates. Portal areas often show some fibrosis, and there may be foci of bridging fibrosis, but the degree of nodularity is out of keeping with the amount of scarring, in contradistinction to cirrhosis.

1.3 Pathogenesis

There are two major theories of pathogenesis.

1.3.1 Neoplastic
Two lines of evidence suggest that NRH is a neoplastic process. First, there is the similarity of the lesions to the nodules produced in experimental animals by a wide variety of experimental carcinogens, such as ethionine, aflatoxin B, 2-acetylaminofluorene, and diethylnitrosamine. These are called "hyperplastic nodules," "hepatocellular foci," or "neoplastic nodules" and are thought to be precursors of hepatocellular carcinoma [21, 22]. Second, there is the association of NRH with numerous chronic diseases, as noted above. These generally require chronic therapy with a variety of drugs, especially steroids and antineoplastic agents. A number of other reported patients had taken long-term oral contraceptives, anticonvulsants, and other drug. Thus it has been suggested that drug therapy may induce

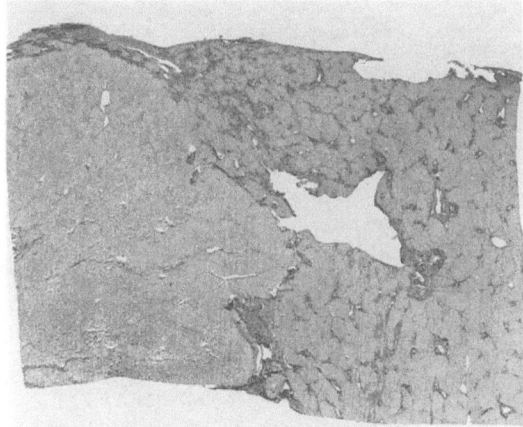

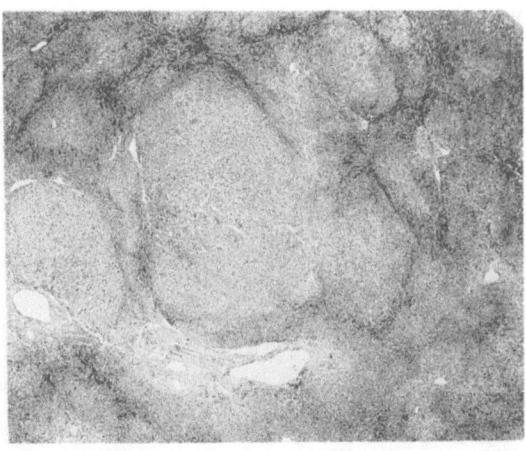

Fig. 8.2. Nodular regenerative hyperplasia. On *left* part of a large, adenomalike nodule formed by confluence of small nodules. *Right* shows numerous small cirrhosislike nodules without intervening fibrosis. Reticulin stain, AFIP neg 86-6973, × 4

Fig. 8.3. Nodular regenerative hyperplasia. Small hyperplastic hepatocellular nodules surrounded by compressed, atrophic liver cell plates. Reticulin stain, AFIP neg 86-6980, × 25

nodules similar to the neoplastic nodules of experimental animals and so cause NRH [5, 23]. Similar hyperplastic foci have also been described in humans exposed to vinyl chloride and Thorotrast [24]. The evidence that NRH is a premalignant lesion in humans is scant, but at least one case of hepatocellular carcinoma following NRH has been described [5], and the presence of hepatocellular dysplasia in some cases suggests that NRH may at least sometimes be the precursor of hepatocellular carcinoma.

1.3.2 Vascular
A vascular pathogenesis of NRH has been proposed by Wanless and co-workers [7, 15, 16]. In morphometric studies, patients with NRH were shown to have smaller portal vein branches than controls as well as a reduced number of small portal vein and hepatic artery branches. This suggested that a reduction in portal blood flow might cause atrophy of the circulatory periphery of the acini or of entire acini and that compensatory hyperplasia of the remaining liver could be the cause of nodule formation. The cause of this "obliterative portal venopathy" was suggested to be thrombosis in cases of hematological disorders, sluggish blood flow in congestive heart failure or macroglobulinemia, or arteritis with secondary involvement of portal vein branches in collagen-vascular diseases [16].

The actual pathogenetic mechanism may be a combination of the two above types. In Asia, Japanese and Indian patients with the disease called idiopathic portal hypertension or noncirrhotic portal fibrosis [25] have markedly reduced portal blood flow and hepatic atrophy with only a minimal number of regenerative nodules. If the vascular theory is correct, these patients should all have typical NRH. In North America, this disease, which is also called hepatoportal sclerosis [26], is extremely rare. It may be, however, that some other factor, either racial, dietary, or chemical (i.e., drug) stimulates nodular regeneration in these patients, producing NRH rather than the pronounced atrophy of hepatoportal sclerosis.

2 Hepatocellular adenoma

Hepatocellular adenoma (HCA) is a benign growth of hepatocytes that usually occurs within an otherwise normal liver. HCA was an extremely rare tumor before the introduction of oral contraceptives in 1960 [2, 27–29]. The current histological criteria for diagnosis were formulated by Edmondson in 1958 [30] based on very limited experience. After the advent of contraceptive steroid therapy, HCA was observed more often. It was still an uncommon tumor, but increasingly larger series of cases were reported, almost exclusively in women taking oral contraceptives [2, 27–29, 31–40], leading to studies demonstrating a causal relationship [27, 28] and generating considerable interest in this tumor. Confusion in terminology and in the distinction

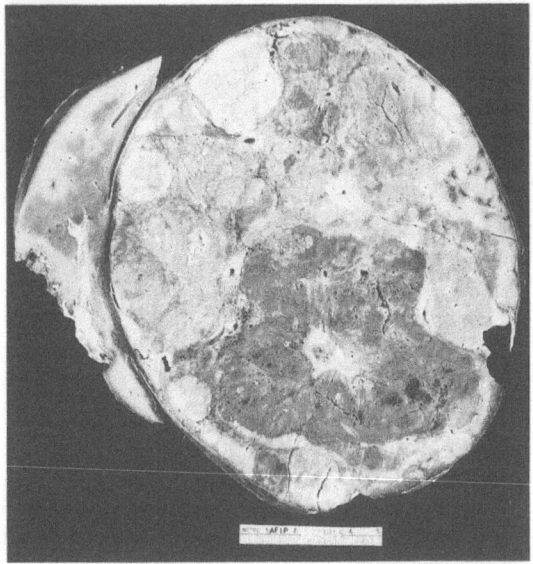

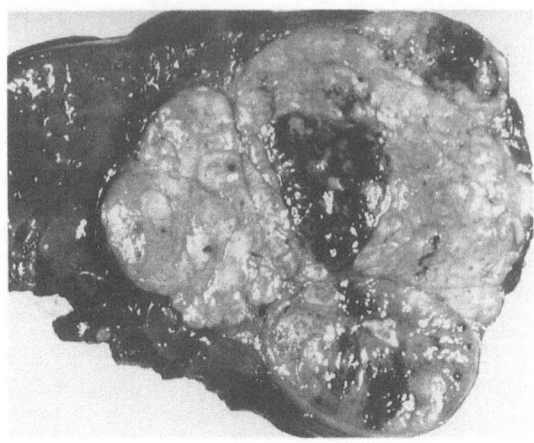

Fig. 8.5. Hepatocellular adenoma after resection. The soft, yellow, unencapsulated tumor has an area of central hemorrhage. AFIP neg 86-7395

Fig. 8.4. Hepatocellular adenoma 15 cm in diameter. Cut surface of resected specimen after formalin fixation has a variegated appearance. The color ranges from yellow to tan to brown. AFIP neg 82-7050

of HCA from focal nodular hyperplasia, from nodular regenerative hyperplasia, and from well-differentiated hepatocellular carcinoma led to confused reports in the 1970s, but much of this has now been resolved. However, many of the cases previously called "benign hepatoma," or "minimal deviation hepatoma" were actually HCA; many cases of "hepatic adenoma" or other similar terms were actually focal nodular hyperplasia; many cases of "multiple adenoma" were actually nodular regenerative hyperplasia. Thus, every report, particularly in the older literature, must be critically evaluated.

2.1 Clinical features

HCA occurs nearly always in women in the reproductive years, ages 15–45, who have taken oral contraceptives (OCs). HCA has been reported in men, children, and women not taking OCs [28, 40–42], but such cases are rare. In two large series, the average age was 30, and most patients were between 20 and 39 years of age [28, 29].

Patients with HCA seek medical attention for several reasons. In approximately 5%–10% of cases the HCA is found incidentally; 25%–35% are aware of an abdominal mass; 20%–25% have chronic or mild episodic abdominal pain; and 30%–40% have acute abdominal pain, due to hemorrhage into the tumor (30%) or into the

peritoneal cavity (70%). Intraperitoneal hemorrhage, the most serious complication, often requires emergency surgery and causes circulatory collapse and death in 20% of patients.

2.2 Pathology

HCA is a solitary nodule, although occasional patients may have more than one. Most cases of multiple adenomas [43–45] or "adenomatosis" [8, 12] are actually examples of nodular regenerative hyperplasia. The tumors are globular or spherical and may measure up to 30 cm in diameter, although the majority are 5–15 cm. Many adenomas bulge from the surface of the liver and often have large blood vessels running across the surface. A few are pedunculated. On cut section, the tumors are well demarcated from the surrounding liver, but usually unencapsulated. The color varies from yellow to tan or brown, and there are usually areas of necrosis and/or hemorrhage (Figs. 8.4, 8.5). Sometimes, irregular scars mark areas of previous necrosis.

Microscopically, HCA is composed of benign hepatocytes arranged in sheets and cords without an acinar architecture (Figs. 8.6, 8.7). The tumor cells are the same size or slightly larger than non-neoplastic hepatocytes and often have a pale cyoplasm due to increased glycogen and/or fat content. The nuclei are uniform and regular, and the nuclear-cytoplasmic ratio is normal; mitoses are almost never seen. Bile is sometimes present in intercellular canaliculi. Thin-walled vascular channels are scattered throughout the tumors, but large arteries are only seen around the periphery. The sinusoids are usually compressed with flattened lining cells, contributing to the sheetlike appearance; sometimes the sinusoids are dilated, a finding which has mistakenly been called "peliosis" [39]. Kupffer cells are present but usually inconspicuous; hematopoietic cells may also be found in sinusoids; and rare cases have noncaseating granulomas in the tumor [46].

Ultrastructural studies have emphasized the similarity of the tumor cells of HCA to normal liver cells [47]. The neoplastic hepatocytes, however, are said to have a "simplified" structure with relatively fewer organelles and bile canaliculi and relatively more cytoplasmic glycogen and fat. Sinusoidal lining cells are similarly decreased in number and complexity [48].

2.3 Pathogenesis

Epidemiological case-control studies have demonstrated a causal relationship between HCA and the use of OC steroids [27, 28]. The incidence is estimated to be 3–4/year/100 000 long-term OC users but only 1/million in nonusers or women who have used OCs for less than 2 years. Furthermore, the risk of developing HCA increases with the durating of OC use and with the potency of the preparations used. The exact mechanism by which adenomas are produced is

not known. Experimental evidence suggests that sex hormones are promotors rather than initiators of hepatocellular neoplasms [49]. This is supported by the clinical observations of regression of tumor size in some women with unresectable HCA after discontinuing OCs [50–52]. Other etiological mechanisms are suggested by the fact that HCA has also been associated with use of noncontraceptive estrogens, virilizing and feminizing ovarian tumors, anabolic (androgenic) steroids, type 1 glycogen storage disease, diabetes mellitus, and iron overload secondary to beta thalassemia [41, 53–55].

2.4 Natural history

If the stimulus to growth of the HCA is removed, the tumors usually regress, at least in those associated with OCs and type I glycogen storage disease [50–52, 56]. Too few other cases have been followed to know whether this is true for HCA not related to OCs or to glycogen storage disease. There are a few reported cases of hepatocellular carcinoma arising in OC-associated HCA, but this is extremely rare [40, 57]. Most reported cases of hepatocellular carcinoma in women taking OCs are probably coincidental [58]. Surgical resection is usually advised for HCA, however, to prevent the possibility of rupture and hemorrhage. Recurrence is unusual if use of the OCs has been discontinued; many cases of recurrent adenoma were probably really NRH in which resection of one large nodule stimulated the growth of other nodules. Preg-

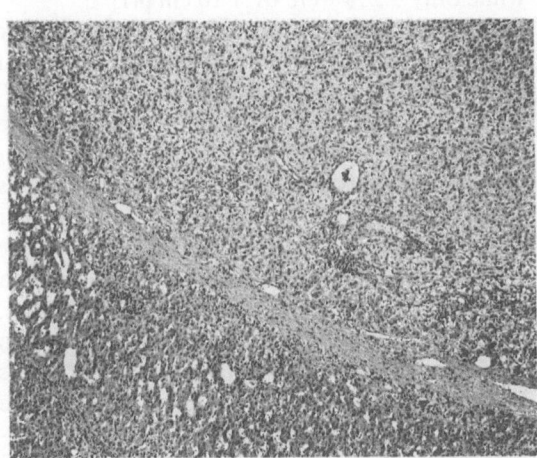

Fig. 8.6. Hepatocellular adenoma. Sheetlike growth of large pale hepatocytes (*upper right*) compressing the normal, darker-staining hepatic parenchyma. H and E, AFIP neg 86-8025, × 60

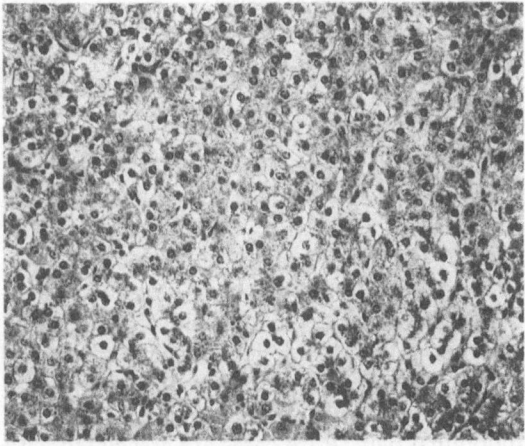

Fig. 8.7. Hepatocellular adenoma. Sheetlike growth of plump, benign hepatocytes with low nuclear-cytoplasmic ratio, abundant pale cytoplasm, and regular round nuclei. H and E, AFIP neg 86-8026, × 250

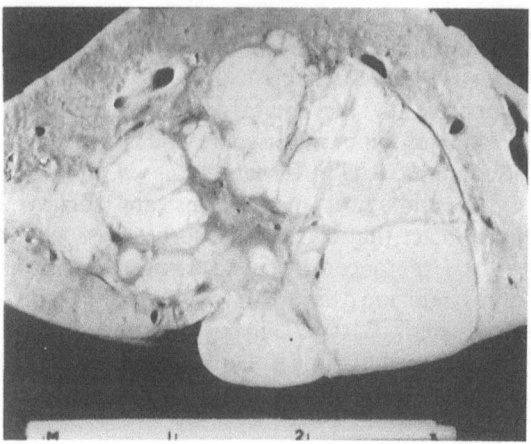

Fig. 8.8. Focal nodular hyperplasia. Cut section shows the central "stellate" scar, producing umbilication of the capsular surface. AFIP neg 86-7405

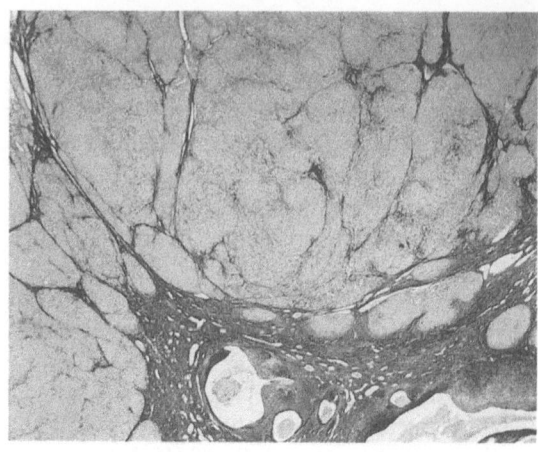

Fig. 8.9. Focal nodular hyperplasia. The central scar (*bottom center*) contains several large arteries. Fibrous septa radiate from the scar, separating the hyperplastic nodules. PAS stain, AFIP neg 86-8027, × 15

nancy is reported to cause unresected HCAs to grow, become symptomatic, and sometimes rupture [59], but women who have had their tumors resected do not have further problems during subsequent pregnancy [28].

3   Focal nodular hyperplasia

Focal nodular hyperplasia (FNH), which has also been called focal cirrhosis, hepatic hamartoma, benign hepatoma, mixed adenoma of the liver, hamartomatous cholangiohepatoma, and "hepatic adenoma" [30], is most notable for its confusion with hepatocellular adenoma. FNH is usually considered to be a tumorlike malformation rather than a neoplasm.

3.1   Clinical features

FNH occurs in both sexes and at all ages [2, 29, 32, 37, 38, 40, 41, 60, 61]. Cases have been reported from infancy to the eighth decade of life, but the greatest number of reported cases have been between 20 and 50 years of age. In every series, females have outnumbered males by 2 or more to 1. Most lesions are incidental findings at surgery or autopsy. Less than 20% cause symptoms, usually awareness of a mass or upper abdominal pain. Rare cases are associated with portal hypertension [2, 37], usually for uncertain reasons. A few patients, almost always women taking OCs, have presented with rupture of the lesion and hemoperitoneum [37, 62].

3.2   Pathology

FNH is usually a solitary nodule with a typical gross appearance (Fig. 8.8). The lesions are well circumscribed but unencapsulated. On the surface of the liver they may appear umbilicated. They are usually a lighter color than the surrounding liver, ranging from yellow to tan or light brown. The cut surface typically contains a central "stellate" scar with radiating fibrous septa, dividing the lesion into nodules. FNH is usually a small lesion, in contrast to HCA. In one large series, 84% were less than 5 cm in diameter, while only 3.2% were over 10 cm [41].

The microscopic features correspond to the gross pathology. A section through the center of lesion nearly always shows the central "stellate" scar (Fig. 8.9). This usually contains one or more large arteries, often with abnormal intimal or medial fibromuscular proliferation. Bile ducts are usually present but of a much smaller caliber than the artery. Fibrous septa of variable size radiate from the central scar. The septa contain a mild to moderate inflammatory cell infiltrate, predominantly lymphocytes. Between the septa are hyperplastic nodules of normal hepatocytes in plates two or more cells thick. Cholestatic features (canalicular bile plugs, pseudoxanthomatous change, copper storage) are usually present to some degree and are occasionally prominent [63]. Proliferating ductules are frequent within the septa and at the junction of the septa and hyperplastic nodules (Fig. 8.10).

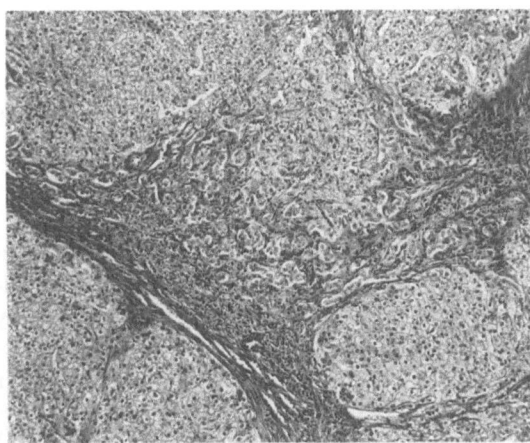

Fig. 8.10. Focal nodular hyperplasia. Fibrous septa containing proliferating ductules and inflammatory cells separate the hyperplastic hepatocellular nodules. H and E, AFIP neg 86-8028, × 100

3.3 Pathogenesis

Most observers have suggested that FNH is a hamartoma or response to a vascular malformation, rather than a neoplasm [47, 61, 64]. Wanless et al. [65] demonstrated that the lesions have an artery larger than would be expected for that part of the liver but no portal vein branches, suggesting that the hyperplastic nodules form as a response to arterialization of the blood supply or increased blood flow in the sinusoids. Most authors have concluded that OCs do not cause FNH, that any apparent association is due to the fact that FNH seems to be more common in women in the reproductive years, and that liver tumors in women taking OCs may be over-reported [38, 40, 41, 60]. However, it is also possible that OCs may have a trophic effect on FNH. Nearly all reported cases of rupture and hemorrhage of FNH have occurred in women taking OCs, and there have ben a few reported cases of FNH that have regressed in size after OCs or estrogens were stopped [37, 62, 66, 67].

3.4 Natural history

FNH is a benign, nonprogressive lesion. Cases of "malignant transformation" probably always represent misdiagnosis; most of these are actually cases of fibrolamellar carcinoma of the liver which grossly can look like FNH [68]. Those few cases of symptomatic FNH can be treated by simple excision, unless the size or location make this unfeasable. Radiological studies can sometimes help distinguish FNH from HCA preoper-

atively [38, 40, 69–72]. Features said to be helpful in differential diagnosis include uptake of colloid on radionuclide scan (more frequent in FNH), a central artery with a "spokewheel pattern" on arteriogram (more frequent in FNH), a central scar on computed tomography (CT) or sonography (more frequent in FNH), or hemorrhage into the tumor (more frequent in HCA).

4 Bile duct adenoma

Other names that have been used for bile duct adenoma (BDA) include "benign cholangioma" and "cholangioadenoma" [30]. BDA is always a small, almost trivial lesion. Its only clinical significance lies in the potential confusion with the equally benign von Meyenburg complex or with an adenocarcinoma.

4.1 Clinical features

These tumors are probably not uncommon, but they have only rarely been described in the literature. Series of 68 [2] and 16 [73] cases have been described. Gold et al. [37] included ten cases in a review of benign liver tumors. This was nearly equal to the number of cases of HCA and about half of the number of cases of FNH in their hospital. All but a few of the reported patients have been over 40 years old. The large series from the Armed Forces Institute of Pathology [2] had a marked male predominance (49/68 cases), while the two smaller series had about equal numbers of men and women. BDA is virtually always an incidental finding at autopsy or in a patient undergoing surgery for some other reason. No symptoms or signs have been attributed to this tumor. When one of these tumors is discovered during surgery for carcinoma of another organ (e.g., colon or stomach), a biopsy may be performed for frozen section diagnosis, and a pathologist who is unaware of this entity may be tempted to call the lesion metastatic adenocarcinoma. However, BDA has no known malignant potential.

4.2 Pathology

BDA is usually a solitary subcapsular nodule, although occasionally livers have more than one. The tumors may grow up to 4 cm in diameter, but this is uncommon and 90% are 1 cm or less. The lesions are firm, white, and discrete, but unencapsulated. Microscopically, they are composed of a proliferation of small, round, normal-

appearing ducts with cuboidal, slightly basophilic cells that have very regular nuclei and
lack any evidence of dysplasia or mitotic figures
(Fig. 8.11). There is always a fibrous supporting
stroma that may be very dense and hyalinized.
Preexisting normal or inflamed portal areas may
be present within the tumor.

5   Von Meyenberg complex (biliary microhamartoma)

This lesion is sometimes confused with bile duct
adenoma, but it is a hamartomatous malformation, part of the spectrum of the fibropolycystic
diseases, rather than a neoplasm. Like bile duct
adenoma, the von Meyenburg complex is sometimes mistaken for metastatic adenocarcinoma
by the unwary.

5.1   Clinical features

The lesions may be single or multiple. When
multiple, the patient may be considered to have a
very mild form of adult-type polycystic liver disease. They may also be found in patients with
other features of polycystic disease (adult or infantile types), congenital hepatic fibrosis, or
Caroli's disease [74, 75]. Most often von Meyenberg complexes are incidental findings at autopsy
or in biopsies done for some other indication,
and consequently they tend to be found in older
individuals. There is no predominance of either
sex. Symptoms, signs, or complications from

these lesions are extremely uncommon. There are
rare reported cases of portal hypertension attributed to multiple von Meyenberg complexes
[75] or of carcinoma arising in a von Meyenberg
complex [74].

5.2   Pathology

The lesions are small, seldom more than 5 mm in
diameter. They are usually multiple and typically are adjacent to a portal area although it may
not be visible in the plane of section. Within a
fibrous or hyalinized stroma, there are irregular
or rounded ductal structures that appear somewhat dilated and have a flattened or cuboidal
epithelium (Fig. 8.12). The lumina contain pro-
teinaceous or bile-stained secretions, but there
are no communications with the biliary system.
The distinction from BDA is usually readily
apparent.

5.3   Pathogenesis

The lesions are considered to be hamartomas
that result from an arrest of development or abnormal remodeling of the primitive ductal plate
that is the precursor of the normal bile duct [76].

6   Biliary cystadenoma

This is a relatively rare tumor which is similar
clinically and histologically to the mucinous cystadenomas of the pancreas [77]. There are less
than 100 reported cases of cystadenomas of the

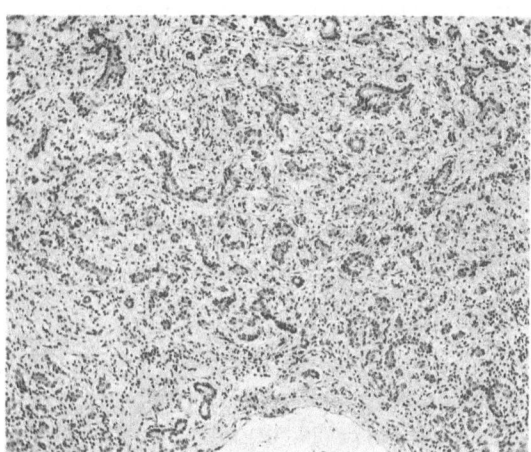

Fig. 8.11. Bile duct adenoma. Small benign bile ducts
in a fibrous stroma. H and E, AFIP neg 68-9426,
× 115

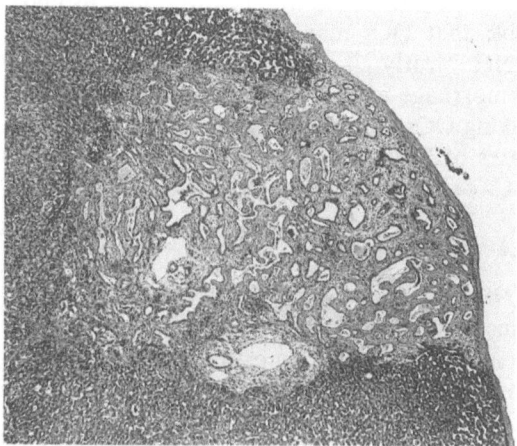

Fig. 8.12. Von Meyenburg complex. Small nodule adjacent to portal area with irregular, serpiginous ducts
in a fibrous stroma. H and E, AFIP neg 86-8030, × 40

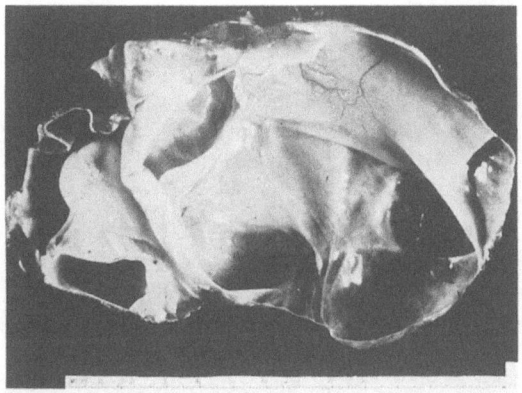

Fig. 8.13. Biliary cystadenoma. Resected specimen showing a collapsed 14-cm multilocular cyst. AFIP neg 75-13649

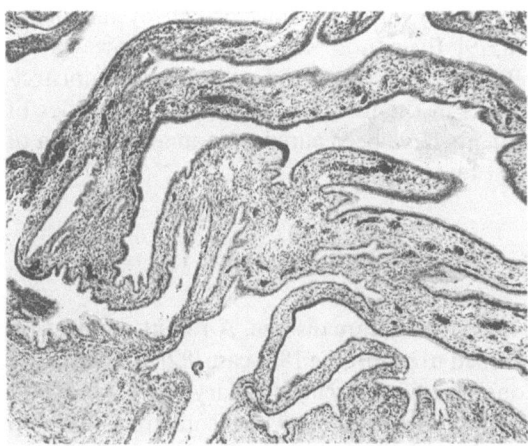

Fig. 8.14. Biliary cystadenoma. Multiple locules lined with mucinous glandular epithelium overlying a compact, cellular stroma. H and E, AFIP neg 86-8031, × 60

liver and bile ducts, and in a critical review of the literature less than half of these were found to be adequately documented and acceptable as examples of this tumor [78].

6.1 Clinical features

This is predominantly a tumor of middle-aged women [78, 79]. Over 85% of reported cases are females, and 80% are over 30 years old with a peak incidence in the fifth decade of life. The tumors are nearly always symptomatic with variable findings depending on size and exact location. Pain and/or abdominal enlargement are most frequent. Occasional patients have biliary obstruction with resultant jaundice or ascending infection. Cases have been reported with rupture of the tumor [80] and with findings or complications attributed to pressure on adjacent organs, including thrombosis of the inferior vena cava [81]. The tumors are slow-growing; some patients have had symptoms for as long as 12 years.

6.2 Pathology

The key feature is that biliary cystadenoma is a *multilocular* cyst (Fig. 8.13). Development cysts are never truly multilocular (although secondary changes occasionally make them seem so). Cystadenomas may occur anywhere in the intra- or extrahepatic bile ducts, but nearly all are partly or totally within the liver. They are usually globular with a smooth external surface. The lesions have ranged in diameter from 2.5 to 25 cm. Most are over 10 cm in diameter. The locules

of the cyst also vary in size. In some cases, the locules are approximately equal in size. In other cases, one locule predominates, giving an appearance of a unilocular cyst. However, even in those cases, examination of the wall reveals other, smaller locules. The fluid within the locules ranges from clear to cloudy, mucinous, or gelatinous and from white to yellow to brown. The lining may be smooth or trabeculated.

Microscopically, biliary cystadenoma has a mucin-secreting columnar epithelium lining the cysts (Fig. 8.14). The lining cells have pale eosinophilic cytoplasm and basally oriented nuclei, typical of biliary-type epithelium. The epithelium is supported by what has been called a "mesenchymal stroma." This is compact and cellular and resembles the stroma of the ovary. The stromal cells are spindled or oval and for the most part resemble fibroblasts, although smooth muscle, fat, and capillary components have also been described [78]. The septa between the cysts often show secondary changes, including foamy or pigmented macrophages, cholesterol clefts, inflammation, scarring, and sometimes calcification.

6.3 Natural history

The origin and exact histogenesis of biliary cystadenoma remain uncertain. Ectopic ovarian tissue and embryonic foregut rests have been suggested as sources of the neoplasms, and the resemblence to embryonic gallbladder has been noted [78]. Biliary cystadenoma is regarded as a premalignant tumor. In the two largest series, 10 of 31 cases had evidence of a cystadenocarcinoma arising in a previous benign cystadenoma [78, 79]. Even those with carcinoma, however, do relatively well compared with other adenocarcinomas in the liver and bile ducts; a number of patients have been cured by primary excision of the tumor.

7   Biliary papillomatosis

This is a very rare disease. A recent publication claimed to report the 18th case [82]. The disorder consists of multicentric biliary tract adenomatous polypoid tumors which sometimes develop invasive adenocarcinoma. Thus, it is similar to polyposis coli.

7.1   Clinical features

Reported cases have ranged from 42 to 72 years in age [82, 86]. Men outnumber women by 2 to 1. Patients present with obstructive jaundice and die within a few years as a result of recurrent ascending cholangitis, liver failure, or carcinoma. In rare cases with limitation to one lobe of the liver, the patient has been cured by radical surgery [86].

7.2   Pathology

The lesions may occur anywhere in the extra- or intrahepatic bile ducts. They are described as being soft, friable, and white to red or tan. They are usually sessile, but are occasionally grossly papillary, and may grow as large as 3 cm. The bile ducts proximal to the tumors are dilated and the livers show inflammatory and cholestatic changes secondary to obstruction. Microscopically, the tumors are papillary adenomas with delicate fibrovascular stalks that have many branches and papillary fronds covered with a glandular epithelium (Fig. 8.15). The epithelial layer is adenomatous, usually with tall cells with a pale eosinophilic cytoplasm and basally oriented nuclei. However, there may be variable degrees of atypia and occasionally carcinoma, either in situ or frankly invasive, may be present.

8   Hemangioma

Small benign vascular tumors are common in many areas of the body, including the liver. Only occasionally do they become large enough to be clinically important. Cavernous hemangioma, sclerosing hemangioma, solitary necrotic nod-

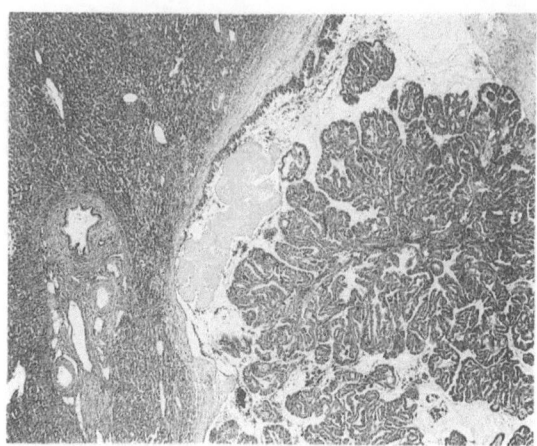

Fig. 8.15. Biliary papillomatosis. A markedly dilated intrahepatic bile duct containing an adenomatous papillary epithelial proliferation. H and E, AFIP neg 86-8032, × 25

ule, and various other synonyms have been used to describe different stages of the development and involution of this lesion [4, 30, 87].

8.1   Clinical features

Hemangiomas of the liver are fairly common. Their reported incidence depends on how vigorously they are sought. Various series report figures ranging from less than 1% to 20% for incidental hepatic hemangiomas found at autopsy [30, 88–91]. Hemangiomas occur at all ages, although they are most often diagnosed in adults. Most series have reported a greater frequency in women than in men, although the figures have ranged from a slight male predominence [30] to a 6 to 1 female predominance [88]. However, it may be that hemangiomas tend to be larger in women and therefore more often symptomatic and diagnosed. A role of sex hormones in the pathogenesis of this tumor has been suggested [2, 4, 30], but there is little evidence to support this.

Hemangiomas less than 4 cm in diameter are rarely symptomatic. About 40% of those 4 cm or larger are associated with symptoms [92]. Pain or discomfort, abdominal enlargement, mass and/or hepatomegaly are most frequent. The pain is rarely severe, and its exact cause is seldom apparent. Since surgically resected hepatic hemangiomas frequently contain organizing thrombi, it may be that recurrent or intermittent thromboses cause the tumors to swell, producing

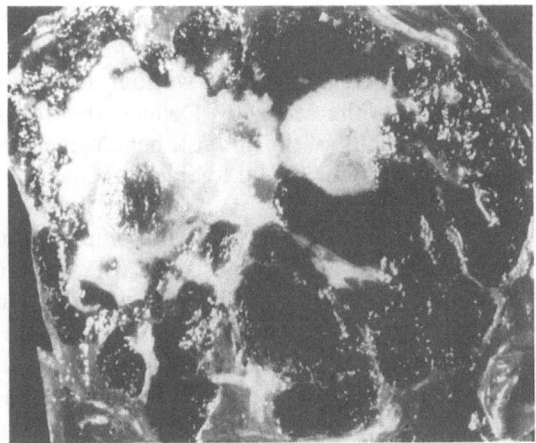

Fig. 8.16. Cavernous hemangioma. Cut section shows a spongy blood-filled mass with white areas of thrombosis and scarring. AFIP neg 86-7391

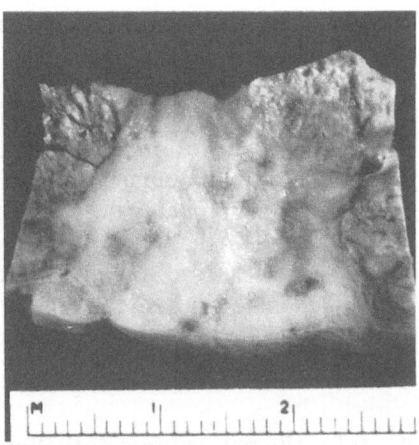

Fig. 8.17. Sclerosed hemangioma. The end result of a hemangioma with thrombosis and scarring, leaving a fibrous nodule. AFIP neg 68-4663

stretching of Glisson's capsule and pain. Rare reported cases have presented with spontaneous rupture of the hemangioma [93], but the true incidence of this complication is not known. Even rarer is the dramatic syndrome of consumptive coagulopathy, thrombocytopenia, and hypofibrinogenemia occasionally associated with large hepatic hemangiomas [94, 95].

The various radiological modalities (Chap. 19–23) have all been reported to have useful roles in the detection and diagnosis of hepatic hemangiomas. This is especially important because needle biopsy of hemangiomas may lead to severe hemorrhage [92]. Characteristic findings are detected by sonography [96], CT [97–99], and arteriography [100].

8.2 Pathology

Hepatic hemangiomas are usually solitary. Only about 10% are multiple [4]. The vast majority are less than 4 cm in diameter, but occasional tumors may be as large as 30 cm. They may occur anywhere in the liver and are sometimes present on the capsular surface. When viewed through the capsule, they appear as red or purple blotches. On cut section, they are spongy with relatively little tissue and a great deal of dark, venous blood (Fig. 8.16). Hemangiomas sometimes undergo regressive changes. Areas of thrombosis (recent or old), scarring, and occasionally calcification may be present in older hemangiomas. They sometimes reach the end stage of this process and resemble a fibrous scar, i.e., a "sclerosed

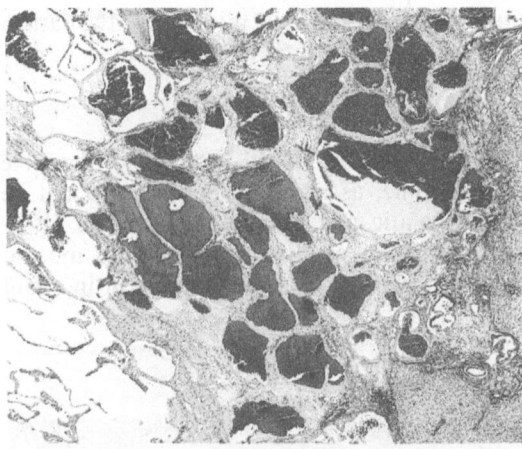

Fig. 8.18. Cavernous hemangioma. Multiple, thin-walled, variable-sized, blood-filled, endothelial-lined vascular spaces comprise the tumor. H and E, AFIP neg 86-8033, × 25

hemangioma," (Fig. 8.17) and may even become entirely calcified.

Microscopically, cavernous hemangiomas are composed of vascular channels of various size lined by flattened endothelial cells (Fig. 8.18). They are usually discrete and well-demarcated from the surrounding liver, although an occasional hemangioma may contain trapped bile ducts or foci of parenchyma. Variable amounts of fibrous tissue separate the vascular channels. Many consist of thin, delicate strands, but large areas of scarring may be present. Fresh and organizing thrombi may be found in the vascular channels. The dynamics of these thrombi are not known, but they are commonly observed in surgically resected hemangiomas. Because of the sluggish blood flow through these tumors, small thrombi probably form and lyse constantly. Fibroblasts can be found growing into a few thrombi and are probably the source of the scarring that results in the "sclerosing hemangioma." In end-stage sclerosed and/or calcified hemangiomas, an underlying vascular pattern can usually still be discerned, providing the clue to the diagnosis.

9   Infantile hemangioendothelioma

This is similar to the capillary hemangiomas of infancy that are relatively common in the skin and mucous membranes. They are rarely diagnosed in the viscera. As in other sites, hepatic hemangioendotheliomas typically undergo stages of proliferation, maturation, and involution and will eventually disappear if the patient does not develop a fatal complication.

9.1   Clinical features

The true incidence of this tumor is impossible to determine, as many small lesions could be asymptomatic and remain undiagnosed [101–107]. Cutaneous capillary hemangiomas, most of which are clinically insignificant, occur in about 0.5% of neonates [108]; it is conceivable that small hepatic hemangioendotheliomas remain clinically occult and regress without attracting attention. In the series by Dehner and Ishak [101], nearly half of the infantile hemangioendotheliomas were incidental findings at surgery or autopsy.

Nearly all cases, both symptomatic and asymptomatic, are diagnosed in the first 6 months of life. A few cases have been reported in adults [103], but these are unusual. Females outnumber males by 2 : 1. Hepatomegaly and/or an abdominal mass is a frequent mode of presentation. Coincidental cutaneous hemangiomas are frequent, being reported in 19%–87% of patients [102, 106, 107]. Some patients, and in some series the majority of symptomatic patients, present with high-output congestive heart failure due to arteriovenous shunting through the tumor [109].

The natural history of this tumor is variable and belies its histologically benign nature. Up to two-thirds of symptomatic patients may die as a result of the tumor. Causes of death include congestive heart failure, hepatic failure, or rupture of the tumor with hemorrhage. Surgical resection may be possible, but is often not since the tumor is frequently multicentric. Hence, hepatic artery ligation or embolization [105, 110–112], radiation [106, 113], and corticosteroids [106, 109, 114] have been suggested as alternative therapies. If life-threatening complications can be avoided,

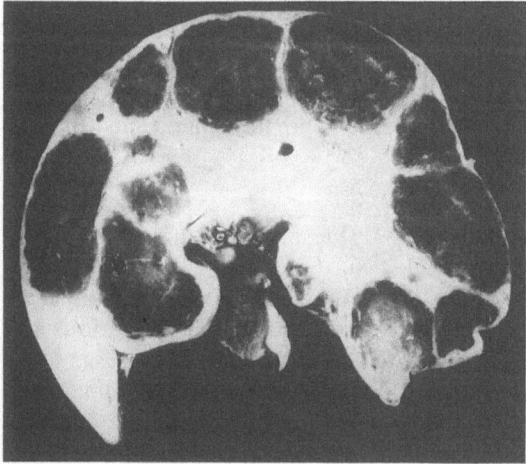

Fig. 8.19. Infantile hemangioendothelioma. Autopsy specimen showing multiple large vascular tumors within the liver. AFIP neg 86-7401

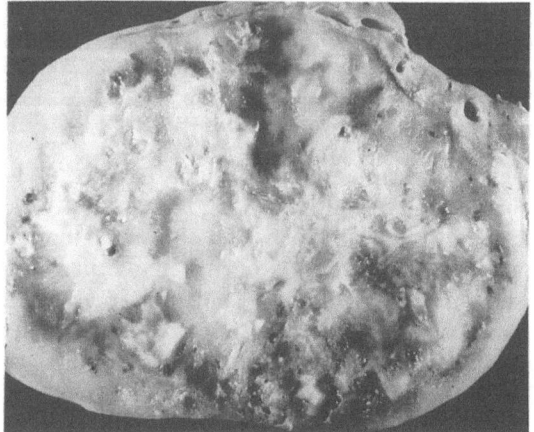

Fig. 8.20. Infantile hemangioendothelioma. Resected specimen showing mottled, laminated appearance. The center has irregular yellow-white areas of necrosis, scarring, and focal calcification, while the periphery, containing the proliferating capillary channels, is reddish-brown and fleshy. AFIP neg 86-7402

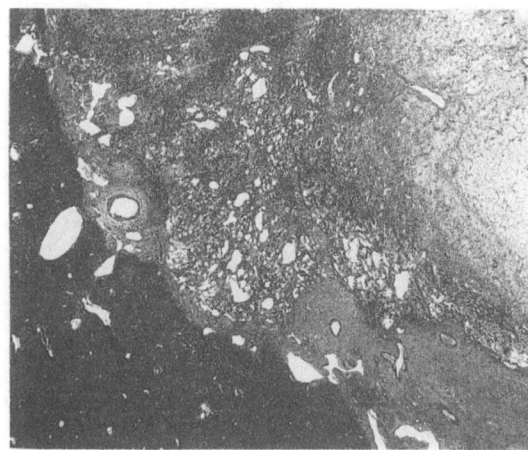

Fig. 8.21. Infantile hemangioendothelioma. The center of the tumor is necrotic (*upper right*) while the edge contains the proliferating vascular channels and trapped portal areas. H and E, AFIP neg 86-8034, × 15

Fig. 8.22. Infantile hemangioendothelioma. Plump endothelial cells line the predominantly capillary-sized vascular channels. Two larger "cavernous" vascular spaces are present and a few small bile ducts are trapped within the tumor. H and E, AFIP neg 86-8035, × 160

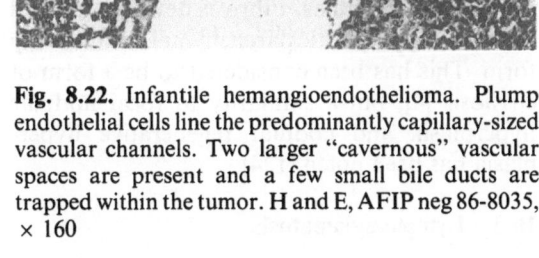

most tumors probably regress, and the patients usually do well. A few cases pursue an aggressive course with metastasis and death from disseminated disease. Dehner and Ishak [101] noted that these appeared histologically more aggressive and termed them type II hemangioendothelioma. Other cases have been reported as angiosarcoma arising in infantile hemangioendothelioma [115–117], but the distinction between cases such as these and type II hemangioendotheliomas is not always clear.

9.2 Pathology

The tumors may be single or multicentric and may occur anywhere in the liver (Fig. 8.19). Individual tumor nodules range from barely visible up to 15 cm in diameter. They are usually well demarcated fom the surrounding liver and appear red, brown, or white, depending on the degree of vascularity and involutional change. Some tumors appear laminated with yellowish-white areas of necrosis and scarring in the center and a reddish, well-vascularized periphery (Fig. 8.20).

Microscopically, the periphery of the tumor is composed of proliferating small vascular channels (capillarylike), which are irregularly shaped and lined by plump endothelial cells (Figs. 8.21, 8.22). There is relatively little fibrous stroma, but bile ducts and hepatocytes are often trapped within the advancing edge of the tumor. Toward the center of the tumor, the amount of stroma increases and number of vascular channels decreases. In many cases, the more centrally located vascular spaces are larger and "cavernous" with a flattened endothelium. Irregular zones of infarction, necrosis, hemorrhage, scarring, and foci of dystrophic calcification are usually present, accounting for the regression of the tumor. The endothelial cells of the proliferating vascular channels at the periphery constitute the neoplastic element. Dehner and Ishak [101] distinguished between type I tumors, in which cytologically bland endothelial cells formed a single layer around the vascular channels, and type II tumors, which had more pleomorphic and hyperchromatic endothelial cells with intravascular budding and branching. The latter were felt to be more aggressive tumors.

10 Other tumorlike vascular lesions

10.1 Peliosis hepatis

This is a very rare lesion characterized by scattered lakes of blood of variable size (1 mm to several centimeters) with or without an endothelial lining. Peliosis was formerly seen primarily at autopsy as a complication of chronic wasting diseases such as tuberculosis and cancer. It is now more often associated with anabolic steroid therapy and occasionally other drugs [118, 119]. The pathogenesis is unknown. Theories which have been proposed include toxic damage to the endothelium [120], focal parenchymal necrosis and cavitation [121], and blockage of the sinusoidal-terminal hepatic venule junction by fibrosis or by hyperplastic hepatocytes [122, 123]. The natural history is variable. Some lesions are incidental autopsy findings, while others are clinically important, causing hepatomegaly, portal hypertension, liver failure, or rupture and hemorrhage [119, 121].

10.2 Hereditary hemorrhagic telangiectasia

This can involve the liver with telangiectases and arteriovenous fistulas. Fibrosis develops around these and hyperplastic parenchymal nodules may form. This has been considered to be a form of cirrhosis [4], but a similarity to focal nodular hyperplasia and nodular regenerative hyperplasia has been noted [124].

10.3 Lymphangiomatosis

This is a rare multisystem disease in which lymphangiomas are present in multiple organs, including the liver [125]. The lesions consist of endothelial-lined lymphatic channels that form spongy fluid-filled lesions up to 5 cm in diameter.

11 Mesenchymal hamartoma

This is a rare tumorlike malformation of the liver that occurs predominantly in young children. Its pathogenesis is unknown, but the most likely cause seems to be an aberration in embryonic development of the liver coupled with secondary degenerative changes. The largest and most definitive series is that of Stocker and Ishak [126], who reported 30 cases and reviewed 42 others from the literature.

11.1 Clinical features

Reported cases have ranged in age from newborn up to 19 years, but approximately 85% are under 2 years of age. About 60% of reported patients are male. In a few cases, the lesions have been incidental findings at autopsy, but most are symptomatic. Nearly all present with abdominal enlargement or an abdominal mass; in a few, pain was present or there was failure to thrive. Radiological studies show a multilocular or multicystic mass, especially evident by sonography or CT [127]. Most cases have been treated by surgical excision of the mass. None have been reported to recur. Those cases which were biopsied but not resected have also done well, and

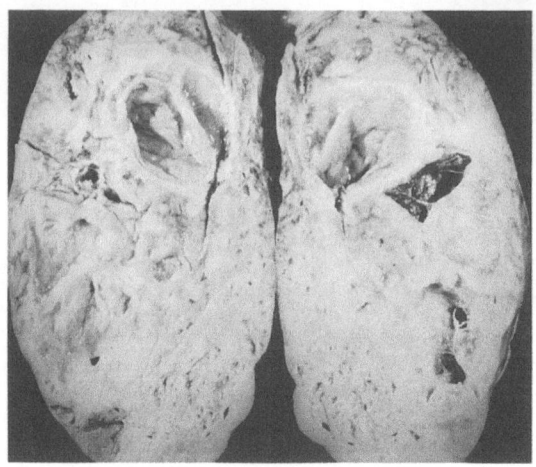

Fig. 8.23. Mesenchymal hamartoma. Bisected resection specimen showing multiple cysts within the firm tan-white mesenchymal tissue. AFIP neg 86-7399

so conservative therapy is recommended in cases where complete excision carries a high operative risk. It has been suggested that the undifferentiated (embryonal) sarcoma of the liver may be the malignant counterpart of mesenchymal hamartoma [128], but there is no direct evidence that mesenchymal hamartoma ever becomes malignant.

11.2 Pathology

The lesions can occur in any part of the liver and may be pedunculated or protrude from surface. They are usually globular or ovoid with irregular borders, sometimes appearing to invade the adjacent liver or to have satellite lesions. Reported cases have ranged 5–29 cm in greatest dimension, often forming an impressive abdominal mass, considering the small size of most of the patients. They typically contain multiple cysts of varying size, ranging from barely visible to 14 cm (Fig. 8.23). Some larger ones appear multilocular. The cysts contain clear, yellow, or gelatinous fluid. The tissue between the cysts can be white and fibrous, yellow and myxoid, tan and firm.

Microscopically, the lesions consist of disorganized arrangements of primitive mesenchyme, bile ducts, and hepatic parenchyma (Fig. 8.24). The mesenchymal element consists of a mixture of stellate cells and collagen in a loose, myxoid stroma. In some areas, the stroma undergoes cystic degeneration, producing the grossly visible cysts and giving rise to areas that resemble a lymphangioma (Fig. 8.25). In other areas, the

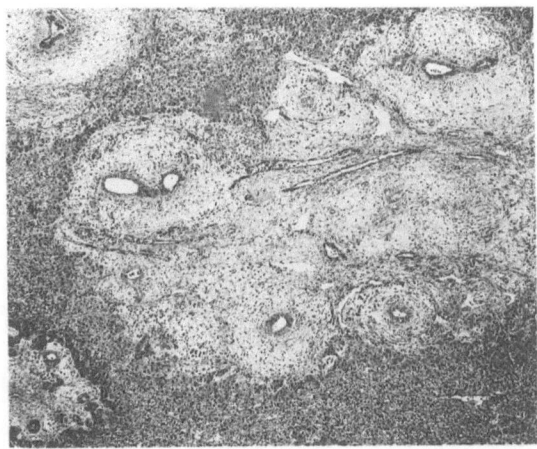

Fig. 8.24. Mesenchymal hamartoma. Masses of primitive loose mesenchyme surround abnormal bile ducts. Cords of hepatocytes are present, but lack lobular architecture. H and E, AFIP neg 86-8036, × 60

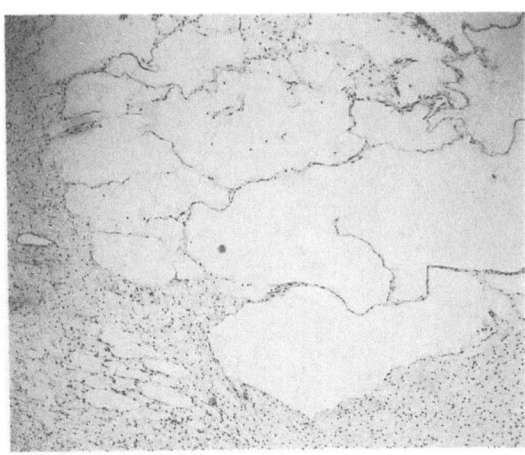

Fig. 8.25. Mesenchymal hamartoma. Lymphangiomalike area of cystic degeneration within the primitive mesenchyme. H and E, AFIP neg 86-8037, × 60

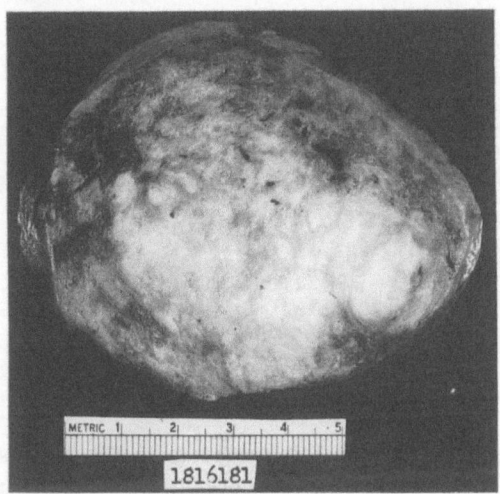

Fig. 8.26. Fibrous mesothelioma. Cut surface of pedunculated tumor from surface of liver, showing whorls of grayish-white fibrous tissue. AFIP neg 82-6029

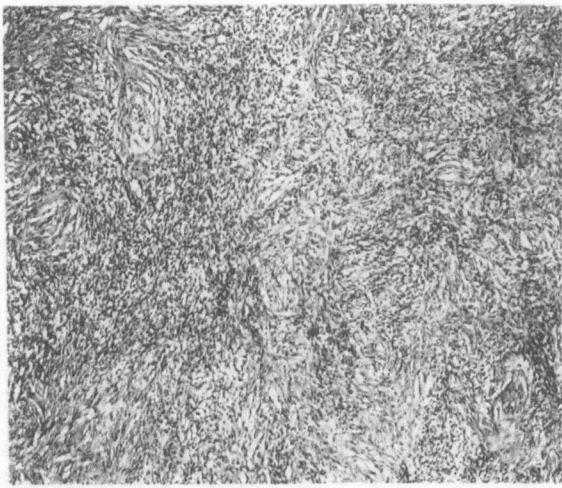

Fig. 8.27. Fibrous mesothelioma. Interlacing bundles of collagen and fibroblastlike spindle cells. H and E, AFIP neg 86-8038, × 60

mesenchyme surrounds bile ducts that often appear abnormal, irregular, and inflamed. Variable numbers of normal-appearing hepatocytes are present in the lesions, but lobular architecture is not present.

12 Other benign tumors and tumorlike lesions

12.1 Leiomyomas

Primary leiomyomas in the liver have been re-ported in three patients [129]. They may reach a large size (up to 3750 g). The histological features are similar to benign smooth muscle tumors at other sites.

12.2 Fibrous mesotheliomas or fibromas

These have been reported as localized tumors on the surface of the liver [4, 130]. Like leiomyomas, they may attain a large size (Fig. 8.26). Their histogenesis is uncertain, but histologically they consist of fibroblastlike spindle cells and collagen (Fig. 8.27).

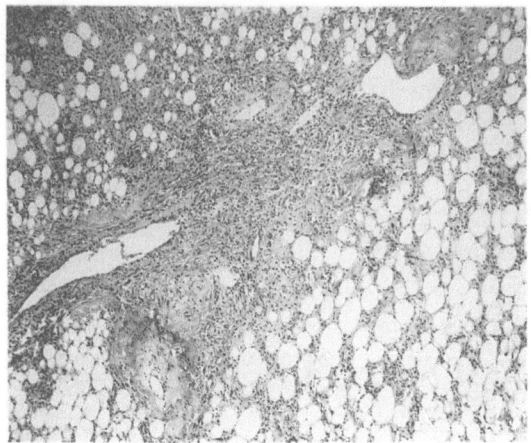

Fig. 8.28. Angiomyolipoma. The tumor is compsed of adipose cells, smooth muscle, and tortuous thick walled blood vessels. H and E, AFIP neg 86-8039, × 60

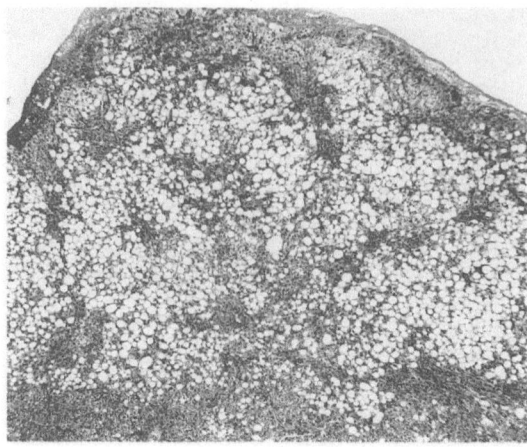

Fig. 8.29. Focal fatty change of the liver. A discrete area of hepatocellular fat accumulation, forming a tumorlike mass. H and E, AFIP neg 86-8040, × 40

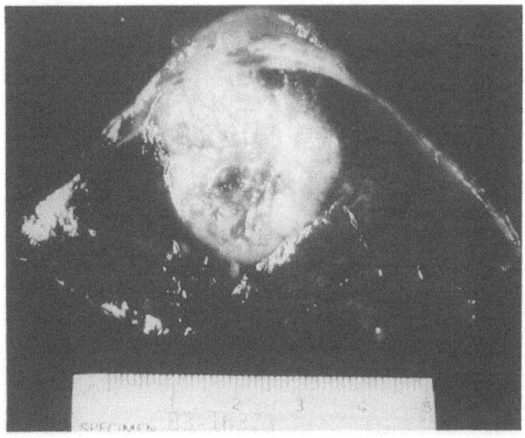

Fig. 8.30. Inflammatory pseudotumor. A discrete, firm white mass within the hepatic parenchyma. AFIP neg 86-7396

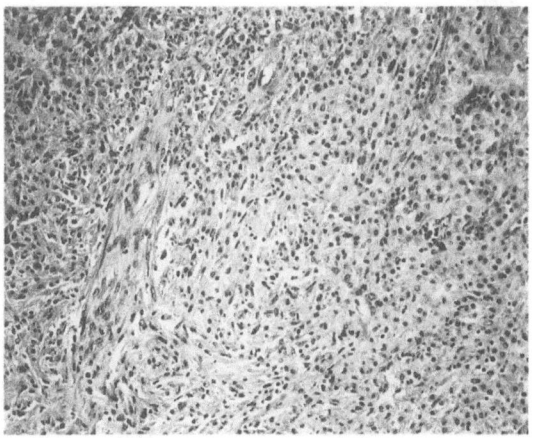

Fig. 8.31. Inflammatory pseudotumor. The mass is composed of a mixture of inflammatory cells, fibroblasts, and foamy macrophages. H and E, AFIP neg 86-8041, × 160

12.3 Lipomatous tumors

Lipomatous tumors of the liver have been rarely reported in the past but will probably be found more frequently in the future due to the ease with which they are detected with CT [131]. Previously reported cases of various lipomatous tumors range in size from less than 1 to 20 cm [4, 132–135]. All have been in adults with no sex predominance. Most have been asymptomatic, usually incidental findings, but a few have presented with abdominal pain from hemorrhage into the tumor. In this category are included *lipomas*, composed entirely of mature fat, *angiolipomas*, composed of fat and blood vessels, *my-* *elolipomas*, composed of fat and hematopoietic tissue, *angiomyelolipomas*, composed of fat, vessels, and hematopoietic cells, *angiomyolipomas*, composed of fat, blood vessels, and smooth muscle (Fig. 8.28), and *angiomyomyelolipomas*, with hematopoietic elements. *Pseudolipomas* (also called coelomic fat ectopia), representing epiploic appendices that become attached to the liver or within the liver parenchyma have also been described. *Focal fatty change* of the liver may also present as a tumorlike lesion noted incidentally at surgery [136] or found by sonography or CT [137]. It consists of a localized area of hepatocellular fat accumulation (Fig. 8.29), the cause of which is unknown.

12.4 Benign teratomas

Benign teratomas of the liver have been reported rarely [138, 139]. Most have been found in infants or young children who presented with an abdominal mass. Microscopically, mature or immature tissues derived from all three germ layers must be present to make the diagnosis, as in teratomas of other more common sites. Skin, bone, and gastrointestinal mucosa are frequent findings.

12.5 Adrenal rest tumors

Adrenal rest tumors, presumably derived from ectopic adrenal tissue, have been reported to have caused Cushing's syndrome and virilization [140]. Histologically, these are identical to adrenal cortical tumors.

12.6 Pancreatic heterotopias

These have rarely presented as hepatic masses [141].

12.7 Inflammatory pseudotumors

Inflammatory pseudotumors of the liver have been reported several times [142, 143] but are probably more frequent than has been recognized. Cases have been reported in children and adults, usually with systemic symptoms and fever. The lesions may be several centimeters in diameter (Fig. 8.30), and histologically they consist of variable amounts of acute and chronic inflammation with an exuberant proliferation of granulation tissue, numerous fibroblasts, and a variable number of foamy macrophages (Fig. 8.31). The mesenchymal proliferation has caused some cases to be mistaken for sarcomas. The cause and pathogenesis of these lesions remain unknown, but the clinical and pathological features suggest that they may be the result of healing abscesses with secondary extravasation of bile into the parenchyma. They bear a histological resemblance to inflammatory pseudotumors of other sites, such as lung and soft tissue, and to the xanthogranulomatous inflammation that sometimes occurs in gallbladders secondary to intramural bile extravasation [144].

References

1. Ishak KG, Goodman ZD (1985) Benign tumors of the liver. In: Berk JE (ed) Bockus gastroenterology, 4th edn. Saunders, Philadelphia, pp 3302–3314

2. Ishak KG, Rabin L (1975) Benign tumors of the liver. Med Clin N Am 59: 995–1013

3. Edmondson HA (1976) Benign epithelial tumors and tumorlike lesions of the liver. In: Okuda K, Peters RL (eds) Hepatocellular carcinoma. Wiley, New York, pp 309–330

4. Ishak KG (1976) Mesenchymal tumors of the liver. In: Okuda K, Peters RL (eds) Hepatocellular carcinoma. Wiley, New York, pp 247–307

5. Stromeyer FW, Ishak KG (1981) Nodular transformation (nodular "regenerative" hyperplasia) of the liver. A clinicopathologic study of 30 cases. Human Pathol 12: 60–71

6. Sherlock S, Feldman CA, Moran B, Scheuer PJ (1966) Partial nodular transformation of the liver portal hypertension. Am J Med 40: 195–203

7. Wanless IR, Lentz JS, Roberts EA (1985) Partial nodular transformation of the liver in an adult with persistent ductus venosus. Arch Pathol Lab Med 109: 427–432

8. Ranstrom S (1953) Miliary hepatocellular adenomatosis. Acta Path Microbiol Scand 33: 225–229

9. Smith JC (1978) Noncirrhotic nodulation of the liver. Arch Pathol Lab Med 102: 398–401

10. Gindhart TD, Cimis RJ, Mosenthal WT, Longnecker DS (1979) Adenomatous hyperplasia of the liver. Arch Pathol Lab Med 103: 34–37

11. Weinbren K, Mutum SS (1984) Pathologic aspects of diffuse nodular hyperplasia of the liver. J Pathol 143: 81–92

12. Flejou JF, Barge J, Menu Y, Degott C, Bismuth H, Potet F, Benhamou JP (1985) Liver adenomatosis. An entity distinct from liver adenoma? Gastroenterology 89: 1132–1138

13. Steiner PE (1959) Nodular regenerative hyperplasia of the liver. Am J Pathol 35: 943–953

14. Blendis LM, Parkinson MC, Shilkin KB, William R (1974) Nodular regenerative hyperplasia of the liver in Felty's syndrome. Quart J Med 43: 25–32

15. Wanless IR, Godwin TA, Allen F, Feder A (1980) Nodular regenerative hyperplasia of the liver in hematologic disorders: A possible response to obliterative portal venopathy. Medicine 59: 367–379

16. Wanless IR, Solt LC, Kortan P, Deck JHN, Gardiner GW, Prokipchuk EJ (1981) Nodular regenerative hyperplasia of the liver associated with macroglobulinemia. A clue to pathogenesis. Am J Med 70: 1203–1209

17. Thorne C, Urowitz MB, Wanless I, Roberts E, Blendis LM (1982) Liver disease in Felty's syndrome. Am J Med 73: 35–40

18. Thung SN, Gerber MA, Bodenheimer HC Jr (1982) Nodular regenerative hyperplasia of the liver in a patient with diabetes mellitus. Cancer 49: 543–546

19. Nakanuma Y, Ohta G, Sasaki K (1984) Nodular regenerative hyperplasia of the live associated with polyarteritis nodosa. Arch Pathol Lab Med 108: 133–135

20. Snover D, Bloomer J, McGlave P (1986) Nodular regenerative hyperplasia: A possible

cause of liver disease following bone marrow transplantation. Lab Invest 54: 60A

21. Stewart HL, Williams G, Keysser CH, Lombard LS, Montali RJ (1980) Histologic typing of liver tumors of the rat. J Natl Cancer Inst 64: 179–206

22. Farber E (1982) Neoplastic transformation. In: Arias I, Popper H, Schachter D, Shafritz DA (eds) The liver: Biology and pathobiology, Raven, New York, pp 811–819

23. Mones JM, Saldana MJ, Albores-Saaverdra J (1984) Nodular regenerative hyperplasia of the liver. Report of three cases and review of the literature. Arch Pathol Lab Med 108: 741–743

24. Popper H, Thomas LB, Telles NC, Falk H, Selikoff IJ (1978) Development of hepatic angiosarcoma in man induced by vinyl chloride, thorotrast, and arsenic. Am J Pathol 92: 349–376

25. Okuda K, Nakashima T, Okudaira M, Kage M, Aida Y, Omata M, Sugiura M, Kameda H, Inokuchi K, Bhusnurmath SR, Aikat BA (1982) Liver pathology of idiopathic portal hypertension. Comparison with non-cirrhotic portal hypertension of India. Liver 2: 176–192

26. Mikkelsen WP, Edmondson HA, Peters RL, Redeker AG, Reynolds TB (1965) Extra- and intrahepatic portal hypertension without cirrhosis (hepatoportal sclerosis). Ann Surg 162: 602–620

27. Edmondson HA, Henderson B, Benton B (1976) Liver-cell adenomas associated with use of oral contraceptives. Engl J Med 294: 470–472

28. Rooks JB, Ory HW, Ishak KG, Strauss LT, Greenspan JR, Hill AP, Tyler CW Jr (1979) Epidemiology of hepatocellular adenoma. The role of oral contraceptive use. JAMA 242: 644–648

29. Christopherson WM, Mays ET, Barrows GH (1980) Liver tumors in young women: A clinical pathologic study of 201 cases in the Louisville Registry. In: Fenoglio CM, Wolff M (eds). Progress in surgical pathology, vol II Masson, New York, pp 187–205

30. Edmondson HA (1958) Tumors of the liver and intrahepatic bile ducts. Atlas of tumor pathology. First Series. Fasc 25. Armed Forces Institute of Pathology, Washington

31. Baum JK, Holtz F, Bookstein JJ, Klein EW (1973) Possible association between benign hepatomas and oral contraceptives. Lancet 2: 926–929

32. Sorensen TIA, Baden H (1975) Benign hepatocellular tumors. Scand J Gastroent 10: 113–119

33. Ameriks JA, Thompson NW, Frey CF, Appelman HD, Walter JF (1975) Hepatic cell adenomas, spontaneous liver rupture, and oral contraceptives. Arch Surg 110: 548–557

34. McAvoy JM, Tompkins RK, Longmire WP Jr (1976) Benign hepatic tumors and their association with oral contraceptives. Arch Surg 111: 761–767

35. Kent DR, Nissen ED, Nissen SE (1977) Liver tumors and oral contraceptives. Int J Gynaecol Obstet 15: 137–142

36. Fechner RE (1977) Benign hepatic lesions and orally administered contraceptives. A report of seven cases and a critical analysis of the literature. Human Pathol 8: 255–268

37. Gold JH, Guzman IJ, Rosai J (1978) Benign tumors of the liver. Pathologic examination of 45 cases. Am J Clin Pathol 70: 6–17

38. Knowles DM, Casarella WJ, Johnson PM, Wolff M (1978) The clinical, radiologic, and pathologic characterization of benign hepatic neoplasms. Alleged association with oral contraceptives. Medicine 57: 223–237

39. Nime F, Pickren JW, Vana J, Aronoff BL, Baker HW, Murphy GP (1979) The histology of liver tumors in oral contraceptive users observed during a national survey by the American College of Surgeons Comission on Cancer. Cancer 44: 1481–1489

40. Kerlin P, Davis GL, McGill DB, Weiland LH, Adson MA, Sheedy PR II (1983) Hepatic adenoma and focal nodular hyperplasia: Clinical, pathologic, and radiologic features. Gastroenterology 84: 994–1002

41. Ishak KG (1979) Hepatic neoplasms associated with contraceptive and anabolic steroids. In: Lingeman CH (ed) Carcinogenic hormones. Springer, Berlin Heidelberg New York, 73–128

42. Wheeler DA, Edmondson HA, Reynolds TB (1986) Spontaneous liver cell adenoma in children. Am J Clin Pathol 85: 6–12

43. Monaco AP, Hallgrimsson J, McDermot WV (1964) Multiple adenoma (hamartoma) of the liver treated by subtotal (90%) resection. Ann Surg 159: 513–519

44. Lui AFK, Hiratzka LF, Hirose FM (1980) Multiple adenomas of the liver. Cancer 45: 1001–1004

45. Chen KTK, Bocian JJ (1983) Multiple hepatic adenomas. Arch Pathol Lab Med 107: 274–275

46. Malatjalian DA, Graham CH (1982) Liver adenoma with granulomas. The appearance of granulomas in oral contraceptive-related hepatocellular adenoma and in the surrounding nontumorous liver. Arch Pathol Lab Med 106: 244–246

47. Phillips MJ, Langer B, Stone R, Fisher MM, Ritchie S (1973) Benign liver cell tumors. Classification and ultrastructural pathology. Cancer 32: 463–470

48. Biolac-Sage P, Lamouliatte H, Saric J, Merlio JP, Balabaud C (1986) Ultrastructure of sinusoidal cells in a benign liver cell adenoma. Ultrastructural Pathol 1986; 10: 49–54

49. Wanless IR, Medline A (1982) Role of estrogens as promoters of hepatic neoplasia. Lab Invest 46: 313–320

50. Edmondson HA, Reynolds TB, Henderson B, Benton B (1977) Regression of liver cell adenomas associated with oral contraceptives. Ann Intern Med 86: 180–182

51. Steinbrecher UP, Lisbona R, Huang SN, Mishkin S (1981) Complete regression of hepatocellular adenoma after withdrawal of oral contraceptives. Dig Dis Sci 26: 1045–1050

52. Buhler H, Pirovino M, Akovbiantz A, Altorfer J, Weitzel M, Maranta E, Schmid M (1982) Regression of liver cell adenoma. A follow-up study of three consecutive patients after discontinuation of oral contraceptive use. Gastroenterology 82: 775–782

53. Howell RR, Stevenson RE, Ben-Menachem Y, Phyliky RL, Berry DH (1976) Hepatic adenomata associated with type 1 glycogen storage disease. JAMA 236: 1481–1484

54. Foster JH, Donohue TA, Berman MM (1978) Familial liver-cell adenomas and diabetes mellitus. N Engl J Med 299: 239–241

55. Cannon RO III, Dusheiko GM, Long JA Jr, Ishak KG, Kapur S, Anderson KD, Nienhuis AW (1981) Hepatocellular adenoma in a young woman with beta-thalassemia and secondary iron overload. Gastroenterology 81: 352–355

56. Parker P, Burr I, Slonim A, Ghishan FK, Greene H (1981) Regression of hepatic adenomas in type Ia glycogen storage disease with dietary therapy. Gastroenterology 81: 534–536

57. Tesluk H, Lawrie J (1981) Hepatocellular adenoma. Its transformation to carcinoma in a user of oral contraceptives. Arch Pathol Lab Med 105: 296–299

58. Goodman ZD, Ishak KG (1982) Hepatocellular carcinoma in women: Probable lack of etiologic association with oral contraceptive steroids. Hepatology 2: 440–444

59. Kent Dr, Nissen ED, Nissen SE, Ziehm, DJ (1978) Effect of pregnancy on liver tumor associated with oral contraceptives. Obstet Gynecol 51: 148–151

60. Knowles DM II, Wolff M (1976) Focal nodular hyperplasia of the liver. A clinicopathologic study and review of the literature. Human Pathol 7: 533–545

61. Stocker JT, Ishak KG (1981) Focal nodular hyperplasia of the liver: A study of 21 pediatric cases. Cancer 48: 336–345

62. Stauffer JQ, Lapinski MW, Honold DJ, Myers JK (1975) Focal nodular hyperplasia of the liver and intrahepatic hemorrhage in young women on oral contraceptives. Ann Intern Med 83: 301–306

63. Butron Vila MM, Haot J, Desment VJ (1984) Cholestatic features in focal nodular hyperplasia of the liver. Liver 4: 387–395

64. Whelan TJ, Baugh JH, Chandor S (1973) Focal nodular hyperplasia of the liver. Ann Surg 177: 150–158

65. Wanless IR, Mawdsley C, Adams R (1985) On the pathogenesis of focal nodular hyperplasia of the liver. Hepatology 5: 1194–1200

66. Ross D, Pina J, Mirza M, Galvan A, Ponce L (1976) Regression of focal nodular hyperplasia after discontinuation of oral contraceptives. Ann Intern Med 85: 203–204

67. Aldinger K, Ben-Menachem Y, Whalen G (1977) Focal nodular hyperplasia of the liver associated with high-dosage estrogens. Arch Intern Med 137: 357–359

68. Craig JR, Peters RL, Edmondson HA, Omata M (1980) Fibrolamellar carcinoma of the liver: A tumor of adolescents and young adults with distinctive clinicopathologic features. Cancer 46: 372–379

69. Fechner RE, Roehm JOF Jr (1977) Angiographic and pathologic correlations of hepatic focal nodular hyperplasia. Am J Surg Pathol 1: 217–224

70. Casarella WJ, Knowles DM, Wolff M, Johnson PM (1978) Focal nodular hyperplasia and liver cell adenoma: Radiologic and pathologic differentiation. Am J Roentgenol 131: 393–402

71. Sandler MA, Petrocelli RD, Marks DS, Lopez R (1980) Ultrasonic features and radionuclide correlation in liver cell adenoma and focal nodular hyperplasia. Radiology 135: 393–397

72. Welch TJ, Sheedy II PF, Johnson CM, Stephens DH, Charboneau JW, Brown ML, May GR, Adson MA, McGill DB (1985) Focal nodular hyperplasia and hepatic adenoma. Comparison of angiography, CT, US, and scintigraphy. Radiology 156: 593–595

73. Govindarajan S, Peters RL (1984) The bile duct adenoma. A lesion distinct from Meyenburg complex. Arch Pathol Lab Med 108: 922–924

74. Ishak KG, Sharp HL (1979) Developmental anomalies and liver disease in childhood. In: MacSween RNM, Anthony PP, Scheuer PJ (eds) Pathology of the liver, Churchill Livingstone, Edinburgh, pp 68–87

75. Summerfield J, Nagafuchi Y, Sherlock S, Cadafalch J, Scheuer PJ (1986) Hepatobiliary fibropolycystic diseases. A clinical and histological review of 51 patients. J Hepatol 2: 141–156

76. Desmet VJ (1985) Intrahepatic bile ducts under the lens. J Hepatol 1: 545–559

77. Compagno J, Oertell JE (1978) Mucinous cystic neoplasms of the pancreas with overt and latent malignancy (cystadenocarcinoma and cystadenoma). A clinicopathologic studies of 41 cases. Am J Clin Pathol 69: 573–580

78. Wheeler DA, Edmondson HA (1985) Cystadenoma with mesenchymal stroma (CMS) in the liver and bile ducts. A clinicopathologic study of 17 cases, 4 with malignant change. Cancer 56: 1434–1445

79. Ishak KG, Willis GW, Cummins SD, Bullock AA (1977) Biliary cystadenoma and cystadenocarcinoma. Report of 14 cases and review of the literature. Cancer 38: 322–338

80. Snedecor PA (1967) Bile duct cystadenoma of the liver. Ann Surg 33: 581–583

81. Case records of the Massachusetts General Hospital (1985) Case 46–1985. N Engl J Med 313: 1275–1282

82. Veloso FT, Ribeiro AT, Teixeira A, Ramalhao J, Saleiro JS, Serrao D (1983) Biliary papillomatosis: Report of a case with 5-year follow-up. Am J Gastroent 78: 645–648

83. Madden JJ Jr, Smith GW (1974) Multiple biliary papillomatosis. Cancer 34: 1316–1320

84. Neumann RD, LiVolsi VA, Rosenthal NS, Bur-

rell M, Ball TJ (1976) Adenocarcinoma in biliary papillomatosis. Gastroenterology 70: 779–782

85. Helpap B (1977) Malignant papillomatosis of the intrahepatic bile ducts. Acta Hepato-Gastroenterol 24: 419–425

86. Gouma DJ, Mutum SS, Benjamin IS, Blumgart LH (1984) Intrahepatic biliary papillomatosis. Br J Surg 71: 72–74

87. Berry CL (1985) Solitary "necrotic nodule" of the liver: a probable pathogenesis. J Clin Pathol 38: 1278–1280

88. O'Donoghue JB, Nicosia AJ (1950) Cavernous hemangioma of the liver. Ill Med J 98: 15–17

89. Ochsner JL, Halpert B (1958) Cavernous hemangioma of the liver. Surgery 43: 577–582

90. Feldman M (1958) Hemangioma of the liver. Special reference to its association with cysts of the liver and pancreas. Am J Clin Pathol 29: 160–162

91. Karhunen PJ (1986) Benign hepatic tumors and tumor like conditions in men. J Clin Pathol 39: 183–188

92. Trastek VF, van Heerden JA, Sheedy PF II, Adson MA (1983) Cavernous hemangiomas of the liver: Resect or observe? Am J Surg 145: 49–53

93. Sewell JH, Weiss K (1961) Spontaneous rupture of hemangioma of the liver: a review of the literature and presentation of illustrative case. Arch Surg 83: 729–733

94. Behar A, Moran E, Izak G (1963) Acquired hypofibrinogenemia associated with a giant cavernous hemangioma of the liver. Am J Clin Pathol 40: 78–82

95. Martinez J, Shapiro SS, Holburn RR, Carabasi RA (1973) Hypofibrinogenemia associated with a giant cavernous hemangioma of the liver. Am J Clin Pathol 59: 192–197

96. Wiener SN, Parulekar SG (1979) Scintigraphy and ultrasonography of hepatic hemangioma. Radiology 132: 149–153

97. Freeny PC, Vimont TR, Barnett DC (1979) Cavernous hemangioma of the liver: Ultrasonography, arteriography, and computed tomography. Radiology 132: 143–148

98. Itai Y, Furui S, Araki T, Yashiro N, Tasaka A (1980) Computed tomography of cavernous hemangioma of the liver. Radiology 137: 149–155

99. Johnson CM, Sheedy PF, Stanson AW, Stephens DH, Hattery RR, Adson MA (1981) Computed tomography and angiography of cavernous hemangioma of the liver. Radiology 138: 115–121

100. McLaughlin MJ (1971) Angiography in cavernous hemangioma of the liver. Am J Roentgenol 113: 50–55

101. Dehner LP, Ishak KG (1971) Vascular tumors of the liver in infants and children. A study of 30 cases and review of the literature. Arch Pathol 92: 101–111

102. McLean RH, Moller JH, Warwick WJ, Satran L, Lucas RV Jr (1972) Multinodular hemangiomatosis of the liver in infancy. Pediatrics 49: 563–573

103. Chowdhury AR, Black M, Lorber SH, Chey WY (1977) Hemangioendotheliomatosis of the liver. A 12-year follow-up. Gastroenterology 72: 157–160

104. Berman B, Lim HWP (1978) Concurrent cutaneous and hepatic hemangiomata in infancy: Report of a case and a review of the literature. J Dermatol Surg Oncol 4: 869–873

105. Larcher VF, Howard ER, Mowat AP (1981) Hepatic hemangiomata: diagnosis and management. Arch Dis Child 56: 7–14

106. Pereyra R, Andrassy RJ, Mahour GH (1982) Management of massive hepatic hemangiomas in infants and children: a review of 13 cases. Pediatrics 70: 254–258

107. Dachman AH, Lichtenstein JE, Friedman AC, Hartman DS (1983) Infantile hemangioendothelioma of the liver: A radiologic-pathologic-clinical correlation. Am J Roentgenol 140: 1091–1096

108. Enzinger FM, Weiss SW (1983) Soft tissue tumors. Mosby, St. Louis, pp 381–383

109. Rocchini AP, Rosenthal A, Issenberg HJ, Nadas As (1976) Hepatic hemangioendothelioma: Hemodynamic observations and treatment. Pediatrics 57: 131–135

110. Vorse HB, Smith I, Luckstead EF, Fraser JF Jr (1983) Hepatic hemangioendotheliomatosis of infancy. Am J Dis Child 137: 672–673

111. Moazam F, Rodgers BM, Talbert JL (1983) Hepatic artery ligation for hepatic hemangiomatosis of infancy. J Pediat Surg 18: 120–123

112. Johnson DH, Vinson AM, wirth FH, Presberg HJ, Harkins G, Nuss D, Walburgh CE, Raff JC (1984) Management of hepatic hemangioendotheliomas of infancy by transarterial embolization: A report of two cases. Pediatrics 73: 546–549

113. Rotman M, John M, Stowe S, Inamdar S (1980) Radiation treatment of pediatric hepatic hemangiomatosis and coexisting cardiac failure. N Engl J Med 302: 852

114. Touloukian RJ (1970) Hepatic hemangioendothelioma during infancy: Pathology, diagnosis and treatment with prednisone. Pediatrics 15: 71–76

115. Falk HF, Herbert JT, Edmonds L, Heath CW Jr, Thomas LB, Popper H (1981) Review of four cases of childhood hepatic angiosarcoma—elevated environmental arsenic exposure in one case. Cancer 47: 382–391

116. Weinberg AG, Finegold MJ (1983) Primary hepatic tumors of childhood. Human Pathol 14: 512–537

117. Noronha R, Gonzalez-Crussi F (1984) Hepatic angiosarcoma in childhood. A case report and review of the literature. Am J Surg Pathol 8: 863–871

118. Ishak KG (1981) Hepatic lesions caused by anabolic and contraceptive steroids. Sem Liv Dis

1: 116–128

119. Zafrani ES, Pinaudeau Y, Dhumeaux D (1983) Drug-induced vascular lesions of the liver. Arch Intern Med 143: 495–502

120. Zafrani ES, Cazier A, Baudelot AM, Feldmann G (1984) Ultrastructural lesions of the liver in human peliosis. A report of 12 cases. Am J Pathol 114: 349–359

121. Bagheri SA, Boyer JL (1974) Peliosis hepatis associated with androgenic-anabolic steroid therapy: A severe form of hepatic injury. Ann Intern Med 81: 610–618

122. Degott C, Rueff B, Kreis H, Duboust A, Potet F, Benhamou JP (1978) Peliosis hepatis in recipients of renal transplants. Gut 19: 748–753

123. Paradinas FJ, Bull TB, Westaby D, Murray-Lyon IM (1977) Hyperplasia and prolapse of hepatocytes into hepatic veins during longterm methyltestosterone therapy: Possible relationships of these changes to the development of peliosis hepatis and liver tumors. Histopathology 1: 225–246

124. Wanless IR, Gryfe A (1986) Nodular transformation of the liver in hereditary hemorrhagic telangectasia. Arch Pathol Lab Med 110: 331–335

125. Van Steenbergen W, Joosten E, Marchal G, Baert A, Vanstapel MJ, Desmet V, Wijnants P, De Groote J (1985) Hepatic lymphangiomatosis. Report of a case and review of the literature. Gastroenterology 88: 1968–1972

126. Stocker JT, Ishak KG (1983) Mesenchymal hamartoma of the liver: Report of 30 cases and review of the literature. Pediatr Pathol 1: 245–267

127. Ros PR, Goodman ZD, Ishak KG, Dachman AH, Olmsted WW, Hartman DS, Lichtenstein JE (1986) Mesenchymal hamartoma of the liver: Radiologic-pathologic correlation. Radiology 158: 619–624

128. Stanley RJ, Dehner LP, Hesker AE (1973) Primary malignant mesenchymal tumors (mesenchymoma) of the liver in childhood. An angiographic-pathologic study of three cases. Cancer 32: 973984

129. Hawkins EP, Jordan GL, McGavran MH (1980) Primary leiomyoma of the liver. Successful treatment by lobectomy and presentation of criteria for diagnosis. Am J Surg Pathol 4: 301–304

130. Kim H, Damjanov I (1983) Localized fibrous mesothelioma of the liver. Report of a giant tumor studied by light and electron microscopy. Cancer 52: 1662–1665

131. Roberts JL, Fishman EK, Hartman DS, Sanders R, Goodman Z, Siegelman SS (1986) Lipomatous tumors of the liver: Evaluation with CT and US. Radiology 158: 613–617

132. Peters WM, Dixon MF, Williams NS (1983) Angiomyelolipoma of the liver. Histopathology 7: 99–106

133. Goodman ZD, Ishak KG (1984) Angiomyolipomas of the liver. Am J Surg Pathol 8: 745–750

134. Wheeler DA, Edmondson HA (1985) Coelomic fat ectopia in the liver. Arch Pathol Lab Med 109: 783–785

135. Karhunen PJ (1985) Hepatic pseudolipoma. J Clin Pathol 38: 877–879

136. Brawer MK, Austin GE, Lewin KJ (1980) Focal fatty change of the liver, a hitherto poorly recognized entity. Gastroenterology 78: 247–252

137. Clain JE, Stephens DH, Charboneau JW (1984) Ultrasonography and computed tomography in focal fatty liver. Report of two cases with special emphasis on changing appearances over time. Gastroenterology 87: 948–952

138. Gonzalez-Crussi F (1982) Extragonadal teratomas. Atlas of tumor pathology. Second Series. Fasc 18. Armed Forces Institute of Pathology, Washington

139. Witte DP, Kissane JM, Askin FB (1983) Hepatic teratomas in children. Pediatr Pathol 1: 81–92

140. Wilkins L, Ravich MM (1952) Adrenocortical tumor arising in the liver of a three-year-old boy with signs of virilism and Cushing's syndrome. Report of a case with cure after partial resection of the right lobe of the liver. Pediatrics 9: 671–680

141. Mobini J, Krouse TB, Cooper DR (1974) Intrahepatic pancreatic heterotopia. Review and report of a case presenting as an abdominal mass. Am J Dig Dis 19: 64–70

142. Someren A (1978) "Inflammatory pseudotumor" of the liver with occlusive phlebitis. Report of a case in a child and review of the literature. Am J Clin Pathol 69: 176–181

143. Chen KTK (1984) Inflammatory pseudotumor of the liver. Human Pathol 15: 694–696

144. Goodman ZD, Ishak KG (1981) Xanthogranulomatous cholecystitis. Am J Surg Pathol 5: 653–659

Chapter 9
Hepatoblastoma*

J. Thomas Stocker[1] and Kamal G. Ishak[2]

1 Introduction

Hepatoblastoma is the most common hepatic tumor of childhood, accounting for nearly 45% of all primary hepatic tumors and tumorlike lesions and 62% of primary malignant tumors [1]. It affects about 1/100 000 children under the age of 15 years in Britain [2] and accounts for about 1/10 000 admissions at Children's Hospital Medical Center in Boston, USA [3].

2 Clinical features

Hepatoblastoma is primarily a tumor of young children. Of 256 cases of hepatoblastoma published between 1976 and 1985, 235 (91.8%) were in children 5 years of age or younger; the majority were less than 2 years of age. All but 3 of the other 21 cases were between 6 and 15 years of age [3–40]. The oldest patients were 27 [23], 58 [12], and 60 years [20] of age. Hepatoblastoma is more frequent in males (1.75 : 1), although in patients over 5 years of age it occurs with nearly equal frequency in males and females (1 : 1.2). Familial occurrence has been noted only in two sisters in one family [41] and a brother and sister in another [7]. The presenting symptom in the majority of patients is an enlarging abdomen. An upper abdominal mass is often noted by a parent or discovered on routine physical examination. Anorexia and weight loss and, less frequently, nausea, vomiting, and abdominal pain may accompany the abdominal enlargement [3, 32]. Jaundice is

noted in less than 6% of cases [9]. Physical examination confirms the presence of a firm, often irregular right upper abdominal mass that may extend across the midline or down to the pelvic brim. Hepatoblastoma has also been noted in association with a variety of other clinical presentations and malformations (Table 9.1).

Some boys with hepatoblastoma may present initially with signs of precocious puberty such as genital enlargement, deepening voice, and pubic hair [13, 14, 21, 33, 38, 42]. These children have increased levels of serum and urinary human chorionic gonadotrophin (HCG), the result of production of HCG by the tumor cells [13, 33]. Serum luteinizing hormone and plasma testosterone levels are also increased in patients with HCG-producing tumors, either secondary to HCG stimulation of the Leydig's cells of the testes [21] or to stimulation of the pituitary gland to produce luteinizing hormone [49].

Cystathionine excretion in the urine has been increased in nearly 50% of patients with hepatoblastoma [45, 47]. Cystathioninuria has also been noted consistently in patients with neuroblastoma and rarely in patients with Hodgkin's disease but not with Wilms' tumor, acute leukemia, soft tissue sarcoma, and a variety of other childhood malignancies. Geiser et al. [45] noted disappearance of the cystathioninuria after excision of the tumor and its reappearance at the time of recurrence. The tumor content of cystathionine is increased in patients with cystathioninuria, implying direct production by the tumor cells [45].

Hepatoblastoma, along with Wilms' tumor, adrenocortical tumor, and hemangioma, has been seen in Beckwith–Wiedeman syndrome [32, 46], and the synchronous appearance of Wilms' tumor and hepatoblastoma has been reported in two patients [3, 4].

A familial association between hepatoblastoma and polyposis coli has been noted in five

---

* The opinions expressed are the private views of the authors and should not be construed as being official or as necessarily reflecting the views of the Department of the Army or the Department of Defense. Department of Pediatric Pathology[1] and Department of Hepatic pathology[2], The Armed Forces Institute of Pathology, Washington, DC 20306, USA

families [2]. No chromosomal abnormality was noted in the peripheral blood lymphocytes of two of the patients and three of the mothers. Cytogenetic studies of the tumor cells in hepatoblastomas, however, demonstrate abnormalities of chromosome 1, most frequently deletion of the short arm, 1p, with formation of isochromosome or trisomy of 1q48. These changes are not specific for hepatoblastoma as they are frequently seen in other solid childhood tumors (Wilms' tumor, Ewing's sarcoma, rhabdomyosarcoma) [48].

Congenital anomalies associated with hepatoblastoma include cleft palate, macroglossia, and dysplasia of the ear lobes [40], absence of the right adrenal gland [44], umbilical hernia [44], and various cardiovascular and renal anomalies (Table 9.1) [29, 43]. Fetal hydrops secondary to tumor compression of the inferior vena cava has been described in a stillborn infant [25]. The incidence of congenital anomalies in four of the larger series of hepatoblastoma totaling 162 cases was 5.5% [2, 32, 40, 44].

3 Laboratory data

With the exception of serum alpha fetoprotein, the laboratory findings in children with hepatoblastoma are of little help. Anemia and jaundice are infrequently present [1]. The common tests of hepatic function (LDH, SGOT, alkaline phosphatase) may be normal or mildly to moderately elevated. Serum cholesterol levels, when elevated, however, have been associated with a poor prognosis [50].

Serum alpha fetoprotein (AFP) is elevated in the majority of patients with hepatoblastoma (75%–96%) [3, 22, 40], with levels occasionally exceeding 1 000 000 ng/ml [38]. AFP levels closely parallel the course of the disease, decreasing or disappearing with regression of the tumor and reappearing or increasing with tumor growth and metastasis. The levels of AFP at the time of diagnosis, however, are apparently of little prognostic significance [32, 38].

4 Imaging studies

Imaging studies of the liver including ultrasound, computerized tomography, and radionuclide scanning may be helpful in diagnosing hepatoblastoma and differentiating it from other liver disorders. Computed tomography demonstrates

Table 9.1. Associations and clinical manifestation of hepatoblastoma

	Reference
Isosexual precocity	13, 14, 21, 33, 38, 42
Hemihypertrophy	43–45
Beckwith-Wiedemann syndrome	32, 46
Synchronous Wilms tumor	3, 4
Osteoporosis	3, 44
Alcohol embryopathy	18
Cystathioninuria	45, 47
Chromosome 1 abnormalities	48
Polyposis coli families	2, 34
Fetal hydrops	25
Cleft palate, macroglossia, dysplasia of ear lobes	40
Absence of right adrenal gland	44
Umbilical hernia	44
Down's Syndrome, malrotation of colon, Meckel's diverticulum, pectus excavatum, intrathoracic kidney, single coronary artery	29
Horseshoe kidney	29
Heterotopic lung tissue	29
Duplicated ureters	29
Heterozygous alpha 1 antitrypsin deficiency	34

a solitary mass (rarely multifocal) with attenuation values between those of water and normal liver parenchyma [35]. Attenuation values of hepatoblastoma and normal liver show a similar increase after intravenous infusion of contrast material [51]. Computed tomography may also display areas of speckled or amorphous calcification more frequently than on conventional radiography [52]. Calcification may be seen in more than 50% of cases using this modality [35, 53].

Ultrasonography of hepatoblastoma displays a solitary mass with increased inhomogeneous echogenicity, occasional cystic areas, and punctate or amorphous calcification [53]. Technetium sulfur-colloid scanning reveals decreased perfusion in most hepatoblastomas [53], but uptake of the radiocolloid has been noted in some instances, thus simulating the pattern seen with focal nodular hyperplasia [28]. Other radionuclides including technetium medronate diphosphonate, technetium iminodiacetic acid, and gallium also display decreased uptake by hepatoblastomas [53].

Conventional radiographic studies such as flat plates of the abdomen, intravenous pyelograms, and barium studies of the upper and lower gastrointestinal tract usually display an upper ab-

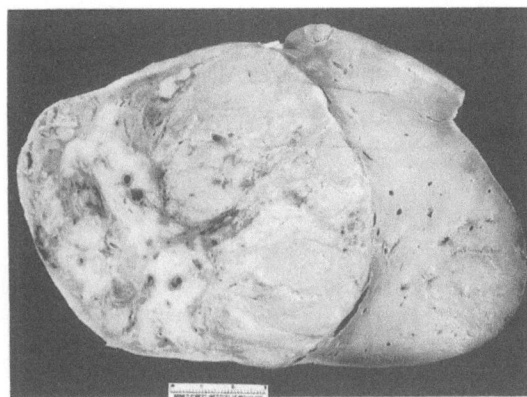

Fig. 9.1. Epithelial hepatoblastoma. A single large mass composed of irregular lobules of pale to focally hemorrhagic tissue occupies a large portion of the right lobe of the liver. AFIP neg 67-5439

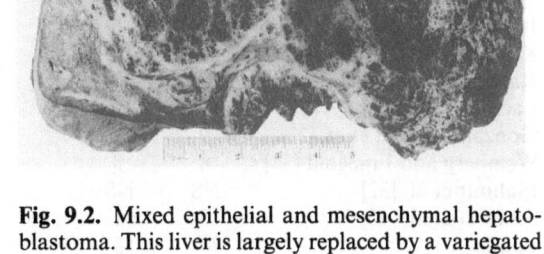

Fig. 9.2. Mixed epithelial and mesenchymal hepatoblastoma. This liver is largely replaced by a variegated light to dark mass subdivided by pale septa. AFIP neg 65-559

dominal mass with or without calcification, but localization of the mass to the liver may not be possible [43].

Angiography may help to localize the lesion and provide information as to whether it can be resected. Hepatoblastomas are usually hypervascular, with distortion and displacement of vessels, pooling of contrast material and an ill-defined irregular tumor margin [43].

5 Experimental studies

Hepatoblastoma cell lines have been established in culture [54, 55] and used for the study of bile acid synthesis [56] and the activity and regulation of low-density lipoprotein receptors [57]. Anti-AFP serum has been shown to suppress proliferation of hepatoblastoma cells in culture [58].

6 Pathology

Hepatoblastomas are usually single masses (approximately 80% of cases) [43]. They vary in size from 5.5 to 17 cm [3, 24] and weigh 180–1300 g [3, 43]. The right lobe alone is involved in 58% of cases and the left in 15%; the remaining 27% have either multiple lesions involving both lobes or a single lesion extending across the midline [3, 40, 43]. The gross appearance is variable but is largely dependent on the presence or absence of different types of mesenchymally derived tissue (osteoid and cartilagenous or fibrous tissue) (Figs. 9.1, 9.2). Externally, the tumor is usually coarsely nodular or lobulated and bulges from

one of the surfaces of the liver. Glisson's capsule remains intact in most cases (intra-abdominal rupture of a tumor has been described) [32, 43], and prominent vascularity can be noted beneath the capsule.

On cut section, the tumors have tan to light brown to green bulging lobules along with frequent areas of hemorrhage and necrosis. This variegated pattern is more prominent with mixed hepatoblastomas than with pure epithelial ones (see below; Fig. 9.2). Tumors may be sharply demarcated by a capsule or may blend imperceptibly with the adjacent liver. Cirrhosis, frequently associated with hepatocellular carcinoma, is rarely present with hepatoblastoma [1].

The classification of hepatoblastoma histologically into epithelial and mixed epithelial and mesenchymal types was proposed in 1967 by Ishak and Glunz [43] and has gained wide acceptance (Table 9.2). Many pathologists (including ourselves) have incorporated Kasai and Watanabe's anaplastic (or undifferentiated) variant into this classification [59]. In addition Gonzalez-Crussi et al. have described a "macrotrabecular" component of some hepatoblastomas, in which broad trabeculae composed of malignant cells resembling hepatocellular carcinoma cells are seen in addition to fetal epithelial cells [29].

The epithelial component (of both the epithelial and the mixed epithelial-mesenchymal types) consists of two cell types, resembling either fetal or embryonic cells. The fetal-type cells (resembling the hepatocytes of the fetus at 6–8 weeks' gestation) are smaller than normal hepatocytes and are arranged in irregular plates two cells thick (Fig. 9.3). The nucleocytoplasmic

Table 9.2. Histological classification of hepatoblastoma

First author	Epithelial			Mixed	Anaplastic	Total no. cases
	Predominantly		Total			
	Fetal	Embryonic				
Ishak and Glunz [43]	10	6	16	19		35
Kasai and Watanabe [59]	20	16	36	11	10	57
Randolph et al. [24]	NS	NS	8	5		13
Lack et al. [3]	13	19	32	12	5	49
Gonzalez-Crussi et al. [29]	9	3	17[a]	4		21
Weinberg and Finegold [34]	8	8	16	9	2	27
Mahour et al. [32]	NS	NS	25	8		33
Schmidt et al. [40]	10	1	11	13		24
Total	70	53	161(62.2%)	81(31.3%)	17(6.5%)	259

NS not stated

[a] Five cases called macrotrabecular (see text)

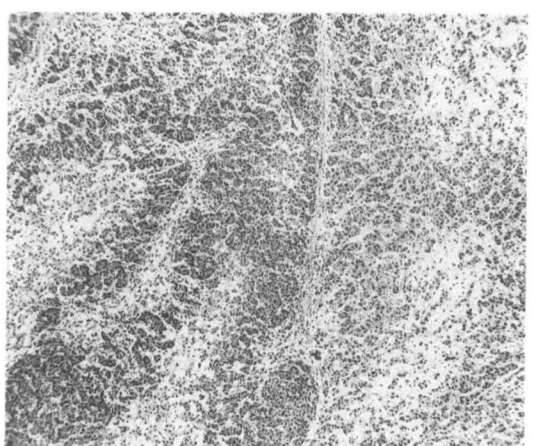

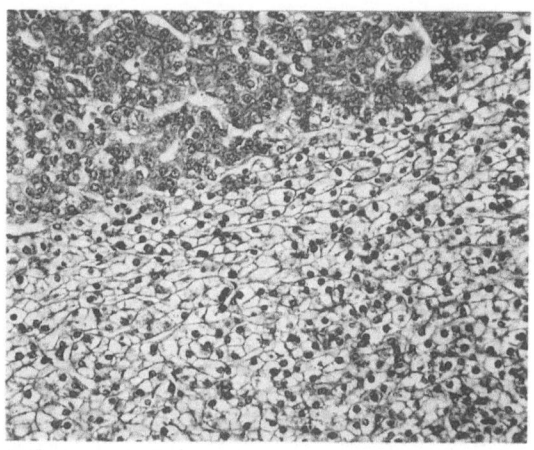

Fig. 9.3. Epithelial hepatoblastoma composed predominantly of fetal-type cells. Small epithelial cells resembling fetal liver cells are arranged in one- to two-cell-thick cords separated by irregular sinusoids. Note the alternating light-dark pattern typical of fetal-type epithelial hepatoblastomas. H and E, AFIP neg 64-1081, × 50

Fig. 9.4. Epithelial hepatoblastoma, fetal-type cells. The light-dark pattern is imparted by the cytoplasmic content of the fetal-type cells. The clear cells (*lower right*) in this formalin-fixed tissue appear to have an empty cytoplasm when compared with the finely granular cytoplasm of the cells at *upper left*. H and E, AFIP neg 81-19082, × 250

ratio is 1 : 2 to 1 : 4 with the round or oval nuclei containing a single nucleolus and fine to coarse nuclear chromatin. Mitotic figures are infrequently seen. Bile canaliculi can be identified between fetal-type cells, and sinusoidal vessels lined by flattened endothelial cells separate the plates. The cells are polyhedral with well-defined outlines and are supported by a poorly defined reticulum network. The cytoplasm may be finely granular and acidophilic or appear largely empty or vacuolated ("pale" cells; Fig. 9.4). Glycogen and neutral fat can be demonstrated by periodic

acid-Shiff and oil red-O (of frozen sections) stains, respectively, in the pale cells which constitute the "light" component of the light/dark pattern typically seen in the fetal areas of hepatoblastomas (Fig. 9.5). Intracytoplasmic bile along with intracanalicular bile plugs may be present.

Foci of extramedullary hematopoiesis composed of clusters of red and white cell precursors and megakaryocytes are consistently associated with the fetal-type cell component in children who have not received prior chemotherapy or irradiation (Fig. 9.6).

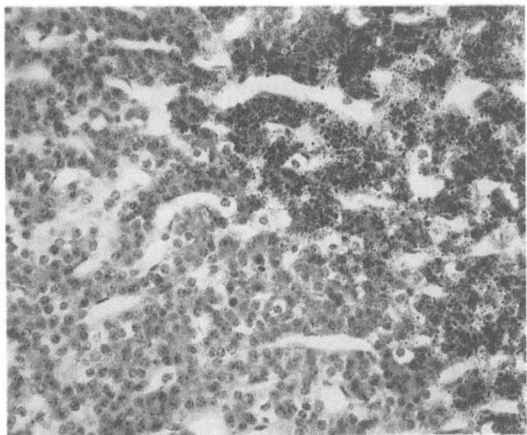

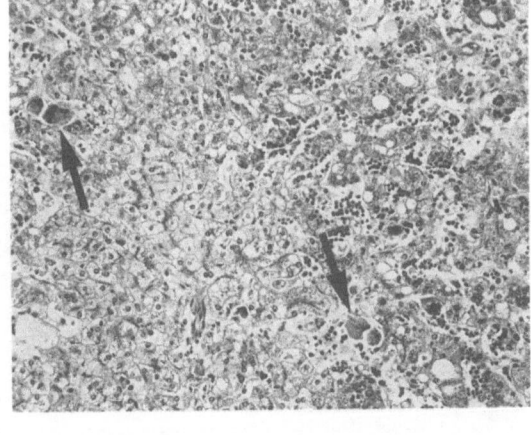

Fig. 9.5. Epithelial hepatoblastoma, fetal-type cells. In this frozen section preparation stained with oil red-O, fat droplets fill the fetal-type cells (*upper right*) but are absent in the fetal-type cells (*lower left*). Oil red-O, AFIP neg 81-19084, × 250

Fig. 9.6. Epithelial hepatoblastoma, fetal-type cells. Clusters of red cell precusors fill the sinusoids between cords of fetal-type cells. Note the megakaryocytes (*arrows*), another component of the extramedullary hematopoiesis. H and E, AFIP neg 86-5276, × 160

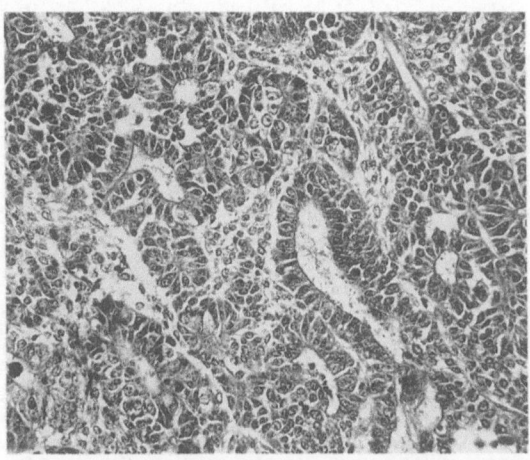

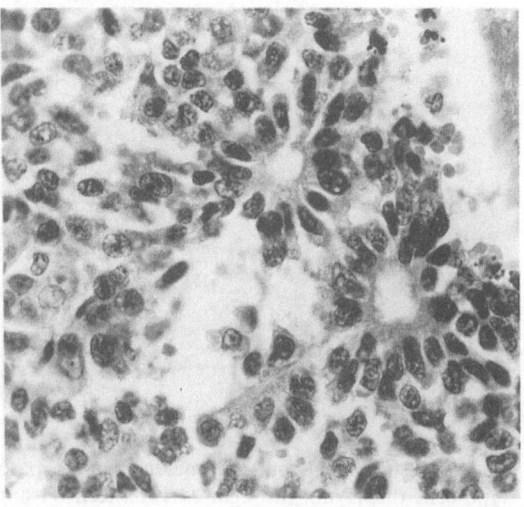

Fig. 9.7. Epithelial hepatoblastoma, embryonic-type cells. Small, elongated, embryonic-type cells with a scanty cytoplasm and hyperchromatic nuclei appear singly or in irregular cords or ribbons. H and E, AFIP neg 81-10216, × 250

Fig. 9.8. Epithelial hepatoblastoma, embryonic-type cells. Embryonic-type cells form rosettelike structures (*right*) with a central clear lumen. Note the lack of cohesiveness of the cells at *left*. H and E, AFIP neg 64-1090, × 575

The *embryonic-type cells* are small, elongated, dark-staining cells with a scanty amphophilic cytoplasm and poorly defined cellular outlines (Fig. 9.7). Cells and nuclei vary considerable in size with a nuclear cytoplasmic ratio of 1 : 1 to 1 : 2. The nucleus, single in each cell, is oval to round with abundant chromatin and a large distinct nucleolus. Mitotic activity is seen much more frequently than in areas with fetal-type cells, and extramedullary hematopoiesis is not present. Embryonic-type cells do not contain fat, glycogen, or bile within their cytoplasm. They may aggregate in rosettelike clusters (often large enough to show tubular patterns), appear as cords or ribbons of loosely cohesive cells, or exist singly in a fibrous stroma (Fig. 9.8). Embryonic- and fetal-type cells are often admixed in the tumor.

The *anaplastic type* of hepatoblastoma, as described by Kasai and Watanabe, is composed of cells resembling those of neuroblastomas that have scanty cytoplasm and hyperchromatic

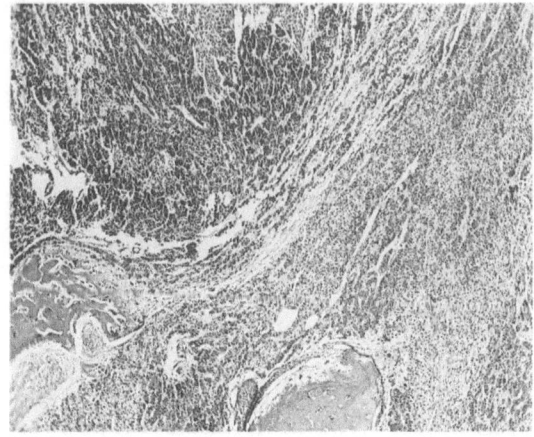

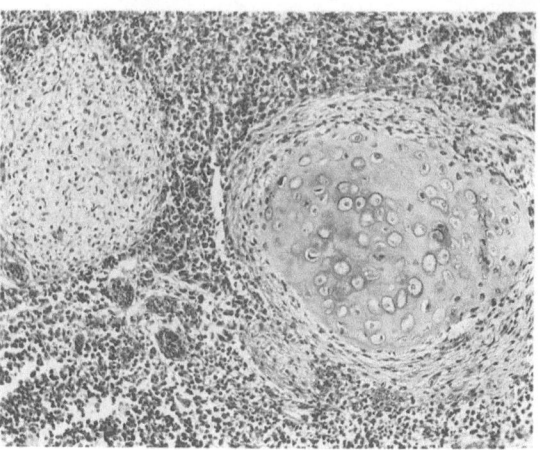

Fig. 9.9. Mixed epithelial-mesenchymal hepatoblastoma. Embryonic type cells (*upper left*), fetal-type cells (*right*), and osteoid tissue (*lower left*) are admixed in this hepatoblastoma. H and E, AFIP neg 64-718, × 50

Fig. 9.10. Mixed epithelial-mesenchymal hepatoblastoma. Islands of cartilage (*right*) and primitive mesenchyme (*left*) are surrounded by loosely cohesive embryonic-type cells. H and E, AFIP neg 64-1292, × 110

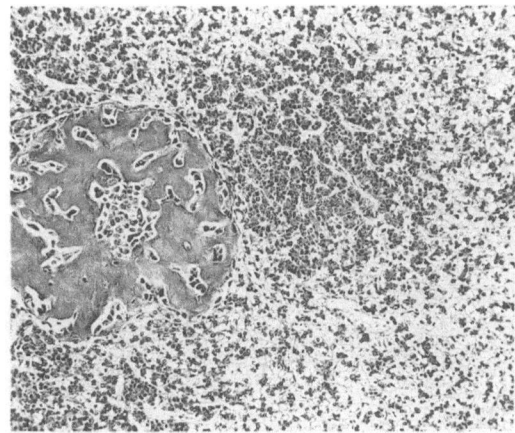

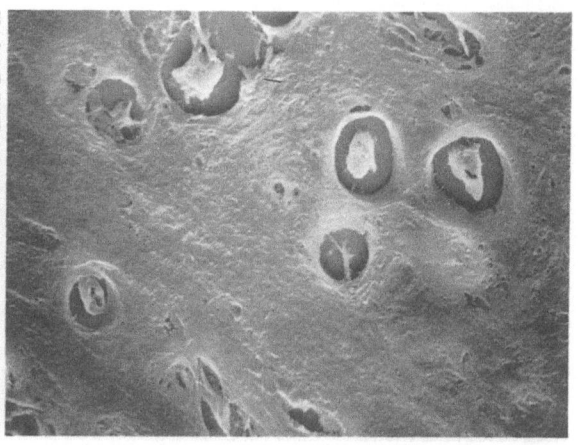

a   b

Fig. 9.11a, b. Mixed epithelial-mesenchymal hepatoblastoma. **a** A focus of osteoid tissue lies adjacent to fetal-type cells displaying the light-dark pattern. H and E, AFIP neg 76-11652, × 110. **b** By scanning electron microscopy, a focus of osteoid tissue displays osteoblasts within lacunae. × 320

nuclei. The cells grow in sheets but can lack cohesiveness. Mitoses are uncommon. As with embryonic-type cells, anaplastic cells do not produce glycogen, fat droplets, or bile pigment, but abortive or incompletely formed bile ductules may be present.

The *mixed epithelial-mesenchymal type* of tumor contains varying amounts of fetal- and embryonic-type cells admixed with primitive mesenchyme and various mesenchymally derived tissues (Fig. 9.9). The highly cellular primitive mesenchyme consists of elongated, spindle-shaped cells with scanty cytoplasm and elongated pump nuclei with rounded ends. Some areas may display parallel orientation of cells

with definite collagen fibers and young fibroblasts, while other areas may have more loosely arranged cells leading to a myxomatous appearance. Mature fibrous septa are also seen along with areas of osteoid and cartilagenous tissue (Figs. 9.10, 9.11). Cells within the osteoid foci have an irregular, angular outline and short processes, which make them indistinguishable from osteoblasts. Foci of calcification may also be seen away from the osteoid tissue and probably represent areas of previous necrosis. Mixed epithelial-mesenchymal hepatoblastomas may also contain foci of squamous cells, some wth keratin pearls (Fig. 9.12).

Unique cases of hepatoblastomas have been

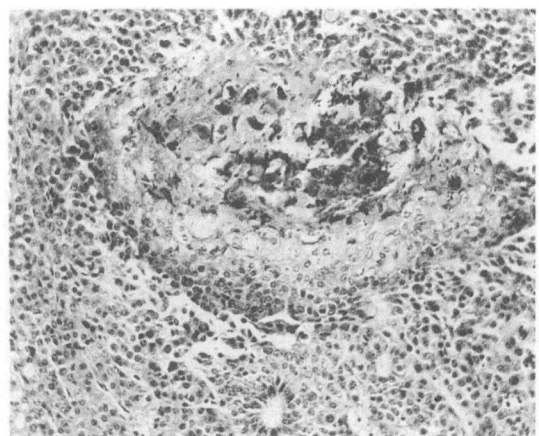

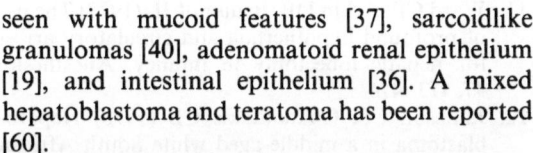

Fig. 9.12. Mixed epithelial-mesenchymal hepatoblastoma. A focus of squamous epithelial cells with central calcification (keratin pearl) is surrounded by embryonic-type (*below*) and fetal-type (*left*) cells. H and E, AFIP neg 64-6342, × 195

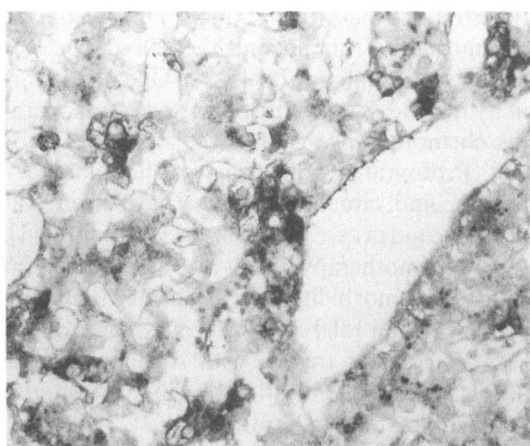

Fig. 9.13. Epithelial hepatoblastoma, fetal-type, shows abundant (black) alpha-fetoprotein production by tumor cells. Peroxidase antiperoxidase technique, × 400

seen with mucoid features [37], sarcoidlike granulomas [40], adenomatoid renal epithelium [19], and intestinal epithelium [36]. A mixed hepatoblastoma and teratoma has been reported [60].

Immunohistochemical studies of hepatoblastoma have identified AFP (Fig. 9.13), keratin, alpha-1-antitrypsin, alpha-1-chymotrypsin, and HCG in tumor cells [33, 40]. AFP was demonstrated in 10 of 12 cases by Schmidt et al. [40], with the two negative cases displaying predominantly embryonic-type cells. Morinaga et al. [33] showed localization of HCG to syncytial-appearing multinucleated tumor giant cells in a predominantly embryonic-type hepatoblastoma in a young boy with sexual precocity. An ultrastructural study of hepatoblastoma in another boy with sexual precocoity displayed dense membrane-bound, secretory granules that were felt to be the source of the HCG in the serum and tumor tissue [13].

Ultrastructural studies of hepatoblastomas have demonstrated lack of differentiation and simple cytoplasmic organelles within the epithelial elements, along with occasional intramitochondrial crystalloids [16, 61, 62]. Small desmosomes and tight junctions are seen along with bile canaliculi with microvilli [62]. Mesenchymal-type cells in regions of osteoid production may resemble undifferentiated epithelial cells or contain dilated rough endoplasmic reticulum in which fibrillar material is present. Dense extracellular bundles of collagen fibrils surround these cells [61].

7 Treatment

Surgical resection, in combination with chemotherapy and/or irradiation, is the primary treatment of hepatoblastoma. At the time of diagnosis, 39%–70% of tumors are considered to be unresectable [3, 32]. Preoperative chemotherapy with Adriamycin in combination with cisplatin [36, 39] or other agents (fluorouracil, vincristine, cytoxan, and/or cyclophosphamide) [10, 63] may reduce tumor size sufficiently to permit resection.

Tumors may be staged according to the Children's Cancer Study Group system as follows [64]:

Group I: Complete resection of tumor by wedge, lobectomy, or extended lobectomy as initial treament

Group IIA: Tumors rendered completely resectable by initial irradiation and chemotherapy

Group IIB: Residual tumor confined to one lobe

Group III: Tumor involving both lobes of the liver

Group IIIB: Regional lymph node involvement with tumor

Group IV: Distant metastases of tumor regardless of the extent of liver involvement

Because of the large size of many of these tumors, their location near vital structures (inferior vena cava), and the need for total resection for long-term survival, operative morbidity (bleeding, cardiac arrest) is high [30], with operative mortality from uncontrolled bleeding or air embolism as high as 22% [3, 34]. Operative mortality may be significantly decreased by preoperative chemotherapy to reduce the size of the tumor [63]. Profound hypothermia, cardiopulmonary bypass, and circulatory arrest have been employed to aid in cases of extensive lobectomy [11].

The chemotherapy used is also associated with significant morbidity. Neutropenia (leukoyte count less than 1500 cm³/ml) occurs in more than 50% of patients treated with Adriamycin and may lead to severe infections, including bacterial pneumonia and fetal septicemia [64]. Thrombocytopenia may also be seen with Adriamycin, and magnesium wasting may occur in patients treated with cisplatin [39].

Long-term survival, which in larger series varies from 15% to 37% [3, 32, 34, 40], is dependent on resectability (initially or following preoperative chemotherapy) and histological type. Children with pure fetal-cell type hepatoblastoma in which surgical excision is achieved (groups I and IIA) have the best prognosis at (75%) [34]. The prognosis by histological type, assuming resectability of the tumor, is as follows: Good—pure fetal-type cell; intermediate—predominantly embryonic-cell type, mixed epithelial-mesenchymal; poor—anaplastic (undifferentiated), macrotrabecular. Anaplastic histology in a hepatoblastoma, on the other hand, is almost uniformly fatal despite resectability or type of chemotherapy used [3]. Lack et al. [3] also noted a younger average age at diagnosis (8 months) for children with anaplastic hepatoblastoma than those with "conventional" histology hepatoblastomas (18 months). The macrotrabecular pattern as described by Gonzalez-Crussi et al. [29] is also associated with a poor outcome. Other histological patterns (embryonic-cell type, mixed epithelial-mesenchymal type) have far less predictive value than the extent of the tumor at the time of diagnosis (i.e., groups I–IV, as described above) [64].

References

1. Dehner LP (1978) Hepatic tumors in the pediatric age group: A distinctive clinicopathologic spectrum. Perspec Ped Pathol 4: 217–268
2. Kingston JE; Herbert A, Draper GJ, Mann JR (1983) Association between hepatoblastoma and polyposis coli. Arch Dis Child 58: 959–62
3. Lack EE, Neave C, Vawter GF (1982) Hepatoblastoma. A clinical and pathologic study of 54 cases. Am J Surg Pathol 6: 693–705
4. Dura W (1976) Coexistence of nephroblastoma and hepatoblastoma in a 5-year-old boy. Pathol Pol 27: 85–90
5. Cameron HM, Warwick GP (1977) Primary cancer of the liver in Kenyan children. Br J Cancer 36: 793–803
6. Fegiz G, Rosati D, Tonelli F, Donfrancesco A (1977) A case report of hepatoblastoma treated by chemotherapy and hepatic lobectomy. World J Surg 1: 407–414
7. Napoli VM, Campbell Jr. WG (1977) Hepatoblastoma in infant sister and brother. Cancer 39: 2647–2650
8. Otten J, Smets R, deJager R, Gerard A, Maurus R (1977) Hepatoblastoma in an infant after contraceptive intake during pregnancy. N Eng J Med 297–222
9. Rosenberg GJ (1977) Hepatoblastoma—case report and literature review. Clin Proc: Child Hosp Nat Med Center 33: 11–19
10. Shafter AD, Selinkoff (1977) Preoperative irradiation and chemotherapy for initially unresectable hepatoblastoma. J Pediatr Surg 12: 1001–1007
11. Ward CF, Arkin DB, Benumof JL (1977) The use of profound hypothermia and circulatory arrest for hepatic lobectomy in infancy. Anesthesiol 47: 473–474
12. Jameson CP, Chatkadakis CB (1978) Hepatoblastoma in a middle-aged white South African Woman. S Afr Med J 53: 143–144
13. Kumar EV, Kumar L, Pethak IC, Dash RJ, Joshi VV (1978) Clinical, hormonal and ultrastructural studies of a virilizing hepatoblastoma. Acta Pediatr Scand 67: 389–392
14. Abbassi V, Hoy G, Weintraub BD (1979) HCG production by hepatoblastoma causing isosexual precocious puberty. Pediatric Res 13: 375–381
15. Chung SS, Pinus J, De Nobrega FJ, Banholzer MCAG, Stump MV, Da Silva GP (1979) Hepatoblastoma em recemnascidoapresentacao de um caso com revisao da literatura. J Ped (Brazil) 47: 41–48
16. Horie A, Kotoo Y, Hayashi I (1979) Ultrastructural comparison of hepatoblastoma and hepatocellular carcinoma. Cancer 44: 2184–2193
17. Ikeda K, Suita S, Nakagawara A, Takabayashi K (1979) Preoperative chemotherapy for initially unresectable hepatoblastoma in children. Arch Surg 114: 203–207
18. Kahan A, Bader JL, Hoy GR, Sinks LF (1979) Hepatoblastoma in child with fetal alcohol syndrome. Lancet 1: 1403–1404
19. Knowlson GTG, Cameron AC (1979) Hepatoblastoma with adenomatoid renal epithelium. Histopathology 3: 201–208
20. Yoshida T, Okazaki N, Yoshino M, Shimamura Y, Miyazawa N, Miyamoto K, Kishi K (1979) A case of hepatoblastoma in adult. Jpn J Clin Oncol 9: 163–168
21. Butenandt O, Knorr D, Hecker WC, Lohrs U (1980) Precocious puberty in a boy with HCG-producing hepatoma. Helv Paediat Acta 3: 155–163

22. Geiser CF, Shin VE (1980) Cystathioninuria and its origin in children with hepatoblastoma. J Pediatr 96: 72–75

23. Honan RP, Haqqani MT (1980) Mixed hepatoblastoma in the adult: case report and review of the literature. J Clin 33: 1058–1063

24. Randolph J, Chandra R, Leiken S (1980) Malignant liver tumor in infants and children. World J Surg 4: 71–82

25. Benjamin E, Lendon M, Marsden HB (1981) Hepatoblastoma as an intrauterine fetal death. Case report. Br J Obstet Gynaecol 88: 329–332

26. Miller JH (1981) The ultrasonographic appearance of cystic hepatoblastoma. Radiology 138: 141–143

27. Demanes DJ, Friedman MA, McKerrow JH, Hoffman PG (1982) Hormone receptors in hepatoblastoma: A demonstration of both estrogen and progesterone receptors. Cancer 50: 1828–1832

28. Diament MJ, Parvey LS, Tonkin IL, Johnson KD, Bernstein R, Webber B (1982) Hepatoblastoma: technetium sulfur colloid uptake simulating focal nodular hyperplasia. AJR 139: 168–171

29. Gonzalez-Crussi F, Upton MP, Maurer HS (1982) Hepatoblastoma: Attempt at characterization of histologic subtypes. Am J Surg Pathol 6: 599–612

30. Price JB, Schullinger JN, Santulli TV (1982) Major hepatic resections for neoplasia in children. Arch Surg 117: 1139–1141

31. Weinblatt ME, Siegel SE, Siegel MM, Stanley P, Weitzman JJ (1982) Preoperative chemotherapy for unresectable primary hepatic malignancies in children. Cancer 50: 1061–1064

32. Mahour GH, Wogu GU, Siegel SE, Isaacs H (1983) Improved survival in infants and children with primary malignant liver tumors. Am J Surg 146: 236–240

33. Morinaga S, Yamaguchi M, Watanabe I, Kasai M, Ojima M, Sasano N (1983) An immunohistochemical study of hepatoblastoma producing human chorionic gonadotropin. Cancer 51: 1647–1652

34. Weinberg AG, Finegold MJ (1983) Primary hepatic tumors of childhood. Human Pathol 14: 512–537

35. Amendola MA, Blane CE, Amendola Bs, Glazer GM (1984) CT findings in hepatoblastoma. J Comput Assist Tomogr 8: 1105–1109

36. Forouhar FA, Quinn JJ, Cooke R, Foster JH (1984) The effect of chemotherapy on hepatoblastoma. Arch Pathol Lab Med 108: 311–314

37. Joshi VV, Kaur P, Ryan B, Saad S, Walters TR (1984) Mucoid anaplastic hepatoblastoma. Cancer 54: 2035–2039

38. Nakagawara A, Ikeda K, Tsuneyoshi M et al (1985) Hepatoblastoma producing both alpha-fetoprotein and human chorionic gonadotropin. Cancer 56: 1636–1642

39. Quinn JJ, Altman AJ, Robinson HJ, Cooke RW, Hight DW, Foster JH (1985) Adriamycin and cisplatin for hepatoblastoma. Cancer 56: 1926–1929

40. Schmidt D, Harms D, Lang W (1985) Primary malignant hepatic tumors in childhood. Virch Arch (Pathol Anat) 407: 387–405

41. Fraumeric JF, Rosen PJ, Hull EW, Barth RF, Shapiro SR, O'Connor JF (1969) Hepatoblastoma in infant sisters. Cancer 24: 1086–1090

42. Beach R, Betts P, Radford M, Millward-Sadler H (1984) Production of human chorionic gonadotrophin by a hepatoblastoma resulting in precocious puberty. J Clin Pathol 37: 734–737

43. Ishak KG, Glunz PR (1967) Hepatoblastoma and hepatocarcinoma in infancy and childhood. Report of 47 cases. Cancer 20: 396–422

44. Fraumeni JF Jr., Miller RW, Hill JA (1986) Primary carcinoma of the liver in childhood: An epidemiologic study. J Natl Cancer Inst 40: 1087–1099

45. Geiser CF, Baez A, Schindler AM, Shik VE (1970) Epithelial hepatoblastoma associated with congenital hemihypertrophy and cystathionuria. Pediatrics 46: 66–70

46. Sotelo-Avila C, Gooch WM III (1976) Neoplasm associated with the Bechwith-Wiedemann Syndrome. Perspect Pediatr Pathol 3: 255–272

47. Helson L, Peterson RHF, Schwartz MK (1973) Cystathionine excess in children with hepatic cancer. Cancer Res 33: 1570–1573

48. Douglass EC, Green AA, Hayes FA, Etcubanas E, Horowitz M, Williams JA (1985) Chromosome 1 abnormalities: a common feature of pediatric solid tumors. JNCI 75: 51–54

49. Behrle FC, Mantz FA, Olson RL, Trambold JC (1963) Virilization accompanying hepatoblastoma. Pediatrics 32: 265–271

50. Muraji T, Woolley MM, Sinatra F, Siegel SM, Isaacs H (1985) The prognostic implication of hypercholesterolemia in infants and children with hepatoblastoma. J Pediatr Surg 20: 228–230

51. Korobkin M, Kirks DR, Sullivan DC, Mills SR, Bowie JD (1981) Computed tomography of primary liver tumors in children. Radiology 139: 431–435

52. Cremin BJ, Nuss D (1974) Calcified hepatoblastoma in a newborn. Pediatr Surg 9: 913–915

53. Miller JH, Greenspan BS (1985) Integrated imaging of hepatic tumors in childhood: I. Malignant lesions (primary and metastatic). Radiology 145: 83–90

54. Helson L, Helson C (1976) Human hepatoblastoma in cell culture. In Vitro 12: 327–328

55. Doi I (1976) Establishment of a cell line and its clonal sublines from a patient with hepatoblastoma. Gann 67: 1–10

56. Amuro Y, Tanaka M, Higashino K, Hayashi E, Endo T, Kishimoto S, Nakabayashi H, Sato J (1982) Bile acid synthesis by long-term cultured cell line established from human hepatoblastoma. J Clin Invest 70: 1128–1130

57. Wu CY, Wu CH, Rifici VA, Stockert RJ (1984) Activity and regulation of low density lipoprotein receptors in a human hepatoblastoma cell line. Hepatology 4: 1190–1194

58. Hata Y, Uchino J, Sasaki F, Une Y, Naito H, Sato K, Kukita K, Sano H, Kasai Y, Tsultada Y, Hirai H (1984) Effect of anti-alpha-fetoprotein serum

on human hepatoblastoma. J Pediatr Surg 19: 573–576
59. Kasai M, Watanabe I (1970) Histologic classification of liver cell carcinoma in infancy and childhood and its clinical evaluation. Cancer 25: 551–563
60. Misugi K, Reiner CB (1965) A malignant true teratoma of liver in childhood. Arch Pathol 80: 409–412
61. Silverman JF, Fu Y, McWilliams NB, Kay S (1975) An ultrastructural study of mixed hepatoblastoma with osteoid elements. Cancer 36: 1436–1443
62. Ordonez NG, Mackay B (1983) Ultrastructure of liver cell and bile duct carcinomas. Ultrastruct Path 5: 201–241
63. Andrassy RJ, Brennan LP, Siegel MM, Weitzman JJ, Siegel SE, Stanley P, Mahour GH (1980) Preoperative chemotherapy for hepatoblastoma in children: report of six cases. J Pediatr Surg 15: 517–522
64. Evans AE, Land VJ, Newton WA, Randolph JG, Sather HN, Tefft M (1982) Combination chemotherapy (vincristine, adriamycin, cyclophosphamide, and 5-fluorouracil) in the treatment of children with malignant hepatoma. Cancer 50: 821–826

Chapter 10
Fibrolamellar Carcinoma of the Liver

DONALD B. ROLFES[1]

1 Introduction

Hepatocellular carcinoma (HCC) usually develops in cirrhotic livers of older adults. Typically, it is widely disseminated or multicentric at the time of diagnosis, unresectable, and has a poor prognosis with survival time measured in months. Fibrolamellar carcinoma (FLC) is a variant of HCC whose separation as a distinct entity is justified by clinicopathological features which sharply contrast with those commonly observed in HCC (Table 10.1). FLC occurs in children and young adults with noncirrhotic livers and has unique histological features from which its name derives. Edmondson first recognized these characteristics in a case he described in 1956 [1], and this was followed by the report of five additional cases by Peters in 1976, who referred to them as HCC with lamellar fibrosis [2]. The existence of this neoplasm was subsequently confirmed by two large series in 1980: In the series of Berman et al. [3] the term HCC of polygonal cell type with lamellar fibrosis was used; the other series was by Craig et al. [4], whose term FLC of the liver has persisted. While this neoplasm constitutes only 1%–2% of all HCC [5], 40% of cases seen in patients under 35 years of age are of this type [6]. At the time of diagnosis, the tumor is frequently localized in the liver, surgically resectable, and potentially curable. The recognition of FLC is consequently of major importance.

2 Clinical aspects

FLC usually develops in patients 5–35 years of age, although it occasionally occurs in older adults. It is seen with equal incidence in males

[1] Department of Hepatic Pathology, Armed Forces Institute of Pathology, Washington, DC 20306, USA

and females. No association with oral contraceptive use has been found [7]. Abdominal pain, malaise, and weight loss are the common presenting complaints. An abdominal mass is palpable in two-thirds of patients. Jaundice is occasionally detected. In one series, these symptoms and signs had been noticed for an average of 11 months prior to diagnosis compared with the 2.8-month delay usually observed with HCC [6].

Liver function tests reveal nonspecific mild to modest elevations of the serum transaminases, alkaline phosphatase, and bilirubin. The serum alpha fetoprotein level is elevated in less than 10% of cases, but other potential tumor markers have been identified. These include increased serum vitamin B_{12} binding capacity and B_{12} levels [8], neurotensin [9], and carcinoembryonic antigen (CEA) [10]. The increased B_{12} binding capacity is due to an abnormal transcobalamin-1 protein, which is either synthesized by the tumor or represents circulating transcobalamin-1 that has been chemically modified by it. While elevated serum vitamin B_{12}-binding capacity and neurotensin are highly correlated with FLC, neither is completely sensitive nor specific for it [8, 11]; they are also occasionally detected in patients with ordinary HCC and patients with other primary neoplasms, particularly when liver metastases are present. These laboratory studies, therefore, cannot be used as substitutes for histological diagnosis.

The most helpful radiographic clue is the presence of calcification within the tumor, an otherwise uncommon finding in untreated HCC [12, 13]. This may be detected on plain films of the abdomen or by computed tomography (Fig. 10.1a, b). These neoplasms produce a defect on sulfur colloid liver-spleen scintigrams and are echogenic with ultrasound and hypodense with unenhanced computed tomography. The latter two imaging modalities may detect a central scar, manifested by areas of increased echogenicity

Table 10.1. Comparison of clinicopathological features of fibrolamellar carcinoma with normal hepatocellular carcinoma

	FLC	HCC
Age-group	5–35 years	50–70 years
Sex distribution	Equal in males and females	Males predominate (3.5:1)
Nonneoplastic liver	Normal	Cirrhotic (75%)
Serum HBsAg	Absent	Present (60%)
Serum alpha fetoprotein	Normal	Elevated (85%)
Histopathology		
Fibrosis	Prominent	Absent
Cytology	Abundant eosinophilic cytoplasm	Variable
Extent of disease in liver at diagnosis	Localized	Widely disseminated
Surgical resectability	50%–75%	10%–20%
Mean survival from time of diagnosis	32–68 months	Less than 6 months

FLC fibrolamellar carcinoma, *HCC* hepatocellular carcinoma

and lower density within the neoplasm, respectively, which can create confusion with focal nodular hyperplasia. Angiograms show a highly vascularized tumor whose arterial phase is characterized by abnormal vessels arranged in a septate fashion (Fig. 10.1c). Early arteriovenous shunting to the hepatic portal vein, if present, is a good clue to the presence of FLC [14].

3 Pathology

FLC usually occurs in a noncirrhotic liver. It is rarely seen in association with chronic liver disease and cirrhosis [4]. Two-thirds of reported cases have been located in the left lobe. Grossly, the tumor is usually a sharply circumscribed solitary mass with a scalloped border. Occasionally, smaller adjacent satellite nodules are present. Fibrous septa course through the tumor, in some instances radiating from a central scar mimicking the appearance of focal nodular hyperplasia (Fig. 10.2). Consequently, it has been suggested that FLC may develop as a result of malignant transformation in focal nodular hyperplasia [3, 15], a theory which has met with some disagreement [4]. The distribution of metastases is similar to that in ordinary HCC with a tendency for abdominal lymph node and peritoneal and pulmonary spread. Endodermal sinus tumors with hepatoid differentiation arising in the ovary have a close histological similarity to FLC and may be confused with metastases [16].

The distinctive histological characteristics of this tumor include both stromal and cytological components. Fibrosis, which is typically incon-

spicuous in HCC, is abundant in FLC. Collagen and fibroblasts are arranged in lamellae about nests, pseudoglands, cords, and sheets of neoplastic cells (Fig. 10.3). This desmoplastic response is also apparent in metastases, though it is often less pronounced. The neoplastic cells have an abundant deeply eosinophilic cytoplasm. Most have a centrally placed vesicular nucleus and a single prominent nucleolus. Mitotic figures are rare. Cytoplasmic pale bodies (Fig. 10.4) and eosinophilic globules (Fig. 10.5), both of which represent various secretory products of the cells, are common. The latter are usually positive with periodic acid-Schiff (PAS) staining following diastase pretreatment and some represent the accumulation of alpha$_1$-antitrypsin [17, 18]. Fibrinogen is often present in the pale bodies [19], which are PAS negative. Copper and copper-binding protein (Fig. 10.5) can frequently be detected with special stains and are distinctive features of this neoplasm [10, 18, 20]. Bile production is common and mucin is occasionally present [21].

FLC is not always a pure pathological entity [22]. The characteristic histological features may vary in degree within a given tumor and on occasion can be absent from wide areas. It is unknown whether the clinical features or survival differ in those patients whose tumors have nonfibrolamellar components.

Ultrastructural descriptions have accompanied many of the reports of this tumor [4, 6, 15, 17, 19, 23–26]. The most outstanding feature has been the presence of abundant mitochondria, which fill the cytoplasm and account for its eosinophilic appearance by light microscopy

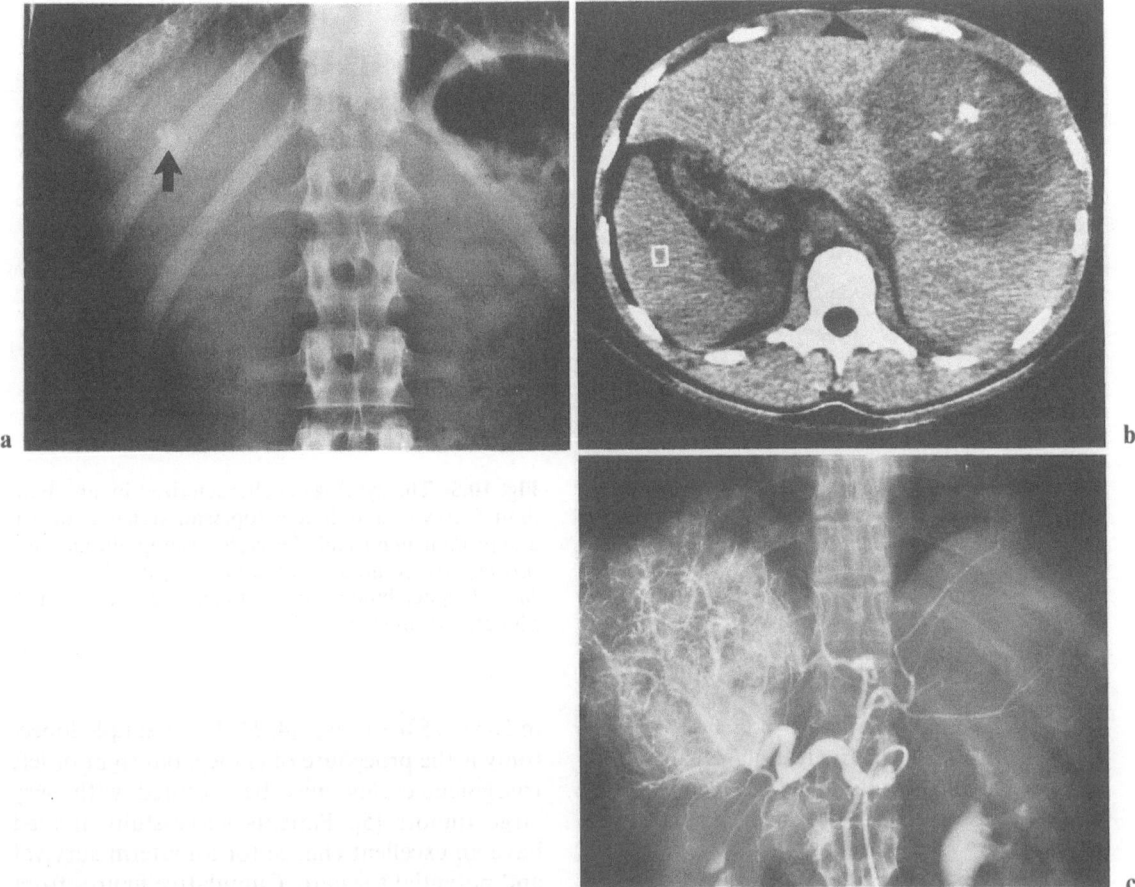

Fig. 10.1. a Supine plain film of abdomen. Note the globular, well-defined calcification in the right upper quadrant (*arrow*). **b** Unenhanced axial computed tomography corresponding to same patient as **a**. There is a well-defined hypodense mass lesion with lobulated borders located in the anterior segment of the right lobe of the liver. Observe the central area of calcification correlating with the plain film. The density of the lesion is otherwise homogeneous. **c** Capillary phase of a selective hepatic artery arteriogram corresponding to the same patient as **a** and **b** reveals a large hypervascular tumor. There is no gross arteriovenous shunting. (Courtesy of Pablo Ross MD, Chief of Gastrointestinal Radiology, Armed Forces Institute of Pathology)

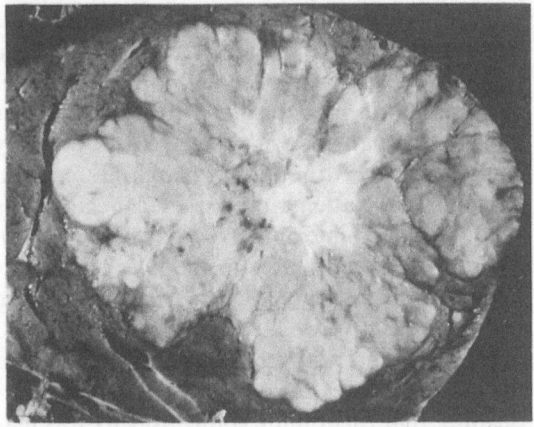

Fig. 10.2. The tumor is sharply circumscribed. Fibrous septa create a gross multinodular appearance and coalesce, centrally mimicking focal nodular hyperplasia

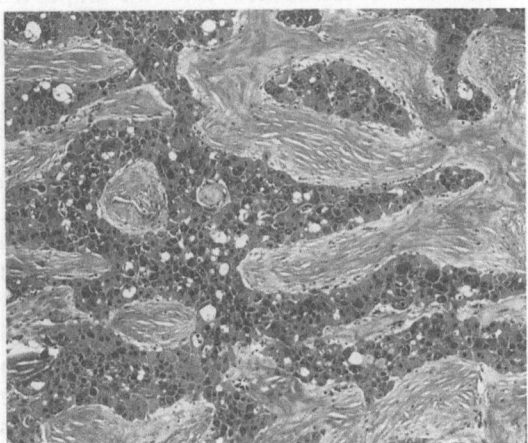

Fig. 10.3. Lamellae of dense connective tissue surround nests and anastomosing cords of neoplastic hepatocytes. H and E, × 60

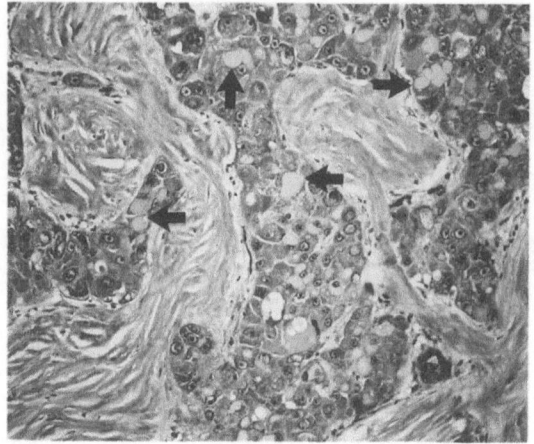

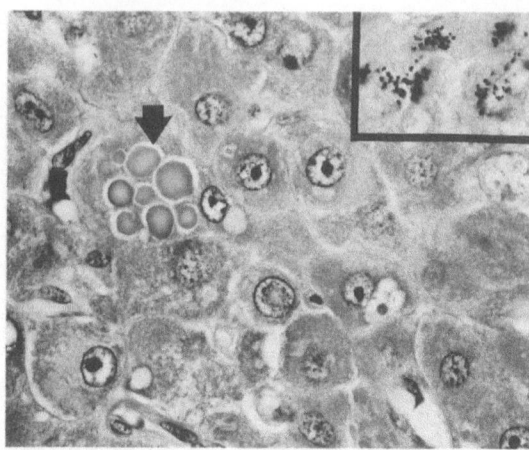

Fig. 10.4. Pale Cytoplasmic inclusions, which mimic the ground glass cells seen in chronic hepatitis B infections, are present in numerous cells (*arrows*). H and E, × 160

Fig. 10.5. The cytology is characterized by an abundant deeply eosinophilic cytoplasm, vesicular nuclei, and prominent nucleoli. Discrete eosinophilic globules (*arrow*) are commonly observed. H and E, × 630. *Inset*: Copper binding protein can often be detected. Shikata orcein stain, × 630

(Fig. 10.6). Tumor cells are attached by well-formed desmosomes. Intercellular spaces lined by microvilli representing bile canaliculi are present. A wide variety of cytoplasmic inclusions are described.

Immunohistological studies show carcinoembryonic antigen lining the canalicular spaces and pseudoglands [10, 21] and globules of alpha$_1$-antitrypsin [17, 18, 21] and ferritin diffusely distributed in the cytoplasm [17]. Alpha fetoprotein is usually not detected. Fibronectin is abundant in the stroma, suggesting that this substance participates in the desmoplastic response to the tumor and is associated with the improved prognosis [27].

4 Treatment and prognosis

The outlook for patients with HCC is bleak with a mean survival of 6 months. In contrast, the average survival of patients with FLC has been reported to be 32–68 months. This improved prognosis is due to multiple factors which include the greater resectability of the tumor and its indolent growth. A more aggressive approach by surgeons influenced by the young age of these patients and the lack of complicating cirrhosis probably also plays a role in the more favorable prognosis.

Complete surgical resection is the basis for treatment of this tumor and can be accomplished

in 50%–75% of cases [4, 22, 28]. A simple lobectomy is the procedure of choice, but right or left trisegmentectomy may be required with very large tumors [5]. Patients successfully treated have an excellent chance for long-term survival and potential for cure. Cumulative figures from four large series [3, 6, 22, 29] involving 37 patients show 24% to be living and free of disease greater than 5 years following complete resection, 19% healthy 2–5 years following surgery, and another 19% healthy less than 2 years after the procedure; 38% developed recurrences or died of the disease. Further extensive efforts are probably justified for those patients with more advanced disease. When primary resection of the tumor is not possible, hepatic transplantation has been employed [29]. Experience with orthotopic liver transplantation for primary liver cancer has shown that patients with FLC benefit most by this procedure. Although the neoplasm recurs in over 50% of patients thus treated, recurrences tend to develop late and grow slowly (chap. 32). Resection of recurrences in the liver and extrahepatic metastases may be beneficial and in some instances curative [3, 22].

Even patients with nonresectable tumors and distant metastases have prolonged survival, indicating that this tumor is intrinsically less malignant than HCC. In one study, such patients survived an average of 24 months [30]. Various chemotherapeutic regimens have been used in this context [10, 29, 30] with partial responses

Fig. 10.6. Electron micrograph shows mitochondria, packed back to back, filling the cytoplasm of the tumor cells. × 12 000

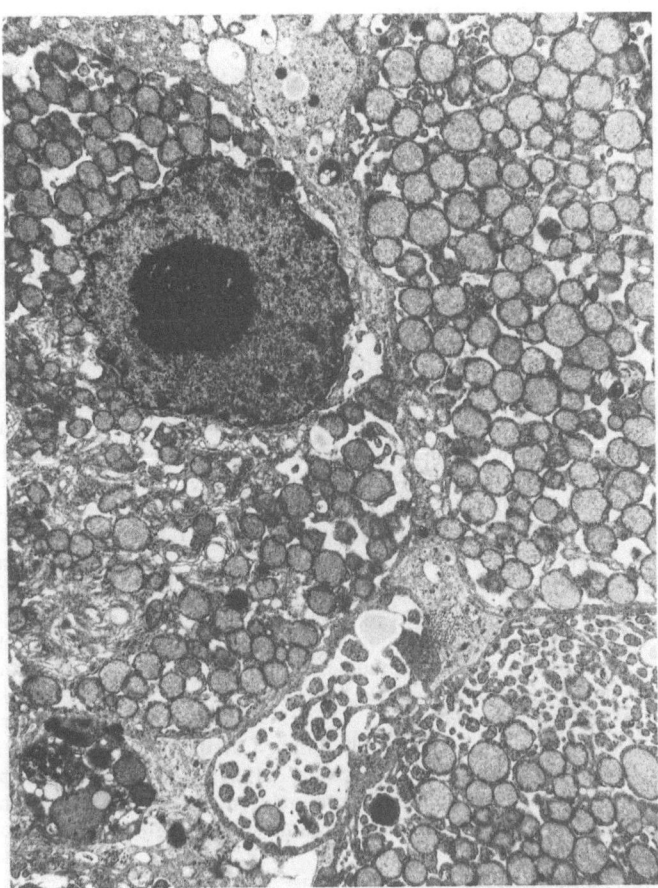

being observed in occasional patients, but they have had little demonstrable impact on survival. There are no reports of radiotherapy having been successfully employed.

References

1. Edmondson HA (1956) Differential diagnosis of tumors and tumor-like lesions of liver in infancy and childhood. Arch Dis Child 1: 168–186
2. Peters RL (1976) Pathology of hepatocellular carcinoma. In: Okuda K, Peters RL (eds) Hepatocellular carcinoma. Wiley, New York, p 107
3. Berman MM, Libbey NP, Foster JH (1980) Hepatocellular carcinoma. Polygonal cell type with fibrous stroma—an atypical variant with a favorable prognosis. Cancer 46: 1448–1455
4. Craig JR, Peters RL, Edmondson HA, Omata M (1980) Fibrolamellar carcinoma of the liver: a tumor of adolescents and young adults with distinctive clinicopathologic features. Cancer 46: 372–379
5. Craig JR, Van Thiel DH (1985) Fibrolamellar carcinoma. In: Ishak KG (ed) Hepatopathology 1985. Syllabus of the postgraduate course of the American Association for the Study of Liver Disease, 3–4 Nov. 1985, Chicago. Available from Slack Inc. Thorocare, New Jersey 08086, pp 361–371
6. Farhi DC, Shikes RH, Murari PJ, Silverberg SG (1983) Hepatocellular carcinoma in young people. Cancer 52: 1516–1525
7. Goodman ZD, Ishak KG (1982) Hepatocellular carcinoma in women: probable lack of etiologic association with oral contraceptive steroids. Hepatology 2: 440–444
8. Paradinas FJ, Melia WM, Wilkinson ML, Portmann B, Johnson PJ, Murray-Lyon IM, Williams R (1982) High serum vitamin B_{12} binding capacity as a marker of the fibrolamellar variant of hepatocellular carcinoma. Br Med J 285: 840–842
9. Collier NA, Bloom SR, Hodgson HJF, Weinbren K, Lee YC, Blumgart LH (1984): Neurotensin secretion by fibrolamellar carcinoma of the liver. Lancet 1: 538–540
10. Teitelbaum DH, Tuttle S, Carey LC, Clausen KP (1985) Fibrolamellar carcinoma of the liver. Review of three cases and the presentation of a characteristic set of tumor markers defining this tumor. Ann Surg 202: 36–41

11. Wood JR, Melia WM, Wood SM, Wilkinson ML, Lee YC, Portmann B, Bloom SR, Williams R (1984) Neurotensin and hepatocellular carcinoma (Letter to the editor). Lancet 1: 687

12. Friedman AC, Lichtenstein JE, Goodman ZD, Fishman EK, Siegelman SS, Dachman AH (1985) Fibrolamellar hepatocellular carcinoma. Radiology 157: 583–587

13. Francis IR, Agha FP, Thompson NW, Keren DF (1986) Fibrolamellar hepatocarcinoma: clinical, radiologic and pathologic features. Gastrointest Radiol 11: 67–72

14. Wong LK, Link DP, Frey CF, Ruebner BH, Tesluk H, Pimstone NR (1982) Fibrolamellar hepatocarcinoma: radiology, management and pathology AJR 139: 172–175

15. Vecchio FM, Fabiano A, Ghirlanda G, Manna R, Massi G (1984) Fibrolamellar carcinoma of the liver: the malignant counterpart of focal nodular hyperplasia with oncocytic change. Am J Clin Pathol 81: 521–526

16. Prat J, Bhan AK, Dickersin GR, Robboy SJ, Scully RE (1982) Hepatoid yolk sac tumor of the ovary (endodermal sinus tumor with hepatoid differentiation). A light microscopic, ultrastructural and immunohistochemical study of seven cases. Cancer 50: 2355–2368

17. Caballero T, Aneiros J, Lopez-Caballero J, Gomez-Morales M, Nogales F (1985): Fibrolamellar hepatocellular carcinoma. An immunohistochemical and ultrastructural study. Histopathology 9: 445–456

18. Lefkowitch JH, Muschel R, Price JB, Marboe C, Braunhut S (1983) Copper and copper-binding protein in fibrolamellar liver cell carcinoma. Cancer 51: 97–100

19. Stromeyer FW, Ishak KG, Gerber MA, Mathew T (1980) Ground-glass cells in hepatocellular carcinoma. Am J Clin Pathol 74: 254–258

20. Sheahan DG (1986) Fibrolamellar carcinoma of the liver: an immunohistochemical study (abstract) Lab Invest 54: 57A

21. Goodman ZD, Ishak KG, Langloss JM, Sesterhenn IA, Rabin L (1985) Combined hepatocellular-cholangiocellular carcinoma. A histologic and immunohistologic study. Cancer 55: 124–135

22. Nagorney DM, Adson MA, Weiland LH, Knight CD, Smalley SR, Zinsmeister AR (1985) Fibrolamellar hepatoma. Am J Surg 149: 113–119

23. An T, Ghatak N, Kastner R, Kay S, Lee HM (1983) Hyaline globules and intracellular lumina in a hepatocellular carcinoma. Am J Clin Pathol 79: 392–396

24. Baithun SI, Pollock DJ (1983) Oncocytic hepatocellular tumor. Histopathology 7: 107–112

25. Farhi DC, Shikes RH, Silverberg SG (1982) Ultrastructure of fibrolamellar oncocytic hepatoma. Cancer 50: 702–709

26. Mierau GW, Orsini EN (1983) Case for diagnosis. Ultrastruct Pathol 5: 273–279

27. Jagirdar J, Ishak KG, Colombo M, Brambilla C, Paronetto F (1985) Fibronectin patterns in hepatocellular carcinoma and its clinical significance. Cancer 56: 1643–1648

28. Lack EE, Neave C, Vawter GF (1983) Hepatocellular carcinoma. Review of 32 cases in childhood and adolescence. Cancer 52: 1510–1515

29. Starzl TE, Iwatsuki S, Shaw BW, Nalesnik MA, Farhi DC, Van Thiel DH (1986) Treatment of fibrolamellar hepatoma with partial or total hepatectomy and transplantation of the liver. Surg Gynecol Obstet 162: 145–148

30. Ihde DC, Matthews MJ, Makuch RW, McIntire KR, Eddy JL, Seeff LB (1985) Prognostic factors in patients with hepatocellular carcinoma receiving systemic chemotherapy. Identification of two groups of patients with prospects for prolonged survival. Am J Med 78: 399–406

Chapter 11
Pathology of Cholangiocarcinoma

SHIGETAKA SUGIHARA and MASAMICHI KOJIRO[1]

Primary liver cancer is roughly divided into hepatocellular carcinoma (HCC) arising from liver cells and cholangiocarcinoma arising from the epithelium of the bile ducts. Of these, the pathological characteristics of cholangiocarcinoma have not yet been elucidated fully because its incidence is low compared with that of HCC and because its differentiation from extrahepatic bile duct cancer is often difficult. Only carcinomas arising from the intrahepatic bile ducts should be classified as cholangiocarcinoma. Carcinomas originating from the right and left hepatic ducts and the area of their junction are generally classified as the hilar type of cholangiocarcinoma, because it is often difficult clinically and pathologically to distinguish the intrahepatic bile duct carcinomas from extrahepatic carcinomas [1–5].

According to "The General Rules for Surgical Studies on Cancer of the Bile Duct" issued by "The Japanese Biliary Surgical Society" [6], the bile duct located on the liver side of the first intraphepatic branch of the right and left hepatic ducts is considered intrahepatic; cancers peripheral to this site are classified as cholangiocarcinoma. However, it is often impossible to identify the first branch of the intraphepatic bile duct in cancer occurring within the liver in autopsy cases and occasionally even in surgical cases. Further, it is often difficult, especially when the cancer is massive, to determine whether it arose from the intrahepatic bile duct.

This chapter deals with the pathological and morphological features of cholangiocarcinoma in 60 autopsy cases examined at the Pathology Department of Kurume University School of Medicine during the past 15 years. They included 41 cases with hilar-type lesions arising from the bifurcation of the right and left hepatic ducts and

their vicinity and 19 cases with peripheral-type lesions. In addition, 22 surgical resection cases are discussed.

1 Historical remarks and definition

Sabourin (1881) and Hanot and Gilbert (1888) are generally held to have been the first to classify primary liver cancers into those originating either from liver cells or from the intrahepatic biliary epithelium. In 1911, Goldzieher and Bockay [7] classified primary liver cancer into carcinoma hepatocellulare and carcinoma cholangiocellulare on the basis of the morphological features of the cells. In the same year, Yamagiwa [8] described in detail the morphology of primary liver cancer and proposed the terms "hepatoma and cholangioma." The term "cholangioma" has since been used worldwide, both for intrahepatic and extrahepatic cancers. Furthermore, it was also used as synonymously for cholangiocellular carcinoma, bile duct carcinoma, intrahepatic bile duct carcinoma, and alveolar carcinoma in Western countries. Accordingly, the term "cholangiocarcinoma" was proposed at the Sixth Meeting of the International Association for the Study of the Liver in 1974 at Acapulco, Mexico [9]. Since then, this term has been used exclusively.

Since cholangiocarcinoma is in the strict sense a cancer arising from the epithelium of the intrahepatic bile duct, other tumors should be designated as extrahepatic bile duct cancer. However, differentiation of intrahepatic bile duct cancers from extrahepatic ones is difficult, as noted above in autopsy cases with massive tumors at the hilum of the liver. Furthermore, it is also difficult to define the intrahepatic bile duct. For such reasons, cancers arising from the bile duct epithelium of the right and left hepatic ducts and the bifurcation are also considered cholangiocar-

---

[1] The First Department of Pathology, Kurume University School of Medicine, Kurume, 830 Japan

cinoma in this chapter. This hilar cholangiocarcinoma includes a special type called "Klatskin's tumor," which occurs relatively often in young males and often requires clinical differentiation from sclerosing cholangitis [9–13]. In surgical cases, cancers occurring in the hilum are often small and can be identified relatively easily as being intrahepatic or extrahepatic in origin. Accordingly, there is a possibility that the clinical and pathological differentiation of intrahepatic and extrahepaptic bile duct cancers will become easier by additional studies of larger numbers of surgically resected cases.

The intrahepatic bile ducts from the small radicles, including the cholangioles or canals of Hering, to the major branches are considered the site of origin of cholangiocarcinoma.

2 Pathogenesis

There are few factors showing an apparent cause-and-effect relationship with cholangiocarcinoma, in contrast to the well-established relationship of HCC to hepatitis B. It is well known that cholangiocarcinoma is the most common of the thorium dioxide (Thorotrast)-related hepatic malignancies [14–17]. In addition, hepatolithiasis, hepatic infestation by *Clonorchis sinensis*, cystic and dysplastic hepatic lesions, and chronic inflammatory bowel disease [18] have been reported as factors etiologically related to cholangiocarcinoma. Furthermore, there is a case report indicating that anabolic steroids might be related to this cancer [19].

2.1 Thorotrast

Thorotrast, a colloidal solution of thorium dioxide (ThO_2), was used worldwide as a contrast medium for X-ray examination in the 1930s and 1940s. Since 1947, when MacMahon et al. [20] reported the first case of Thorotrast-related hepatic angiosarcoma, many malignant tumors have been reported. Of the Thorotrast-related hepatic malignancies, cholangiocarcinoma, angiosarcoma, and HCC are the most common. In the epidemiological study conducted by Mori [15], deaths from hepatic malignancies accounted for 66.6% of the total deaths in Thorotrast cases, with cholangiocarcinoma being the most common. In our study of 35 cases of Thorotrast-related cholangiocarcinomas, we found no essential histological differences between them and non-Thorotrast cases [21]. However, there was a remarkable difference in tumor location: Most

Thorotrast-related cholangiocarcinomas were located in the liver. Furthermore, small to medium-sized papillary growths of the bile duct epithelium and proliferation of bile ductules around Glisson's capsule were notable changes in the noncancerous liver parenchyma. These changes are not specific to Thorotrast-related disease but are considered to reflect marked active changes in the bile duct epithelium [16]. Rubel et al. [17] termed an atypical change in the bile duct epithelium "duct dysplasia, carcinoma in situ" and considered that it might be a precancerous change.

2.2 Hepatolithiasis

Carcinoma of the gallbladder is often associated with cholelithiasis, and there are many reports concerning this relationship. On the other hand, it has been suggested that cholangiocarcinoma is rarely complicated by hepatolithiasis [22]. However, the number of cholangiocarcinomas associated with hepatolithiasis has increased recently; thus, hepatolithiasis is now observed in 5.7%–17.5% of cholangiocarcinomas [23–25].

Repeated bouts of inflammation of the bile duct epithelium due to hepatolithiasis may be a contributory cause of cholangiocarcinoma. Sanes and MacCallum [26] reported various degrees of papillary changes and adenomatous hyperplasia of the bile duct epithelium in the vicinity of stones in two such cases [24, 27]. Nakanuma et al. [28] focused attention on chronic proliferative cholangitis, especially atypical epithelial hyperplasia, observed in the stone-bearing bile duct in hepatolithiasis.

In our series, hepatolithiasis was noted in 4 of 19 peripheral-type (21.1%) and in 3 of 41 hilar-type (7.3%) cholangiocarcinomas, i.e., in a total of 7 (11.7%) of 60 cases. On the other hand, cholelithiasis was found in three peripheral-type and nine hilar-type cases, a total of 12 cases.

2.3 Parasites

There are many reports of cholangiocarcinoma associated with liver fluke infection in the Orient [29], for example *Clonorchis sinensis* in Hong Kong [30–32] and Canton and *Opisthorchis viverrini* in Thailand [33]. Furthermore, there is a report concerning experimental carcinogenesis in *Clonorchis sinensis* infection. However, no direct contributory factor has been demonstrated in any case.

Infections caused by *Schistosoma mansoni*, *Schistosoma japonicum*, and *Fasciola hepatica* are well-recognized parasitic diseases of the liver not causally related to cholangiocarcinoma. The prevalence of *Schistosoma japonicum* infection is high in the Kurume district. Although chronic schistosomiasis japonica is relatively often complicated by HCC [34], cholangiocarcinoma was noted in only 1 of 60 cases (1.7%).

2.4 Cystic and dysplastic hepatic lesions

Cholangiocarcinoma is a recognized complication of congenital liver disorders, such as congenital dilatation of the intrahepatic bile duct [35, 36], congenital cysts [37, 38], Carolis' disease [39], and congenital hepatic fibrosis [40].

3 Incidence

The proportion of cholangiocarcinoma to HCC ranges from 2.6% to 35.5%. In the United States [1, 3, 41–44], this proportion varies slightly between 17.8% and 35.5%, but it is about 20% according to many reports from England (20.8%) [45] and Mexico (18.9%) [46]. On the other hand, it is low in Africa (2.6%, 6.7%) [4, 47], Singapore (9%) [48], Japan (10%) [49], China (10.3%) [50], and Hong Kong (15%) [51]. In our series, HCC and cholangiocarcinoma were noted in 462 and 60 cases, respectively, and the proportion of cholangiocarcinoma was as low as 11.5%, which was almost the same as that for the rest of Japan. The proportion of cholangiocarcinoma to HCC is relatively low in Asian and African countries because of the high incidence of HCC [23]. The incidence of cholangiocarcinoma tends to be slightly higher in the Orient, but it does not show the marked regional differences of HCC [9].

4 Sex and age

The incidence of HCC is much higher in males. In contrast, there is generally no, or little, difference in the sex incidence of cholangiocarcinoma [1, 4, 42, 43, 45, 52]. Thus, the sex ratio is 4.0–8.3 : 1 for HCC but 1–2.2 : 1 for cholangiocarcinoma. In some reports, the number of female patients with cholangiocarcinoma is higher than that of males [41, 46]. In our series, the male to female ratio was 1.6 : 1. There is no difference in sex ratio between extrahepatic bile duct carcinoma and cholangiocarcinoma [53–55].

The age of patients with cholangiocarcinoma

is higher than that of patients with HCC in all reports [1, 4, 42, 46, 49]. In most cases, this difference is partly ascribable to the lack of associated cirrhosis. In the series of Edmondson and Steiner [1], patients with the hilar type were slightly younger (56.1 years) than those with the peripheral type (60.0 years) of carcinoma. In our series, however, there was no age difference (average age 62.8 years) between the peripheral (62.4 years) and hilar (63.0) types. Additionally, the majority of patients were in their 60s, followed by those in their 50s and 70s.

5 Symptoms and prognosis

The initial symptoms of the peripheral type are abdominal pain, generalized malaise, loss of appetite, and fever; the incidence of jaundice is low. On the other hand, the initial presentation of the hilar type is mainly one of obstructive jaundice, as well as generalized malaise.

In five surgically treated cases of the peripheral type, palpable abdominal masses and upper abdominal pain and discomfort were observed as initial symptoms, but jaundice was not noted. Conversely, jaundice was the initial symptom regardless of the site of the tumors (intrahepatic bile duct and vicinity of the junction) in 16 of 17 patients with the hilar type. (One patient experienced pain in the upper right quadrant.) Jaundice also develops with time in the peripheral type; it is rapidly progressive if no appropriate measures are taken [1, 12, 43, 56]. Fever also occurs in many patients during the course of disease.

According to Okuda et al [23], the clinical features of the peripheral type fall between those of HCC and the hilar type of cholangiocarcinoma. The clinical symptoms of the hilar type are very similar to those of extrahepatic bile duct carcinoma [53, 55].

Since early detection of cholangiocarcinoma, especially the peripheral type, is difficult, its prognosis in unfavorable. In conjunction with recent rapid advances in diagnostic imaging techniques, such as ultrasonography [57, 58], computed tomography [59], percutaneous transhepatic cholangiography (PTC) [60, 61], endoscopic retrograde cholangiopancreatography (ERCP) [62, 63], and peritoneoscopy [64, 65], however, the frequency of relatively early detection of cholangiocarcinoma has increased, as has the number of cases undergoing surgery.

In our series, the survival time after the appearance of initial symptoms averaged 7.2 months. It was slightly longer in the peripheral type (7.7 months) than in the hilar type (7.0 months). Moreover, the asymptomatic stage is generally longer in the peripheral type, while symptoms tend to appear relatively early in the hilar type. Accordingly, the survival time after actual carcinogenesis is considered longer in the peripheral type.

The average survival time for the past 15 years (calculated for each 5-year period) has increased gradually from 5.3 to 7.6 and 9.0 months. These results are probably attributable to improved diagnostic and therapeutic techniques. The most common cause of death in our series was hepatic failure, followed by cachexia, gastrointestinal bleeding, and infection.

6 Gross features

Grossly, cholangiocarcinoma is a gray to gray-white tumor, which is firm and solid because of abundant fibrous stroma. When a mass is present on the surface of the liver, umbilication may be present. Cholangiocarcinoma is usually classified macroscopically into three types—massive, nodular, and diffuse types—according to Eggel's classification of 1901 [66]. Unlike HCC, cholangiocarcinoma is rarely complicated by liver chirrhosis, and the liver is often enlarged.

On the basis of the growth patterns, we have proposed the following gross classification.

6.1 Infiltrative type

The tumor is not well-demarcated (Fig. 11.1). It is usually large enough to occupy the entire right or left lobe, but it is small in some cases. This type corresponds to the massive type in Eggel's classification. It is usually gray to gray-white in color. Metastatic foci are scattered within the liver in most cases.

6.2 Nodular type

This type of tumor is relatively well-demarcated but is not encapsulated (Fig. 11.2). It is uniformly gray-white. More cases consist of a single nodule than multiple nodules; small metastatic foci are often noted around the tumor nodule(s).

6.3 Diffuse type

Small tumor nodules are distributed uniformly over the entire liver; they are less than 1 cm in diameter (Fig. 11.3). In general, the nodules are not sharply demarcated from the nonneoplastic parenchyma.

6.4 Periductal type

The tumor infiltrates and proliferates along the extrahepatic bile duct, which is thickened in many cases (Fig. 11.4). Mass formation is minimal and there is thickening and enlargement of the portal region. The infiltration in the liver has an arborescent appearance. Extensive parenchymal infiltration is also observed in most cases.

No gross differences are observed between the shapes of peripheral and hilar tumors. However, dilatation of the intrahepatic bile ducts is not observed in the noncancerous areas of the peripheral type, but it is often prominent in the hilar type. Furthermore, the incidence of biliary fibrosis is higher in the hilar type. The cut surface of the tumors is gray to gray-white, a reflection of the abundant interstitial connective tissue. A fibrous capsule, commonly seen in HCC [67], is not present in cholangiocarcinoma. This is presumably because the basic growth pattern of cholangiocarcinoma is infiltrative. This characteristic leads to ill-defined boundaries between the cancerous and noncancerous parts in the nodular and infiltrative types.

Differences in growth patterns between HCC and cholangiocarcinoma are also reflected by the lack of gross invasion of the portal vein in the latter tumor.

In our cases, the proportion of the infiltrative pattern in the peripheral and hilar types was 57% and 52%, while that of the nodular type was 29% and 14%, respectively. The periductal type was noted only in patients with hilar carcinomas. However, in future, this type may also be detectable in patients with early peripheral-type lesions with advances in diagnostic imaging techniques, such as ultrasonography, angiography, and computed tomography.

There is no difference in the proportion of each gross type between Thorotrast- and non-Thorotrast-related cholangiocarcinomas, but there is a marked difference in the tumor location. The incidence of the peripheral type is remarkably high (89.2%) and that of the hilar type is low. This result is in contrast to the peripheral- to hilar-type ratio of 19:41 in non-Thorotrast cases. There are two possible explanations for this. First, the peripheral bile ducts are preferentially affected by Thorotrast. Second, a large number of extrahepatic bile duct cancers

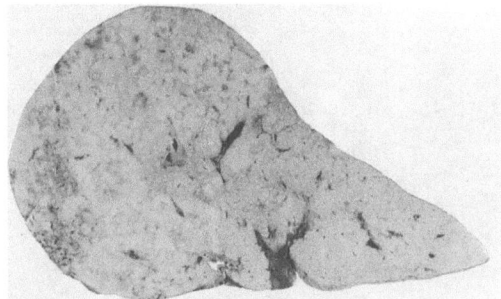

Fig. 11.1. Infiltrative type. Tumor-nontumor boundary is not clear. Tumor shows infiltrative growth

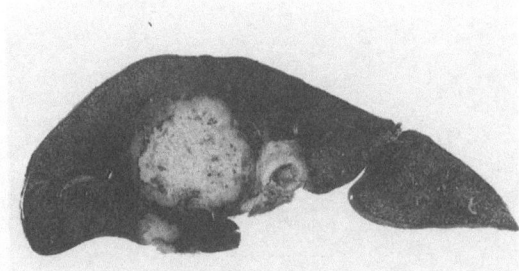

Fig. 11.2. Nodular type. Tumor is well-demarcated, but not encapsulated

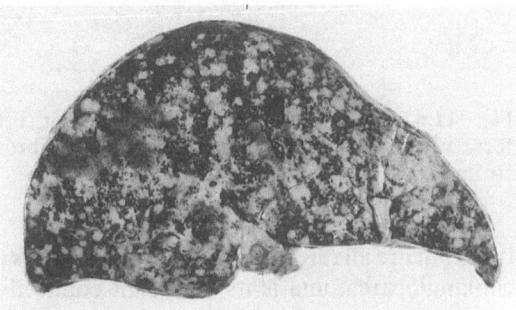

Fig. 11.3. Diffuse type. Numerous small tumor nodules are scattered throughout the liver

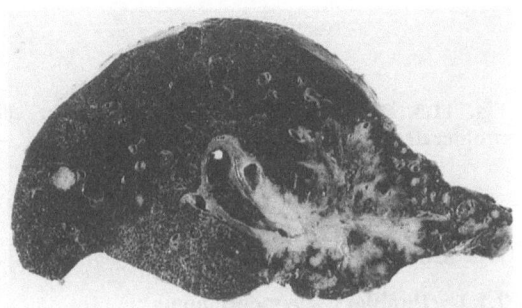

Fig. 11.4. Periductal type. Tumor proliferates along the bile duct in an infiltrative fashion

may be included in the cases of the hilar type of non-Thorotrast bile duct cancer.

Okuda (unpublished data) noted that the deposition of Thorotrast is more prominent in the periphery of the liver than in the hilar portion and suggested that it might explain the high incidence of the peripheral type of cholangiocarcinoma.

The macroscopic changes in Thorotrast cases are almost identical to those of the non-Thorotrast ones. However, tumors showed a "maplike" spread (though demarcated relatively sharply) in some cases of the infiltrative type.

7 Histology

Cholangiocarcinoma is an adenocarcinoma arising from the intrahepatic biliary epithelium. It is usually a differentiated tubular adenocarcinoma with an abundant fibrous stroma and often presents a relatively uniform histological picture. However, various degrees of differentiation or different histological patterns are occasionally noted, even in the same case. Tumor cells are

cuboidal or columnar; the cytoplasm is usually clear but is sometimes granular. The nucleus is small compared with that in HCC and contains abundant chromatin granules. The nucleolus is usually less prominent than that of HCC. Mucous production can usually be identified, but bile production is never observed.

The histological classification is as follows:

Common type
  Papillary adenocarcinoma
  Tubular adenocarcinoma
    Well-differentiated type
    Moderately differentiated type
  Poorly differentiated adenocarcinoma
    Pleomorphic type
    Acinar type
    Signet-ring-cell type
  Mucinous carcinoma
Specific type
  Adenosquamous carcinoma
  Mucoepidermoid carcinoma
  Squamous cell carcinoma
  Carcinoid tumor
  Undifferentiated carcinoma

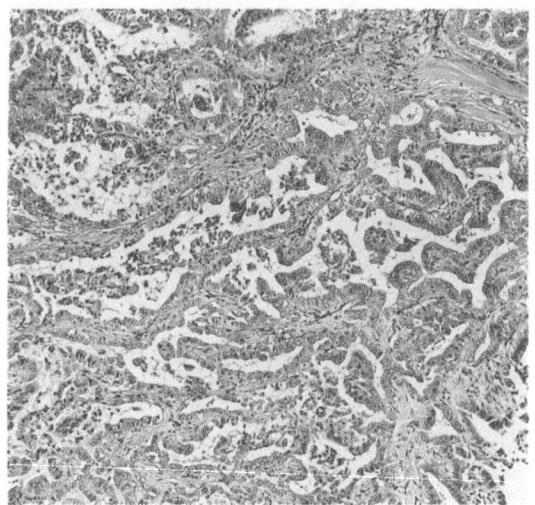

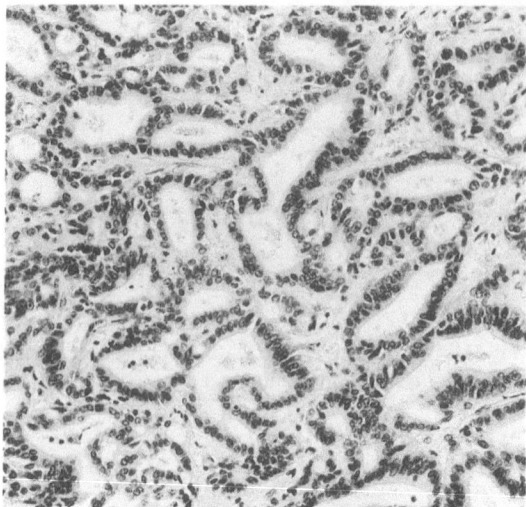

Fig. 11.5. Papillary adenocarcinoma. Tumor cells proliferate in a papillary pattern

Fig. 11.6. Tubular adenocarcinoma. Tumor cells form variously sized tubules with abundant fibrous stroma

7.1 Common types

7.1.1 Papillary adenocarcinoma
Most tumors of this type are morphologically papillotubular adenocarcinoma with a predominant papillary pattern (Fig. 11.5). There is a scanty fibrous stroma.

7.1.2 Tubular adenocarcinoma
Tumors characterized by relatively abundant atypical cells and irregularly sized tubules are classified as moderately differentiated, while tumors consisting mainly of less atypical tubular structure are classified as well-differentiated (Fig. 11.6). Many cholangiocarcinomas are of this histological type.

7.1.3 Poorly differentiated adenocarcinoma
The tumors consist mainly of pleomorphic cells (Fig. 11.7a), signet-ring cells (Fig. 11.7b), or cells showing an acinar structure (Fig. 11.7c), but tubule formation is observed occasionally.

7.1.4 Mucinous carcinoma
Mucin is present within the cells and lumina (Fig. 11.8). In addition, large amounts of mucin are noted extracellularly.

7.2 Specific types

Adenosquamous carcinoma [68, 69], mucoepidermoid carcinoma [70, 71], squamous cell carcinoma [72, 73], carcinoid tumor [74, 75], and undifferentiated carcinoma are included as specific types but are all rare. One of the characteristics of cholangiocarcinoma is its abundant connective tissue stroma, which when excessive permits designation of the tumor as a scirrhous or sclerosing carcinoma [13, 76].

In our series, there was no marked difference in histological pattern between the peripheral and hilar types. Tubular adenocarcinoma was observed most frequently (as also reported in the literature), accounting for 66.7% of cases of the peripheral type and 78% of the hilar type; papillary adenocarcinoma was noted in 5.3% (one case) of the peripheral type and 17% of the hilar type. The latter might include tumors arising from a large hepatic duct showing a papillary proliferation into the duct. In surgical hilar-type cases, the papillary pattern was often present in the area where tumor cells proliferated into the lumen of a large bile duct, but the degree of differentiation tended to be low in the area where tumor cells infiltrated the wall, even in the same case. Mucinous carcinoma was noted in only one hilar-type case, but the mucinous pattern was partially observed in many cases of the peripheral and hilar types. There were no cases with bile in the cytoplasm of tumor cells. However, bile was retained around the margin of tumors in cases with severe bile stasis. Tumor calcification was noted in one case.

Adenosquamous carcinoma was noted in one case each in the peripheral and hilar types (Fig. 11.9), but no other specific type was observed.

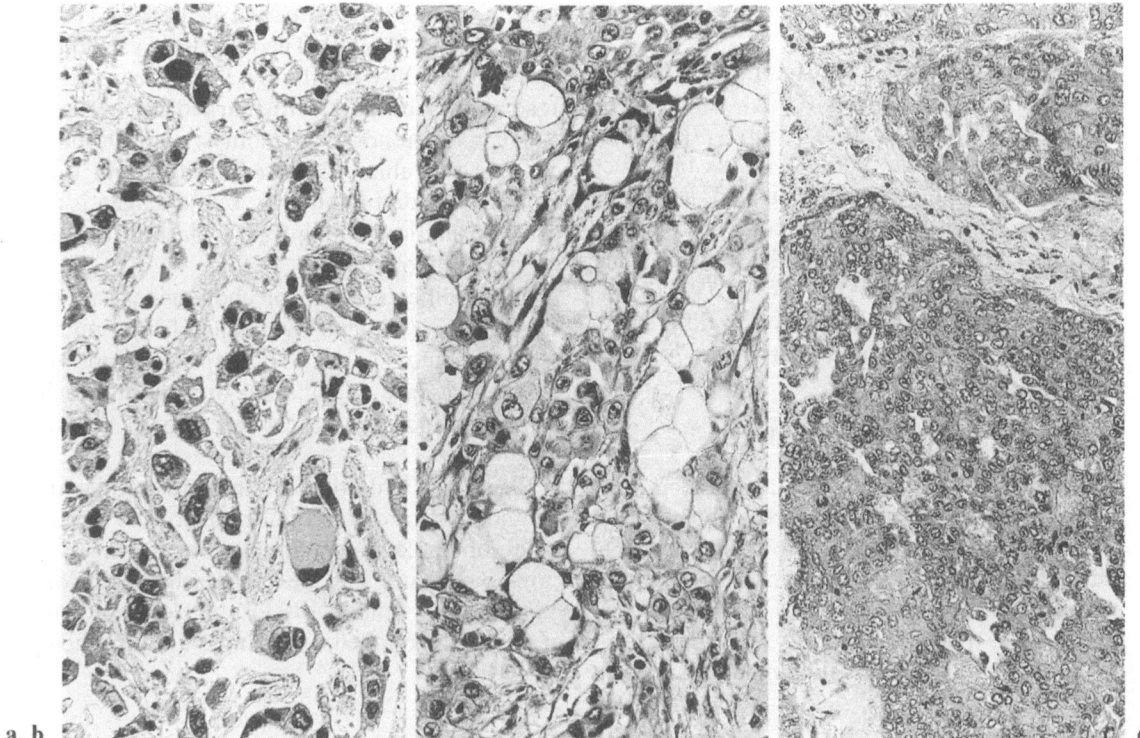

a, b   c

Fig. 11.7a–c. Poorly differentiated adenocarcinoma. **a** Pleomorphic type; **b** Signet-ring cell type; **c** Acinar type

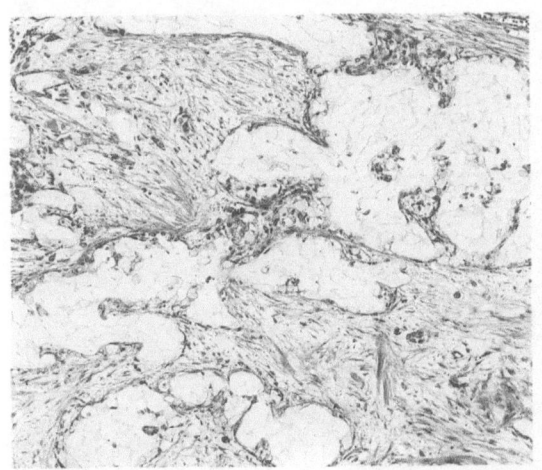

Fig. 11.8. Mucinous carcinoma. Cancerous glands are filled with mucin. Mucin is also observed outside the glands

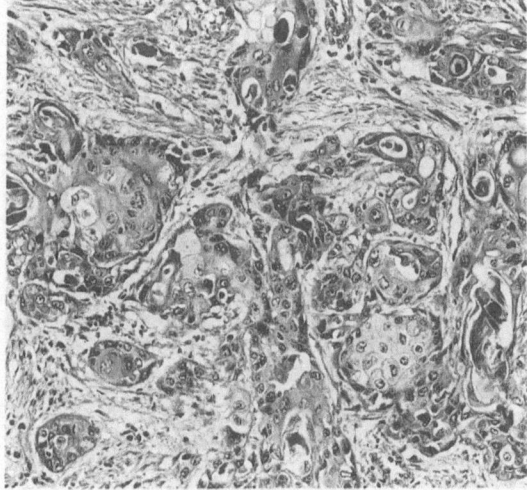

Fig. 11.9. Adenosquamous carcinoma. Tumor consists of squamous cell carcinoma with keratinization and tubular adenocarcinoma. This figure shows a part of the squamous carcinoma component

8 Tumor markers

In the present study, alpha-fetoprotein (AFP), carcinoembryonic antigen (CEA), and carbohydrate antigen 19-9 (CA 19-9) [77], which are known to be elevated in various bile duct disorders [78, 79], were investigated immunohistologically by the avidin-biotin peroxidase complex (ABC) method [80]. The positive rates for CEA, CA 19-9, and AFP were 97.7%, 73.6% and 0%, respectively; there were no differences between the peripheral and hilar types.

9 Electron-microscopic features

Ultrastructural studies of cholangiocarcinoma reveal cuboidal or columnar cells forming irregular glands. Microvilli are found toward the lumen, and a basement membrane is noted (continuously or discontinuously) at the base of the glands (Fig. 11.10a). The cells are closely apposed and many junctional complexes are pre-sent. Interdigitation of the cell membrane is often marked (Fig. 11.10b). The nucleus is variable in size and usually oval, though the nuclear margin is sometimes irregular with marked indentations. Small mitochondria, lysosomes, smooth endoplasmic reticulum, Golgi apparatus, and ribosomes are found in all cells, but glycogen is absent. Formation of an intracytoplasmic lumen is occasionally observed.

While differentiation of cholangiocarcinoma from HCC is difficult by means of light microscopy, the ultrastructural diagnosis is supported by the presence of cuboidal or columnar cells forming glands that have a basement membrane [81].

Electron-microscopic findings are useful in the diagnosis of carcinoid tumor, one of the specific types of cholangiocarcinoma. A diagnosis of carcinoid tumor can be made when electron-microscopic study discloses electron-dense granules surrounded by a single limiting membrane [82].

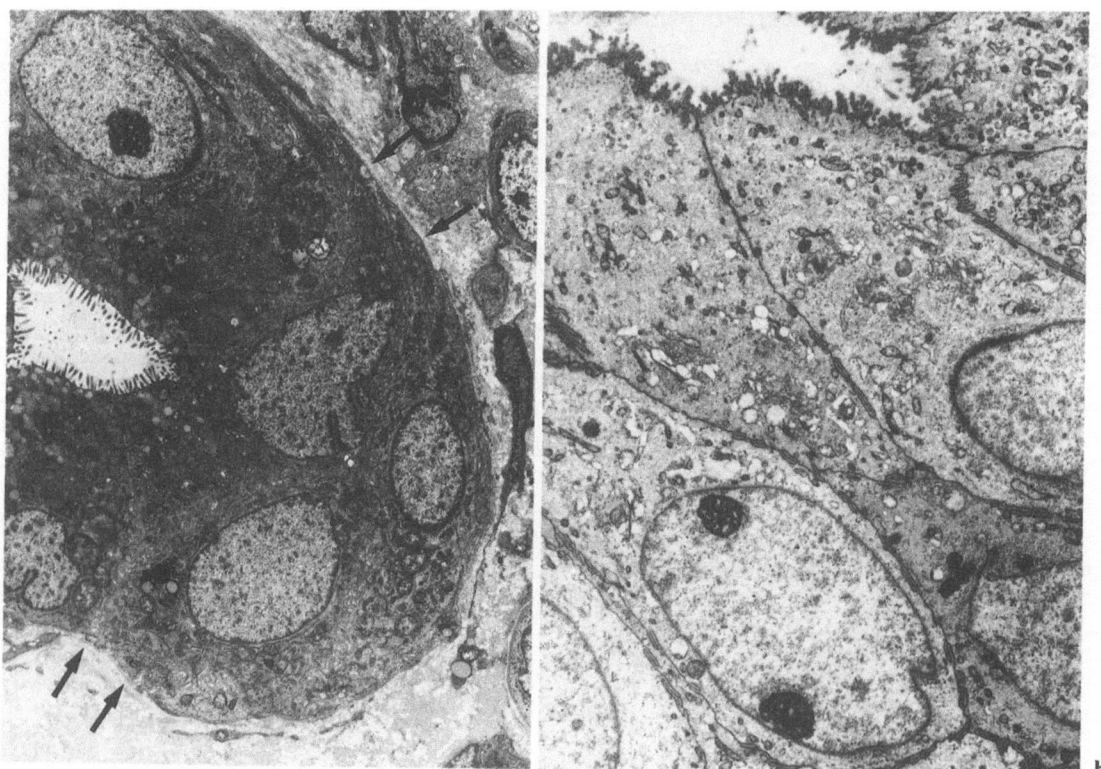

Fig. 11.10a, b. Ultrastructural findings of cholangiocarcinona. **a** Microvilli project into the lumen and the basement membrane (*arrows*) is clearly observed. × 2700. **b** Plasma membranes show marked interdigitation. × 4100

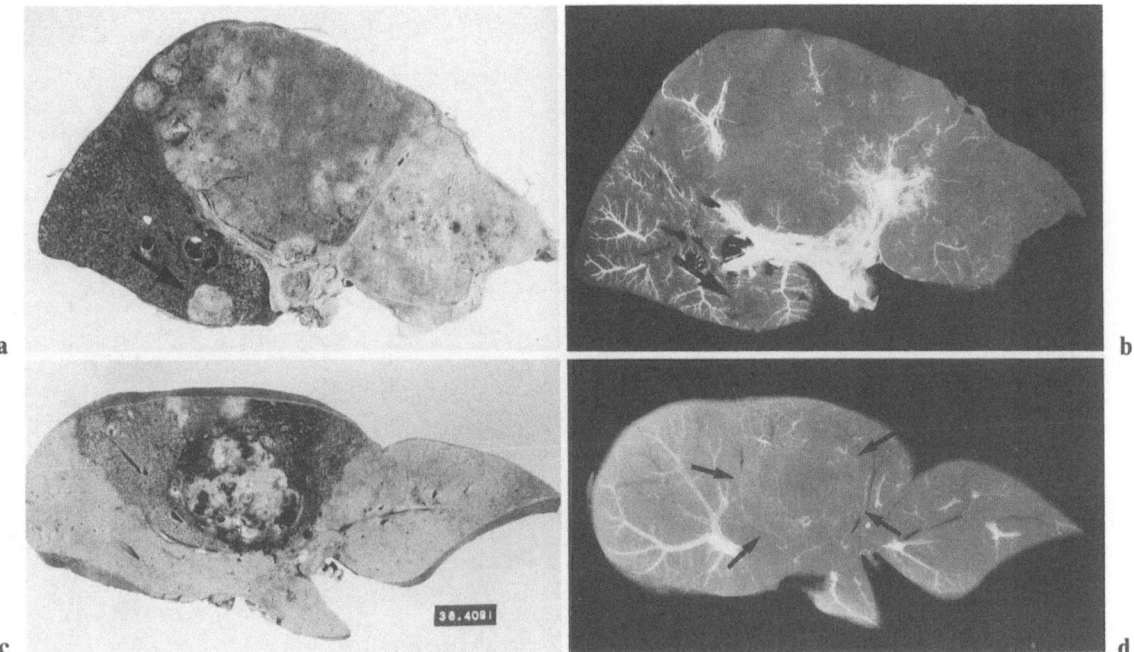

Fig. 11.11a–d. Angioarchitecture of cholangiocarcinoma. **a** Gross picture of an infiltrative cholangiocarcinoma. **b** Soft X-ray finding of the infiltrative type. Both primary and daughter lesions (*arrow*) are hypovascular. **c** Gross picture of a nodular type cholangiocarcinoma. **d** Soft X-ray finding of the nodular type. Tumor is hypervascular (*arrows*) but avascular in the center because of necrosis. *Scale* in centimeters

10   Angioarchitecture

Based on angiographic studies, cholangiocarcinoma is generally considered a hypovascular tumor, unlike HCC which is hypervascular [83–85]. However, almost no systematic studies of the angioarchitecture of cholangiocarcinoma have been conducted. The angiographic findings consist mainly of irregularity, stenosis, and encasement of the hepatic artery and the tumors themseleves are often hypovascular [86–88]. However, according to the results of a statistical analysis conducted by the Liver Cancer Study Group of Japan [49], 38% of cholangiocarcinomas are hypervascular. It is difficult to diagnose hilar-type cholangiocarcinoma by angiography when the tumor is small.

Postmortem angiographic studies indicate that some cholangiocarcinomas are hypovascular while others are hypervascular. In the hypovascular cases, intrahepatic metastatic foci are also hypovascular, and the hepatic artery is encased by tumor. In the hypervascular cases, fine blood vessels are abundant in the marginal area but scanty in the center of the tumors (Fig. 11.11).

11   Histological growth patterns

Since cholangiocarcinoma is a tumor arising from the bile ducts, the tumor cells can proliferate along large portal tracts (Glisson's sheath) as well as in the liver parenchyma, unlike HCC which proliferates only in the parenchyma.

11.1   Parenchymal proliferation

Tumor cells in cholangiocarcinoma can grow along the sinusoids (sinusoidal growth; Fig. 11.12), but it is sometimes difficult to observe areas where tumor cells directly infiltrate the sinusoids. Because of the abundant fibrous stroma at the leading edge of tumor growth, the cells usually have a tubular structure or show poor mutual contact as they infiltrate the sinusoids. Bile can be retained between tumor cells or in their cytoplasm at the junction of the tumor with normal parenchyma. Bile is retained as a result of neoplastic destruction of normal cholangioles containing bile or by entrapment of normal bile-containing liver cells.

As a result of infiltrative proliferation of tumor cells, Glisson's sheath can be observed around

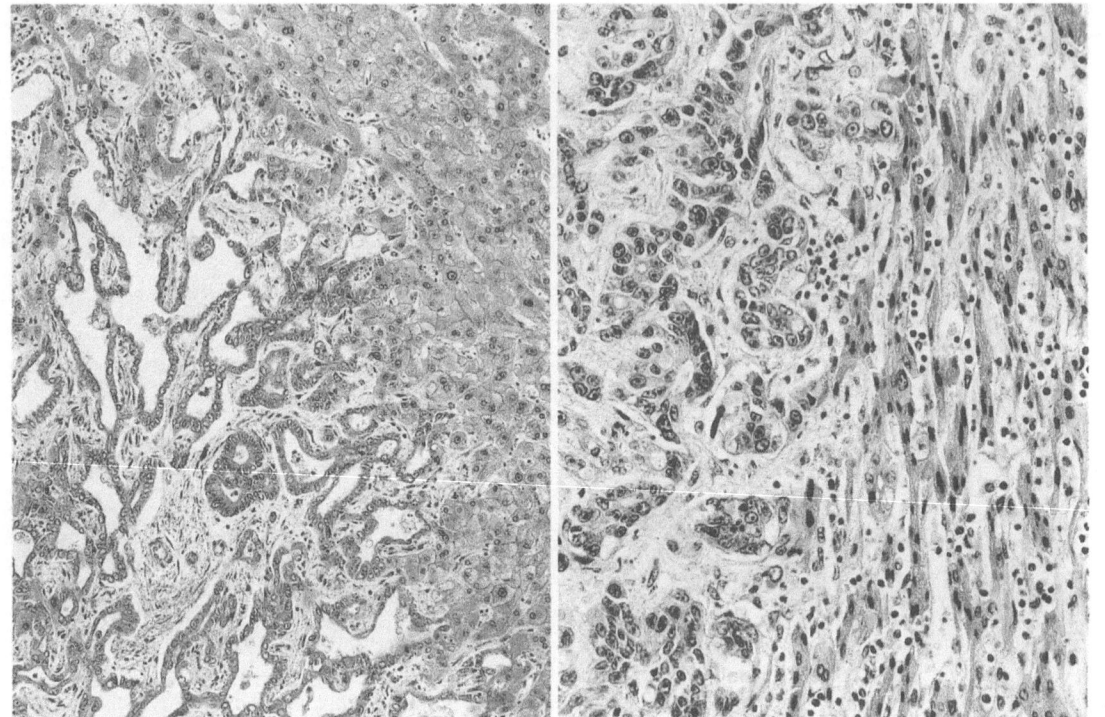

Fig. 11.12a, b. Tumor cells have grown in the sinusoids in an infiltrative fashion. **a** Papillary adenocarcinoma. **b** Poorly differentiated adenocarcinoma

the boundary. In the more central parts of the tumor, it appears as a tract of dense connective tissue.

11.2 Proliferation along Glisson's sheath

The large portal tract is infiltrated by tumor cells which show a tubular structure, poor mutual contact, and abundant fibrous stroma. Infiltration of tumor cells is also noted in the wall of the bile duct and all over the interstitium of the portal tract. The epithelium of the bile duct occasionally exhibits a hyperplastic change but usually shows no atypia. The tumor-nontumor boundary is often serrated and tumor cells infiltrate into the liver parenchyma (Fig. 11.13). Continuous cancer growth is also confirmed in serial sections. Vascular infiltration within the portal tract is often observed simultaneously.

11.3 Intrahepatic metastatic lesions

A portal tract is often noted in the center of small intrahepatic metastatic lesions. It is assumed from this finding that tumor cells infiltrate the liver parenchyma through the area, with vascular infiltration within the portal tract, to form intrahepatic metastatic lesions.

Necrosis, proliferation of connective tissue, and hyalinization are noted in the center of large intrahepatic metastases. Sinusoidal growth is noted at the edges of both intrahepatic metastases and the primary foci.

11.4 Tumor spread along the major bile duct

The incidence of this growth pattern is high in the hilar type. Tumors expand as papillary to well-differentiated adenocarcinoma toward the lumen of the major bile duct. However, tumor cells infiltrating the wall of the duct in a scirrhous pattern are less differentiated; such tumor spread has been referred to as "ductal spread."

11.5 Vascular invasion

In general, it has been stated that the lymphatics are located around the edge of the portal tract and that the portal vein branches are within the tract. However, it is often difficult to differentiate tumor thrombi of the portal vein from tumor casts of the lymphatics within the portal tract.

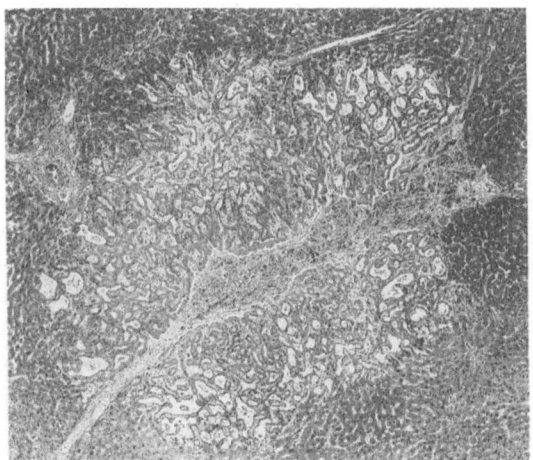

Fig. 11.13. Tumor extends into the parenchyma from Glisson's sheath in an infiltrative fashion

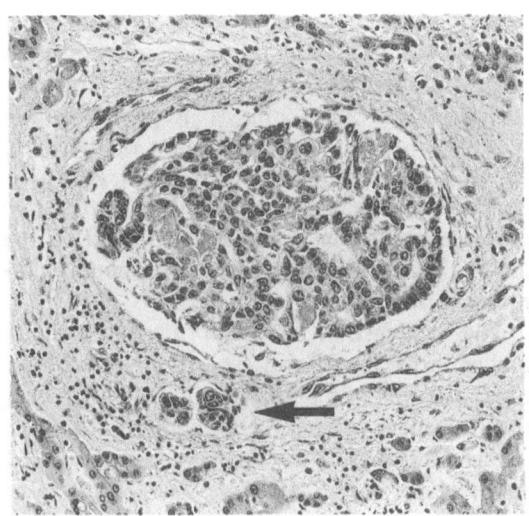

Fig. 11.14. Tumor thrombus of the portal vein and tumor cast of the lymphatics (*arrow*) in Glisson's sheath

For this reason both have been designated as "vascular invasion" in this chapter (Fig. 11.14). Furthermore, it is occasionally difficult to distinguish tumor casts of well-differentiated tubular adenocarcinoma in small branches of the portal vein and lymphatics from noncancerous bile ducts and/or proliferated bile ductules.

Vascular invasion in the peripheral and hilar types is as frequent as 89.5% (17/19) and 90.2% (37/41), respectively. In surgical cases, the incidence of vascular invasion is also as high as 86.4% (19/22). These findings indicate that vascular invasion occurs at a high rate at a relatively early stage in cholangiocarcinoma.

12 Histological features of noncancerous area

It is apparent from many reports that HCC is often complicated by liver cirrhosis, in contrast to cholangiocarcinoma [1, 4, 41–43, 46, 52]. However, the reported incidence of liver cirrhosis in cholangiocarcinoma varies from less than 10% to about 40%. Tull [89] reported an extremely high incidence of liver cirrhosis in cholangiocarcinoma (23 of 35 cases). Postnecrotic or posthepatitic cirrhosis and nutritional cirrhosis are noted in HCC [90], though there are regional differences in the type of cirrhosis. In contrast, biliary fibrosis is generally noted in cholangiocarcinoma [1, 3, 4, 23, 43, 89].

In our series, cirrhosis was noted in 8 of 60 cases of cholangiocarcinoma (13.3%). Posthepatitic or postnecrotic cirrhosis and biliary fibrosis were noted in four patients each; all patients with biliary fibrosis had cholangiocarcinoma of the hilar type. If mild cases are included, biliary fibrosis was found in 31 of 41 cases (75.6%) of the hilar type. On the other hand, biliary fibrosis was noted in only 3 of 19 cases (15.8%) of the peripheral type. In addition, various degrees of biliary fibrosis were observed in the noncancerous areas of the liver.

Proliferation of bile ductules around the portal area was more frequent in the hilar type (23 of 41 cases or 56.1%) than in the peripheral type (4 of 19 cases or 21.1%), and the incidence of severe bile stasis was also greater in the hilar type. Edmondson [2] has proposed that proliferation of bile ductules is elicited by the influence of bile stasis. Tateno et al. [16] noted a relationship between the periportal proliferation of bile ductules and deposits of Thorotrast in Thorotrast-related bile duct cancers, but this finding is not specific.

13 Metastases

The incidence of metastases, particularly to lymph nodes, is higher in cholangiocarcinoma than in HCC [2, 32, 41, 43, 46]. Metastases are classified by mode of spread into three types—hematogenous, lymphatic, and infiltrative or disseminated. Hematogenous metastases are often noted in the lungs, adrenal glands, and intestinal tract and to a lesser extent in the pancreas, spleen, bone, and kidneys. Regional lymph nodes such as those in the hilum of the liver, posterior part of the pancreatic head, and peri-aortic region are most often involved. Infiltrative or disseminated metastases were noted in the gallbladder, intestinal tract, peritoneum, diaphragm, and pouch of Douglas.

The incidence of metastases by any route is higher in the peripheral type than in the hilar type. This may be partly ascribable to the fact that the survival time of the peripheral type is longer than that of the hilar type, as described subsequently (Chap. 31).

14   Other related types of cancer

14.1   Cholangiolocellular carcinoma

The term "cholangiolocellular carcinoma" was used for the first time by Steiner in 1957 [91]. Steiner and Higginson [92] presented 11 cases of this type to establish the concept. They reported that cholangiolocellular carcinoma was a specific type of primary liver cancer derived from the cholangioles or canals of Hering and accounted for 1% of cases of primary liver cancer. However, the cellular origin of this type has not yet been

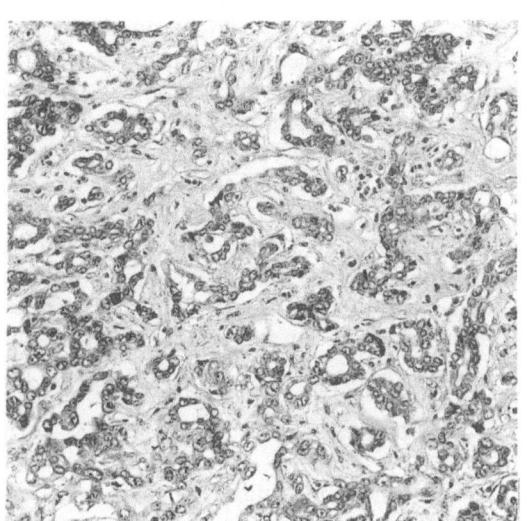

Fig. 11.15. Cholangiolocellular carcinoma. Tumor consists of the anastomosing ductules resembling cholangioles

elucidated and, therefore, this cancer is sometimes classified as a specific type of HCC [93].

As described by Steiner [91], the most characteristic feature of cholangiolocellular carcinoma is the tendency for the neoplastic cells to be arranged in small cords. The neoplastic cells are fairly uniform and show no apparent tendency to differentiate to HCC or cholangiocarcinoma [94]. This type is also characterized by an abundant fibrous stroma. The cytoplasm of the neoplastic cells is scanty and pale. Each cell has an oval nucleus and less marked nucleoli and is very similar to the epithelial cell of cholangioles (Fig. 11.15).

14.2   Bile duct cystadenocarcinoma

Bile duct cystadenocarcinoma is defined as a malignant cystic tumor lined by mucus-secreting epithelium with papillary infoldings [9, 95]. Histologically, it is similar to bile duct cystadenoma except for the transition from benign to malignant epithelial proliferation in a papillary growth.

Problems often arise during its differentiation from bile duct cystadenoma. Infiltration of the underlying fibrous stroma as well as cellular pleomorphism, the presence of bizarre giant cells, anaplasia, and abnormal mitoses are considered the most important features in differentiation [96].

The course of bile duct cystadenocarcinoma is longer than that of ordinary malignant tumors arising from the liver. It is characterized by a more frequent occurrence in middle-aged females; the male to female ratio is 1 : 4–5.

The clinical symptoms of this cancer are the same as those of bile duct cystadenoma or other hepatic cysts: Bulging and palpable masses and pain and discomfort in the right hypochondrium and upper abdomen appear slowly with increasing size of the cysts.

In a patient under our care, surgery was performed after the diagnosis of adenocarcinoma was confirmed by needle cytodiagnosis of a cystic tumor (Fig. 11.16). Accordingly, it is expected that the definitive diagnosis of this cancer will be made more frequently in the future with increased application of ultrasound-guided puncture.

References

1. Edmondson HA, Steiner PE (1954) Primary carcinoma of the liver. A study of 100 cases among 48,900 necropsies. Cancer 7: 462–503

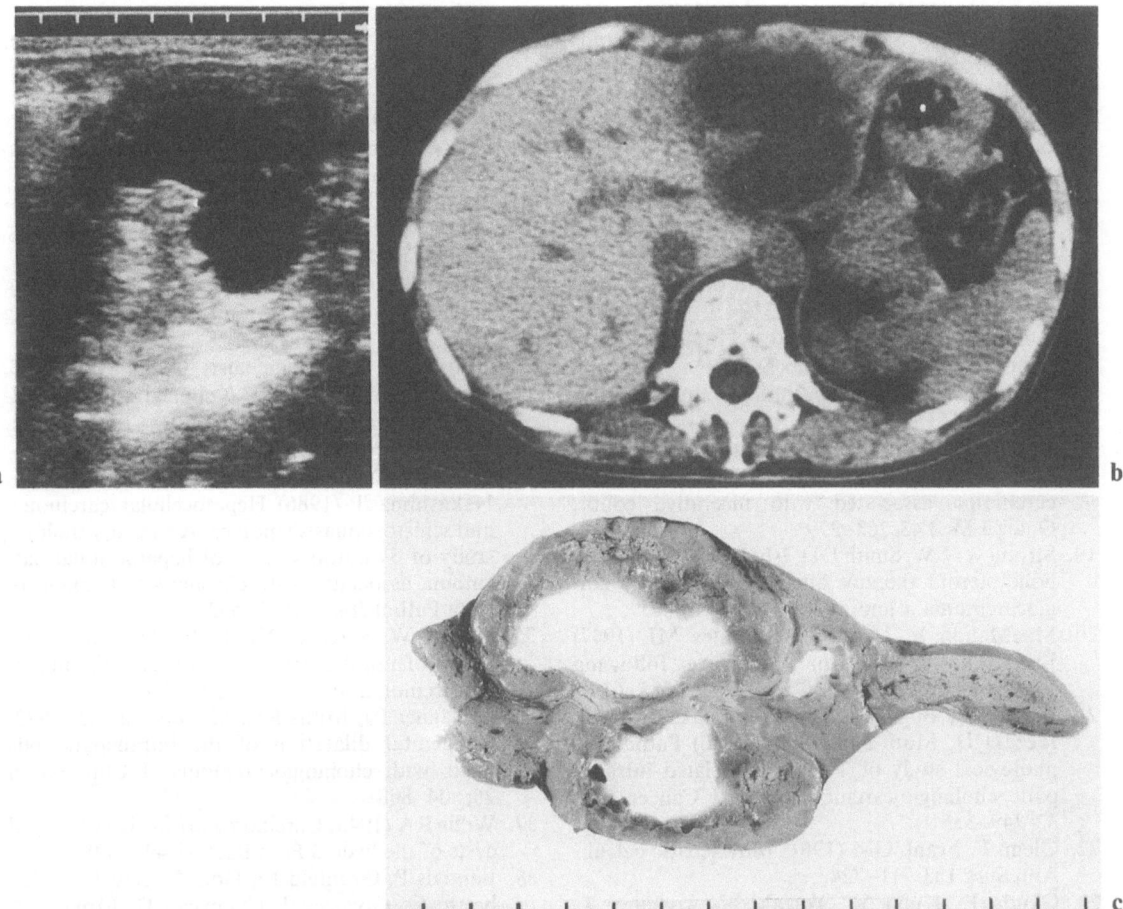

Fig. 11.16a–c. Bile duct cystadenocarcinoma. **a** Cystic tumor is found by ultrasonography. Cyst wall shows irregular thickening. **b** Abdominal computed tomography disclosed the irregular low-density mass corresponding to the lesion. **c** Gross finding. The cyst wall is irregularly thickened (Scale, 1 cm)

2. Edmondson HA (1958) Tumors of the liver and intrahepatic bile duct. Fascicle 24. Armed Forces Institute of Pathology, Washington
3. Gall EA (1960) Primary and metastatic carcinoma of the liver. Relationship to hepatic cirrhosis. Arch Pathol 70: 226–232
4. Anthony PP (1972) Primary carcinoma of the liver. A study of 282 cases in Ugandan Africa. J Pathol 110: 37–48
5. Mori W, Nagasako K (1976) Cholangiocarcinoma and related lesions. In: Okuda K, Peters RL (eds) Hepatocellular carcinoma. Wiley, New York, pp 227–246
6. Japanese Biliary Surgical Society (1981) General rules for surgical studies on cancer of biliary tract, Kanehara Shuppan, Tokyo
7. Goldzieher M, Bockay Z (1911) Der primäre Leberkrebs. Virchows Arch A (Pathol Anat) 203: 75–131
8. Yamagiwa K (1911) Zur Kenntnis des primären parenchymatosen Leber Karzinoma (Hepatoma) Virchows Arch A (Pathol Anat) 206: 437–467

9. Leevy CM, Popper H, Sherlock S (1974) Disease of the liver and biliary tract. Standardization of nomenclature, diagnostic criteria, and diagnostic methodology, Fogarty International Center Proceedings no. 22, 6th Meeting. IASL, Acapulco
10. Klatskin G (1965) Adenocarcinoma of the hepatic duct at its bifurcation within the porta hepatis. An unusual tumor with distinctive clinical and pathological features. Am J Med 38: 241–256
11. Alvarez AF (1958) Carcinoma of the main hepatic ducts within the liver. A report of two cases, treated by intra-hepatic cholangiojejunostomy. Ann Surg 148: 773–782
12. Meyerowitz BR, Aird I (1962) Carcinoma of the hepatic ducts within the liver. Br J Surg 50: 178–184
13. Altemeier WA, Gall EA, Culbertson WR, Inge WW (1966) Sclerosing carcinoma of the intrahepatic (hilar) bile ducts. Surgery 60: 191–200
14. Takahashi S, Kitabatake T, Yamagata S, Miyagawa T, Masuyama G, Mori T, Tanaka T, Hibino S, Miyagawa M, Kaneda H, Okajima S,

Komiyama K, Hashizume M, Adachi T, Koga Y, Hashimoto Y, Sakuragi S (1966) Statistical study on Thorotrast-induced cancer of the liver. Nippon Act Radiol 25: 13–21

15. Mori T (1984) Epidemiological study of late effect of Thorotrast administration. Annual report of research on thorium fuel. Ministry of Education Science and Culture, Tokyo

16. Tateno H, Hosoda S, Yamada S, Kido C (1984) Proliferative lesions in Thorotrast-deposited livers pertaining to development of primary cancers. Jpn J Cancer Clin 30: 23–34

17. Rubel LR, Usn CMC, Ishak KG (1982) Thorotrast-associated cholangiocarcinoma. An epidemiologic and clinicopathologic study. Cancer 50: 1408–1415

18. Ritchie JK, Allan RN, Macartney J, Thompson H, Hawley PR, Cooke WT (1974) Biliary tract carcinoma associated with ulcerative colitis. Quart J Med 43: 263–279

19. Stromeyer FW, Smith DH, Ishak KG (1979) Anabolic steroid therapy and intrahepatic cholangiocarcinoma. Cancer 43: 440–443

20. MacMahon E, Murphy AS, Bates MI (1947) Endothelial cell sarcoma of the liver following Thorotrast injections. Am J Pathol 25: 585–613

21. Kojiro M, Sugihara S, Ito Y, Nakashima T, Ikezaki H, Mori T, Kido C (1986) Pathomorphological study of Thorotrast related intrahepatic cholangio-carcinoma. Jpn J Cancer Clin 32: 349–355

22. Glenn F, Frank GM (1961) Intrahepatic calculi. Ann Surg 153: 711–724

23. Okuda K, Kubo Y, Okazaki N, Arishima T, Hashimoto M, Jinnouchi S, Sawa Y, Shimokawa Y, Nakajima Y, Noguchi T, Nakano M, Kojiro M, Nakashima T (1977) Clinical aspects of intrahepatic bile duct carcinoma including hilar carcinoma. A study of 57 autopsy-proven cases. Cancer 39: 232–246

24. Kinami Y, Noto H, Miyazaki I, Matsubara F (1978) A study of hepatolithiasis associated with cholangiocarcinoma. Acta Hepatol Jpn 19: 578–583

25. Yamamoto K, Tsuchiya R, Ito T, Harada N, Yoshino R, Tsunoda T, Noda T, Izawa K, Yamaguchi T, Oribe T, Motoshima K, Tomioka T, Chiba K, Koga M, Matsumoto M (1984) A study of cholangiocarcinoma coexistent with hepatolithiasis. Jpn J Gastroenterol Surg 17: 601–609

26. Sanes S, MacCallum JD (1942) Primary carcinoma of the liver. Cholangioma in hepatolithiasis. Am J Pathol 18: 675–687

27. Falchuk KR, Lesser RB, Galdabini JJ, Isselbacher KJ (1976) Cholangiocarcinoma as related to chronic intrahepatic cholangitis and hepatolithiasis. Am J Gastroenterol 66: 57–61

28. Nakanuma Y, Terada T, Tanaka Y, Ohta G (1985) Are hepatolithiasis and cholangioma aetiologically related? A morphological study of 12 cases of hepatolithiasis associated with cholangiocarcinoma. Virchows Arch A (Pathol Anat)

406: 45–58

29. Gibson JB (1971) Parasites, liver disease and liver cancer. In: Liver cancer, IARC Scientific publications, no. 1. WHO, Lyon, pp 42–59

30. Hou PC (1956) The relationship between primary carcinoma of the liver and infestation with chlonorchis sinensis. J Path Bact 72: 239–246

31. Belamaric J (1972) Intrahepatic bile duct carcinoma and C. sinensis infection in Hong Kong. Cancer 31: 468–473

32. Chou ST, Chan CW (1976) Mucin-producing cholangiocarcinoma. An autopsy study in Hong Kong. Pathology 8: 321–328

33. Juttijudata P, Chiemchaisri C, Palavatana C, Churnratanakul S (1982) A clinical study of cholangiocarcinoma caused cholestasis in Thailand. Surg Gynecol Obstet 155: 373–376

34. Kojiro M, Yano H, Tsumagari J, Kenmochi K, Nakashima T (1986) Hepatocellular carcinoma and schistosomiasis japonica. A clinicopathologic study of 59 autopsy cases of hepatocellular carcinoma associated with chronic schistosomiasis. Acta Pathol Jpn 36: 525–532

35. Jones AW, Shreeve DR (1970) Congenital dilatation of intrahepatic biliary ducts with cholangiocarcinoma. Br Med J 2: 277–278

36. Gallagher PJ, Millis RR, Mitchinson MJ (1972) Congenital dilatation of the intrahepatic bile ducts with cholangiocarcinoma. J Clin Pathol 25: 804–808

37. Willis RA (1943) Carcinoma arising in congenital cysts of the liver. J Path Bact 55: 492–495

38. Landais P, Grünfeld JP, Dorz D, Drüeke T, Albouze G, Gogusev J, Chauveau D, Moynot A (1984) Cholangiocellular carcinoma in polycystic kidney and liver disease. Arch Intern Med 144: 2274–2276

39. Phinney PR, Austin GE, Kadell BM (1981) Cholangiocarcinoma arising in Carolis' disease. Arch Pathol Lab Med 105: 194–197

40. Daroca PJ Jr, Tuthill R, Reed RJ (1975) Cholangiocarcinoma arising in congenital hepatic fibrosis. A case report. Arch Pathol 99: 592–595

41. Hoyne RM, Kernohan JW (1947) Primary carcinoma of the liver. A study of thirty-one cases. Arch Intern Med 79: 532–554

42. MacDonald RA (1957) Primary carcinoma of the liver. A clinicopathologic study of one hundred eight cases. Arch Intern Med 99: 226–279

43. Patton RB, Horn RC Jr (1964) Primary liver carcinoma. Autopsy study of 60 cases. Cancer 17: 757–768

44. El-Domeri AA, Huvos AG, Goldsmith HS, Foote FW (1971) Primary malignant tumors of the liver. Cancer 27: 7–11

45. Cruickshank AH (1961) The pathology of 111 cases of primary hepatic malignancy collected in the Liverpool region. J Clin Pathol 14: 120–130

46. Lopez-Corella E, Ridaura-Sanz R, Albores-Saavedra J (1968) Primary carcinoma of the liver in Mexican adults. Cancer 22: 678–685

47. Steiner PE (1960) Cancer of the liver and cirrhosis in trans-Saharan Africa and United States of

America. Cancer 13: 1085–1166

48. Shanmaugaratnam K, Tye CY (1970) Liver cancer differentials in immigrant and local-born Chinese in Singapore. J Clin Dis 23: 443–448

49. Okuda K, The liver cancer study group of Japan (1980) Primary liver cancer in Japan. Cancer 45: 2663–2669

50. Ying YY, Ma CC, Hsu Y, Lei HH, Liang SF, Lin C, Ku CY (1963) Primary carcinoma of the liver. Chinese Med J 82: 279–294

51. Ong GB, Chan PW (1976) Primary carcinoma of the liver. Surg Gynecol Obstet 143: 31–38

52. MacSween RNM (1974) A clinicopathological review of 100 cases of primary malignant tumors of the liver. J Clin Pathol 27: 669–682

53. Kuwayti K, Baggenstoss AH, Stauffer MH, Priestley JT (1957) Carcinoma of the major intrahepatic and the extrahepatic bile ducts exclusive of the papilla of Vater. Surg Gynecol Obstet 104: 357–366

54. Sako K, Seitzinger GL, Garside E (1957) Carcinoma of the extrahepatic bile ducts. Surgery 41: 416–437

55. Thorbjarnarson B (1959) Carcinoma of the bile ducts. Cancer 12: 708–713

56. Foster JH, Berman MM (1977) Solid liver tumors. Major problems in clinical surgery, vol. 23. Saunders, London, pp 62–104

57. Dewbury KC, Joseph AEA, Hayes S, Murray C (1974) Ultrasound in the evaluation and diagnosis of jaundice. Br J Radiol 52: 276–280

58. Nakano T, Tsuchiya Y, Ohto M, Unosawa T, Tsunetomi S, Kobayashi T, Iino Y (1982) Ultrasonic appearance of cholangiocarcinoma. JSUM Proceedings 40: 113–114

59. Itai Y, Araki T, Furui S, Yashiro N, Ohtomo K, Iio M (1983) Computed tomography of primary intrahepatic biliary malignancy. Radiology 147: 485–490

60. Flemma RJ, Schauble JF, Gardner CE Jr, Anlyan WG, Capp MP (1963) Percutaneous transhepatic cholangiography in the differential diagnosis of jaundice. Surg Gynecol Obstet 116: 559–568

61. Okuda K, Tanikawa K, Emura T, Kuratomi S, Jinnouchi S, Urabe K, Sumikoshi T, Kaneda Y, Furuyama J, Musha H, Mori H, Shimokawa Y, Yakushiji F, Matsuura Y (1974) Non-surgical percutaneous transhepatic cholangiography: Diagnostic significance in medical problems of the liver. Am J Dig Dis 19: 21–36

62. Takagi K, Ikeda S, Nakagawa Y, Sakaguchi N, Takahashi T, Kumakura K, Murayama M, Someya N, Nakano H, Takada T, Takekoshi T, Kin T (1970) Retrograde pancreatography and cholangiography by fiber duodenoscope. Gastroenterology 59: 445–452

63. Okuda K, Someya N, Goto A, Kunisaki T, Emura T, Yasumoto M, Shimokawa Y (1973) Endoscopic pancreato-cholangio graphy. A preliminary report on technique and diagnostic significance. Am J Roentgenol 117: 437–445

64. Jori GP, Peschle C (1972) Combined peritoneoscopy and liver biopsy in the diagnosis of hepatic neoplasm. Gastroenterology 63: 1016–1019

65. Reynolds TB, Lowan RE (1979) Peritoneoscopy. In: Wright R, Alberti KGMM, Karrans S, Millward-Sadler GH (eds) Liver and biliary disease. Saunders, Philadelphia, pp 543–556

66. Eggel H (1901) Ueber das Carcinom der Leber. Beitr z Path Anat u z allgem Pathol. 30: 506–604

67. Nakashima T, Sakamoto K (1977) A study of hepatocellular carcinoma among Japanese from the point of view of morphodevelopmental pathology. Gross anatomical types classified in relation to capsule formation. Kurume Med J 24: 43–62

68. Barr RJ Hancock DE (1975) Adenosquamous carcinoma of the liver. Gastroenterology 69: 1326–1330

69. Tokunaga S, Matsuo T, Shimokawa I, Maeda H, Ikeda T, Yamamoto K (1985) An autopsy case of adenosquamous carcinoma of the liver. Gastroenterol Surg 8: 1657–1660

70. Pianzola LE, Drut R (1971) Mucoepidermoid carcinoma of the liver. Am J Clin Pathol 56: 758–761

71. Katsuda S, Kajikawa K (1984) Mucoepidermoid carcinoma of the liver. Acta Pathol Jpn 34: 153–157

72. Greenwood N, Orr WM (1972) Primary squamous-cell carcinoma arising in a solitary non-parasitic cyst of the liver. J Pathol 107: 145–148

73. Bloustein PA, Silverberg SG (1976) Squamous cell carcinoma originating in an hepatic cyst. Case report with a review of the hepatic cyst-carcinoma association. Cancer 38: 2002–2005

74. Shiffman MA, Juler G (1964) Carcinoid of the biliary tract. Arch Surg 89: 1113–1115

75. Weichert RF (1970) The neural ectodermal origin of the peptide-secreting endocrine glands. A unifying concept for the etiology of multiple endocrine adenomatosis and inappropriate section of peptide hormones by non-endocrine tumors. Am J Med 49: 232–241

76. Axiotis CA, Walker Smith GJ (1982) Seclerosing carcinoma of the right hepatic duct at the porta hepatis. Anicteric presentation of early hilar cholangiocarcinoma. Am J Gastroenterol 77: 414–418

77. Koprowski H, Herlyn M, Steplewski Z (1981) Specific antigen in serum of patients with colon carcinoma. Science 212: 53–55

78. Inoue Y, Sato M, Kurosawa T, Takikawa Y, Suzuki A, Kano A (1984) Clinical evaluation of a new tumor maker (CA 19-9) in malignant disease. J Iwate Med Assoc 36: 211–217

79. Hora K, Oguchi H, Kawa S, Tamura Y, Hirabayashi H, Shimakura K, Shirai T, Yonekura H, Kamijyo K, Nagata A, Homma T, Furuta S (1984) Clinical evaluation of a new tumor maker, CA 19-9. Shinshu Med J 32: 225–230

80. Hsu SM, Raine L, Fanger H (1981) Use of avidin-biotion-peroxidase complex (ABC) in immunoperoxidase techniques. A comparison between ABC and unlabeled antibody (PAP) procedures. J Histochem Cytochem 29: 577–580

81. Schaffner F (1972) Electron microscopy in the

study of human liver disease. Hum Pathol 3: 293–294

82. Alpert LI, Zak FG, Westhamer SW, Bochetto JF (1974) Cholangiocarcinoma. A clinicopathologic study of five cases with ultrastructural observation. Hum Pathol 5: 709–728

83. Boijsen E, Abrams HL (1965) Roentgenologic diagnosis of primary carcinoma of the liver. Acta Radiol Diagn 3: 257–277

84. Yu C (1967) Primary carcinoma of the liver (Hepatoma). Its diagnosis by selective celiac arteriography. Am J Roentgenol 99: 142–149

85. Kido C, Sasaki T, Kaneko M (1971) Angiography of primary liver cancer. Am J Roentgenol Rad Therapy and Nuclear Med 113: 70–81

86. Kaude J, Rian R (1971) Cholangiocarcinoma. Radiology 100: 573–580

87. Bree RL, Reuter SR (1974) Angiographic findings in patients with choledocholithiasis and obstructive jaundice. Radiology 112: 291–295

88. Walter JF, Bookstein JJ, Bouffard EV (1976) Newer angiographic observations in cholangiocarcinoma. Radiology 118: 19–23

89. Tull JC (1932) Primary carcinoma of the liver. A study of one hundred and thirty-four cases. J Path

Bact 35: 557–562

90. Mori W (1967) Cirrhosis and primary cancer of the liver. Comparative study in Tokyo and Cincinnati. Cancer 20: 627–631

91. Steiner PE (1957) Carcinoma of liver in United States. Acta Unio Internat. Contra Cancrum 13: 628–645

92. Steiner PE, Higginson J (1959) Cholangiolocellular carcinoma of the liver. Cancer 12: 753–759

93. Popper H, Schaffner F (1977) Primary hepatic carcinoma. In: Popper H, Schaffner F (eds) Liver: Structure and function. Blakiston, New York, pp 593–612

94. Peters RL (1976) Pathology of hepatocellular carcinoma. In: Okuda K, Peters RL (eds) Hepatocellular carcinoma. Wiley, New York, pp 107–168

95. Gibson JB (1978) Histological typing of tumours of the liver, biliary tract and pancreas. International histological classification of tumours, no. 20, WHO, Geneva

96. Ishak K, Willis GW, Cummins SD, Bullock AA (1977) Biliary cystadenoma and cystadenocarcinoma. Report of 14 cases and review of lietarature. Cancer 38: 322–338

Chapter 12
Malignant Mesenchymal Tumors of the Liver*

Kamal G. Ishak[1]

Primary malignant mesenchymal tumors of the liver are much rarer than epithelial neoplasms, but figures regarding their incidence are quite limited. Of the 405 primary malignant tumors collected by Edmondson and Peters [1] 1.2% were sarcomas. A survey of death certificates, notoriously unreliable, in the United States from 1966 to 1973 disclosed 205 hepatic sarcomas [2]; the cases included angiosarcoma (36%), leiomyosarcoma (12%), fibrosarcoma (7%), and unspecified sarcomas (44%).

Primary sarcomas of the liver usually develop in a noncirrhotic liver, although various degrees of fibrosis may be present in cases of angiosarcoma related to prior exposure to Thorotrast or vinyl chloride. Sarcoma and carcinoma occurring simultaneously in a cirrhotic liver are exceptionally rare [3]. The diagnosis should be made with caution since hepatocellular carcinoma can show a spindle cell (pseudosarcomatous) pattern. Carcinosarcomas (admixtures of carcinoma, either hepatocellular or cholangiocellular, and various sarcomatous elements) are also rare.

The clinical course of some sarcomas, such as epithelioid hemangioendothelioma is unpredictable but, in general, the sarcomas are rapidly growing and uniformly fatal. Therapy remains unsatisfactory, although some progress has been made in the treatment of childhood sarcomas, such as undifferentiated sarcoma and embryonal rhabdomyosarcoma. Etiological factors for sarcomas are unknown, except for angiosarcoma that has been linked to Thorotrast, vinyl chloride, and arsenic exposure.

The major part of this chapter is devoted to the primary malignant mesenchymal tumors that occur relatively frequently in the liver. They include epithelioid hemangioendothelioma, angiosarcoma, undifferentiated (embryonal) sarcoma, and rhabdomyosarcoma. Rare tumors, such as fibrosarcoma, leiomyosarcoma, malignant fibrous histiocytoma, and Kaposi's sarcoma, will be briefly alluded to.

1 Epithelioid hemangioendothelioma

This recently reported hepatic neoplasm [4, 5] also occurs in the lung, where it has been termed "intravascular bronchioloalveolar tumor" [6], soft tissue [7–9], and bone [9]. Since the publication of a series of 32 cases involving the liver by Ishak et al. [4, 5], seven other cases have been reported [10–12]. It is very likely that many more cases will be identified in the future with increasing awareness of this entity.

The age at presentation ranges from the second to the eighth decades of life, with an average of approximately 50 years. Two-thirds of the affected patients are women. Symptoms and signs include weakness, anorexia, nausea, episodic vomiting, upper abdominal aching and pain, jaundice, and hepatosplenomegaly [4, 5]. An acute abdomen from rupture of the tumor with hemoperitoneum [4, 5] and a Budd-Chiari-like syndrome [10] are rare presentations.

Tests of hepatic function do not offer clues to the diagnosis, although increased serum alkaline phosphatase activity is demonstrable in about two-thirds of the patients [4, 5]. One of the cases reviewed at the Armed Forces Institute of Pathology (AFIP) had elevated serum factor VIII levels. Hepatic scintigraphy generally reveals "filling defects" throughout the liver. Multifocal areas of decreased density are noted by computed tomography [4, 12].

---

* The opinions or assertions contained herein are the private views of the author and are not to be construed as official or as reflecting the views of the Department of the Army or the Department of Defense.
[1] Department of Hepatic Pathology, Armed Forces Institute of Pathology, Washington, DC 20306, USA

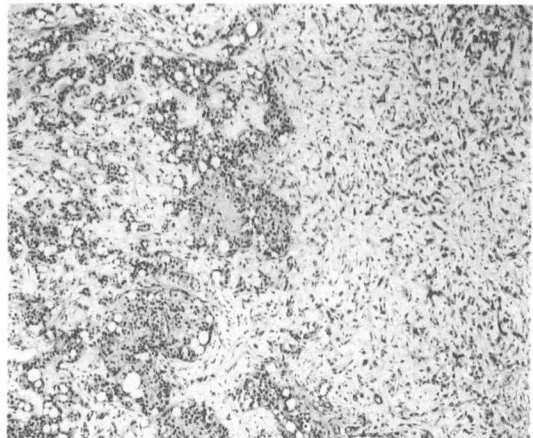

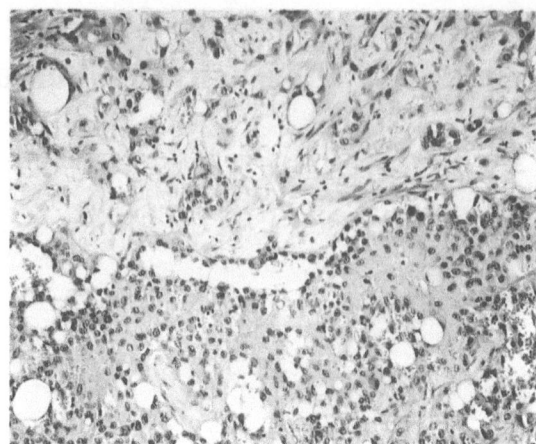

Fig. 12.1. Epithelioid hemangioendothelioma. Tumor has destroyed hepatic parenchyma and shows epithelioid nests (*left*) and dendritic cells (*right*). H and E, × 60

Fig. 12.2. Higher magnification of case illustrated in Fig. 11.1 shows loosely arranged dendritic cells (*top*) and more compact epithelioid cells (*bottom*). "Vacuoles" represent intracellular vascular lumens formed by tumor. H and E, × 160

Calcification may be evident in plain films of the abdomen. Hepatic arteriography in one reported case disclosed diffuse stretching and distortion of the intrahepatic branches of the common hepatic artery [12]. There were large areas of hypovascularity, slow sinusoidal clearing, and only limited areas of normal capillary filling. At the present time, a definitive diagnosis of epithelioid hemangioendothelioma can only be established by liver biopsy.

Grossly, epithelioid hemangioendothelioma usually consists of multiple lesions involving the entire liver; the lesions vary from a few millimeters to several centimeters in diameter. The neoplastic tissue is tan to white in color, firm in consistency, and sometimes has a gritty texture when sectioned. The tumor generally does not arise on a background of chronic liver disease, but one reported case occurred in a cirrhotic liver [4]. Some cases are associated with nodular regenerative hyperplasia [4].

Histopathologically, the tumor nodules are ill-defined and often involve mutiple contiguous acini. In actively proliferating lesions, the acinar landmarks such as terminal hepatic venules (THV) and portal areas, are readily recognized despite extensive infiltration by the tumor. The tumor cells grow along preexisting sinusoids, THV, and portal vein branches and often invade Glisson's capsule. Growth within the acini is associated with gradual atrophy and eventual disappearance of liver cell plates (Figs. 12.1, 12.2). Intravenous growth may be in the form of a solid plug or as polypoid or tuftlike projections (Fig.

12.3). Neoplastic cells are either "dendritic," with irregular shapes and multiple interdigitating processes (Figs. 12.1, 12.2, 12.4), or "epithelioid," with a more rounded shape and abundant cytoplasm; nuclear atypia and mitoses are mainly observed in the epithelioid cells (Figs. 12.1, 12.2). Cytoplasmic vacuoles, representing intracellular vascular lumina, are often identified and may contain erythrocytes (Fig. 12.2). The tumor cells synthesize a factor VIII-related antigen, which can be demonstrated in the cytoplasm or in the neoplastic vascular lumina (Fig. 12.5). The stroma of actively proliferating lesions has a myxoid appearance due to an abundance of sulfated mucopolysaccharide. A basement membrane can be demonstrated around the cells by the periodic acid-Schiff (PAS) stain as well as ultrastructurally. As the lesions develop, they are associated with progressive fibrosis and calcification (Fig. 12.6). Eventually, tumor cells (and indeed, the vascular nature of the lesion) may be difficult if not impossible to recognize in the densely sclerosed areas.

The histopathological differential diagnosis, which includes other benign and malignant vascular tumors (Table 12.1) and epithelial tumors (e.g., cholangiocarcinoma) as well as nonneoplastic conditions, is discussed in detail elsewhere [4, 9].

Ultrastructurally, the cells of epithelioid hemangioendothelioma have many of the characteristics of endothelial cells. These include a basal lamina, pinocytotic vesicles, and Weibel-Palade bodies. Unlike normal endothelial cells, the tu-

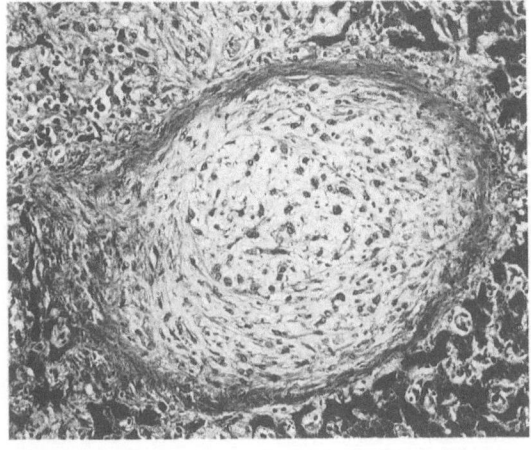

Fig. 12.3. Growth of epithelioid hemangioendothelioma has completely blocked lumen of terminal hepatic venule. Masson trichrome, × 250

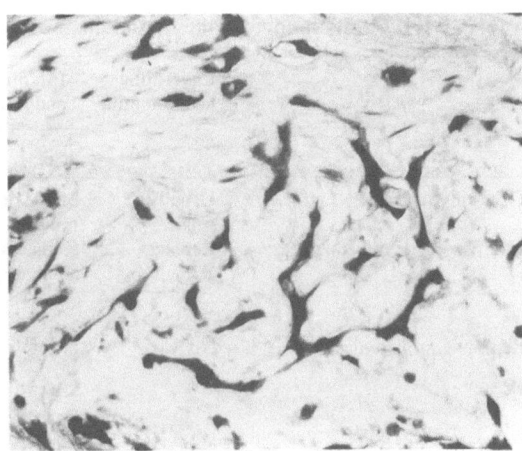

Fig. 12.4. Dendritic cells with interdigitating process (darkly stained) are embedded in an abundant stroma that was found to contain large amounts of sulfated mucopolysaccharide. Masson trichrome, × 400

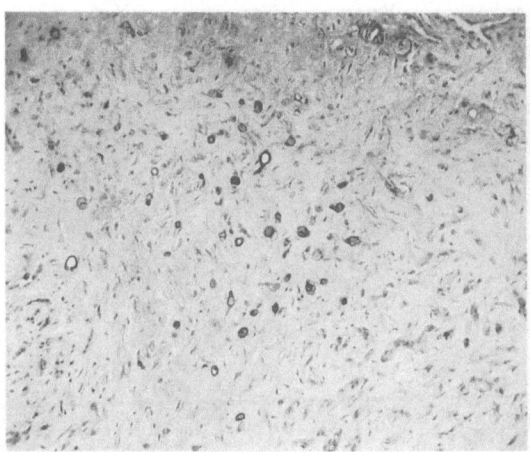

Fig. 12.5. Factor VIII-related antigen (black) is demonstrated in center of field within vascular lumens of the tumor. Peroxidase-antiperoxidase, × 160

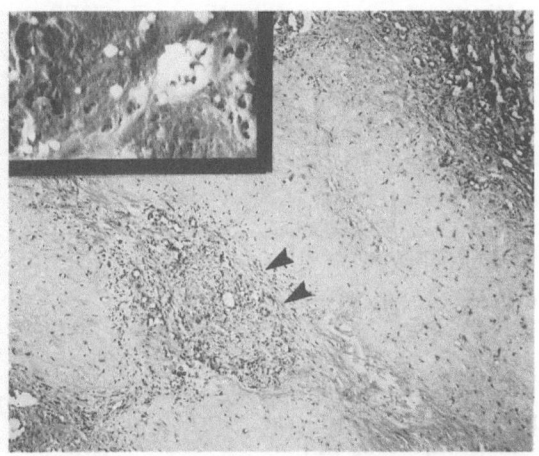

Fig. 12.6. Extensive fibrosis in epithelioid hemangioendothelioma. A residual portal area (*arrowheads*) is still recognizable despite extensive involvement by the tumor. H and E, × 60. Calcospherules (*inset*) in the fibrotic stroma are identified by scanning electron microscopy. × 1280. X-ray microanalysis (not shown) revealed both calcium and phosphorous in the calcospherules

mor cells contain a large number of intermediate filaments, which account for their "epithelioid" appearance under light microscopy; dense bodies may also be present.

The prognosis of epithelioid hemangioendothelioma is unpredictable. About 28% of the tumors metastasize [4, 5], but the development of metastases does not preclude a long survival. Follow-up information on 17 of the 32 cases reported by Ishak et al. [4, 5] is available; 8 of the 17 patients died, but only six of the deaths (35%) were attributable to the tumor [9]. The deaths

occurred within 2 years of diagnosis with the exception of one patient who died of metastatic disease 10 years after diagnosis. Of the 17 patients, 12 have survived more than 3 years (range 3–28 years; average 9.8 years). Only 3 of the 12 surviving patients have been treated: one, who survived 3 years, was treated by radiation and chemotherapy; a second patient, who survived 9 years, underwent a lobectomy; the third patient is still alive 15 years after hepatic transplantation. Another patient treated by hepatic transplantation was alive and well 9 months postoperatively [12].

Table 12.1. Histopathological differential diagnosis of vascular neoplasms of the liver

	Cavernous hemangioma	Infantile hemangio-endothelioma		Kaposi's sarcoma	Epithelioid hemangio-endothelioma	Angio-sarcoma
		Type 1	Type 2			
Gross involvement	Usually single	Single or multiple	Single or multiple	Multiple	Usually multiple	Usually multiple
Microscopic involvement	Replaces acini	Replaces acini	Replaces acini	Grows in portal areas	Infiltrates and partially destroys acini	Infiltrates and destroys acini
Remnants of hepatic acini	No	No	No	No (tumor within portal areas)	Yes	No
Infiltration of preexisting sinusoids	No	No	Yes (rare)	No	Yes	Yes
Invasion of veins (terminal hepatic venules, portal vein branches)	No	No	Yes (rare)	No	Yes	Yes
Invasion of capsule	No	No	No	No	Yes	Yes
Cells lining neoplastic vessels						
Pleomorphism	No	No	Yes	No	Yes	Yes
Mitoses	No	No	Yes	Yes	Yes	Yes
"Epithelioid" change	No[a]	No	No	No	Yes	Yes (rare)
Multinucleation and giant cells	No	No	Yes (rare)	No	Yes (rare)	Yes
"Dendritic" cells	No	No	No	No	Yes	No
Factor VIII-related antigen in tumor cells	Yes	Yes	Yes	Only in cells lining blood vessels	Yes	Yes
Bile ducts in tumor (excluding those in preexisting portal areas)	No	Yes	Yes	No	No	No
Collagenous matrix	Yes (in sclerosed type)	Yes (central)	Yes (central)	Yes (rare)	Yes (diffuse)	No
Inflammation (other than in necrotic foci)	No	No	No	Yes	Yes	No
Hemosiderin (other than in old hemorrhages or infarcts)	No	No	No	Yes	No	No
Extramedullary hematopoiesis in neoplastic vessels	No	Yes	Yes	No	No	Yes
Nodular regenerative hyperplasia in non-neoplastic liver	No	No	No	No	Yes (some cases)	Yes (some cases)
Extrahepatic metastases	No	No	Yes (lung, lymph nodes)	Simultaneous foci in skin, GI tract, etc.	Yes (lung, pleura, peritoneum, lymph nodes, spleen)	Yes (lung, spleen, lymph nodes, bone marrow)

GI gastro intestinal

a Except for the "histiocytoid type of hemangioma" (Rosai J, Gold J, Landy R (1979) The histiocytoid hemangiomas. Hum Pathol 10: 707–730) which is exceptionally rare in the liver

2 Angiosarcoma

Although rare, this malignant vascular tumor is the commonest sarcoma arising in the liver. Worldwide, over 200 cases are diagnosed annually [2, 13]. The peak age incidence for angiosarcoma is in the sixth and seventh decades of life, with a male to female ratio of 3:1 [14]. In my experience [15], the modes of presentation include: (1) symptoms and signs indicative of liver disease (62%), such as hepatomegaly, ascites, abdominal pain, anorexia, nausea, and occasional vomiting, weight loss, and fever; (2) signs and symptoms of an acute abdomen from hemoperitoneum due to rupture of the tumor (15%); (3) splenomegaly, with or without pancytopenia

(5%); (4) symptoms or signs referable to metastases to distant organs such as the skeleton or lungs (9%). The diagnosis is best established by open liver biopsy following suggestive radiographic studies.

Laboratory data include anemia and sometimes a microangiopathic hemolytic anemia, leukocytosis (65%) or leukopenia (22%), and thrombocytopenia (62%) [15]. Disseminated intravascular coagulopathy is a rare complication [16]. Tests of hepatic function show abnormal results in about two-thirds of the patients [14, 15]. The most consistent abnormalities are bromosulfophthalein (BSP) retention (100%) an increased serum alkaline phosphatase value (83%) and a prolonged prothrombin time (72%). Hyperbilirubinemia develops in about 60% of cases, while mild to modest aminotransferase elevations are found in less than half the cases.

Chest roentgenograms reveal elevation of the diaphragm (32% of cases) or, much less frequently, right pleural effusions, atelectasis, or pleural masses [14]. Plain films of the abdomen in Thorotrast-related angiosarcomas invariably disclose opacification of the liver, spleen, and abdominal lymph nodes [17]. Hepatic scans are abnormal in the majority of cases, but definite filling defects are recorded in only 70% cases [14]. Computed tomography (CT) has been utilized in diagnosis [17–19] as well as in detecting rupture of the tumor [18]. The smallest tumor detected by CT in the large series of van Kaick et al. [19] was 3 cm in diameter. Angiographic studies are considered to yield valuable information in angiosarcoma [14, 20]. The abnormal vascular pattern, with a persistent peripheral tumor stain and a central radiolucent area, is thought to be highly suggestive of angiosarcoma [20].

The majority of patients with angiosarcoma die less than 6 months after diagnosis, usually from liver failure or abdominal bleeding. Surgical excision is generally not feasible, but some prolongation of survival has been achieved by chemotherapy [14, 20].

Gross examination of the liver involved by angiosarcoma reveals grayish-white tumor tissue alternating with hemorrhagic foci (Fig. 12.7). Large cavities filled with liquid blood may be observed. A reticular pattern of fibrosis is often seen in cases associated with Thorotrast or prior exposure to vinyl chloride. Typically, the entire liver is involved. The spleen is usually large, except in Thorotrast-related angiosarcoma, when it is atrophic. Cut sections of the spleen and

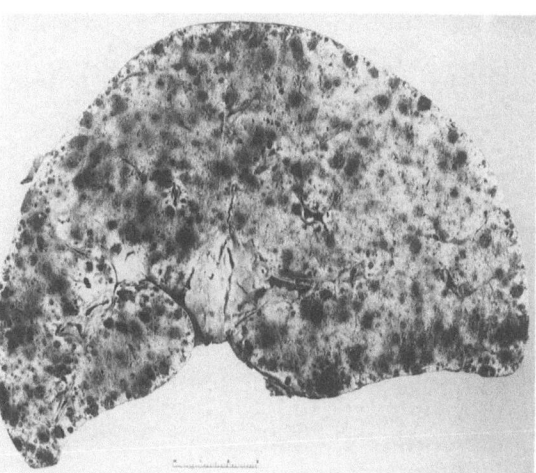

Fig. 12.7. Cut surface of liver shows multifocal involvement of right and left lobes by angiosarcoma

abdominal lymph nodes have a chalky white appearance in cases with a previous history of Thorotrast exposure. A true cirrhosis, regardless of etiology, is exceptionally rare in my experience, but in the review of Locker et al. [14] it was recorded in 20% of cases.

Microscopically, the tumor is composed of malignant endothelial cells that are spindle-shape or irregular in outline and have ill-defined borders (Figs. 12.8, 12.9). The cytoplasm is lightly eosinophilic, and nuclei are hyperchromatic and elongated or irregular in shape. Nucleoli can be small or large and eosinophilic. Large, bizarre nuclei and multinucleated cells may be seen, and mitotic figures are frequently identified (Fig. 12.10). In my experience and that of others [21, 22], factor VIII-related antigen may be identified in tumor cells by immunohistological techniques (Fig. 12.11), although it was reported to be negative in the series of Kojiro et al. [23]. Immunostaining with *Ulex europaeus* is more sensitive though less specific than that for factor VIII [24].

The tumor cells grow along preformed vascular channels, viz. sinusoids, THV, and portal vein branches (Figs. 12.9, 12.12). Sinusoidal growth is associated with progressive atrophy of liver cells and disruption of the plates, formation of larger and larger vascular channels, and, eventually, the development of cavitary spaces of varied size (Fig. 12.13). These cavities have ragged walls lined by tumors cells (sometimes with polypoid or papillary projections) and are filled with clotted blood and tumor debris (Fig. 12.13). Invasion of THV and portal vein

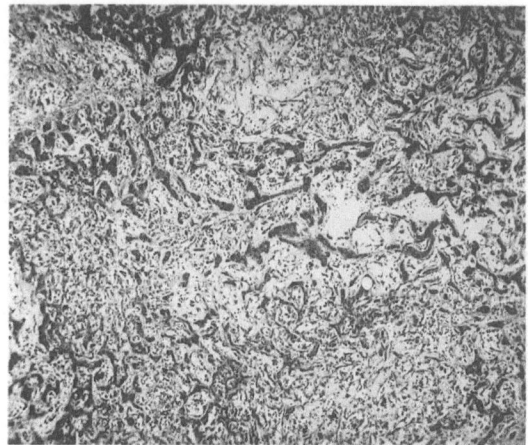

Fig. 12.8. Vinyl chloride-related angiosarcoma reveals infiltration of the hepatic parenchyma, with disruption and destruction of the liver cell plates. H and E, × 60

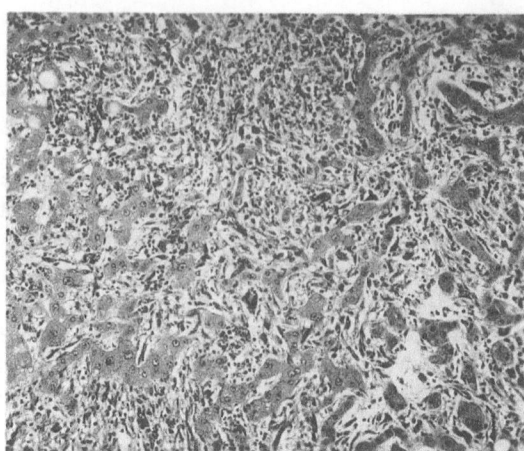

Fig. 12.9. Higher magnification of case illustrated in Fig. 11.8 demonstrates infiltration of hepatic sinusoids by the sarcoma cells. H and E, × 160

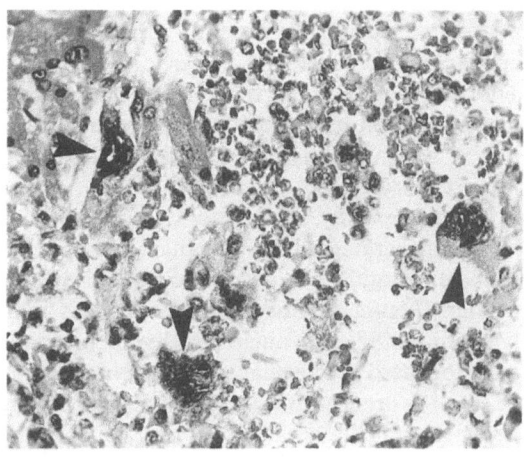

Fig. 12.10. Angiosarcoma cells are bizarre and multinucleated (*arrowheads*). (HE × 350)

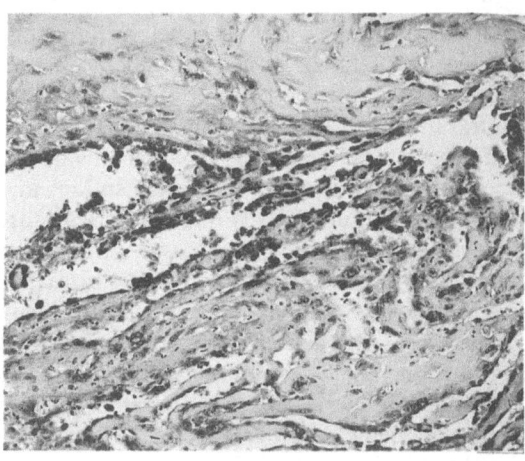

Fig. 12.11. Angiosarcoma cells reveal strong immunoreactivity (black) to antibody to factor VIII-related antibody. Peroxidase-antiperoxidase technique, × 160

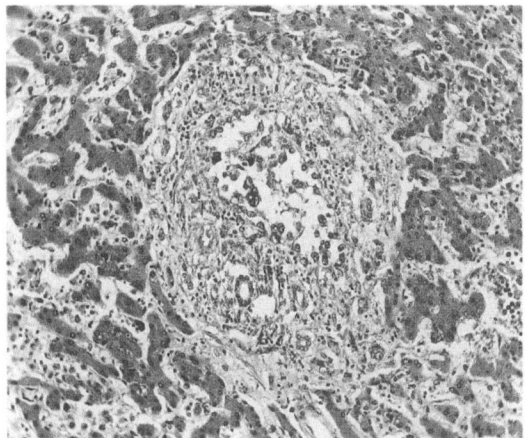

Fig. 12.12. Vein in a portal area is lined and partly filled by angiosarcoma cells. H and E, × 130

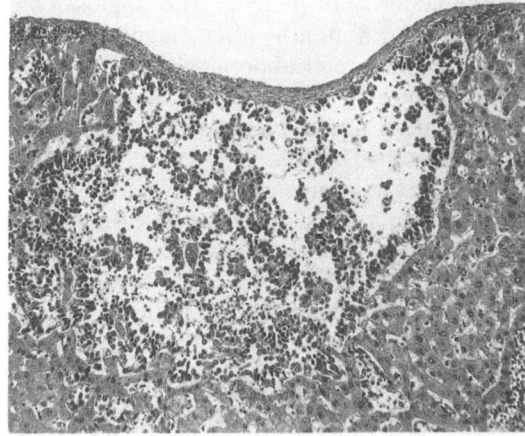

Fig. 12.13. Subcapsular cavity of angiosarcoma is lined with tumor cells which have also formed papillary fronds partially filling the lumen. H and E, × 120

branches leads to progressive obstruction of the lumen and readily explains the frequently encountered areas of hemorrhage, infarction, and necrosis. The tumor cells are sometimes packed solidly in nodules that resemble fibrosarcoma (Fig. 12.14). Hematopoietic activity (Fig. 12.15) is observed in the majority of tumors [15], although it was considered to be a feature most typical of Thorotrast-related cases in one study [25].

A precursor stage in the development of angiosarcoma has been observed in cases etiologically related to vinyl chloride, Thorotrast, and arsenic [25–29]. It is characterized by foci of simultaneous activation of both hepatocytes and sinusoidal lining cells, with associated lesions in the sinusoids and perisinusoidal spaces. In my experience, the most striking precursor lesion is that affecting isolated sinusoidal lining cells that are hypertrophied and have large irregular

and hyperchromatic nuclei. In the case of vinyl chloride, the lesions in exposed humans are quite comparable with those induced experimentally in rodents [30]. Additional light-microscopic and ultrastructural studies of hepatic lesions in workers exposed to vinyl chloride (but who did not have angiosarcoma) have been reported [31, 32].

Cases related to Thorotrast and vinyl chloride are often associated with considerable periportal and subcapsular fibrosis, and cirrhosis has been etiologically related to these two agents as well as to arsenic. In Thorotrast-induced angiosarcomas, the Thorotrast deposits are readily recognized in reticuloendothelial cells or lying free in portal areas, Glisson's capsule or the wall of THV (Fig. 12.16). The deposits are colorless and refractile, but in sections stained with H and E they usually have a pink-brown hue; they are not birefringent but can be illuminated by phase-

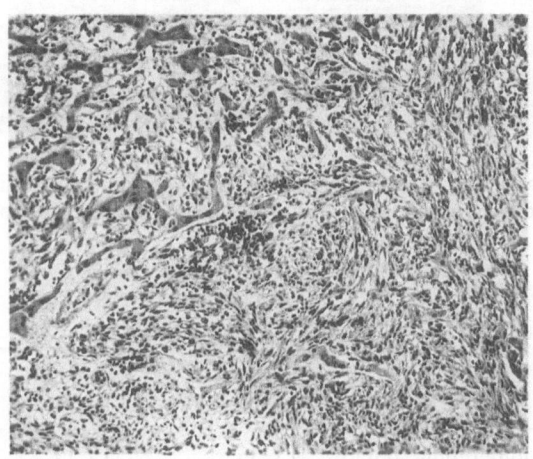

Fig. 12.14. Solid fibrosarcomalike growth in angiosarcoma. H and E, × 160

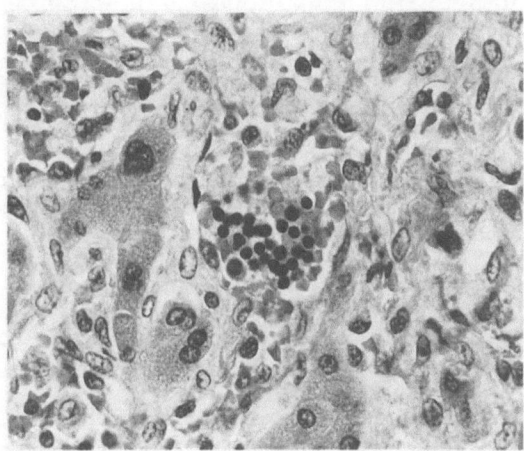

Fig. 12.15. Cluster of nucleated erythrocytes and an erythroblast are present in a sinusoid. H and E, × 575

Fig. 12.16. Darkly stained clusters of Thorotrast (*arrowheads*) are scattered throughout the photographic field. H and E, × 35

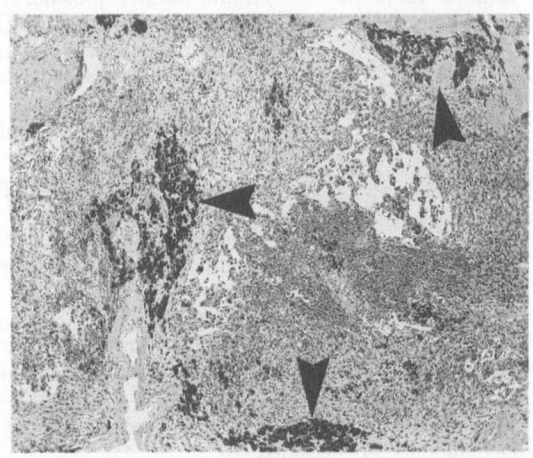

contrast microscopy. The alpha emissions of the thorium doxide can be captured by autoradiography, appearing as short, dotted tracks. The particles are readily visualized by scanning electron microscopy of a paraffin section (Fig. 12.17), and the element thorium can be definitively identified by energy dispersive X-ray microanalysis (Fig. 12.18) [33–36].

In the majority of hepatic angiosarcomas, the cause is unknown. A survey of angiosarcomas in the United States from 1964 through 1974 by Falk et al. [2] disclosed 168 cases; 75% of these were of uncertain etiology while the remainder were related to vinyl chloride, Thorotrast, inorganic arsenic, and androgenic/anabolic steroids. Etiological factors implicated in angiosarcoma in humans, together with pertinent references, are listed in Table 12.2.

Angiosarcoma occurs rarely in children. Most cases are believed to arise from infantile heman-

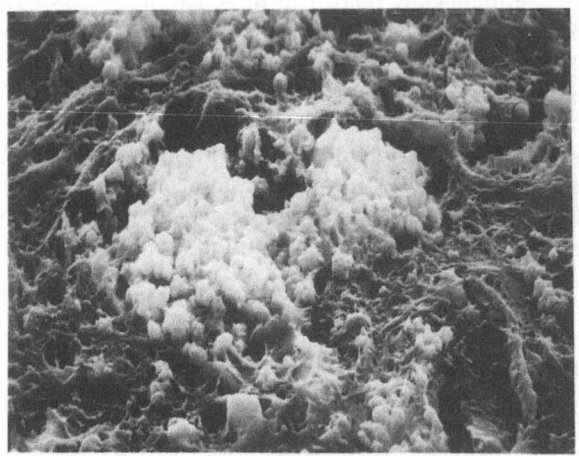
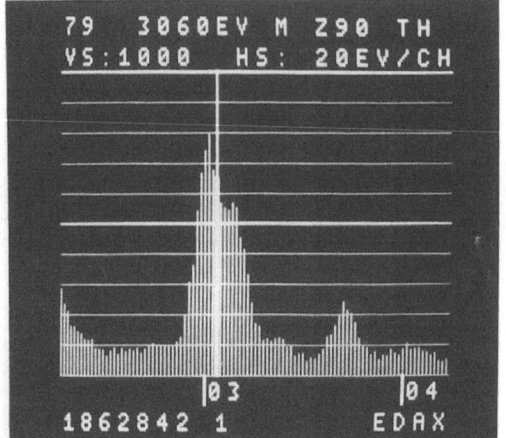

Fig. 12.17. Three-dimensional appearance of Thorotrast particles embedded in fibrous tissue. Scanning electron micrograph, × 640

Fig. 12.18. Energy-dispersive X-ray microanalysis of particles in Fig. 11.17 identifies one peak of element thorium

Table 12.2. Etiology of angiosarcoma

Physical/ chemical injury	Circumstances of exposure	Latent period (years)	Reference
Thorotrast	Used as contrast medium for radiographic studies	15–36	2, 15, 19, 23, 25, 28, 37–41
Radium	Radium needle implanted for treatment of breast carcinoma (1 case)	3	42
External radiation	Atomic bomb explosion, Hiroshima (1 case)	36	43
Vinyl chloride	Industrial exposure during manufacture of polyvinyl chloride; exposure to sprays containing vinyl chloride as propellant	12–28	2, 20, 21, 26–28, 44–46
Inorganic arsenic	Insecticide for spraying of vineyards; medical use of Fowler's solution; high levels of arsenic in drinking water	6–33	47–55
Copper	Use of copper sulfate for spraying of vineyards (1 case)	35	56
Iron	Idiopathic hemochromatosis in cirrhotic stage	?	57–59
Androgenic/anabolic steroids	Treatment of Fanconi's anemia and other disorders	2–35	60–61
Contraceptive steroids	Birth control (1 case)	10	62
Diethylstilbestrol	Treatment of prostatic cancer (1 case)	13	63
Phenelzine	Reason for therapy not stated (1 case)	6	64

Cases arising in preexisting benign vascular tumors, such as infantile hemangioendothelioma and cavernous hemangioma, are excluded

gioendothelioma [65–69] and were referred to in one study as type 2 hemangioendothelioma [69]. Etiological factors implicated in these childhood angiosarcomas include androgenic/anabolic steroids [60] and, possibly, environmental exposure to arsenic [52]. A unique case of an angiosarcoma arising in a calcified cavernous hemangioma in an adult has been reported [70].

Note should also be made of the co-existence of angiosarcoma with one or more malignant tumors (hepatocellular carcinoma and/or cholangiocarcinoma). This has been reported with both Thorotrast- [71–74] and vinyl chloride-associated [45, 75] angiosarcomas.

3 Kaposi's sarcoma

This entity has assumed importance in recent years because of its association with the acquired immune deficiency syndrome (AIDS), but cases apparently not related to AIDS occur sporadically in Europe and Africa [76]. Involvement of the liver has been reported in about a quarter of fatal cases of AIDS [77–80] but does not appear to contribute to the morbidity and mortality of the disease. Definite functional hepatic impairment has not been recorded.

Kaposi's sarcoma in the liver is visible grossly as irregular, variably sized, red-brown spongiform lesions that resemble capillary hemangiomas (Fig. 12.9). Histopathologically, the changes are generally confined to the portal connective tissue (Fig. 12.20) and resemble those seen in

the skin, gastrointestinal tract, and other sites. The exact origin of the Kaposi's sarcoma cell is disputed; some immunohistological studies suggest that it originates in the blood vessel endothelium [76, 81], while others support an origin from the lymphatic endothelium [82]. Monoclonal antibodies generated against soft-tissue sarcomas may help to clarify the nature of Kaposi's sarcoma cell [83].

4 Embryonal rhabdomyosarcoma

This tumor arises in the extrahepatic bile ducts but can extend into the liver. Most patients are less than 5 years of age, but occasional tumors have been diagnosed in older children and adults [84–88]. A primary intrahepatic rhabdomyosarcoma, forming a "collision" tumor with a hepatocellular carcinoma, was recently reported in a 62-year-old man [89]. In children, embryonal rhabdomyosarcoma affects males and females equally.

Patients with embryonal rhabdomyosarcoma usually present with intermittent obstructive jaundice, often with fever and hepatomegaly. A mistaken diagnosis of viral hepatitis can lead to delays in definitive therapy [87]. In patients with the suggestive symptomatology, ultrasonography and computed tomography generally demonstrate a mass in the porta hepatis. Transhepatic cholangiography has been utilized in preoperative diagnosis [90].

Initial therapy should consist of resection of

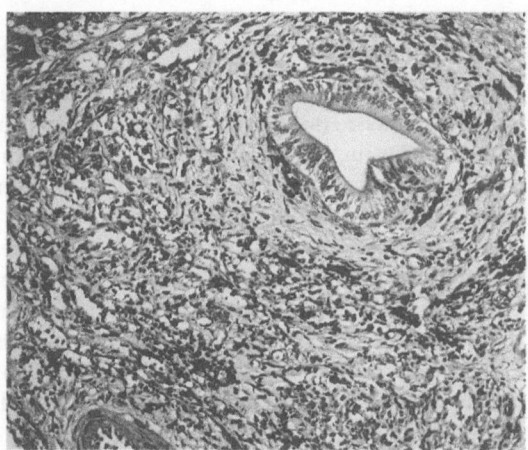

Fig. 12.19. Kaposi's sarcoma involving portal area connective tissue. Note bile duct in *upper right corner*. H and E, × 160

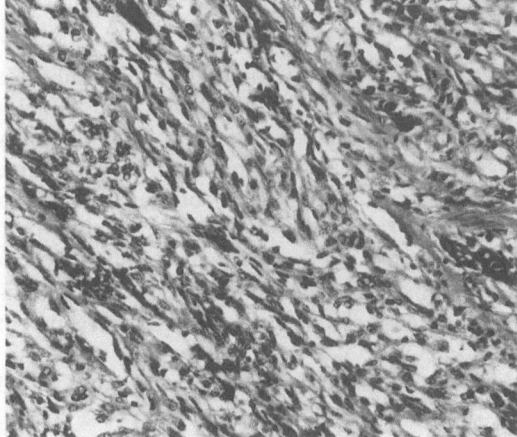

Fig. 12.20. Higher magnification of case illustrated in Fig. 11.19 reveals spindle cells and slitlike spaces. H and E, × 160

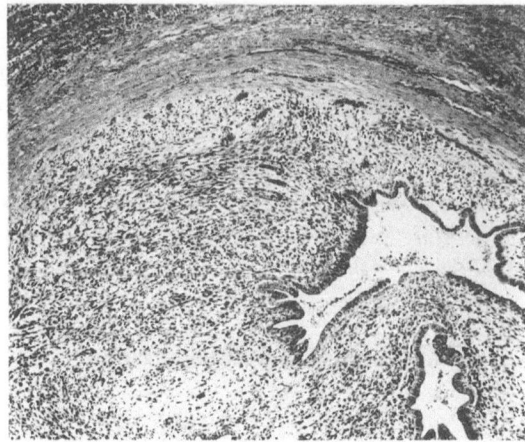

Fig. 12.21. Embryonal rhabdomyosarcoma involves entire thickness of bile duct wall, with marked narrowing of the lumen. H and E, × 60

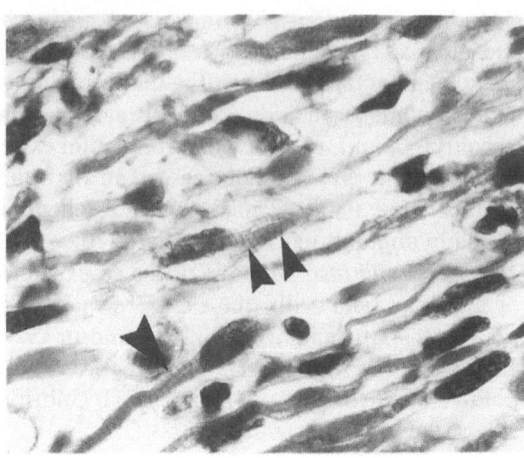

Fig. 12.22. Same case illustrated in Fig. 11.21 reveals cross-striations (*arrowheads*) in tumor cells. H and E, × 1000

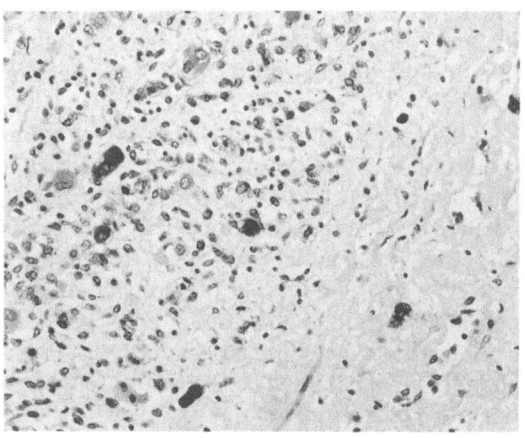

Fig. 12.23. Several well-differentiated rhabdomyosarcoma cells (darkly stained) express myoglobin. Peroxidase-antiperoxidase, × 250

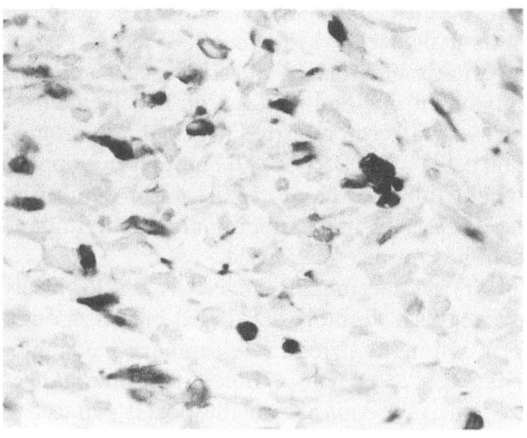

Fig. 12.24. Rhabdomyosarcoma cells (darkly stained) express desmin. Peroxidase-antiperoxidase, × 630

the mass with only microscopic or minimal gross residual tumor; continuity of bile flow is maintained by variations of a Roux-en-Y jejunostomy [87]. Operative cholangiography is invaluable in demonstrating the site of obstruction and in verifying a functioning drainage procedure [87]. Postoperative therapy includes multidrug chemotherapy and radiotherapy. Re-exploration is important in evaluating residual or recurrent disease. Of 10 cases treated by the aforementioned multidisciplinary approach advocated by the Intergroup Rhabdomyosarcoma Study, three patients survived 3, 6¼, and 6½ years after diagnosis [87].

Affected bile ducts grossly have a thick wall with narrowing of the lumen. Cut sections reveal

a white glistening tumor. Soft or gelatinous grapelike masses (sarcoma botryoides) may project into the lumen. Bile ducts proximal to the occluded segment are dilated, and the liver often has a green color from cholestasis.

Microscopically, the polypoid tumor masses projecting into the lumen are covered by bile duct epithelium, but the surface may be ulcerated and inflamed (Fig. 12.21). A dense mass of tumor cells ("cambium layer") lies immediately subjacent to the epithelium. Tumor cells may be round, spindled, or strap-shaped. The nuclei are hyperchromatic, elongated, and have blunt ends. Mitotic figures are usually abundant. Cross-striations are generally identified with difficulty (Fig. 12.22). Ultrastructural studies reveal both thick and thin myofilaments with recognizable Z bands in some cells [86]. Tumor cells are usually set in loose myxoid stroma containing a large amount of acid mucopolysaccharide. Areas of inflammation, necrosis, and hemorrhage may be seen.

Myoglobin (Fig. 12.23), myosin, and desmin (Fig. 12.24) may be identified in tumor cells immunohistologically [91–93]. Desmin is the best marker for the poorly differentiated tumors (Fig. 12.24).

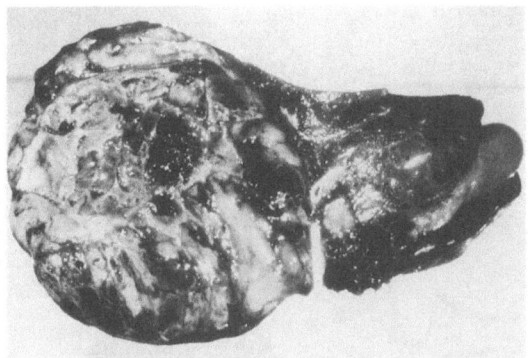

Fig. 12.25. Cut surface of liver shows involvement of right lobe by a solid and cystic tumor

5 Undifferentiated sarcoma

This tumor has been referred to by a variety of synonyms such as primary sarcoma, embryonal sarcoma, and malignant mesenchymoma [94]. The term malignant mesenchymoma used by a number of authors [95, 96] is justified only if there is evidence of differentiation into two or more mesenchymal elements (other than fibrosarcoma), which is rarely the case [97–101].

Undifferentiated sarcoma is quite rare; in the AFIP files (up to 1978) it constituted 13% of all primary hepatic neoplasms in the pediatric age-group [94]. In a survey of 1237 primary hepatic tumors in childhood culled from the literature (up to 1983) by Weinberg and Finegold, 6% were sarcomas [102].

The majority of patients (52%) with undifferentiated sarcoma are between 6 and 10 years of age [94]. Abdominal swelling, with or without a palpable mass, and pain are the usual presenting findings. Some patients complain of various nonspecific gastrointestinal symptoms, fever, and weight loss. Rarely, the tumor invades the inferior vena cava and grows into the right atrium, presenting clinically as a primary intracardiac tumor [100]. Leukocytosis with a shift to the left is a common finding. Tests of hepatic function are abnormal in a third to half of patients, the most frequent being a slight increase of the serum alkaline phosphatase activity. Alphafetoprotein values are normal.

Radiological findings reflect the spectrum of solid and cystic features characteristic of the tumor [103]. Sonography typically demonstrates a large mass that may be predominantly solid, with many small anechoic spaces, or cystic. Computed tomography reveals a hypodense mass with hyperdense septa of variable thickness and a dense peripheral rim corresponding to the fibrous pseudocapsule. Angiographically, the tumor is usually hypovascular, but hypervascular

and avascular patterns occur infrequently. The radiological differential diagnosis from mesenchymal hamartoma may be difficult. The older age and more frequent symptomatic presentation of patients with undifferentiated sarcoma are helpful in differential diagnosis. A definitive diagnosis requires liver biopsy, which is generally performed at laparotomy. One reported case was diagnosed at peritoneoscopy by guided biopsy [104].

The prognosis of undifferentiated sarcoma is very poor with a median survival of less than 1 year after diagnosis [94]. A recent report of a 5-year survival after excision, irradiation, and doxorubicin therapy [105] holds promise of longer survival after combined modality therapy. An initially unresectable tumor in a 7-year-old girl was successfully excised following treatment with cisplatin and doxorubicin [106]. A good response to palliative treatment (hepatic artery ligation and chemotherapy) has been reported [107].

The majority of undifferentiated sarcomas are located in the right lobe of the liver. Most measure 10–20 cm in diameter, with an average weight of 1310 g [94]. They are usually globular and well-demarcated, but encapsulation is uncommon. The cut surface is variegated, with solid, glistening, gray-white tumor tissue, alternating with cystic gelatinous areas and/or red and yellow areas of hemorrhage and necrosis (Fig. 12.25).

Microscopically, a fibrous pseudocapsule may separate the tumor from the adjacent compressed parenchyma. The more peripheral areas of the tumor typically contain entrapped bile ducts, which can be dilated (Fig. 12.26), and sometimes hepatic parenchymal elements. The

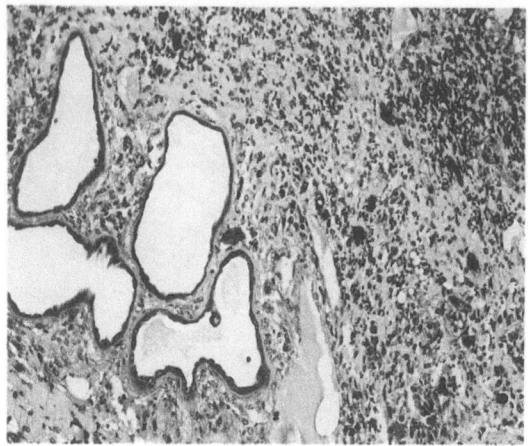

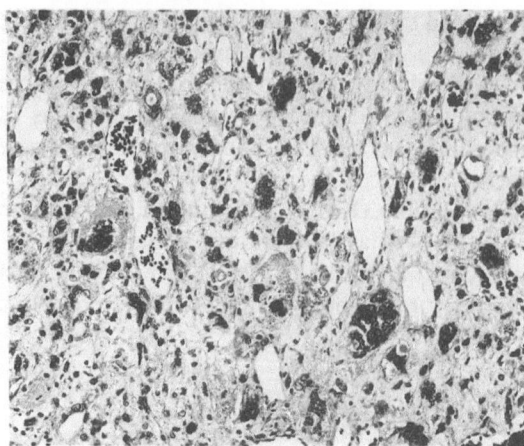

Fig. 12.26. Undifferentiated sarcoma (*right*) and several dilated bile ducts (*left*) near the junction of the tumor with the adjacent liver (not shown). H and E, × 160

Fig. 12.27. Cells of undifferentiated sarcoma exhibit marked pleomorphism and multinucleation. H and E, × 250

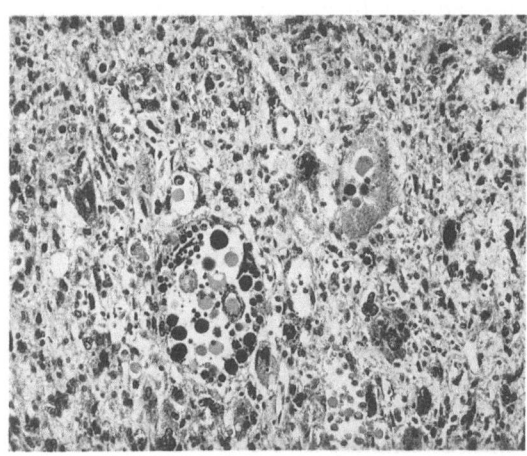

Fig. 12.28. Darkly stained globules are present in degenerating tumor cells. PAS with diastase predigestion, × 160

tumor cells are stellate or spindle-shaped and have ill-defined outlines (Figs. 12.26, 12.27). They may be compactly or loosely arranged, with an abundant mucopolysaccharide matrix, but areas with a more fibrous stroma are also seen in most tumors. Tumor cells often show marked anisonucleosis with hyperchromasia and sometimes bizarre giant cells; mitoses are usually abundant (Fig. 12.27). A characteristic feature is the presence of multiple, varying-size eosinophilic globules in the cytoplasm; these are PAS-positive and resist diastase digestion (Fig. 12.28). Hematopoietic activity is present in half the tumors. Hemorrhages and necrosis are often present. The neoplastic cells may be reactive to antibodies to alpha$_1$-antitrypsin, alpha$_1$-antichymotrypsin, and vimentin [108–110]. There is no evidence of cellular differentiation under the light microscope, but ultrastructural studies in isolated cases have shown fibroblastic, lipoblastic, leiomyoblastic, and/or myofibroblastic differentiation [99–101, 110].

Little is known of possible inducing or promoting factors in undifferentiated sarcoma, other than one report of a 19-year-old patient who had been exposed prenatally to phenytoin [111].

6 Other malignant mesenchymal tumors

Fibrosarcoma is a rare tumor of the liver [15, 112–121]. The ages of the patients range from 30 to 73 years (median 55 years), most of whom (85%) are males. Symptoms and signs are nonspecific and the diagnosis is established by biopsy. The tumor may be associated with severe hypoglycemia [2, 114]. Hemoperitoneum from

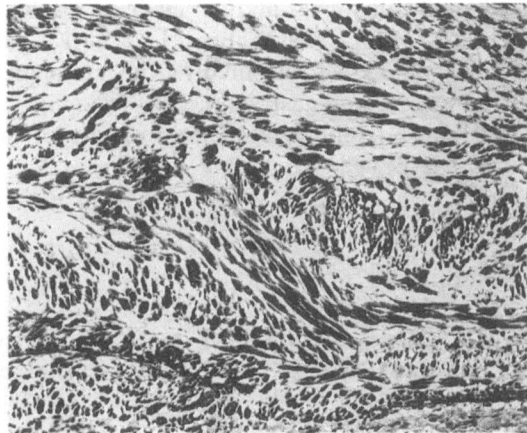

Fig. 12.29. Primary leiomyosarcoma of the liver reveals intersecting bundles of elongated or rounded cells. Masson trichrome, × 160

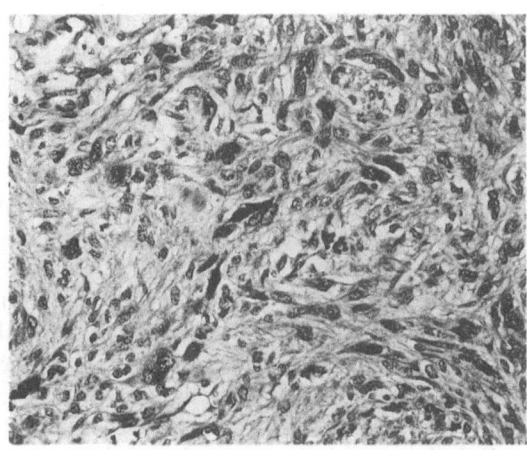

Fig. 12.30. Cells (darkly stained) of case illustrated in Fig. 12.29 demonstrate desmin immunoreactivity. Peroxidase-antiperoxidase, × 250

rupture is rare. The prognosis is very poor, although several patients have survived 1–3 years following resection and/or radiation therapy.

Fibrosarcoma is often large at the time of diagnosis; one of the largest tumors weighed more than 7 kg [15]. The cut surface reveals grayish-white tissue, which can display a whorled appearance. Foci of necrosis and hemorrhage, sometimes with cystic degeneration, are often seen. Microscopically, the tumor is composed of spindle-shaped cells arranged in interlacing bundles, with the typical "herringbone" pattern in some areas. Varying numbers of collagen and reticulin fibers arise from and intermingle with the tumor cells. The nuclei are hyperchromatic and elongated and have pointed ends; mitotic activity is variable.

Leiomyosarcoma is also a very rare tumor of the liver; some 24 cases have been reported [1, 15, 122–128]. It occurs more frequently in women. The man age of presentation is 52 years. Symptoms and signs include an upper abdominal swelling or mass, abdominal pain, and weight loss. Leiomyosarcomas arising in the hepatic veins lead to the Budd-Chiari syndrome [129, 130]. The prognosis of leiomyosarcomas arising in the hepatic outflow tract is worse than that of the tumors that are intrahepatic; the latter, in turn, have a worse prognosis than leiomyosarcomas arising in the ligamentum teres [15, 128]. The mean survival of intrahepatic leiomyosarcoma is 20 months [124], the longest survival being 6.5 years after surgical extirpation [122].

Primary leiomyosarcomas of the liver are usually solitary and can attain a large size; one tumor weighed over 11 kg [122]. They are usually firm in consistency. The cut surface is pinkish-white with yellow areas of necrosis or dark red hemorrhagic foci. Histopathologically, the tumor is composed of intersecting bundles of elongated, spindle-shaped cells (Fig. 12.29). The lightly eosinophilic cytoplasm may display faint longitudinal striations. Nuclei are hyperchromatic and elongated and have blunt ends. Mitotic activity is frequently observed. Tumor cells express desmin, which can be identified by the peroxidase anti-peroxidase (PAP) method (Fig. 12.30). Ultrastructurally, myofilaments, cytoplasmic dense bodies, and marginal dense plaques are seen [123].

Malignant fibrous histiocytoma is an exceptionally uncommon primary tumor of the liver. Only two cases have been reported to date [131, 132]. A possible relationship of this tumor to undifferentiated sarcoma has been raised in one recent case report [110].

Histiocytosis X, also referred to as Langerhan's cell histiocytosis [133], is of unknown etiology and pathogenesis [133–137]. The liver is frequently involved, and jaundice and portal hypertension are well-documented findings [135–137]. Both obstructive and hepatocellular dysfunction occurs. Patients who survive after chemotherapy develop severe fibrosis or cirrhosis with manifestations of portal hypertension [136]. Uncommon complications include sclerosing cholangitis [138] and hepatocellular carcinoma [136].

Microscopically, there is infiltration of portal areas (and to a lesser extent acini) by aggregates of histiocytes and some inflammatory cells (mononuclear cells, eosinophils). Kuppfer cells are prominent and often vacuolated, but there is little or no erythrophagocytosis [135, 137]. Ultrastructurally, Langerhan's cells with typical Birbeck's granules and trilaminar membranous loops are characteristic of the disorder, but the cells may be difficult to identify in the liver [133, 135, 137]. Recent enzyme histochemical and immunohistochemical studies support the concept that histiocytosis X is a proliferative disorder of cells of Langerhans lineage [139, 140].

Familial erythrophagocytic lymphohistiocytosis is characterized by a mixed histiocytic and lymphocytic infiltrate in sinusoids and portal areas, in addition to marked erythrophagocytosis by Kupffer's cells and portal macrophages. Recent immunophenotypic, immunohistochemical, and ultrastructural studies suggest that the condition may represent an uncontrolled proliferation of sinusoidal histiocytes [141].

Malignant histiocytosis (also known as histiocytic medullary reticulosis and the disseminated form of histiocytic sarcoma) can involve the liver [133, 142–145]. The mean survival after diagnosis in one series was 7.6 months, but complete remissions have been achieved in a few patients by aggressive chemotherapy [144]. Occasional patients with this entity present with fulminant hepatic disease [146]. One group of investigators considered liver biopsy very useful in antemortem diagnosis [143].

Histopathologically, portal and periportal areas are infiltrated by atypical as well as well-differentiated histiocytes; lymphocytes and plasma cells are also present in the infiltrates [113, 143, 144]. The atypical histiocytes have lightly stained abundant cytoplasm and very irregular hyperchromatic nuclei with clumped chromatin and one or more large nucleoli. Mitoses are frequently identified. Ultrastructural features are nonspecific, but the presence of lysosomes, phagolysosomes, and phagosomes is helpful in diagnosis [145]. The tumor cells do not contain Langerhans's granules [133]. The well-differentiated histiocytes exhibit phagocytic activity (to erythrocytes and other cellular elements) and stain positively for lysozyme, acid phosphatase, nonspecific esterase, vimentin, and alpha$_1$-antitrypsin [143–145].

Primary lymphoma of the liver is exceptionally rare. Ten cases were reported recently by Osborne et al. [147], who also reviewed 19 previously published cases. Since then, another case associated with a micronodular cirrhosis has been reported [148]. That patient had AIDS and Kaposi's sarcoma that involved his abdominal lymph nodes and gastric mucosa. The majority of primary lymphomas of the liver are of the diffuse large-cell type.

References

1. Edmondson HA, Peters RL (1982) Neoplasms of the liver. In: Schiff L, Schiff ER (eds) Diseases of the liver, 5th edn. Lippincott, Philadelphia, pp 1101–1157
2. Falk H, Herbert J, Crouley S (1981) Epidemiology of hepatic angiosarcoma in the United States: 1964–1974. Environ Hlth Persp 41: 107–113
3. Shin P, Ohmi S, Sakurai M (1981) Hepatocellular carcinoma combined with hepatic sarcoma. Acta Pathol Jpn 31: 815–824
4. Ishak KG, Sesterhenn IA, Goodman ZD, Rabin L, Stromeyer FW (1984) Epithelioid hemangioendothelioma of the liver: A clinicopathologic and follow-up study of 32 cases. Hum Pathol 15: 839–852
5. Ishak KG, Sesterhenn IA, Goodman ZD, Rabin L, Stromeyer (1985) Hepatic epithelioid hemangioendothelioma. In: Brunner H, Thaler H (eds) Hepatology: A Festschrift for Hans Popper. Raven, New York, pp 183–189
6. Dail DH, Liebow AA, Gmelich JT, Friedman PJ, Miyai K, Myer W, Patterson SD, Hannar SP (1983) Intravascular, bronchiolar and alveolar tumor of the lung: An analysis of twenty cases of a peculiar sclerosing endothelial tumor. Cancer 51: 452–464
7. Weiss SW, Enzinger FM (1982) Epithelioid hemangioendothelioma: A Vascular tumor often mistaken for a carcinoma. Cancer 50: 970–981
8. Ellis GL, Kratichvil FJ (1986) Epithelioid hemangioendothelioma of the head and neck: A clinicopathologic report of twelve cases. Oral Surg, Oral Med, Oral Pathol 61: 61068
9. Weiss SW, Ishak KG, Dail DH, Sweet DE, Enzinger FM (1986) Epithelioid hemangioendothelioma and related lesions. Diagnositc Histopathol 3: 259–287
10. Fukayama M, Nihei Z, Takizawa T, Kawaguchi K, Harada H, Koike M (1984) Malignant epithelioid hemangioendothelioma of the liver, spreading through the hepatic veins. Virch Arch (Pathol Anat) 404: 275–287
11. Dean PJ, Haggitt RC, O'Hara CJ (1985) Malignant epithelioid hemangioendothelioma of the liver in young women: Relationship to oral contraceptive use. Am J Surg Pathol 9: 695–704
12. Clements D, Hubscher S, West R, Elias E, McMaster P (1986) Epithelioid hemangioendothelioma: A case report. J Hepatol 2: 441–449
13. Anonymous (1981) Angiosarcoma of the liver: A growing problem? Br Med J 282: 504–505

14. Locker GY, Doroshow JH, Zwelling LA, Chabner BA (1979) The clinical features of hepatic angiosarcoma: A report of four cases and a review of the English Literature. Medicine 58: 48–64

15. Ishak KG (1976) Mesenchymal tumors of the liver. In: Okuda K, Peters RL (eds) Hepatocellular carcinoma. Wiley, New York, pp 247–307

16. Truell JE, Peck SD, Reiquam CW (1973) Hemangiosarcoma of the liver complicated by disseminated intravascular coagulation: A case report. Gastroenterology 65: 936–942

17. Levy DW, Rindsberg S, Friedman AC, Fishman EK, Ros PR, Radecki PD, Siegelman SS, Goodman ZD, Pyatt RS, Grumbach K (1986) Thorotrast-induced hepatosplenic neoplasia: CT identification. AJR 146: 997–1004

18. Mahony B, Jeffrey RM, Federle MP (1982) Spontaneous rupture of hepatic and splenic angiosarcoma demonstrated by CT. AJR 138: 965–966

19. Van Kaick G, Siegert A, Luhrs H, Lieberman D (1986) Der Beitrag der Computertomographie zur Qunatifizierung der Thorotrastose und zur thorotrastinduzierter Lebertumoren. Radiologe 26: 123–128

20. Dannaher CL, Tamburro CL, Yam LT (1981) Occupational carcinogenesis: The Louisville experience with vinyl chloride-associated hepatic angiosarcoma. Am J Med 70: 279–287

21. Fortwengler HP, Jones D, Espinosa E, Tamburro CL (1981) Evidence for endothelial cell origin of vinyl chloride-induced hepatic angiosarcoma. Gastroenterology 80: 1415–1419

22. Manning JT, Ordonez NG, Barton JH (1983) Endothelial cell origin of thorium oxide-induced angiosarcoma of liver. Arch Pathol Lab Med 107: 456–458

23. Kojiro M, Nakashima T, Ito Y, Ikezaki H, Moni T, Kido C (1985) Thorium dioxide-related angiosarcoma of the liver: Pathomorphologic study of 29 autopsy cases. Arch Pathol Lab Med 109: 853–857

24. Miettinen M, Holhofer H, Lehto V-P, Miettinen A, Virtanen I (1983) Ulex europaeus 1 lectin as a marker for tumors derived from endothelial cells. Am J Clin Pathol 79: 32–36

25. Telles NC, Thomas LB, Popper H, Ishak KG Falk H (1979) Evolution of Thorotrast-induced hepatic angiosarcomas. Environ Res 18: 74–78

26. Thomas LB, Popper H, Berk PD, Selikoff I, Falk H (1975) Vinyl-chloride-induced liver disease. From idiopathic portal hypertension (Banti's syndrome) to angiosarcomas. N Engl Med 292: 17–22

27. Berk PD, Martin JF, Young RS, Creech J, Selikoff IJ, Falk H, Watanabe P, Popper H, Thomas L (1976) Vinyl chloride-associated liver disease. Ann Intern Med 84: 717–731

28. Popper H, Thomas LB, Teller NC, Falk H, Selikoff IJ (1978) Development of hepatic angiosarcoma induced by vinyl chloride, Thorotrast and arsenic: Comparison with cases of unknown etiology. Am J Pathol 92: 349–376

29. Tamburro CH, Makk L, Popper H (1984) Early hepatic histologic alterations among chemical (vinyl monomer) workers. Hepatology 4: 413–418

30. Popper H, Maltoni C, Selikoff IJ (1980) Vinyl chloride-induced hepatic lesions in man and rodents. A comparison. Liver 1: 7–20

31. Gedigk P, Muller R, Bechtelsheimer H (1975) Morphology of liver damage among polyvinyl chloride production workers: A report of 51 cases. Ann NY Acad Sci 246: 278–285

32. Schattenberg PJ, Totovic V, Gedigk P, Marsteller HJ (1977) Die Ultrastruktur der Leberschädigung bei der chronischen Vinylchlorid-Intoxikation. Virch Arch (Pathol Anat) 373: 233–247

33. Terzakis JH, Sommers SC, Snyder RW, Sabbath M (1974) X-ray microanalysis of hepatic thorium depositions. Arch Pathol 98: 241–242

34. Bowen JH, Woodward BH, Mossler JA, Ingram P, Shelburne JD (1980) Energy dispersive X-ray detection of thorium dioxide. Arch Pathol Lab Med 104: 459–461

35. Irie H, Mori W (1984) Long term effects of thorium dioxide (Thorotrast) administration on human liver: Ultrastructural localization of thorium dioxide in human liver by analytical electron microscopy (1984) Acta Pathol Jpn 34: 221–228

36. Ishak KG (1986) Applications of scanning electron microscopy to the study of liver disease. Prog Liver Dis 8: 1–32

37. Falk H, Telles NC, Ishak KG, Thomas LB, Popper H (1979) Epidemiology of Thorotrast-induced hepatic angiosarcoma in the united States. Environ Res 18: 65–73

38. Da Motta CL, Da Silva Horta J, Tavares MH (1979) Prospective epidemiological study of Thorotrast-exposed patients in Portugal. Environ Res 18: 152–173

39. Baxter PJ, Langlands AO, Anthony PP, MacSween RNM, Scheuer PJ (1980) Angiosarcoma of the liver: A marker tumour for the late effects of Thorotrast in Great Britain. Br J Cancer 41: 446–452

40. Van Kaick G, Muth H, Kaul A, Immich H, Lieberman D, Lorenz D, Lorenz WJ, Luhrs H, Scheer KE, Wagner G, Wegener K, Wesch H (1984) Results of the German Thorotrast study. Prog Cancer Res 26: 253–262

41. Yamada S, Hosoda S, Tateno H, Kido C, Takahashi S (1983) Survey of Thorotrast-associated liver cancers in Japan. J Natl Cancer Inst 70: 31–35

42. Ross JM (1932) A case illustrating the effects of prolonged action of radium. J Pathol Bacteriol 35: 899–912

43. Miyake S, Onoue K, Ueda M, Kohno H, Araki F, Iwasaki K (1982) Clinical studies on two cases of hepatic angiosarcoma. Acta Hepatol Jap 23: 1326–1333

44. Falk H, Creech JL, Heath CW, Johnson MN, Key MM (1974) Hepatic disease among workers at a vinyl chloride polymerization plant. JAMA

230: 59–63

45. Pialat J, Pasquier B, Pahn M, Kopp N (1979) Pathologie hépatique du chlorure de vinyle monomère (CVM): Huit observations anatomocliniques personnelles. Arch Anat Cytol Pathol 27: 361–375

46. Forman D, Bennett B, Stafford J, Doll R (1985) Exposure to vinyl chloride and angiosarcoma of the liver: A report of the register of cases. Br J Ind Med 42: 750–753

47. Roth F (1957) The sequelae of chronic arsenic poisoning in Moselle vintners. Ger Med Mon 2: 211–217

48. Regelson W, Kim U, Ospina J, Holland JF (1968) Hemangioendothelial sarcoma of the liver from chronic arsenic introxication by Fowler's solution. Cancer 21: 514–522

49. Rennke H, Prat GA, Etcheverry RB, Katz RU, Donoso S (1971) Hemangioendothelioma maligno del higado y arsenicismo chronica. Rev Med Chil 99: 664–668

50. Lander JJ, Stanley RJ, Sumner HW, Boswell D, Asch RD (1975) Angiosarcoma of the liver associated with Fowler's solution. Gastroenterology 68: 1582–1586

51. Brady J, Liberatore F, Harper P, Greenwald P, Burnett W, Davies JNP, Bishop M, Polan A, Vianna N (1977) Angiosarcoma of the liver: An epidemiologic study. J Natl Cancer Inst 59: 1383–1385

52. Falk H, Herbert JT, Edmonds L, Heath CW, Thomas LB, Popper H (1981) Review of four cases of childhood hepatic angiosarcoma-elevated environmental arsenic exposure in one case. Cancer 47: 382–391

53. Falk H, Caldwell GG, Ishak KG, Thomas LB, Popper H (1981) Arsenic-related hepatic angiosarcoma. Am J Ind Med 2: 43–50

54. Roat JW, Wald A, Mendelow H, Pataki KG (1982) Hepatic angiosarcoma associated with short-term arsenic ingestion. Am J Med 73: 933–936

55. Kasper ML, Schoenfield L, Strom RL, Theologides A (1984) Hepatic angiosarcoma and bronchioloalveolar carcinoma induced by Fowler's solution. JAMA 252: 3407–3408

56. Pimentel JC, Menezes AP (1977) Liver disease in vineyard sprayers. Gastroenterology 72: 275–283

57. Baker HC, Paget GE, Davson J (1956) Haemangioendothelioma of the liver. J Pathol Bacteriol 72: 173–182

58. Kwittken J, Tartow LR (1966) Haemochromatosis and Kupffer cell sarcoma with unusual localization of iron. J Pathol Bacteriol 92: 571–573

59. Sussman EB, Nydick I, Gray G (1974) Hemangioendothelial sarcoma of the liver and hemochromatosis. Arch Pathol 97: 39–42

60. Falk H, Thomas LB, Popper H, Ishak KG (1979) Hepatic angiosarcoma associated with androgenic-anabolic steroids. Lancet 2: 1120–1123

61. Nordsten M (1985) Hemangiosarcoma hepatis associeret med brug of androgene steroider. Ugeskr Laeger 147: 2615–2616

62. Shi ECP, Fischer A, Crouch R, Ham JM (1981) Possible association of angiosarcoma with oral contraceptive agents. Med J Aust 1: 473–474

63. Hoch-Ligeti C (1978) Angiosarcoma of the liver associated with diethylstilbesterol. JAMA 240: 1510–1511

64. Daneshmend TK, Scott GL, Bradfield JWB (1979) Angiosarcoma of liver associated with phenelzine. Br M J 6: 1679

65. Kirchner SG, Heller RM, Kasselberg AG, Greene HL (1981) Infantile hemangioendothelioma with subsequent malignant degeneration. Pediatr Radiol 11: 42–45

66. Strate SM, Rutledge JC, Weinberg AG (1984) Delayed development of angiosarcoma in multinodular infantile hepatic hemangioendothelioma. Arch Pathol Lab Med 108: 943–944

67. Noronha R, Gonzalez-Crussi F (1984) Hepatic angiosarcoma in childhood: A case report and review of the literature. Am J Surg Pathol 8: 863–871

68. Alt B, Hafez GR, Trigg M, Shahidi N, Gilbert EF (1985) Angiosarcoma of the liver and spleen in an infant. Ped Pathol 4: 331–339

69. Dehner LP, Ishak KG (1971) Vascular tumors of the liver in infants and children. Arch Pathol Lab Med 92: 101–111

70. Bertrand L, Puyeo J, Pages A, Ciurana AJ, Blanc F, Kitschke B (1980) Hemangiosarcoma du foie secondaire a un angiome caverneux calcifie: Mort en coagulopathie de consommation. Ann Gastroenterol Hépatol 18: 19–27

71. Winberg CD, Ranchod M (1979) Thorotrast induced hepatic cholangiocarcinoma and angiosarcoma. Hum Pathol 10: 108–112

72. Wegener K, Leipolz-Angermuller S (1979) Double tumors of the liver following intravenous Thorotrast injection: Patho-anatomic report on two cases. Virch Arch (Pathol Anat) 382: 63–71

73. Kojiro M, Kawano Y, Kawasaki H, Nakashima T, Ikezaki H (1982) Thorotrast-induced hepatic angiosarcoma, and combined hepatocellular and cholangiocarcinoma in a single patient. Cancer 49: 2161–2164

74. Sakai K, Shiina M, Ishihara N, Kato Y (1984) Thorotrast-induced multiple primary malignant tumors of the liver—cholangiocarcinoma and malignant hemangioendothelioma. Jpn Clin Oncol 14: 411–416

75. Delorme FC (1978) Association d'un angiosarcome du foie et d'un hépatome, chez un ouvrier du chlorure de vinyle. Ann Anat Pathol 23: 105–113

76. Leu HJ, Odermatt B (1985) Multicentric angiosarcoma (Kaposi's sarcoma): Light and electron microscopic and immunohistological findings of idiopathic cases in Europe and Africa and of cases associated with AIDS. Virch Arch (Pathol Anat) 408: 29–41

77. Reichert CM, O'Leary TJ, Levens DL (1983) Autopsy pathology in the acquired immune deficiency syndrome. Am J Pathol 112: 357–382

78. Welch K, Finkbeiner W, Alpers CE (1984) Autopsy findings in the acquired immune deficiency syndrome. JAMA 252: 1152–1159

79. Guarda LA, Luna MA, Smith IL (1984) Acquired immune deficiency syndrome: Postmortem findings. Am J Clin Pathol 81: 549–557

80. Niedt G, Schinella RA (1985) Acquired immunodeficiency syndrome: Clinicopathologic study of 56 autopsies. Arch Pathol Lab Med 109: 727–734

81. Bendelac A, Kenitakis J, Chouvet B, Viac J, Thivolet J (1985) Sarcome de Kaposi: Étude immunohistochimique comparative et intérêt histogénétique des marqueurs endothéliaux. Ann Pathol 5: 45–52

82. Beckstead JH, Wood GS, Fletcher V (1985) Evidence for the origin of Kaposi's sarcoma from lymphatic endothelium. Lab Invest 52: 6A

83. Bartal AH, Lichtig C, Friedman-Birnbaum R, Avraham Z, Spivak N, Fass B, Feit C, Robinson E, Hirshaut Y (1985) The interaction of Kaposi's sarcoma with monoclonal antibodies to human sarcoma and connective tissue differentiation antigens. Cancer 56: 1071–1074

84. Davis GL, Kissane JM, Ishak KG (1969) Embryonal rhabdomyosarcoma (sarcoma botryoides) of the biliary tree. Cancer 24: 333–342

85. Mori H, Matsubara N, Fuji M (1979) Alphafetoprotein producing rhabdomyosarcoma of the adult liver. Acta Pathol Jap 29: 485–491

86. Lack EE, Perez-Atayada AR, Schuster SR (1981) Botryoid rhabdomyosarcoma of the biliary tract: Report of five cases with ultrastructural observations and literature review. Am J Surg Pathol 5: 643–652

87. Ruymann FB, Raney B, Crist WM, Lawrence W, Lindberg RD, Soule EH (1985) Rhabdomyosarcoma of the biliary tree in childhood: A report from the intergroup rhabdomyosarcoma study. Cancer 56: 575–581

88. Aldabagh SM, Shibata CS, Taxy JB (1986) Rhabdomyosarcoma of the common bile duct in an adult. Arch Pathol Lab Med 110: 547–550

89. Morimoto H, Takade Y, Akita T, Kato Y, Tanigawa N, Muraoka R, Urata Y (1986) A resected case of the collision tumor of hepatocellular carcinoma and primary liver rhabdomyosarcoma. J Jpn Surg Soc 87: 456–463

90. Cannon PM, Legge DA, O'Donnell B (1979) The use of percutaneous transhepatic cholangiography in case of embryonal rhabdomyosarcoma. Br J Radio 52: 326–327

91. Brooks JJ (1982) Immunochemistry of soft tissue tumors: Myoglobin as a tumor marker for rhabdomyosarcoma. Cancer 50: 1757–1783

92. Tsokos M (1986) The role of immunocytochemistry in the diagnosis of rhabdomyosarcoma. Arch Pathol Lab Med 110: 776–778

93. Scupham R, Gilbert EF, Wilde J, Wiedrich TA (1986) Immunohistochemical studies of rhabdomyosarcoma. Arch Pathol Lab Med 110: 818–821

94. Stocker JT, Ishak KG (1978) Undifferentiated embryonal sarcoma of the liver. Cancer 42: 336–348

95. Stanley RJ, Dehner LP, Hesker AE, (1973) Primary malignant mesenchymal tumors (mesenchymoma) of the liver in childhood. Cancer 32: 973–984

96. Cozzutto C, De Bernardi B, Comelli A, Soave F (1981) Malignant mesenchymoma of the liver in children: A clinicopathologic and ultrastructural study. Hum Pathol 12: 481–485

97. Sumiyoshi A, Nicho Y (1971) Primary osteogenic sarcoma of the liver: Report of an autopsy case. Acta Pathol Jpn 21: 305–312

98. Lagacé R, Delage C, Robert J (1974) Le mésenchymome primitif du foie: Étude ultrastructural. Ann Anat Pathol 19: 275–286

99. Gonzalez-Crussi F (183) Undifferentiated (embryonal) liver sarcoma of childhood: Evidence of leiomyoblastic differentiation. Ped. Pathol 1: 281–290

100. Gallivan MVE, Lack EE, Chun B, Ishak KG (1983) Undifferentiated ("embryonal") sarcoma of the liver: Ultrastructure of a case presenting as a primary intracardiac tumor. Ped Pathol 1: 291–300

101. Pieterse AS, Smith M, Smith LA, Smith P (1985) Embryonal (undifferentiated) sarcoma of the liver: Fine-needle aspiration cytology and ultrastructural findings. Arch Pathol Lab Med 109: 677–680

102. Weinberg AG, Finegold MJ (1983) Primary hepatic tumors of childhood. Hum Pathol 14: 512–537

103. Ros PR, Olmstead WW, Dachman AH, Goodman ZD, Ishak KG, Hartman DS (1986) Undifferentiated (embryonal) sarcoma of the liver: Radiologic-pathologic correlation. Radiology 161: 141–145

104. Esposito R, Pollavini G, de Lalla F (1976) A case of primary undifferentiated sarcoma of the liver diagnosed by peritoneoscopy and guided biopsy. Endoscopy 8: 108–110

105. Smithson WA, Telander RL, Carney JA (1982) Mesenchymoma of the liver in childhood: Five-year survival after combined modality treatment. J Ped Surgery 17: 70–72

106. Harris MB, Shen S, Weiner MA, Bruckner JG, Dasgupta I, Bleicher M, Fortner H, Deleiko NS, Becker N, Rose J, Kasen L (1984) Treatment of primary undifferentiated sarcoma of the liver with surgery and chemotherapy. Cancer 54: 2859–2862

107. Tanner AR, Bolton PM, Powell LW (1978) Primary sarcoma of the liver: Report of a case with excellent response to hepatic artery ligation and infusion chemotherapy. Gastroenterology 74: 121–123

108. Abramowsky CR, Cebelin M, Choudhury A, Izant RJ (1980) Undifferentiated (embryonal) sarcoma of the liver with alph$_1$-antitrypsin deposits: Immunohistochemical and ultrastructural studies. Cancer 45: 3108–3113

109. Ellis IO, Cotton RE (1983) Primary malignant mesenchymal tumor of the liver in an elderly female. Histopathology 7: 113–121

110. Keating S, Taylor GP (1985) Undifferentiated (embryonal) sarcoma of the liver: Ultrastructural and immunohistochemical similarities with malignant fibrous histiocytoma. Hum Pathol 16: 693–699

111. Blattner WA, Henson DE, Young RC, Fraumeni JF (1977) Malignant mesenchymoma and birth defects: Prenatal exposure to phenytoin. JAMA 238: 334–335

112. Shallow TA, Wanger FB (1947) Primary fibrosarcoma of the liver. Ann Surg 125: 439–446

113. Simpson HM, Baggenstoss AH, Stauffer MH (1955) Primary sarcoma of the liver: A report of three cases. South Med J 48: 1177–1182

114. Snapper I, Schraft WC, Ginsberg DM (1964) Severe hypoglycemia duc to fibrosarcoma of the liver. Maendschr Kindergenees 32: 337–347

115. Ojima A, Sugiyama T, Takeda J (1964) Six cases of rare malignant tumors of the liver. Acta Pathol Jpn 14: 95–102

116. Totzke HA, Hutcheson JB (1965) Primary fibrosarcoma of the liver. South Med J 58: 236–238

117. Balouet G, Destombes P (1967) À propos de quelques tumeurs mesenchymateuses hépatiques d'apparence primitive. Ann Anat Pathol 12: 273–286

118. Cavallo T, Lichewitz B Rozov T (1968) Primary fibrosarcoma of the liver: Report of a case. Rev Hosp Clin Med Sao Paulo 23: 44–69

119. Smith D, Rele SR (1972) A case of primary fibrosarcoma of the liver. Postgrad Med J 48: 62–63

120. Walter VE, Bodner E,Lederer B (1972) Primäres Fibrosarkom der Leber. Wieh Klin Wochenschr 84: 808–810

121. Alrenga DP (1974) Primary fibrosarcoma of the liver: Case report and review of the literature. Cancer 36: 446–449

122. Fong JA, Ruebner BH (1974) Primary leiomyosarcoma of the liver. Hum Pathol 5: 115–119

123. Bloustein PA (1978) Hepatic leiomyosarcoma: Ultrastructural study and review of the differential diagnosis. Hum pathol 9: 713–716

124. Chen KTK (1983) Hepatic leiomyosarcoma. J Surg Oncol 24: 325–328

125. Callego MM, Merlo RR, Pascual BG (1984) Leiomyosarcoma hepatico primario. Gastroenterol Hepatol 7: 77–81

126. O'Leary MR, Hill RB, Levine RA (1982) Peritonescopic diagnosis of primary leiomyosarcoma of liver. Hum Pathol 13: 76–78

127. Hara T, Nakata H, Tsujimoto M, Nakatani T, Nishioka S, Yataka I, Tobuse K, Shoji S, Katsumi M, Gen E (1983) Primary leiomyosarcoma of the liver. Acta Hepatol Jpn 24: 1040–1046

128. Tomaszewski M-M, Kuenster T, Hartman K (1986) Leiomyosarcoma of ligamentum teres of liver: Case report. Ped Pathol 5: 147–156

129. Koberle F, Pfleger R (1940) Lebervenenges chevulst mit dem Symptomenbild einer Endophlebitis obliterans hepatica. Wien Arch Intern Med 34: 73–85

130. MacMahon HE, Ball HG (1971) Leiomyosarcoma of hepatic vein and the Budd-Chiari syndrome. Gastroenterology 61: 239–243

131. Alberti-Flor JJ, O'Hara MF, Weaver F, Evans J, McClure R, Dunn GD (1985) Malignant fibrous histiocytoma of the liver. Gastroenterology 89: 890–893

132. Conran RM, Stocker JT (1985) Malignant fibrous histiocytoma of the liver—A case report. Amer J Gastroenterol 80: 813–815

133. Basset F, Nezelof C, Ferrans VJ (1983) The histiocytoses. In: Sommers SL, Rosen PR (eds) Pathology annual, part 2, vol 18. Appleton-Century-Crofts, Norwalk, pp 27–28

134. Broadbent V, Pritchard J (1985) Histiocytosis X—Current controversies. Arch Dis Child 60: 605–607

135. Favara BE, McCarthy RC, Mierau GW (1986) Histiocytosis X. In: Finegold M (ed) Pathology of neoplasia in children and adolescents. Saunders, Philadelphia, pp 126–144

136. Grosfeld JL, Fitzgerald JG, Wagner VM, Newton WA, Brehner RL (1976) Portal hypertension in infants and children with histiocytosis X. Am J Surg 131: 108–113

137. Favara BE, McCarthy RC, Mierau GW (1983) Histiocytosis X. Hum Pathol 14: 663–676

138. Thompson HH, Pitt HA, Lewin KG, Longmire WP (1984) Sclerosing cholangitis and histiocytosis X. Gut 25: 526–530

139. Harrist TH, Bhan AK, Murphy GF, Soto S, Berman RS, Gellis SE, Freedman S, Mihin MC (1983) Histiocytosis X: In situ characterization of cutaneous infiltrates with monoclonal antibodies. Am J Clin Pathol 79: 294–300

140. Beckstead, JH, Wood GS, Turner RR (1984) Histiocytosis X cells and Langerhans cells: Enzyme histochemical and immunologic similarities. Hum Pathol 15: 826–833

141. Wieczorek R, Greco MA, McCarthy K, Bonetti F, Knowles DM (1986) Familial erythrophagocytic, lymphohistiocytosis: Immunophenotypic, immunohistochemical and ultrastructural demonstration of the relation to sinus histiocytes. Hum Pathol 17: 55–63

142. Gupta SM, Kranioinkel RN, Herrera NE (1980) Pathogenesis of jaundice in histiocytic medullary reticulosis: A correlative scintigraphic, histologic and biochemical study. Am J Gastroenterol 73: 500–502

143. Jurco S, Starling K, Hawkins EP (1983) Malignant histiocytosis in childhood: Morphologic considerations. Hum Pathol 14: 1059–1065

144. Ducatman BS, Wick MR, Morgan TW, Banks PM, Pierre RV (1984) Malignant histiocytosis: A clinical, histologic and immunohistochemical study of 20 cases. Hum Pathol 15: 368–377

145. Van der Volk P, Meijer CJLM (1985) Histiocytic sarcoma: Clinical picture, morphology, markers, differential diagnosis. In: Sommers SC, Rosen PP, Fechner RE (eds): Pathology annual, part 2, vol 20. Appleton-Century-Crofts, Norwalk, pp 1–28

146. Colby TV, LaBreque DR (1982) Lymphoreticular malignancy presenting as fulminant hepatic disease. Gastroenterology 82: 339–345

147. Osborne BN, Butler JJ, Guarda LA (1985) Primary lymphoma of the liver: Ten cases and a review of the literature. Cancer 56: 2902–2910

148. Caccamo D, Pervez NK, Marchevsky A (1986) Primary lymphoma of the liver. Arch Pathol Lab Med 110: 553–555

Chapter 13

Comparative Study of the Three Nodular Lesions in Cirrhosis

Adenomatoid Hyperplasia, Adenomatoid Hyperplasia with Intermediate Lesion, and Small Hepatocellular Carcinoma

GOROKU OHTA and YASUNI NAKANUMA[1]

1 Introduction

A large number of livers bearing hepatocellular carcinoma (HCC) show cirrhosis [1], suggesting a close relationship between hepatocarcinogenesis and regenerative nodules [1–3]. Attempts to identify intermediate lesions between HCCs and regenerative nodules, particularly adenomatoid hyperplasia, have not been successful. Peters [1] in studying alcoholic cirrhosis with multifocal HCCs suggested that a carcinoma arises as a nodular lesion in a regenerative nodule. Anthony [2] reported that liver cell dysplasia, which is frequently found in liver cirrhosis associated with HCC, especially in hepatitis B surface antigen (HBsAg)-positive patients, might be a potential preoplastic lesion. Other investigators [4] also proposed that iron-resistant areas within regenerative nodules have a preneoplastic significance in man as well as in experimental animals. Clustering of small dysplastic liver cells or Mallory's body-containing cells in regenerative nodules might also have the same significance in nonalcoholics [3–5].

Recently, Arakawa et al. [6] studied surgically resected small-mass lesions and found that there was a lesion equivalent to a malignancy within adenomatoid hyperplasia [7] in posthepatitic cirrhosis; they proposed that this represented a transition from adenomatoid hyperplasia to HCC. Adenomatoid hyperplasia [7] refers to marked enlargement of a regenerative nodule or an assembly of the nodules in cirrhosis. It usually consists of normal-appearing hepatocytes with a thickness of many cells, which occasionally have a basophilic cytoplasm. The lesion seems to have a greater regenerative activity than the common regenerative nodules in cirrhosis but is distinguishable from HCC.

The aim of this study is to evaluate the morphological characteristics of HCC at an early developmental stage and the intermediate lesion within adenomatoid hyperplasia, and to distinguish histologically one from the other.

2 Materials and methods

2.1 Collection of single HCCs smaller than 1 cm

Pathological reports of autopsies in our department (1973–1985; the total number of autopsies and cases of HCC and liver cirrhosis without HCC were 1939, 95, and 56, respectively), Kanazawa National Hospital (1979–1981; 176, 5, and 4, respectively), and Fukui Prefectural Hospital (1979–1981; 354, 11, and 8, respectively) were reviewed and six autopsied cirrhotic livers with solitary HCC, smaller than 1 cm in their greatest diameter, were collected. The other two cases in the series were found after microscopic examination of whole-liver slices of 25 autopsied livers with cirrhosis from our recent autopsy material.

2.2 Collection of adenomatoid hyperplasia with "intermediate lesion between HCC and regenerative nodule" and of adenomatoid hyperplasia alone

One to several whole-liver slices of autopsied cirrhotic livers (with or without HCC) in these institutes during the same periods mentioned above were examined macroscopically. Small or large regenerative nodules with areas of discoloration and giant regenerative nodules which somewhat compressed the surrounding tissue were all removed. The nodules appeared more or less different from the surrounding regenerative nodules; all were examined histopathologically. The majority of the nodules were consistent with the usual regenerative nodule in cirrhosis and

---

[1] Second Department of Pathology, Kanazawa University School of Medicine, Kanazawa, 920 Japan

178   G. Ohta, Y. Nakanuma

were excluded from the present study. Three cases of cirrhosis and six cases of cirrhosis with HCC contained a total of 19 nodules showing adenomatoid hyperplasia that had the histological features resembling, but not identical to, those of HCC (intermediate lesions) described below. In addition, ten cases of cirrhosis and three cases of cirrhosis with HCC disclosed a total of 17 nodules of adenomatoid hyperplasia lacking "intermediate lesions." All of these adenomatoid hyperplasias with or without the intermediate lesions lacked a marked coagulation necrosis or autolytic changes and so detailed histological and cytological examinations were available.

HCC was histologically graded as "trabecular (sinusoidal)," "pseudoglandular," "compact," and "scirrhous" patterns according to the World Health Organization classification [8] and HCC was graded from I to IV according to Edmondson and Steiner [9]. The pattern of the tumor growth at the boundaries was classified as being either of the "replacing" or "compressing" type [10]. In the replacing type, tumor cells were seen

replacing hepatocytes within the liver cell plates. The compressing type was characterized by HCC compressing the neighboring nonneoplastic parenchyma, resulting in a smooth edge at the periphery of the tumor. The fibrous capsule of HCC was defined grossly as a markedly thick and gray white band surrounding the HCC tissue in order to distinguish it from collapsed stroma of cirrhosis [11].

2.3 Tissue-processing

All tissue specimens were fixed in 10% formalin and embedded in paraffin. After deparaffinization, the 5-μm sections were stained with H and E, Azan-Mallory, Gomori's reticulin, and Perls' iron stains [12].

3 Results

The main clinicopathological features of the eight patients with a single, small HCC arising in a cirrhotic liver, the nine patients with one to

Table 13.1. Presentation of eight cases bearing single small HCC

Case no.	Age(yrs)	Sex	Tumor size(cm)	Type	Nontumor portion	Liver weight(g)	Etiology
1	68	Male	0.3 × 0.3	Expansive	Micronodular LC	710	Alcoholic
2	67	Male	0.3 × 0.4	Expansive	Micronodular LC	630	HBsAg (+) and alcoholic
3	68	Female	0.7 × 0.8	Expansive	Mixed nodular LC	580	HBsAg (+)
4	52	Male	0.7 × 0.8	Expansive	Macronodular LC	740	HBsAg (+)
5	60	Male	0.5 × 0.7	Infiltrative	Mixed nodular LC	1460	Alcoholic
6	49	Male	0.7 × 0.9	Infiltrative	Macronodular LC	950	HBsAg (+)
7	61	Male	0.7 × 0.8	Infiltrative	Mixed nodular LC	910	Alcoholic
8	45	Male	0.7 × 0.8	Infiltrative	Mixed nodular LC	950	Cryptogenic

LC liver cirrhosis

Table 13.2. Presentation of nine cases bearing adenomatoid hyperplasia with intermediate lesions

Case no.	Age(yrs)	Sex	No. of tumors	Hepatic pathology	Etiology
1	40	Male	1	Micronodular LC	Alcoholic
2	46	Male	1	Mixed nodular LC	Cryptogenic
3	56	Female	2	Macronodular LC	Cryptogenic
4	63	Male	3	Mixed nodular LC with HCC	HBsAg (+)
5	51	Male	3	Mixed nodular LC with HCC	Alcoholic
6	57	Female	3	Mixed nodular LC with HCC	Cryptogenic
7	65	Male	2	Mixed nodular LC with HCC	Cryptogenic
8	73	Male	1	Mixed nodular LC with HCC	Cryptogenic
9	75	Female	3	Mixed nodular LC with HCC	Cryptogenic

LC liver cirrhosis

Table 13.3. Presentation of 13 cases with adenomatoid hyperplasia alone

Case no.	Age(yrs)	Sex	Type of cirrhosis	Complication of HCC	Suspected etiology	No. of adenomatoid hyperplasias
1	63	Male	Mixed nodular	−	HBsAg (+)	1
2	68	Male	Mixed nodular	+	HBsAg (+)	1
3	50	Male	Mixed nodular	−	Alcoholic	3
4	48	Male	Micronodular	−	Alcoholic	3
5	66	Male	Macronodular	−	HBsAg (+)	1
6	57	Female	Macronodular	−	HBsAg (+)	1
7	44	Male	Mixed nodular	−	HBsAg (+)	1
8	52	Male	Mixed nodular	+	Cryptogenic	1
9	48	Male	Mixed nodular	−	HBsAg (+)	1
10	43	Male	Macronodular	−	Alcoholic	1
11	49	Male	Macronodular	−	Alcoholic	1
12	63	Male	Mixed nodular	+	HBsAg (+)	1
13	49	Female	Mixed nodular	−	HBsAg (+)	1

three adenomatoid hyperplasias with intermediate lesions, and the 13 patients with one to three adenomatoid hyperplasias alone are shown in Tables 13.1–13.3.

3.1 Small solitary HCCs less than 1 cm

These eight were all found incidentally at autopsy. The size of the HCC ranged from 0.3 × 0.3 cm to 0.9 × 1.0 cm (Table 13.1). These HCCs consisted of green nodules or white nodules, with a dark green hue or spots; their borders were sometimes sharp, sometimes ill-defined (Fig. 13.1). There was no fibrous capsule surrounding the nodules. The patients with these HCCs were clinically diagnosed as having decompensated liver cirrhosis. Four cases showed a single, expansive nodule and the lack of distinct fibrous septa within the HCC nodule (Fig. 13.2). There was no infiltration of the carcinoma into the neighboring regenerative nodules, which were more or less compressed by the HCC nodule (Fig. 13.3). In these four cases, there was replacement or compression of the neighboring hepatic parenchyma by the HCC (Figs. 13.4, 13.5). In case 1, HCC was localized within a regenerative nodule as a type of "nodule within a nodule" [1, 13] (Fig. 13.2), and the entire circumference was rimmed directly by nonneoplastic parenchyma. In cases 2 and 3, the HCC had replaced most of the regenerative nodule. In case 4, an expansive HCC nodule was devoid of a nonneoplastic rim or had not infiltrated the surrounding regenerative nodules; it was demarcated by thin fibrous tissue, seemingly consisting of collapsed cirrhotic stroma (Fig. 13.6).

The remaining four cases showed infiltration into the surrounding regenerative nodules. They were composed of a cluster of two to several carcinoma nodules, each of which was associated

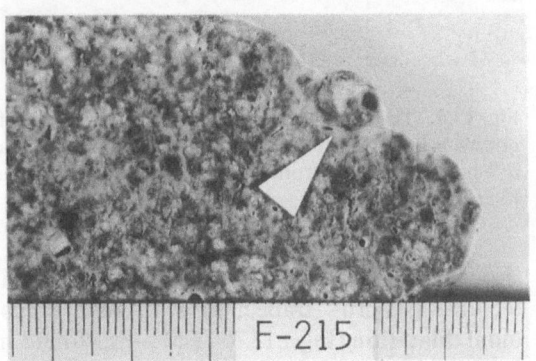

Fig. 13.1. Single small HCC (*white arrowhead*) in liver cirrhosis. There is no fibrous capsule. *Scale* in millimeters

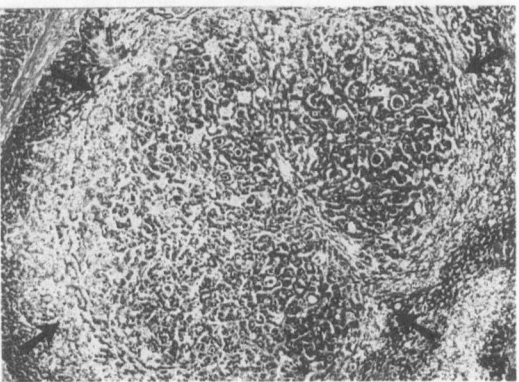

Fig. 13.2. HCC (*arrows*) within a regenerative nodule. H and E, × 40

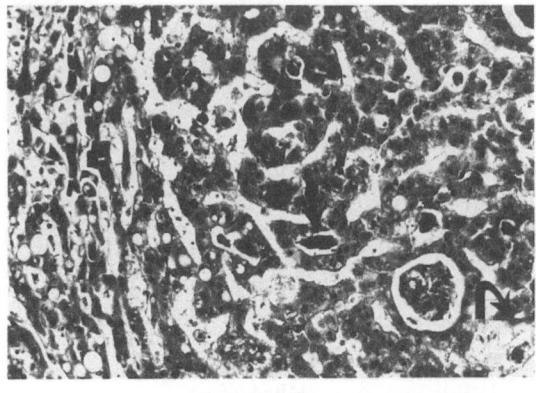

Fig. 13.3. HCC with trabecular pattern compresses the nonneoplastic parenchyma (*left*). *Arrow* bile plugs, *curved arrow* feathery degeneration. H and E, × 180

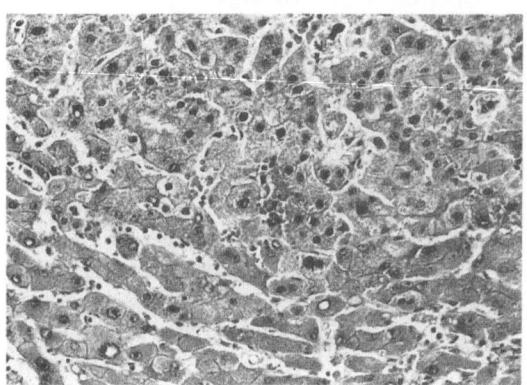

Fig. 13.4. The boundary between HCC (*upper half*) and nonneoplastic parenchyma (*lower half*) is of the replacing type. H and E, × 375

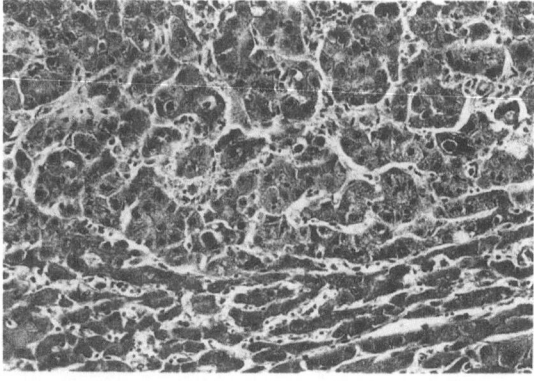

Fig. 13.5. The boundary between HCC (*upper left*) and nonneoplastic parenchyma (*lower right*) is of the compressing type. H and E, × 350

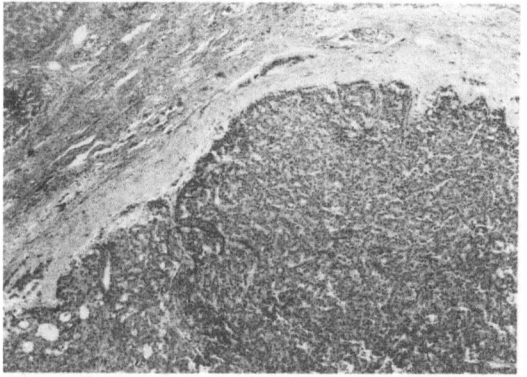

Fig. 13.6. There is collapsed cirrhotic stroma around HCC (*upper half*). H and E, × 40

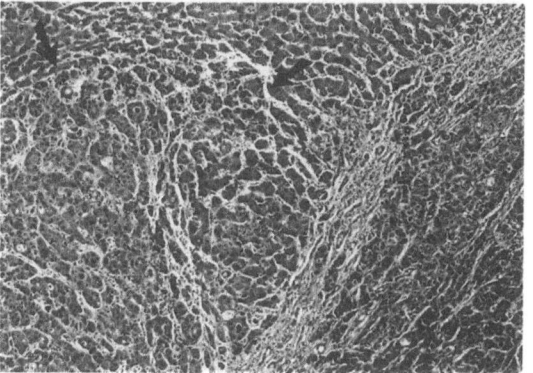

Fig. 13.7. The right nodule is a carcinoma and the left nodule is an infiltrating carcinoma within the regenerative nodule. *Arrows* front of infiltration of carcinoma. H and E

with distinct fibrous septa (Fig. 13.7). Some of the septa contained portal tracts. The boundaries revealed replacing and compressing types, as mentioned above, in various proportions in all four cases.

The tumor cells were generally well-differentiated (grades I + II or II). The main structural patterns and cytoplasmic expression are shown in Table 13.4. The most frequent architectural pattern—trabecular with mild sinusoidal dilatation (Figs. 13.3, 13.5)—was found in seven cases. A pseudoglandular pattern was also recognized in four cases, but it was usually focal (Fig. 13.8). Two HCCs that revealed cords or thin trabeculae surrounded by a small amount of fibrous tissue (Figs. 13.9, 13.10) were regarded as

Table 13.4. Comparison of structural and cytoplasmic features between small HCCs and adenomatoid hyperplasia with and without intermediate lesions

| | Small HCCs/HCCs | | Adenomatoid hyperplasia | | | |
| | | | With intermediate lesions | | Without intermediate lesions | |
	Number	Percentage	Number/ nodule	Percentage	Number/ nodule	Percentage
Prominent bile production	7/8	87.5	10/19	52.6	12/17	63.2
Marked fatty change	1/8	12.5	6/19	31.6	4/17	23.5
Iron resistance	2/2[a]	100	3/3[b]	100	0	
Clustering of Mallory's bodies	4/8	50	8/19	42.1	1/17	5.9
Ground-glass change unrelated to HBsAg	0/8	0	1/19	5.3	0	
Reduction of reticulin fibers	5/8	62.5	9/19	47.4	0	
Small-cell clustering	2/8	25	9/19	47.4	0	
Trabecular pattern	7/8	87.5	13/19	68.4	2/17	11.8
Pseudoglandular pattern	4/8	50	4/19	21.5	0	
Scirrhous pattern	2/8	25	0		0	

[a] Diffuse
[b] Focal

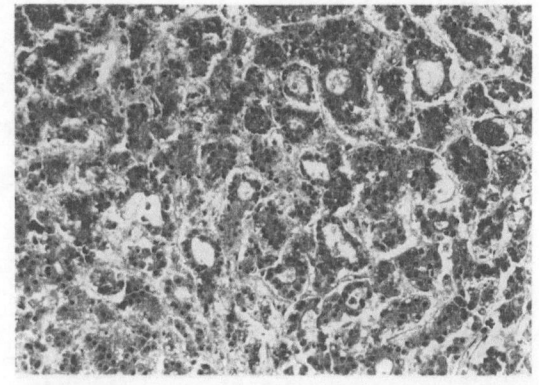

Fig. 13.8. HCC shows a trabecular as well as a pseudoglandular pattern. H and E, × 100

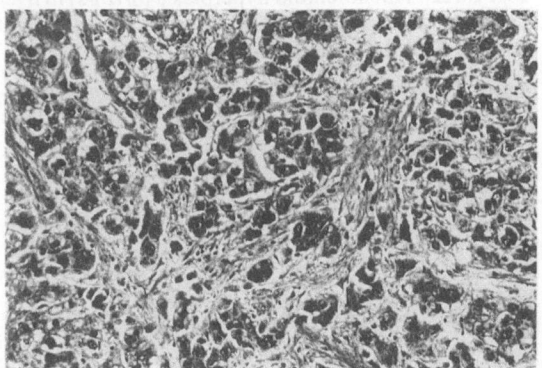

Fig. 13.9. Small cords of HCC are surrounded by fibrous tissue. Scirrhous type. H and E, × 170

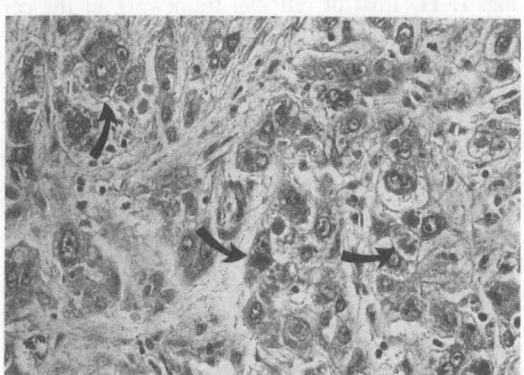

Fig. 13.10. Small cords of HCC containing Mallory's bodies (*arrows*) are surrounded by fibrous tissue. Scirrhous type. H and E, × 375

having a scirrhous, though not altogether typical, pattern [1, 8]. Two tumors revealed a predominantly compact pattern. The following cytoplasmic features were found: highly inspissated bile in the tumor tissue showing areas of feathery degeneration (Fig. 13.3) in seven cases, marked fatty changes in one case, absence of hemosiderin deposition in two HCCs in hemochromatotic livers, clustering of Mallory's body-containing cells in four cases (Fig. 13.10), loss or decrease of reticulin fibers (Fig. 13.11) in five cases, and clustering of small carcinoma cells in two cases. Focal coagulation necrosis was found in two cases.

3.2 Adenomatoid hyperplasia with intermediate lesions

These lesions were found incidentally at autopsy. Their number in a liver varied from one to three (Table 13.2) and they were discrete; the size

ranged from 0.8×1.0 to 2.0×2.0 cm. There was no fibrous capsule around them (Fig. 13.12). Some were deeply green and others were whitish, rusty-colored, or a mixture of green and white. Their borders were sharp or ill-defined. Microscopically, all but one disclosed the presence of well-formed portal tracts within the lesion and an assembly of several nodules subdivided by fibrous septa in which the portal tracts and small hepatic veins were incorporated (Fig. 13.13), a feature similar to that of cirrhosis. The remaining lesion revealed an expansive parenchymal nodule.

In general, the lesions seemed to be composed of different parenchymal cell populations. They showed a more or less expansive growth of the parenchyma within the nodules in which they had arisen, and the adjoining regenerative nodules, fibrous septa, and vascular channels were compressed to some degree. At the boundaries of the expansive growth areas, the adjoining

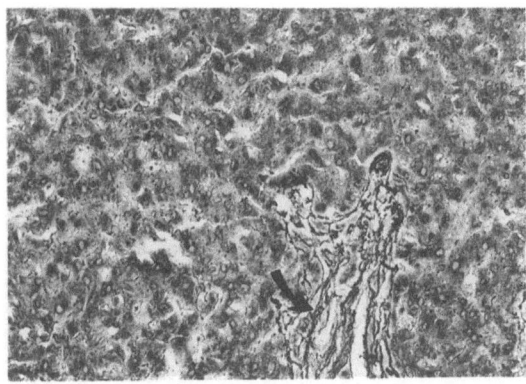

Fig. 13.11. Loss of reticulin framework in the carcinoma. *Arrow* fibrous septa. Gomori's reticulin, × 170

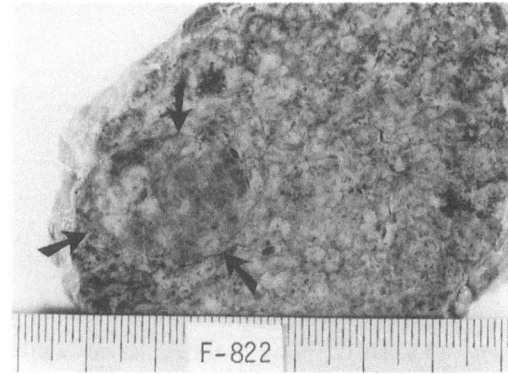

Fig. 13.12. Adenomatoid hyperplasia (*arrows*) in liver cirrhosis associated with HCC. Carcinoma is not shown. *Scale* in millimeters

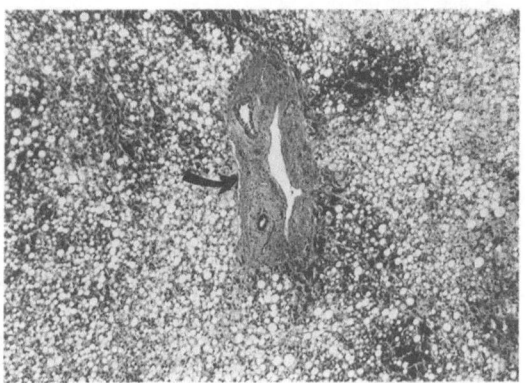

Fig. 13.13. A well-formed portal tract (*arrow*) is seen in the adenomatoid hyperplasia showing prominent fatty change. H and E, × 60

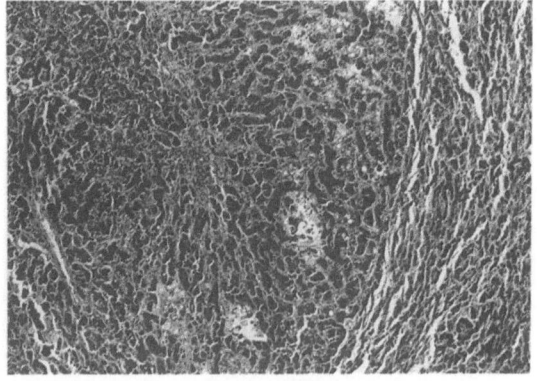

Fig. 13.14. A hyperplastic area (*left* and *middle*) compresses the neighboring parenchyma (*right*). H and E, × 60

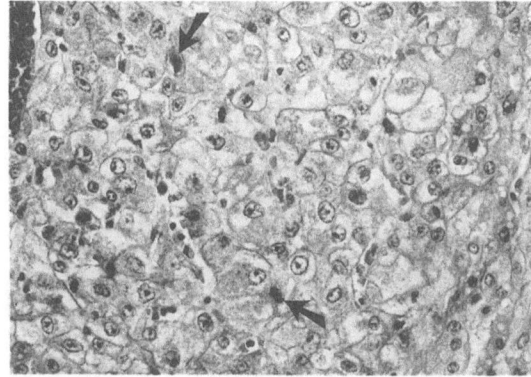

Fig. 13.15. Bile plugs (*arrows*) and a mild degree of nuclear atypia within a mass of adenomatoid hyperplasia. H and E, × 350

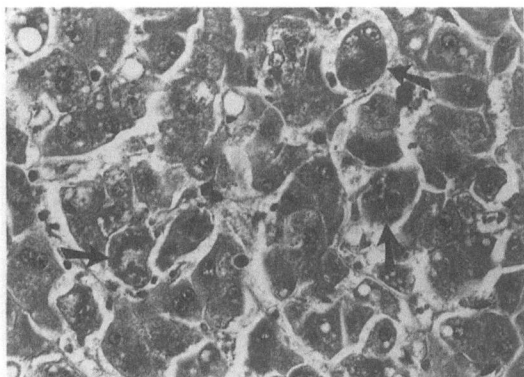

Fig. 13.16. Clustering of Mallory's bodies (*arrows*) is seen. Adenomatoid hyperplasia. H and E, × 375

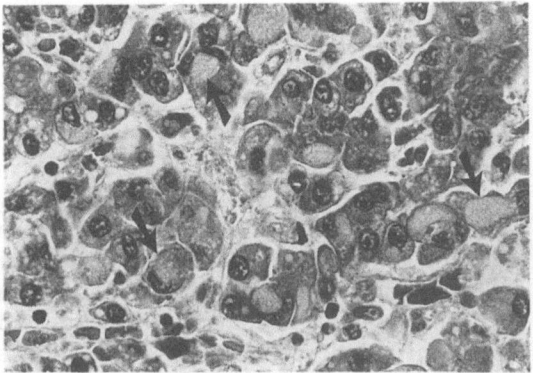

Fig. 13.17. Many ground-glass inclusions (*arrows*) are seen. Adenomatoid hyperplasia. H and E, × 375

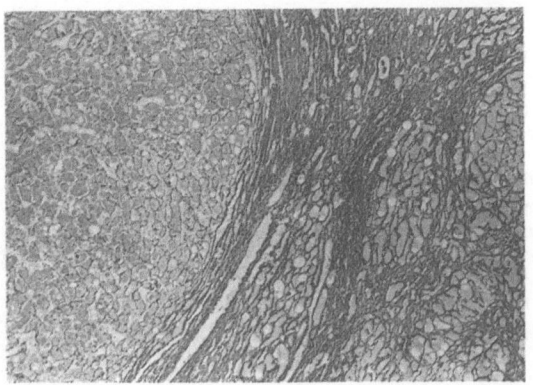

Fig. 13.18. Reduction of reticulin fibers in the adenomatoid hyperplasia (*left*) is evident compared with the surrounding regenerative nodules. Gomori's reticulin stain, × 60

hepatocytes within some areas of the adenomatoid hyperplasia were compressed in a circular or partly circular fashion, giving the appearance of a "nodule within a nodule" (Fig. 13.14). This appearance suggests heterogeneous proliferating activities within the adenomatoid hyperplasia. In some instances, there was a smooth transition from the adjoining hepatocytes to the hyperplastic areas without apparent compression. In all of these adenomatoid hyperplasias, there were areas showing mild nuclear atypia (Fig. 13.15) as well as cytoplasmic or structural abnormalities compared with the surrounding parenchyma. As shown in Table 13.5, there was prominent bile production (Fig. 13.15) with or without feathery degeneration in ten nodules, marked fatty changes (Fig. 13.13) in six nodules, iron "resistance" in three nodules in a hemosiderotic liver, clustering of Mallory's body-containing hepatocytes (Fig. 13.16) in eight nodules, ground-

glass inclusions not related to HBsAg [1, 14] (Fig. 13.17) in one nodule, loss or decrease of reticulin fibers (Fig. 13.18) in nine nodules, small-cell clusters (Fig. 13.19) in nine nodules, a trabecular pattern (Figs. 13.16, 13.20) in 13 nodules, and a pseudoglandular pattern in one nodule. All of these changes tended to be seen in the adenomatoid hyperplasia having highly hyperplastic areas that we termed "intermediate lesions." The intermediate lesions occurred in varying admixtures, and their extent and degree were variable from nodule to nodule, but they were usually focal when present. Three adenomatoid hyperplasias from case 9 revealed preferential hemosiderin deposition compared with the surrounding regenerative nodules.

In addition to three adenomatoid hyperplasias with intermediate lesions, case 9 disclosed another adenomatoid hyperplasia (2.5 cm), in the center of which an HCC (0.7 cm in diameter) was

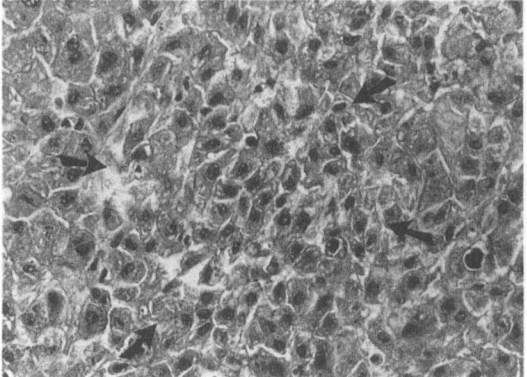
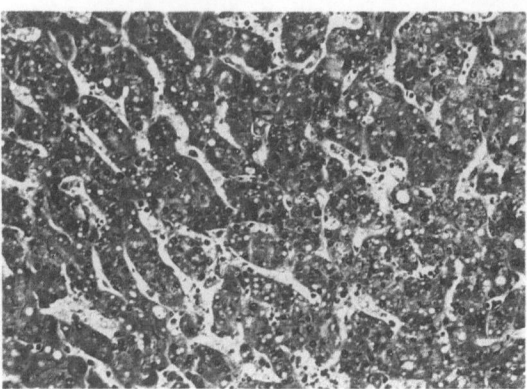

Fig. 13.19. Small-cell clustering with mild nuclear hyperchromasia is seen in the center (*arrows*). Adenomatoid hyperplasia. H and E, × 180

Fig. 13.20. Trabecular pattern is evident. Adenomatoid hyperplasia. H and E, × 180

noted (Fig. 13.21). This hyperplasia was composed of many regenerative nodules, some of which showed areas of small-cell clustering (Fig. 13.22), pseudogland formation, and foci of hepatocytes having a moderate degree of nuclear atypia and, less often, an alpha-fetoprotein-positive cytoplasm (Fig. 13.23). All of these did not fulfill the WHO criteria for HCC and were interpreted as intermediate lesions between malignancy and benignity.

3.3 Adenomatoid hyperplasia alone

These lesions were found incidentally at autopsy. The number of the lesions in a liver was from one to three (Table 13.3), they were discrete, and the size ranged from 0.8 × 0.8 to 1.8 × 1.8 cm. The

gross appearance of the lesion was similar to that of adenomatoid hyperplasia with intermediate lesions. Microscopically, there were some differences between them, as shown in Table 13.5; there was an absence of small-cell clustering in the adenomatoid hyperplasia alone, suggesting lesser activity of hepatocytic regeneration than in the lesion with intermediate features. The other differences included lack of reduction of reticulin fibers, hemosiderin resistance or pseudogland formation, and the rare occurrence of Mallory's body-containing hepatocytes in the adenomatoid hyperplasia alone.

On the other hand, prominent bile production with occasional feathery degeneration was seen in 12 nodules, marked fatty changes in four, and preferential hemosiderin deposition in three.

Table 13.5. Morphology of small HCC, adenomatoid hyperplasia with intermediate lesions, and adenomatoid hyperplasia alone

	Small HCC	Adenomatoid hyperplasia with intermediate lesion	Adenomatoid hyperplasia alone
Portal tract elements within nodule	Rare	Always	Always
Parenchyma appearing nonneoplastic within nodule	Absent	Always	Always
Trabecular pattern	Frequent	Frequent (focal)	Rare
Pseudoglandular pattern	Frequent (focal)	Infrequent (focal)	Absent
Scirrhous pattern	Frequent	Infrequent	Absent
Resistance to hemosiderin deposition	Always	Frequent (focal)	Absent
Preferential hemosiderin deposition	Absent	Infrequent	Frequent
Clustering of Mallory's body-containing cells	Frequent	Frequent (focal)	Rare
Reduction of reticulin framework	Frequent	Frequent (focal)	Absent
Direct transition to neighboring regenerative nodules	Frequent (replacing type)	Frequent	Absent
Direct compression of neighboring regenerative nodules	Frequent (compressing type)	Frequent	Absent

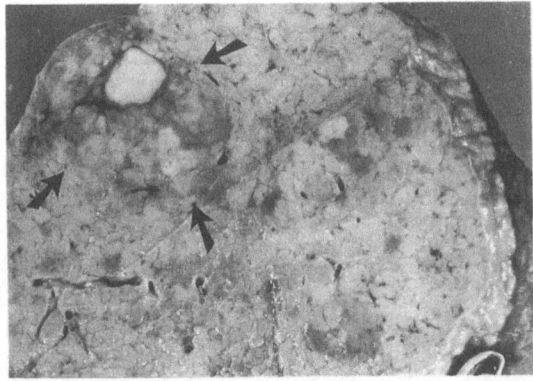

Fig. 13.21. Adenomatoid hyperplasia (*arrows*) of case 9 contains white-gray areas of small HCC, most areas of which have undergone ischemic necrosis

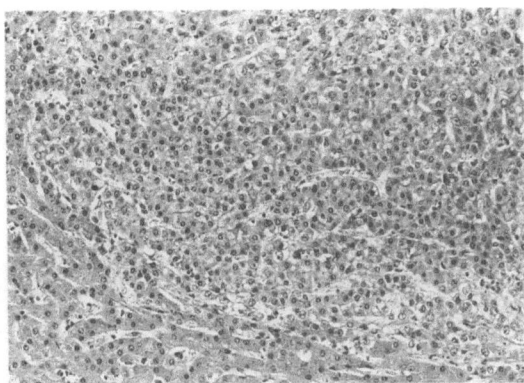

Fig. 13.22. Small-cell clustering with compression of the adjacent hepatic columns is seen in the adenomatoid hyperplasia of Case 9. H and E, × 180

These changes revealed the same prevalence in the adenomatoid hyperplasia with intermediate lesions.

3.4 Differentiation of the three nodular lesions

Macroscopically, differentiation between the three nodular lesions was impossible, except when the small HCCs underwent large areas of necrosis, occasionally encountered in livers following treatment with the recently developed embolization technique. The other two hyperplastic lesions, however, did not show such necrosis, even with the same treatment. The small HCCs were susceptible to ischemia, and the necrotic areas of the HCCs were yellowish gray in color, with or without greenish, brownish, or reddish discoloration. Microscopically (Table 13.5), the histological pattern of the small HCCs was basically trabecular with narrowed sinusoidal spaces and scanty fibrous tissue, while the other two hyperplasias showed large areas of plates that were two or more cells in thickness, separated by slitlike (normal-appearing) sinusoids without fibrous elements. Nuclear and cytoplasmic atypia of neoplastic hepatocytes in small HCCs, when severe, was most helpful in differential diagnosis. However, when the change was mild, difficulty was encountered in distinguishing HCC from nonneoplastic atypical hepatocytes in the adenomatoid hyperplasia. Bile production, Mallory's body formation, pseudoglandular formation, iron resistance, and reduction of reticulin fiber, when present separately or in combination, were found more diffusely in the small HCC, while each of them was distributed only focally in a minority of the two types of hyperplastic lesion. Therefore, these features are not markers of ma-

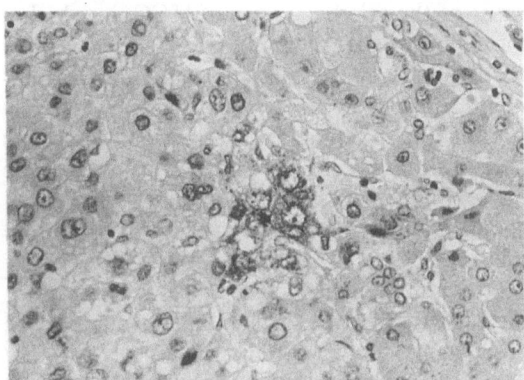

Fig. 13.23. The same hyperplasia as shown in Fig. 13.22 reveals alpha-fetoprotein-positive hepatocytes with nuclear atypia, stained with alpha-fetoprotein antibody by ABC method. × 350

lignancy but are worthy of note in differential diagnosis.

There were a varying number of normal-appearing hepatocytes, together with the unusual hepatocytes mentioned before, in the two hyperplastic lesions, whereas the small HCCs were composed only of neoplastic hepatocytes. An outstanding characteristic of the small HCCs was the tendency to invade and grow along blood vessels when microinvasion from the parent regenerative nodule occurred.

With reference to the morphological difference between adenomatoid hyperplasias with and without intermediate lesions, the trabecular, scirrhous, and pseudoglandular patterns, resistance to hemosiderin deposition, clustering of Mallory's body-containing cells, and reduction of reticulin frameworks were variably present in some hyperplasias with intermediate lesions, but they were absent or minimally present in those without. Furthermore, compression of hyperregenerative areas consisting of small-cell clustering to the surrounding parenchyma within the lesion were seen here and there in adenomatoid hyperplasia with intermediate lesions but were absent in adenomatoid hyperplasia alone.

4 Discussion

We have described the morphology of eight small HCCs less than 1 cm in size that were nonencapsulated. Briefly, the majority were well-differentiated and trabecular, with narrowed and inconspicuous sinusoidal spaces associated with scanty connective tissue fibers. There were two cases of the scirrhous type of HCC, in which a loose fibrous stroma lacking sinusoids separated cords of the tumor cells that contained prominent Mallory's bodies. Cytologically, severe bile production, pseudogland formation, Mallory's body formation, iron resistance in a siderotic background, small-cell clustering, and fatty changes were found in varying degrees and mixtures.

Among the eight HCCs, three were morphologically suggestive of the initial and subsequent growth pattern of carcinoma in the cirrhotic liver. Thus, they showed an expansive carcinoma nodule within a regnerative nodule, the carcinoma being rimmed by the apparently nonneoplastic parenchyma. Such a regenerative nodule is referred to as a parent nodule from which the carcinoma arises.

Another case showed a single HCC nodule without a rim of nonneoplastic tissue. This indicates that the HCC had completely replaced the parent nodule without microinvasion. Thus, it is conceivable that an initial carcinoma could have started within a regenerative nodule as a single nodular lesion and then grown to occupy the entire parent nodule.

There were four other HCCs with a multinodular pattern, in which collagenous septa separated small nodules of the carcinoma. Such septa appeared to consist of the preexisting cirrhotic stroma, which had previously divided the adjacent regenerative parenchyma. It seems, therefore, likely that the invasion of the carcinoma into the neighboring regenerative parenchyma was eventually followed by its carcinomatous replacement, resulting in the multinodular pattern of the HCCs.

The next problem is whether putative preneoplastic lesions in regenerative nodules precede the formation of HCC. There have been several reports linking hepatocarcinogenesis to certain morphological lesions in the regenerative nodules of cirrhosis: foci of liver cell dysplasia [2], hemosiderin-free areas in severely hemosiderotic livers [5], clustering of Mallory's body-containing cells [3], and paraplastic changes (nodular hyperplasia in a regenerative nodule) [1] or small round foci in regenerative nodules [4]. However, there has been as yet no convincing evidence that the cells in such lesions actively divide and dramatically transform into HCC. The present study disclosed some of the above-mentioned features in small HCCs less than 1.0 cm in size—clustering of Mallory's body-containing carcinoma cells with fibrosis, resistance to hemosiderin deposition, and a nodular lesion in a regenerative nodule. Thus, there seem to be features in common between small HCCs and some regenerative nodules with the putative preneoplastic lesions. A careful search was made for such lesions in adenomatoid hyperplasia, since hyperplastic regenerative nodules are easily detectable with the naked eye. Fortunately, there was a case of adenomatoid hyperplasia (2.5 cm) which proved instructive; in its center we noted an HCC (0.7 cm in diameter). This lesion was composed of many regenerative nodules, some of which showed areas of small-cell clustering, pseudogland formation, and foci of hepatocytes having a moderate degree of nuclear atypia and, less often, an alpha-fetoprotein-positive cytoplasm. All of these features did not fulfill the WHO criteria of HCC [8] and were interpreted as intermediate lesions between a malignancy and benignity. In the same liver, there were three other adenomatoid hyperplasias without HCC in which some nodules revealed the same intermediate lesions to a lesser degree. These observations led us to speculate that: (1) hepatic carcinogenesis takes place within part of the adenomatoid hyperplasia and (2) the intermediate lesions found in the adenomatoid hyperplasia are presumably preneoplastic in nature, though direct proof is lacking.

In our survey of 16 other adenomatoid hyperplasias in cirrhosis, we found six that contained the aforementioned intermediate lesions as well as an additional pattern—a trabecular pattern with conspicuous sinusoidal dilatation; the lesions occurred focally in varying admixtures. This also supports the previous concept concerning the carcinogenesis from adenomatoid hyperplasia. The fact that such cellular and histological expression in the adenomatoid hyperplasias varied greatly implies that there may be multistep processes in carcinogenesis.

Differentiation between small HCC and adenomatoid hyperplasia, with or without the intermediate lesions, was impossible with the naked eye. However, when the small HCCs underwent ischemic necrosis they were yellowish gray in color (with or without partial discoloration) and were macroscopically distinguishable from the adenomatoid hyperplasia. The latter is resistant to ischemia, even following embolization therapy. It is difficult to determine whether adenomatoid hyperplasia with circumscribed areas of clustered small cells that have some degree of cellular atypia is malignant or benign.

Highly differentiated HCC, as seen in androgenic steroid-induced HCC looking like a hepatocellular adenoma [15], was not found in our series of small HCCs; this type of HCC is usually huge. It is worth noting for purposes of differential diagnosis that the adenomatoid hyperplasia tended to consist of heterogeneous populations of normal-appearing hepatocytes and hepatocytes of varying abnormality, referred to as intermediate lesions. The distribution of the unusual hepatocytes was often focal. Small HCCs, however, consisted exclusively of atypical neoplastic cells and had to a greater extent and degree some of the cytoplasmic features that were basically similar to those of the intermediate lesions found in the adenomatoid hyperplasia. Small HCCs sometimes occurred in a regenerative nodule with a sharp boundary between the tumor and nodular parenchyma and lacked a fibrous capsule. When microinvasion occurred, small HCCs grew along the adjacent sinusoidal spaces, a change not present in adenomatoid hyperplasia with or without the intermediate lesions.

Finally, it is not known whether adenomatoid hyperplasias with intermediate lesions in cirrhosis progress to small HCC. Only one case of adenomatoid hyperplasia containing a small HCC nodule is presented here. In this context, the presence of the intermediate lesions in many adenomatoid hyperplasias also supports the concept that some of the hyperplasias develop into carcinoma. By contrast, the possibility that some of the hyperplasias remain unchanged for a long period of time and eventually disappear cannot be ruled out.

Acknowledgment. This study was in part supported by a Research Grant from the Japanese Education Ministry (no. 480710115256)

References

1. Peters RL (1976) Pathology of hepatocellular carcinoma. In: Okuda K, Peters RL (eds) Hepatocellular carcinoma. Wiley, New York, pp 107–168
2. Anthony PP (1976) Precursor lesions for liver cancer in humans. Cancer Res 36: 2579–2583
3. Nakanuma Y, Ohta G (1985) Is Mallory body formation a pre-neoplastic change? A study of 181 cases of liver bearing hepatocellular carcinoma and 92 cases of cirrhosis. Cancer 55: 2400–2405
4. Watanabe S, Okita K, Harada T, Kodama T, Numa Y, Takemoto T, Takahashi T (1983) Morphologic studies of the liver cell dysplasia. Cancer 51: 2197–2205
5. Hirota N, Hamazaki M, Williams GM (1982) Resistance to iron accumulation and presence of hepatitis B surface antigen in preneoplastic and neoplastic lesions in human hemochromatic livers. Hepato-Gastroenterol 29: 49–51
6. Arakawa M, Sugihara S, Kenmochi K, Kage M, Nakashima T, Nakayama T, Tashiro S, Hiraoka T, Suenaga M, Okuda K (1986) Transition from benign adenomatous hyperplasia to hepatocellular carcinoma? J Gastroenterol Hepatol 1: 3–14
7. Edmondson HA (1976) Benign epithelial tumors and tumor-like lesions of the liver. In: Okuda K, Peters RL (eds) Hepatocellular carcinoma. Wiley, New York, pp 309–330
8. Gibson JB, Sobin H (1978) Histological typing of tumors of the liver, biliary tract and pancreas: no. 20. World Health Organization, Geneva, pp 19–25
9. Edmondson HA, Steiner PE (1954) Primary carcinoma of the liver: study of 100 cases among 48,700 necropsies. Cancer 7: 462–503
10. Nakashima T, Kojiro M, Kawano Y, Shirai F, Takemoto N, Tomimatsu H, Kawasaki H, Okuda H (1982) Histologic growth pattern of hepatocellular carcinoma: relationship to orcein (hepatitis B surface antigen)-positive cells in cancer tissue. Hum Pathol 13: 563–568
11. Okuda K, Musha H, Nakajima Y, Kubo Y, Shimokawa Y, Nagasaki Y, Sawa Y, Jinnouchi S, Kaneko T, Obata H, Hisamatsu T, Motoike Y, Okazaki N, Kojiro M, Sakamoto K, Nakashima T (1977) Clinicopathologic features of encapsulated hepatocellular carcinoma. A study of 26 cases. Cancer 40: 1240–1245
12. Sano Y (1976) Histological technics: Theoretical and applied, 5th edn Nanzando, Tokyo
13. Popper H (1977) Pathologic aspects of cirrhosis—a review. Am J Pathol 87: 228–264
14. Nakanuma Y, Kono N, Ohta G, Shirasaki S, Takeshita H, Watanabe K, Tsuda S, Yoshizawa H (1982) Pale eosinophilic inclusions simulating ground-glass appearance of cells of hepatocellular carcinoma. Acta Pathol Jap 32: 71–81
15. Anthony PP (1975) Hepatoma associated with androgenic steroids. Lancet 1: 685–686

Chapter 14
Hepatocellular Carcinoma in Hemochromatosis

ROBIN A. BRADBEAR, JUNE W. HALLIDAY, MARK L. BASSETT, W. GRAHAM COOKSLEY, and LAWRIE W. POWELL[1]

1 Introduction and historical aspects

The term "hemochromatosis" has been used in the past to refer to disorders in which excessive iron intake (enteral or parenteral) or absorption leads to an increase in body iron stores, with deposition of iron primarily in the parenchymal cells of the liver, heart, and other organs leading eventually to organ failure. Genetic hemochromatosis is an inherited disease in which an inappropriately high iron absorption from the small intestine is associated with a progressive increase in body iron stores. Hemochromatosis is now widely used to refer to this inherited disease, and the term "secondary iron overload" is used to refer to iron overload resulting from hematological defects or blood transfusions.

Von Recklinghausen introduced the term "hemochromatosis" in 1889, but the syndromes of diabetes mellitus, hyperpigmentation, and cirrhosis had been the subject of a case report by Trousseau in 1865. Sheldon [1] in 1935 reviewed the literature to that date and proposed that the disease was due to an inherited inborn error of iron metabolism. Iron accumulation resulting from anemia associated with hemolysis and ineffective erythropoiesis, e.g., thalassemia major, can lead to a similar clinicopathological disorder (secondary iron overload). However, such patients differ from hemochromatosis subjects in many ways, including the degree and duration of iron loading, the duration of cirrhosis, if present, and the frequent predominance of reticuloendothelial (as opposed to parenchymal) iron storage. Furthermore, the incidence of hepatocellular carcinoma (HCC) is not increased. The potential importance of these fac-

tors with respect to the subsequent development of HCC will be discussed later in this chapter.

2 Aspects of hemochromatosis relevant to HCC

The major complications of hemochromatosis are hepatic cirrhosis, diabetes mellitus, arthritis, hypogonadism, cardiomyopathy, and HCC. The deposition of iron in the liver occurs early in the course of the genetic disease and is predominantly periportal. Hepatic dysfunction is usually mild and cirrhosis develops slowly after many years of excess iron deposition [2–4]. Although liver disease is a major feature of hemochromatosis and liver tissue is used for quantitation of the degree of iron overload, iron deposition eventually occurs in virtually all organs, the notable exceptions being the brain and testis [1, 5]. Not all complications are due solely to increased tissue iron. For example, there is some evidence that the glucose intolerance seen in up to 60% of patients with advanced hemochromatosis is not due purely to pancreatic islet cell destruction but is also related to the presence of cirrhosis and genetic diabetes mellitus [6, 7]. Similarly, the arthropathy which affects up to one-quarter of patients is due usually to deposition of calcium pyrophosphate in the synovium and articular cartilage (chondrocalcinosis). It may precede overt evidence of hemochromatosis and often responds poorly to removal of iron by phlebotomy.

The development of the hepatic fibrosis and cirrhosis, however, appears to be related to the degree and duration of iron deposition within the liver. The classical dense portal fibrosis in a "holly-leaf" pattern occurs where the iron is most heavily deposited. Recent studies have shown that fibrosis was not apparent until the hepatic iron concentration exceeded 400

[1] The Liver Unit, Departments of Medicine and Biochemistry, University of Queensland, Brisbane, Australia

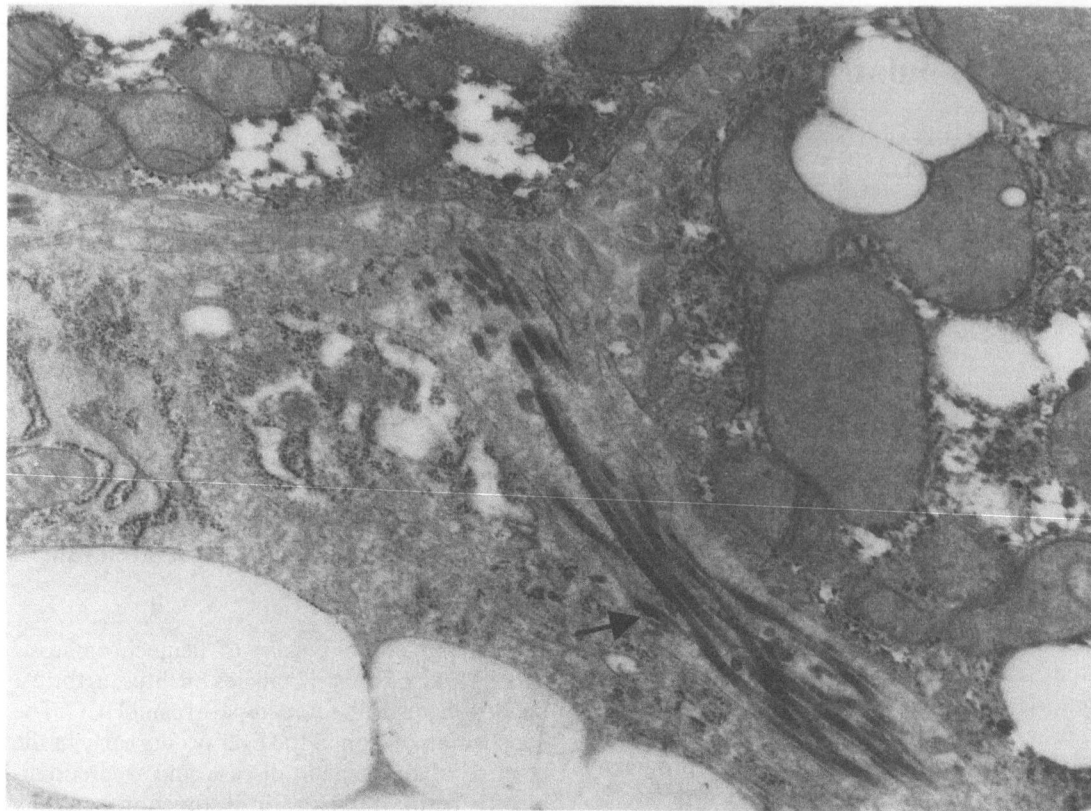

Fig. 14.1. Electron micrograph of rat liver after 42 days of dietary carbonyl iron (2.5%). *Arrow* shows collagen fibrils in the space of Disse. × 27 000

μmol/g dry weight [8]. Bacon and colleagues have recently described an animal model for the study of hepatic iron toxicity using oral carbonyl iron administration [9]. The heavy parenchymal iron loading in their model resulted in mitochondrial and microsomal injury, lipid peroxidation, and fibrosis [10]. Using this model, we (Irving et al., unpublished observations) have demonstrated the stimulation of collagen deposition by isolated hepatocytes from iron-loaded rats. We have also observed collagen deposition in the intact animal; Fig. 14.1 shows the ultrastructure of the liver from a rat treated with oral carbonyl iron (2.5% w/w) for 42 days. Collagen deposition can be seen in the space of Disse.

In subjects detected and treated before hepatic architectural distortion or other complications occur, it seems likely that life and health expectancy are normal, but this supposition has not been investigated in a controlled study. In a recent study by Niederau et al. [11], the survival and causes of death were analyzed in a group of 163 hemochromatosis subjects of whom 51 were noncirrhotic. Survival in noncirrhotic hemochroma-

tosis subjects was not significantly different from that in a normal population, while survival in hemochromatosis patients who were cirrhotic was significantly reduced compared with both normal and noncirrhotic hemochromatosis subjects [11].

2.1 Genetics of hemochromatosis

Although the basic metabolic defect(s) and responsible gene(s) are at present unknown, a major advance in the study of hemochromatosis occurred with the discovery of the association between the hemochromatosis gene and the HLA antigen system [12, 13]. The early observations by Simon et al. in 1975 indicated an increase in HLA-A3 as compared with the general population [12]. Several groups have now demonstrated linkage between this disease and the HLA-A locus on chromosome 6 and the inheritance of hemochromatosis as a recessive trait [14–17]. Family studies have suggested that the gene frequency is 0.08 in Queensland, 0.05 in Brittany, and 0.03 in Utah [14, 18]. The estimated homozygote frequency from several studies is about 0.0025–0.005 [14, 15]; however, many homozygous subjects, especially females, remain undiagnosed. The incidence of complications in these subjects detected by family studies is impossible to document, since there is no genetic marker of hemochromatosis at present; thus, only somatic manifestations can be used to diagnose the disorder. The diagnosis of hemochromatosis is made by liver biopsy in the majority of patients and by quantitative phlebotomy in the remainder [3]. These subjects, detected by family studies of known cases of hemochromatosis, may have a normal hepatic morphology apart from increased deposition of iron [19]. Most subjects detected by family studies have somewhat milder disease than probands, but severe clinical disease and cirrhosis is common and HCC has also occurred in this group. Whether a single mutant gene is responsible for determining disease susceptibility is not established. A recent study suggests that the disease may be heterogeneous [20], but this heterogeneity has not been established as being genetic in origin. The question is of considerable importance in the search for a marker of the disease independent of iron overload.

3 Documentation of HCC in hemochromatosis

HCC is a frequent complication of hemochromatosis, and this association has been recognized for many years. Mallory, in a study of postmortem examinations performed on patients with cirrhosis who died at the Boston City Hospital between 1897 and 1932 [21], reported an incidence of HCC in hemochromatosis at autopsy of 8.2%. A systematic study of 108 autopsied cases of HCC at the same hospital between 1917 and 1954 showed an incidence of HCC in hemochromatosis of 7.7%, compared with an incidence of HCC in all types of cirrhosis of 3.4% [22]. Berk and Lieber [23] reviewed 1989 cases of cirrhosis reported in the literature up to 1941 and noted an overall incidence of HCC of 4.5%, although in 436 cases of hemochromatosis the incidence was 7.3%. Similar figures were obtained by Stewart in 1922 [24]. This incidence of HCC in hemochromatosis was also reflected in surveys of patients with hemochromatosis. Sheldon [1] noted that HCC was the cause of death in 8 of 119 cases (6.3%) in the literature prior to 1935. Similar results were found by Finch and Finch [25] in 1955. However, it should be

Table 14.1. Reported causes of death in hemochromatosis over 50 years

Cause of death	1935[a] (%)	1955[b] (%)	1975[c] (%)	1985[d] (%)
Diabetes mellitus	51	0	0	6
Hepatic failure	11	30	27.2(0)	19
Pneumonia	9	12	9.1(12.5)	0
Tuberculosis	8			0
Cancer of liver	6.7	14	36.4(37.5)	30.2
Heart disease	0	30	18.1(12.5)	13
Cancer of other sites	—	—	—	13
Miscellaneous	13	—	0 (12.5)	19
Valid cases (n)	119	—	19	53

[a] From Sheldon [1]
[b] From Finch and Finch [25]
[c] From Powell [62]; numbers in parenthesis represent figures for nonalcoholic patients with hemochromatosis
[d] From Niederau et al. [11]

noted that these various studies were published before effective therapy for hemochromatosis and its complications was instituted, and some were from cases largely treated in the days before insulin was given. In more recent times the pattern has altered. Table 14.1 shows the cause of death in four studies of hemochromatosis over 50 years. In several other large series, HCC accounted for 20%–36% of deaths in hemochromatosis [26–29]. The changing pattern is presumably due to longer survival in hemochromatosis as a result of more effective therapy of the complications, such as diabetes mellitus, cardiac failure, and hepatic failure, and presumably also as a result of the removal of excess iron by phlebotomy therapy [26, 30]. This incidence of HCC in hemochromatosis contrasts with that in cirrhosis of other causes, where figures are usually in the range of 5%–15% [28, 29, 31, 32].

We have examined the risk of HCC and other internal malignancies in patients with hemochromatosis by examining the records of 208 patients on the hemochromatosis register in the Department of Medicine, University of Queensland from the time of diagnosis to June 1983 [27]. All cancer diagnoses were based on histological findings. Skin cancers (basal cell carcinoma and squamous cell carcinoma) were not included in the survey. In order to derive expected values for the development of cancer, incidence data for each sex over the peroid 1977–1981 were obtained from the South Australian Cancer Registry [33], which is regarded as accurate and comprehensive. Recent estimates of the South Australian resident population [34] were used to compute average annual rates in 5-year age-groups. Cubic splines with minimal smoothing were fitted and the resulting estimated rates by year of age were converted to probabilities in the manner of survival probabilities [35]. In addition, cancers occurring in a comparison group of 148 subjects with other chronic nonalcoholic liver diseases were determined. Among the hemochromatosis group, the 208 subjects comprised 171 males (mean age at diagnosis 47.6 years; range 17–71) and 37 females (mean age at diagnosis 46.3 years; 16–81). The mean follow-up for men was 7.9 years (range 0–33) and for women 7.9 years (0–22). Liver biopsy reports were available for 150 subjects, and cirrhosis was documented in 80 of these. During follow-up 53 deaths were observed.

The number of patients with observed cancers was 24. In 16 of these HCC was present. Of the eight cases of nonhepatic primary cancer, four were of the large bowel, two of the lung, and one each of Hodgkin's disease and squamous cell carcinoma of the pyriform fossa. Two subjects with colorectal cancer were sisters; the mother of these sisters, also in the hemochromatosis group, was one of the cases with HCC.

The expected number of cancers is compared with observed values in Table 14.2. Confidence limits are calculated under the Poisson assumption for numbers of cases [36]. The 16 cases of HCC reflect a 200-fold excess risk (95% confidence limits 138–390). In our data, there appeared to be no increased risk of other malignancies in this disease, although the small numbers of cancers made this estimate less certain (95% confidence limits 0.30–1.37).

The Swiss study of Ammann and co-workers [37] confirmed a high frequency of HCC (five cases in 36 subjects monitored for a mean of 8 years). The London study of Bomford and Williams [26] of 111 patients observed for a mean of 7 years is a survey of the authors' experience of hemochromatosis and includes some cases in which the definitive diagnosis was made at autopsy. In a recent study from Düsseldorf [11], the survival and causes of death were analyzed in 163 hemochromatosis patients followed for a mean period of 10.5 ± 5.6 years. Analysis of the cause of death (53 deaths observed) showed that HCC was present in 16 patients. This represented a marked excess, similar to our results, with an O/E ratio of 219 (95% confidence limits

Table 14.2. Occurrence of cancer

Cancer site	Observed no. of cases	Expected no. of cases	Ratio (O/E)	95% conf. limits of ratio (O/E)
Hemochromatosis cases				
HCC	16	0.067	240	138–390
All except HCC	8	11.52	0.69	0.30–1.37
Colorectal	4	1.79	2.2	0.61–5.8
Lung	2	2.24	0.89	0.11–3.2
Chronic liver disease cases				
HCC	1	0.012	84	2.1–468
All except HCC	1	2.9	0.34	0.01–1.9

125–340). These authors also found no evidence of increased risk of nonhepatic tumors in patients with hemochromatosis.

4   Pathophysiology of cancer occurrence in hemochromatosis

The mechanisms underlying HCC occurrence in hemochromatosis are unclear. The factors which have been considered to be most relevant are: (1) cirrhosis, (2) male sex, (3) iron and/or other metals, and (4) hepatitis B virus. The possible contribution of each will be discussed in the following sections.

4.1   Cirrhosis

As detailed in chapter 7 in this volume, HCC is associated with cirrhosis of any cause, particularly macronodular cirrhosis [28]. Cirrhosis is clearly an important risk factor for the development of HCC in hemochromatosis. Indeed, to our knowledge, there has been no reported case of HCC in a patient with hemochromatosis in the absence of cirrhosis. However, the development of cirrhosis in hemochromatosis is highly correlated with other factors such as hepatic iron concentration (see above), making it difficult to draw conclusions about the independent role of cirrhosis.

4.2   Male sex

All studies of HCC in patients with cirrhosis have emphasized the marked diference in sex incidence, with males predominating. Consecutive series of patients with HCC from the United States and Britain suggest that about 80% of subjects are male [28, 38]. The precise cause for the male preponderance is unclear. In one paper where hemochromatosis subjects were compared with other cirrhotic subjects, the risk of HCC was approximately equal in males in each group. This may suggest that male sex is an independent risk factor for HCC [29]. This sex difference has not been found in HCC in noncirrhotic livers. For example, a study from London [31] found that noncirrhotic patients with HCC were significantly younger and more often female than cirrhotic patients with HCC. This trend was also observed in the recent series of Okuda et al. [39]. Few reports of HCC in hemochromatosis have given details of patient sex; hemochromatosis patients in the early series were predominantly male. A London study of 111 patients included only one female [26]. In our own recent series [27], all 16 cases of HCC in hemochromatosis were in males, although in the overall group 37 of 208 subjects were female. However, male sex is a particular risk factor for the development of overt hemochromatosis because of the lesser physiological requirement for iron in males, and male sex is highly correlated with greater degrees of iron overload.

4.3 Iron and/or other metals

Iron has been associated with malignancy in experimental studies and in humans. At the site of injection of iron dextran in rats, 16 of 23 animals developed sarcoma within 16 months [40]. Sarcomas developing in humans have been attributed to the same cause [41–43]. Exposure to inhaled iron oxide has been shown to be cocarcinogenic in hamsters [44]. Studies of miners exposed to inhaled iron oxide have suggested that a similar effect occurs in humans [45], but some doubt has been cast on this finding [43]. In addition, iron overload may be associated with malignancy in general, because of the important role of iron as a nutrient of the cancer cell [46].

Evidence that iron plays a role in the increased incidence of HCC in hemochromatosis comes from a recent study [11], which found that hemochromatosis patients dying from HCC had significantly higher amounts of mobilizable iron (as determined during phlebotomy therapy) than patients dying from other causes. However, this study also showed that patients who died from any cause during the study had higher amounts of mobilizable iron than the survivors. Our pre-

vious study, unlike two other studies [26, 37], showed no increased risk of other internal malignancy in hemochromatosis. The Düsseldorf group [11] confirmed a lack of excess risk for nonhepatic malignancy in hemochromatosis. In view of the lack of excess risk of malignancies in other organs which also undergo excessive iron deposition in hemochromatosis, it appears that the cause likely involves a specific hepatic factor.

Experimentally, increased hepatic concentrations of iron have been shown to produce tissue injury and fibrosis. The precise mechanisms are uncertain but evidence has accumulated in favor of free radical damage, lipid peroxidation, and lysosomal injury with intracellular release of lysosomal enzymes [9, 47, 48]. This damage progresses to collagen deposition [10]. We (Irving and colleagues, unpublished observations) found increased collagen synthesis in hepatocytes and increased collagen deposition in the space of Disse in iron-loaded rats, suggesting a direct effect of iron on hepatic collagen synthesis (Fig. 14.1).

A further mechanism by which iron may predispose to HCC is through its effects on the immune system. An increasing body of evidence from several groups suggests that iron may have an adverse effect on the host's cell-mediated immune defence mechanisms [49–55]. We have studied the immunological effects of iron and ferritin in vitro using clonal assays which allow the analysis of single-cell function [56–58]. These studies have revealed several effects of iron on lymphocyte function in vitro as outlined below.

We have shown (unpublished observations): (1) that iron significantly inhibited the differentiation of cytotoxic T-lymphocyte precursors to cytotoxic T-lymphocytes but did not affect the growth of cytotoxic T-lymphocytes per se. This inhibition was mediated by low concentrations of nontransferrin-bound iron at similar levels to those reported in the serum of patients with iron overload. (2) Iron significantly enhanced the function of suppressor T-lymphocyte clones while not inhibiting the differentiation of suppressor T-lymphocyte precursors to suppressor T lymphocytes. (3) Iron had no effect on the cloning efficiency of helper T-lymphocyte precursors but significantly reduced the size of the clones that did develop.

The effect of in vivo iron overload was also studied in the murine system, using techniques leading predominantly to hepatocyte iron loading (dietary carbonyl iron) or monocyte-macrophage loading (parenteral injection of iron dextran). Specific cytotoxicity was reduced, and this was shown to result from a reduction in helper T lymphocytes. Iron loading caused an actual deletion of helper T lymphocytes from the spleen.

We have also studied the effect or iron and normal human liver ferritin on the proliferative response of normal human lymphocytes to a specific antigen, tetanus toxoid. Iron affected the initiation of clone development and reduced significantly the cloning efficiency of precursor T cells. Clone size was also reduced when iron was present during culture. Normal human liver ferritin had no effect on lymphocyte proliferation, contrary to reports from some other investigators [52]. In addition, no difference in the function of NK cells, which are thought to be important as a surveillance mechanism against certain tumors, was demonstrated in our studies in patients with hemochromatosis.

These studies indicate that low concentrations of nontransferrin-bound iron can affect lymphocytes stimulated both antigenically and mitogenically; they support the hypothesis that nontransferrin-bound iron may have an immunoregulatory role in cell-mediated immunity. However, while of considerable interest, the relevance of these observations to the development of HCC in patients with hemochromatosis remains to be determined.

The possible oncogenic role of other metals in hemochromatosis is even more conjectural than that of iron. The tissue concentrations of some metals, particularly copper, is increased in the advanced cirrhotic stages of the disease [1]. Sheldon noted that the hepatic copper concentration was more than four times the normal level in advanced hemochromatosis but that the increase was less than that for iron and of the same order as occurs in cirrhosis from other causes [1]. In addition, tissue calcium concentrations were found to be elevated, especially in the liver, pancreas, and spleen. Hepatic concentrations rose to eight times the normal level. There appears to have been no recent systematic study of tissue metal composition in hemochromatosis with and without HCC despite detailed analysis of normal and cirrhotic livers [59].

4.4 Hepatitis B virus

HCC in Caucasoid patients is often associated with serum or tissue markers of the hepatitis B virus (HBV), but in 8 of 24 consecutive patients, no such evidence was found [38]. The role of HBV in the development of HCC in humans and related hepadna viruses in HCC in animals, together with the 200-fold risk of HCC in hemochromatosis (a figure virtually identical to that for HBsAg carriers), has raised the question as to whether the HBV may be reponsible for HCC in patients with hemochromatosis. It has even been suggested that a high serum ferritin level predisposes to hepatitis B infection becoming chronic, at least in hemodialysis patients [60].

Although the incidence of serological markers for HBV infection is not increased in patients with hemochromatosis compared with control subjects, an increased incidence of HBV-DNA sequences has been reported in tumors from hemochromatotic patients without serological markers of HBV. Brechot and co-workers [61] studied liver samples from 14 nonalcoholic patients with primary hemochromatosis and HCC using the Southern blot technique and an HBV-DNA probe. Autopsy, surgical, and needle-biopsy samples were, respectively, obtained in nine, four, and two cases. Tumorous and non-tumorous liver samples were analyzed in eight patients. For six subjects, only tumorous or non-tumorous samples were available. All the subjects were HBsAg negative in the serum by standard radioimmunoassay; two were anti-HBc and anti-HBs positive, one was anti-HBs positive only, and four patients had no HBV markers; the presence of anti-HBs and anit-HBc could not be tested in the remaining five cases. HBV-DNA sequences were detected in 8 of 14 cases tested including four patients lacking any conventional serological HBV markers; in many cases weak bands only could be detected. The authors concluded that their results suggested that HBV chronic infection was present despite the absence of detectable HBsAg in the serum, and thus HBV may play a role in liver carcinogenesis in patients with hemochromatosis.

In a recent study of four patients of our own, only one had integrated HBV-DNA sequences. This patient had evidence of previous exposure to HBV as demonstrated by anti-HBs and anti-HBc in his serum. Thus, we were unable to find evidence of HBV-DNA in HCC in hemochromatosis in the absence of serological evidence of previous or current viral infection. There are a number of possible reasons for these different findings in the two studies. Firstly, the number of subjects studied was small. Secondly, there may have been differences in the frequency of HBV infection in the two populations, although the available evidence does not support this conclusion. Thirdly, our HBV-DNA probe may not be detecting HBV-DNA sequences because of the extensive reorganization, duplication, and deletion of portions of the genome. This is unlikely since our probe is similar to that used by Brechot and colleagues and sequences as small as 50 base pairs are usually sufficient to give a positive signal on hybridization. The most likely explanation is the uncertain interpretation of weak bands. Brechot et al. found that their HBV-DNA bands were weak (approximately 0.1 copy/cell). While this could be due to the loss of HBV genetic material from the tumor cells, it may be unrelated to HBV, e.g., the base-sequence homology between the P gene of HBV and genetic material from retrovirus. Until these bands have been cloned and sequenced, the interpretation of these bands remains in doubt, as does the role of HBV in HCC of hemochromatosis. Meanwhile, the question arises as to whether patients with hemochromatosis should receive vaccination against HBV in view of this increased risk of HCC and the need for repeated phlebotomy. It would clearly be of considerable interest to compare the development of HCC in such subjects prospectively with nonvaccinated subjects with hemochromatosis. One such prospective study at least is currently being undertaken [63]. Unfortunately, the answers from such a study may take decades to obtain.

Acknowledgments. This study was supported in part by the Clive and Vera Ramaciotti Medical Research Foundations and the National Health and Medical Research Council of Australia

References

1. Sheldon JH (1935) Haemochromatosis. Oxford University Press, London
2. Powell LW, Bassett ML, Halliday JW (1980) Haemochromatosis—1980 Update. Gastroenterology 78: 374–81
3. Grace ND, Powell LW (1974) Iron storage disorders of the liver. Gastroenterology 64: 1257–83
4. Milder MS, Cook JD, Stray S, Finch CA (1980) Idiopathic hemochromatosis, an interim report. Medicine 59: 34–49
5. Jacobs A (1980) The pathology of iron overload. In: Jacobs A, Worwood M (eds) Iron in biochemistry and medicine: II. Academic Press, London, pp 428–61
6. Stocks AE, Powell LW (1973) Carbohydrate intolerance in idiopathic haemochromatosis and cirrhosis of the liver. Quart J Med 42: 733–49
7. Walsh CH, Malins JM, Bloom SR (1978) Diabetes mellitus in idiopathic haemochromatosis. Br Med J 2: 1267–8
8. Bassett ML, Halliday JW, Powell LW (1986) Value of hepatic iron measurements in early hemochromatosis and determination of the critical iron level associated with fibrosis. Hepatology 6: 24–29
9. Bacon BR, Tavill AS, Brittenham GM, et al (1983) Hepatic lipid peroxidation in vivo in rats with chronic iron overload. J Clin Invest 71: 429–39
10. Park CH, Stassen WN, Bacon BR, Brittenham GM, Louis L, Tavill AS (1985) Hepatic fibrosis in rats with chronic dietary iron overload. Hepatology 5: 950 (abstr)
11. Niederau C, Fischer R, Sonnenberg A, Stremmel W, Trampisch HJ, Strohmeyer G (1985) Survival and causes of death in cirrhotic and in noncirrhotic patients with primary hemochromatosis. N Engl J Med 313: 1256–62
12. Simon M, Pawlotsky Y, Bourel M, Fauchet R, Genetet B (1975) Hemochromatose idiopathique: maladie associee a l'antigene tissulaire HL-A3? La Nouvelle Presse Medicale 4: 1432
13. Simon M, Bourel M, Fauchet R, Genetet B (1976) Association of HLA-A3 and HLA-B14 antigens with idiopathic hemochromatosis. Gut 17: 332–334
14. Cartwright GE, Edwards CQ, Kravitz K, Skolnick M, Amos DB, Johnson A, Buskjaer L (1979) Hereditary hemochromatosis: phenotypic expression of the disease. N Engl J Med 301: 175–9
15. Bassett ML, Doran TJ, Halliday JW, Bashir HV, Powell LW (1982) Idiopathic hemochromatosis: demonstration of homozygous-heterozygous mating by HLA typing of families. Hum Genet 60: 352–6
16. Simon M, Bourel M, Genetet B, Fauchet R (1977) Idiopathic hemochromatosis: demonstration of recessive transmission and early detection by family HLA typing. N Engl J Med 297: 1017–21
17. Bassett ML, Halliday JW, Powell LW (1984) Genetic Hemochromatosis. In: Seminars in liver disease Berk PD (ed) Thieme-Stratton, New York
18. Doran TJ, Bashir HV, Trejaut J, Bassett ML, Halliday JW, Powell LW (1981) Idiopathic haemochromatosis in the Australian population: HLA linkage and recessivity. Hum Immunol 2: 191–200
19. Bassett ML, Halliday JW, Ferris RA, Powell LW (1984) Diagnosis of hemochromatosis in young subjects: predictive accuracy of biochemical screening tests. Gastroenterology 87: 628–33
20. Muir WA, McLaren GD, Braun W, Askari A (1984) Evidence for heterogeneity in hereditary hemochromatosis: evaluation of 174 persons in nine families. Am J Med 76: 806–14
21. Mallory FB (1932) Cirrhosis of the liver. N Engl J Med 206: 1231–9
22. MacDonald RA (1957) Primary carcinoma of the liver: a clinicopathological study of one hundred and eight cases. Arch Int Med 99: 266–79
23. Berk JE, Lieber, MM (1941) Primary carcinoma

of liver in hemochromatosis. Am J Med Sci 202: 708–714

24. Stewart MJ (1922) Carcinoma of the liver in cirrhosis and hemochromatosis Br Med J 2: 1066

25. Finch SC, Finch CA (1955) Idiopathic hemochromatosis, an iron storage disease: A. Iron metabolism in hemochromatosis. Medicine (Baltimore) 34: 381–430

26. Bomford A, Williams R (1976) Long term results of venesection therapy in idiopathic haemochromatosis. Quart J Med 45: 611–23

27. Bradbear RA, Bain C, Siskind V, Schofield FD, Webb S, Axelsen EM, Halliday JW, Bassett ML, Powell LW (1985) Cohort study of internal malignancy in genetic hemochromatosis and other chronic nonalcoholic liver disease. J Nat Cancer Inst 75: 81–4

28. Purtillo DT, Gottlieb LS (1973) Cirrhosis and hepatoma occurring at Boston City Hospital (1917–1968). Cancer 32: 458–62

29. MacSween RNM (1974) A clinicopathological review of 100 cases of primary malignant tumors of the liver. J Clin Pathol 27: 669–82

30. Powell LW (1970) Changing concepts of haemochromatosis. Postgrad Med J 46: 200–209

31. Melia WM, Wilkinson ML, Portmann BC, Johnson PJ, Williams R (1984) Hepatocellular carcinoma in the non-cirrhotic liver: a comparison with that complicating cirrhosis. Quart J Med 53: 391–400

32. Powell LW, Mortimer R, Harris OD (1971) Cirrhosis of the liver: A comparative study of the four major aetiological groups. Med J Australia 1: 941–50

33. South Australian Central Cancer Registry unit (1983) Cancer in South Australia—Incidence, mortality and survival, 1977–81—Incidence and mortality 1981. South Australian Health Commission, Adelaide

34. Australian Bureau of Statistics (1983) Estimated resident population by sex and age: States and Territories of Australia, June 1977 to June 1982. Australian Government Publishing Service, Canberra

35. Ford JR (1981) Australian life tables 1975–1977. Office of the Australian Government Actuary, Canberra

36. Bailar JC (III) (1964) Significance factors for the ratio of a Poisson variable to its expectation. Biometrics 20: 639–43

37. Ammann RW, Muller E, Bansky J, Schuler G, Hacki WH (1980) High incidence of extrahepatic carcinomas in idiopathic hemochromatosis. Scand J Gastroenterol 15: 733–6

38. Bassendine MF, Chadwick RG, Lyssiotis T, Thomas HC, Sherlock S, Cohen BJ (1979) Primary liver cell cancer in Britain—a viral aetiology? Br Med J 1: 166

39. Okuda H, Obata H, Saito A, Tomimatsu M, Hisamitsu T, Takasaki T, Kobayashi S (1986) Hepatocellular carcinoma not associated with cirrhosis. A clinicopathological study in 41 patients including 29 resected cases. J Gastroent Hepatol 1: 129–137

40. Richmond HG (1959) Induction of sarcoma in the rat by iron-dextran complex. Br Med J 1: 947–9

41. Greenberg G (1976) Sarcoma after intramuscular iron injection. Brit Med J 1: 1508–9

42. Weinbren K, Salm R, Greenberg G (1978) Intramuscular injections of iron compounds and oncogenesis in man. Br Med J 1: 683–5

43. Weinberg ED (1981) Iron and neoplasia. Biol Trace Elem Res 3: 55–80

44. Nettesheim P, Creasia DA, Mitchell TJ (1975) Carcinogenic and cocarcinogenic effects of inhaled synthetic smog and ferric oxide particles. J Natl Cancer Inst 55: 159–69

45. Antoine D, Braun P, Cervoni P, Schwartz P, Lamy P (1979) Le cancer bronchique des mineurs de fer de Lorraine—peut-il etre considere comme une maladie professionelle? A propos de 270 nouveaux cas observes de 1964 a 1978. Rev Fr Mal Respir 7: 63–5

46. Weinberg ED (1984) Iron withholding: a defense against infection and neoplasia. Physiol Rev 64: 65–102

47. Selden C, Owen M, Hopkins JMP, Peters TJ (1980) Studies on the concentration and intracellular localization of iron proteins in liver biopsy specimens from patients with iron; overload with special reference to their role in lysosomal disruption. Br J Haematol 44: 593–603

48. Selden C, Seymour CA, Peters TJ (1980) Activities of some free-radical scavenging enzymes and glutathione concentrations in human and rat liver and their relationship to the pathogenesis of tissue damage in iron overload. Clin Sci 58: 211–9

49. Bergeron RJ, Streiff RR, Elliott GT (1985) Influence of iron in vivo proliferation and lethality of L1210 cells. J Nutr 115: 369–74

50. Van Asbeck BS, Verbrugh HA, Van Oost BA, Marx JJM, Imhoff HW, Verhoef J (1982) Listeria monocytogenes meningitis and decreased phagocytosis associated with iron overload. Br Med J 284: 542–4

51. De Sousa M, Nishiya K (1978) Inhibition of E-rosette formation by two iron salts. Cell Immunol 38: 203–8

52. Matzner Y, Hershko C, Polliack A, Konijn AM, Izak G (1979) Suppressive effect of ferritin on in vitro lymphocyte function. Br J Haematol 42: 345–53

53. Bryan CF, Nishiya K, Pollack MS, Dupont B, De Sousa M (1981) Differential inhibition of the MLR by iron: association with HLA phenotype. Immunogenetics 12: 129–40

54. Nishiya K, De Sousa M, Tsoi E, Bognacki JJ, De Harven E (1980) Regulation of expression of a human lymphoid cell surface marker by iron. Cell Immunol 53: 71–83

55. Keown P, Descamps-Latscha B (1983) In vitro suppression of cell-mediated immunity by ferroproteins and ferric salts. Cell Immunol 80: 257–66

56. Good MF, Halliday JW, Powell LW (1985) A

method for analysing the clonal precursors of con-canavalin A-induced suppressor cells. J Immunol Meth 80: 163–175

57. Good MF, Halliday JW, Powell LW (1984) Natural killer cell function and clonal analysis of immune responses in hemochromatosis and experimental iron overload. Hepatology 4(5): 1021 (abstract)

58. Good MF, Chapman D, Rudd M, Halliday JW, Powell LW (1985) The immunoregulatory effect of non-transferrin-bound iron and iron-overload. Hepatology 5(5): 983 (abstr)

59. Milman N, Laursen J, Podenphant J, Asnaes S (1986) Trace elements in normal and cirrhotic human liver tissue: I. Iron, copper zinc, selenium, manganese, titanium and lead measured by X-ray fluorescence spectrometry. Liver (in press)

60. Lustbader ED, Hann H-WL, Blumberg BS (1983) Serum ferritin as a predictor of host response to hepatitis B virus infection. Science 220: 423–5

61. Brechot C, Pasquinelli C, Saadi P, Deugnier Y, Simon M, Brissot P, Bourel M (1985) Liver hepatitis B virus DNA sequences in the liver of patients with hepatocellular carcinoma and primary haemochromatosis. Hepatology 5: 970 (abstr)

62. Powell LW (1975) The role of alcoholism in hepatic iron storage disease. Am NY Acad Sci 252: 124–134

63. Saddi RS, Ebelin P, Pouliquen A, Gautreau C, Durand J, Jammet P, Courouce AM, Brechot C Franco D, Thibult N (1985) Hepatitis B vaccination and idiopathic haemochromatosis. Lancet 2: 1061–1062

Chapter 15

Clinical Manifestations and Paraneoplastic Syndromes of Hepatocellular Carcinoma

Michael C. Kew[1]

1 Introduction

Hepatocellular carcinoma presents clinically in many diverse ways. The variety of the presentations stems partly from the different biological characteristics of hepatocellular carcinoma in high- and low-incidence regions and partly from the wide range of paraneoplastic phenomena which may precede the local manifestations of the tumor.

Whatever the presentation, hepatocellular carcinoma is almost always in an advanced stage when the patient is first examined. Apart from the rapid growth rate of the tumor, which in some instances has a doubling time of as little as 10 days [1], several explanations may be advanced to account for this phenomenon. The large size of the liver means that the tumor must reach a substantial size before it can be felt or before it invades adjacent structures; the considerable reserves of the liver ensure that jaundice and other evidence of hepatic failute do not appear until a large part of the organ has been replaced by the tumor; spread of hepatocellular carcinoma to distant sites usually occurs late in the course of the disease. Consequently, hepatocellular carcinoma is insidious in onset and runs a silent course in its early stages, making early diagnosis difficult. The absence of pathognomonic symptoms and signs, the position of the liver deep under the lower ribs rendering it relatively inaccessible to the examining hand, and the dearth of specific changes in biochemical tests of hepatic function combine to delay diagnosis further. The resulting large tumor at the time when treatment can be instituted contributes in no small measure to the poor prognosis of hepatocellular carcinoma.

The facility with which the diagnosis of hepatocellular carcinoma is made is determined in part by the prevalence of the tumor in a particular region. In countries in which hepatocellular carcinoma is common, a high level of awareness of the tumor and the various ways in which it may present is responsible for the diagnosis being made far more easily than in countries where the tumor is rarely seen. Nevertheless, even in high-risk populations, because of the generally more rapid growth rate of the tumor, hepatocellular carcinoma is usually advanced when the diagnosis is made. In low-risk populations, lack of familiarity with the tumor and its many guises has in the past often resulted in the diagnosis being made only at necropsy. Fortunately, during recent years, a better understanding of the clinical features of hepatocellular carcinoma, as well as the introduction of alpha fetoprotein as a tumor marker and the availability of improved imaging modalities, has lessened the frequency with which this occurs. For example, in a recent series from the United States, a histological diagnosis was made during life in 84% of patients [2]; in another series from Great Britain, a definitive diagnosis was made during life in 63% of patients, and in a further 20% the condition was strongly suspected although for a variety of reasons a tissue diagnosis was not made ante mortem [3].

In spite of the advanced stage of the tumor when the patient is first seen, the history obtained is often of short duration, sometimes remarkably so. This phenomenon is more evident in, although not confined to, patients in high-incidence regions of hepatocellular carcinoma. In rural southern African Blacks, for example, the mean duration of symptoms before diagnosis is only 5 weeks [4]. A short history is, however, not an invariable feature in these regions as shown by a series of Ugandan patients in whom symptoms had been present on average for 5.8

[1] Department of Medicine, University of the Witwatersrand Medical School and Johannesbury and Baragwanath Hosptials, Johannesburg, South Africa

months before admission [5], a duration not dissimilar to that occurring in patients in the United States (24 weeks) [6].

An important difference in the general mode of presentation of hepatocellular carcinoma between high- and low-risk regions concerns the relation of the tumor to cirrhosis. In countries in which hepatocellular carcinoma is uncommon (and also in Japan), the tumor frequently manifests against a background of clinically apparent cirrhosis or, less often, chronic hepatitis: A patient known for some years to have cirrhosis, usually alcoholic in origin, develops one or more new symptoms or signs which signal that a tumor has supervened in the cirrhotic liver. This sequence of events occurred in one-quarter of British [3] and one-fifth of North American patients [2]. Alternatively, the patient may show all or some of the typical features of cirrhosis when he or she is examined. It may be extremely difficult to recognize the presence of a small hepatocellular carcinoma in a patient with advanced cirrhosis, and these tumors are the ones most likely to be discovered only at necropsy. By contrast, in countries in which hepatocellular carcinoma occurs commonly, the tumor usually develops in individuals who were previously apparently healthy, even though cirrhosis is frequently found to coexist with the hepatocellular carcinoma [4, 5, 7]. The cirrhosis is either discovered coincidentally during the course of investigation of the symptoms attributable to the tumor or is detected at necropsy. The two extremes of the range of clinical presentations and courses of hepatocellular carcinoma are represented, on the one hand, by a previously well young male Black with a short history of pain in the right hypochondrium who is found to have a massively enlarged tender liver and who dies within a few weeks and, on the other hand, by an elderly white male known for years to have cirrhosis in whom a small hepatocellular carcinoma is found to have developed, but who continues to live for several years with few if any additional symptoms.

In countries in which hepatocellular carcinoma is uncommon, important differences in the clinical presentation of the tumor between patients with and without coexisting cirrhosis have been described [8]. These include a greater frequency of jaundice, ascites, and gastrointestinal hemorrhage in patients with cirrhosis.

A variety of hepatocellular carcinoma with distinct pathological features has recently been recognized. Fibrolamellar hepatocellular carcinoma (chap. 11) tends to occur predominantly in young people, particularly women, arise in a noncirrhotic liver, be unassociated with alpha fetoprotein production and markers of hepatitis B virus infection, and have a better prognosis than is usual with hepatocellular carcinoma [9]. The clinical features in these patients are, however, similar to those of other patients with hepatocellular carcinoma unassociated with cirrhosis.

With the very poor prognosis which pertains when hepatocellular carcinoma presents spontaneously, more and more attention has been focused during recent years on detecting the tumor at an early stage when it is still amenable to resection or, if not, at least more responsive to nonoperative modalities of treatment. Small or "minute" hepatocellular carcinomas are being sought in surveillance programs of individuals at high risk of developing this tumor (chronic carriers of the hepatitis B virus and patients with cirrhosis, chronic hepatitis, or hemochromatosis). Individuals in whom tumors are detected in this way are almost always asymptomatic (the term "subclinical hepatocellular carcinoma" has been used to describe these tumors [10]); in the few with symptoms, these are nonspecific and cannot be directly attributed to the tumor.

The ways in which hepatocellular carcinoma typically presents will first be described before discussing the less common presentations, including those resulting from various paraneoplastic phenomena.

2 Common symptoms

2.1 Abdominal pain

The commonest symptom as well as the most frequent initial complaint in populations with a high risk of hepatocellular carcinoma is abdominal pain. In sub-Saharan Blacks, this symptom is almost invariably present (reported prevalence ranges from 89%–95%) [4, 5, 11], with slightly lower frequencies (74%–84%) recorded in Chinese patients [7, 12]. A notable exception are Japanese patients, only a minority of whom (42%) have abdominal pain [13]. In 50% or more of Black and Chinese patients, pain is the first symptom. Abdominal pain is generally less prevalent (53%–58%) in populations with a low risk of hepatocellular carcinoma [2, 3, 6, 14, 15]. A plausible explanation for the different frequencies of this symptom is to be found in the parallel that exists between abdominal pain and the tumor size in Black, Chinese, white, and Japanese patients: The tumorous liver has an average weight of 3960 g in Blacks, 3046 g in Chinese, 2615 g in whites, and 2036 g in Japanese.

Pain is most often felt in the right hypochondrium or epigastrium, although it is sometimes experienced in the left hypochondrium, lower in the abdomen, or in the back. The pain may also radiate into the back or, rarely, be referred to the tip of the right shoulder. The pain is usually a constant, dull ache, although it may become more severe in the later stages of the illness, and it may be aggravated in certain positions and by jolting movements. In Black and Chinese patients, the pain is more frequently severe from the outset. Severe pain *de novo* is less likely in low-incidence regions, e.g., it occurred in only 10% of patients in a British series [3].

Occasionally, right hypochondrial pain accompanied by fever and mild jaundice might initially suggest a diagnosis of acute cholecystitis.

The onset of unexplained upper abdominal pain in a patient known to have cirrhosis should arouse suspicion that hepatocellular carcinoma has supervened.

2.2 Abdominal mass or distension

In patients with hepatocellular carcinoma, the pain may draw their attention to an upper abdominal mass. Other patients may notice a mass in the absence of pain. The latter occurred, for example, in about one-third of the patients in three US studies [2, 15, 16]. In some instances, especially in high-risk regions, the tumor may be so large that the patient cannot fail to be aware of it.

In other patients, increasing abdominal girth or generalized abdominal distension is noticed. This results from the accumulation of moderate or large amounts of ascitic fluid. Abdominal distension is slightly more prevalent in low-incidence populations, reflecting the greater frequency of ascites and well-established cirrhosis in these patients.

In patients known to have cirrhosis, unexplained enlargement of the liver or the appearance of ascites (especially when ths is blood-stained) should alert the clinician to the possibility of hepatocellular carcinoma formation.

2.3 Weakness and malaise

Patients with hepatocellular carcinoma may experience weakness and malaise, although the prominence afforded these symptoms varies in different series of patients not necessarily geographically determined. In Hong Kong Chinese, weakness and malaise are the most common complaints (present in 73% of cases) [7] and they are also frequent in Taiwanese patients (50%) [12]. By contrast, only one-third of southern African Blacks [4] and one-quarter of British patients [3] cite these symptoms.

2.4 Weight loss

Loss of weight is another symptom which varies in frequency in reported series, with no obvious differences between high- and low-incidence populations. Thus, in whites, 71% and 18% of patients in two series complained of loss of weight [3, 6], as did 59% and 19% in two series of Chinese patients [7, 12] and 34% and 54% of sub-Saharan Blacks [4, 5]. Less than 5% of Japanese patients had this symptom [13]. The explanation for these surprising differences is not known, but certainly in the later stages of the illness weight loss is almost invariable.

Unexplained loss of weight in a cirrhotic patient may be the first evidence that a tumor has developed.

2.5 Anorexia or fullness in upper abdomen after meals

This symptom also varies in prominence in different series of patients. It is most frequent in Chinese patients (more than 60%) [12] and least comon in British patients (28%) [3] and southern African Blacks (25%) [4].

Other gastrointestinal symptoms such as constipation, nausea, vomiting, and indigestion may be present, but they are too nonspecific to be of any diagnostic use.

Whereas the typical presentation of hepatocellular carcinoma is one of upper abdominal pain accompanied by varying frequencies and different combinations of weakness, malaise, anorexia, weight loss and abdominal distension, or an awareness of an upper abdominal mass, unusual presentations do occur. Lack of awareness of these may result in the diagnosis being delayed or even missed.

3 Unusual presentations

3.1 Jaundice

Jaundice is an infrequent but important presenting complaint in patients with hepatocellular carcinoma. In some patients, especially those already suffering from advanced cirrhosis, the jaundice is of the hepatocellular type. This jaundice is usually mild at the time of admission to hospital but often deepens as the disease progresses. In the remainder of cases, the jaundice is obstructive in type and is accompanied by other evidence of cholestasis, particularly pruritus. Obstructive jaundice is the initial complaint in 1%–12% of patients with hepatocellular carcinoma [17]. Five mechanisms have been described [17–20]: obstruction of the main intrahepatic bile ducts by the primary tumor; obstruction of the common hepatic duct by malignant glands in the porta hepatis; extensive infiltration into the biliary radicles by the tumor, with subsequent growth into and obstruction of the major bile ducts; necrosis of a tumor mass adjacent to a major bile duct, resulting in escape of malignant tissue into the duct; and hemobilia. The last two, however, are rare. With the first two mechanisms, the jaundice is unremittingly progressive. Less often, free-floating tumor plugs or debris within the lumen of larger bile ducts cause episodic jaundice, which may be accompanied by colicky upper abdominal pain.

3.2 Acute abdominal crisis

A small number of patients with hepatocellular carcinoma present for the first time with a sudden onset of severe abdominal pain and an "acute surgical abdomen"—boardlike rigidity of the anterior abdominal wall accompanied by shock and pallor. This is caused by an acute hemoperitoneum, which results from rupture of the tumor. Rupture is usually spontaneous (or follows inapparent trauma), but it may follow obvious blunt abdominal trauma. This presentation occurred in 2 of 508 Thai patients [21], 1 of 151 Taiwanese [12], and 7 of approximately 2000 southern African Blacks. More commonly, rupture of the tumor occurs later in the course of the disease and is a frequent cause of death. For example, tumor rupture was the terminal event in 12% of Thais [21], 17% of Hong Kong Chinese [7], and 18.6% of rural southern African Blacks [17]. Tumor rupture is appreciably less common in urbanized Blacks (6.7%) [17]. The tumors are smaller in these patients (2956 $\pm$ 1189 g) than in rural Blacks (3914 $\pm$ 1436 g), and this offers a possible explanation for the difference in the prevalence of tumor rupture. However, tumors that had ruptured were not found to be larger than those without this complication, nor was the prevalence of cirrhosis different in those with and without rupture.

3.3 Hematemesis

Patients with hepatocellular carcinoma occasionally present with hematemesis or melena. One would imagine that this presentation would be more likely to occur in those patients known to have advanced cirrhosis and that ruptured esophageal varices would be the source of the bleeding. However, the recorded prevalence of gastrointestinal bleeding in patients with hepatocellular carcinoma ranges from 1.5% to 19% [2, 4–7, 13], the higher figures being reported in Ugandans and Hong Kong Chinese and the lower in southern African Blacks and Japanese.

3.4 Bone pain

Between 3% and 12% of patients with hepatocellular carcinoma experience bone pain, although the prevalence of osseous metastases at necropsy may be as high as 20% [17, 22, 23]. In some patients, bone pain is the sole or initial symptom, but in others it accompanies or follows other symptoms attributable to the primary tumor. When the primary liver tumor is asymptomatic, the osseous metastasis may appear to be a primary tumor and the liver pathology may be overlooked. Hepatocellular carcinoma may also be missed if both the bony lesion and the enlarged liver are attributed to metastases.

Bone metastases may be solitary or multiple. The bones most commonly affected are the vertebrae, ribs, long bones of the limbs (especially the femur), skull bones, sacrum, and clavicle. Vertebral metastases are particularly problematic because of the frequency with which they are complicated by paraplegia or nerve root compression [22, 24]. Metastases in other bones may cause pathological fractures.

3.5 Acute respiratory symptoms

Respiratory symptoms are a rare presenting complaint in patients with hepatocellular carcinoma, e.g., in 1% of Hong Kong Chinese [7]. Less infrequently, respiratory symptoms are present but they are overshadowed by the symptoms attributable to the primary tumor. Respiratory symptoms may be caused by multiple pulmonary metastases (dyspnea, cough, hemoptysis), a markedly raised right (or rarely left) hemidiaphragm (nonproductive cough, dyspnea), and a large pleural effusion (dyspnea, nonproductive cough) [17]. Some of these intrathoracic complications are not infrequent in hepatocellular carcinoma, for example, pulmonary metastases occur in 25% and an elevated right hemidiaphragm in 30% of southern African Blacks with this tumor [25]. Large pleural effusions are less comon, occurring in 1%–2% of Black patients [25].

Very rarely, multiple tumor emboli to the pulmonary microvasculature may result in pulmonary arterial hypertension [26]. These patients do not have radiological evidence of pulmonary metastases and the pulmonary hypertension may be thought to be "primary."

In spite of the wide variety of presentations possible with hepatocellular carcinoma, some patients are asymptomatic. This is more likely to occur when a small tumor arises in a liver with well-established cirrhosis; however, rarely, larger tumors in noncirrhotic livers may also be without symptoms. In a group of US patients, 29% were asymptomatic [15]. In most of these patients, the tumor was discovered at necropsy, but in one it was found during evaluation of another intra-abdominal malignancy.

Physical findings will obviously depend upon the stage of the disease when the patient is first examined. At an early stage, the only abnormality may be a slightly or moderately enlarged liver. More frequently, however, the disease is far advanced when the patient is first seen and the physical findings are obvious.

4 Physical signs

4.1 Hepatomegaly

Enlargement of the liver is the most frequent physical finding in patients in both high- and low-incidence regions of hepatocellular carcinoma. However, hepatomegaly tends to be both more frequent and present to a greater degree in high-incidence regions (91%–98% in Black and Chinese patients) [4, 5, 7, 12] than in Whites (56%–74% in the United States [6, 16], although 93% of patients in a series from Great Britain had an enlarged liver [3]). Japanese patients are similar in this respect to North American patients [13]. The liver may be massively enlarged, especially in Blacks; this is in keeping with the tumor weights (up to 8780 g) which have been recorded at necropsy in the latter patients [17]. In general, in low-incidence regions, hepatic metastases are responsible for a greater degree of hepatic enlargement than is hepatocellular carcinoma, whereas the reverse is true in high-incidence regions.

The surface of the liver may be smooth, but more often it is irregular or even nodular. Focal

or generalized tenderness may be elicited. In some patients, the tenderness is extreme and mimics that characteristically seen with amebic hepatic abscesses. Indeed, with a short history of pain in the upper abdomen and the finding of an enlarged tender liver and fever, it may be very difficult to distinquish clinically between these two diseases. The enlarged liver feels firm and may be stony hard. In some patients, focal, less firm areas may be felt, presumably as a result of tumor necrosis or hemorrhage into the tumor. Tumorous enlargement of the liver may elevate the right (or occasionally the left) hemidiaphragm [25], and this can often be elicited clinically.

In the absence of an obvious primary lesion, it may be extremely difficult to distinguish between hepatocellular carcinoma and hepatic metastases.

4.2 Hepatic arterial bruit

A bruit arising from hepatocellular carcinoma must be distinguished from that resulting from compression of the aorta in the supine position by the enlarged tumorous liver. The latter is a short decrescendo bruit which is loudest in the midline and becomes progressively softer as the stethoscope is moved away from the midline in each direction. Bruits associated with hepatocellular carcinoma can be heard anywhere over the liver (although they are focal) and they are longer, louder, and "rougher" than bruits transmitted from the aorta. A lack of awareness of bruits and their diagnostic significance in hepatocellular carcinoma may explain why the frequency with which they are reported varies so considerably. In Blacks in southern Africa and Zimbabwe and in British patients, a hepatic bruit was heard in 23%, 29% and 25% of cases, respectively [3, 4, 11], whereas in other series no mention at all is made of bruits; bruits were present in 6.5% of Ugandan patients [5].

Rarely, a friction rub is heard over hepatocellular carcinoma. This physical sign must be looked for before undertaking a percutaneous liver biopsy, because the latter may itself produce a friction rub. Rubs are more likely to be heard over the liver when amebic hepatic abscesses or metastases are present.

4.3 Ascites

Ascites is present slightly more often in White (55%–61%) [3, 6, 14] than in Black and Oriental patients (35%–51%) [4, 5, 11, 12]; this difference probably reflects the greater prevalence of well-established cirrhosis in the former patients. It is usually of slight or moderate degree but tense ascites may be present. Fluid accumulation tends to become progressively more troublesome as the disease progresses. Ascitic fluid is often blood-stained. In patients previously known to have cirrhosis, the finding of blood-stained ascitic fluid strongly suggests the presence of hepatocellular carcinoma.

Microscopic examination of the ascitic fluid for malignant cells has not proved to be useful in the diagnosis of hepatocellular carcinoma.

Two mechanisms may be responsible for ascites formation in these patients, viz. portal hypertension and malignant invasion of the peritoneum. Portal hypertension is either secondary to the coexisting cirrhosis when the latter is long-standing or may result from tumorous invasion of the tributaries of either the portal or hepatic veins.

4.4 Splenomegaly

Splenomegaly was recorded most frequently in a British series (48%) [3], although only 15% of Whites in another series of patients (from the United States) were reported to have an enlarged spleen [14]. The prevalence in Blacks and Orientals ranges between 27% and 42% [4, 5, 11, 12]. Massive enlargement, particularly of the left lobe of the liver, may make it difficult to palpate an enlarged spleen or it may be mistaken for the spleen. Likewise, tense ascites may prevent an enlarged spleen from being palpated. Splenomegaly results from portal hypertension. This is usually secondary to coexisting cirrhosis and is long-standing. Enlargement of the spleen over a short period of time should suggest the possibility of portal vein occlusion by a tumor; in very rare instances, multiple splenic metastases are responsible [27].

4.5 Muscle wasting

Evidence of muscle wasting may already be apparent at the time of hospital admission. This is more likely with rapidly growing, large tumors. For example, 25% of southern African Blacks showed obvious signs of muscle wasting when they were first seen [4]. Slight degrees of wasting may easily be overlooked. As the disease runs it course, progressive muscle wasting is the rule, and in the terminal stages the patients are frequently emaciated.

4.6 Fever

A surprisingly high proportion of patients with hepatocellular carcinoma have fever. In some of these patients, an infection or other cause of fever is identifiable, but a significant number remain with unexplained persistent mild or moderate elevation of the body temperature. The exact number varies from series to series, with low-risk populations generally having lower frequencies of fever—about 10% in the United States [2, 16] and 24% in Great Britain [3]. Fever is present in 54% of Chinese patients [7] and 38% of Blacks [4]. A possible explanation for the higher prevalence in high-incidence populations is that large tumors are more likely to undergo necrosis, releasing pyrogenic substances into the circulation. Very rarely, patients with hepatocellular carcinoma may present as a "pyrexia of unknown origin" [28].

Although low-grade fever may be present in patients with cirrhosis, the finding of a persistently raised temperature should suggest the possibility of a hepatic neoplasm.

4.7 Jaundice

Patients with hepatocellular carcinoma may be jaundiced when first seen. This is more likely to occur in those in whom the tumor develops against a background of well-established cirrhosis, e.g., 44% of British patients [3] compared with 25% of southern African Blacks [4], although 39% of Taiwanese patients were noted to be jaundiced [12]. Icterus is usually of slight or moderate degree when the patient is first examined, but it tends to become progressively deeper (or it may appear for the first time) with progression of the disease. The jaundice is usually hepatocellular in origin, although in 1%–12% of patients it is obstructive in type [17–19]. Rarely, the clinical course of hepatocellular carcinoma may be mistaken for that of hepatitis or subacute massive hepatic necrosis.

4.8 Dilated abdominal veins

Dilated veins may be visible on the anterior abdominal wall of patients with hepatocellular carcinoma. These usually take the form of a "caput medusae" secondary to longstanding portal hypertension. Rarely, in Japanese and Black patients, collateral vessels resulting from chronic occlusion of the inferior vena cava by a congenital web or an atretic segment may be present [29, 30].

4.9 Signs of chronic liver disease

In patients in whom hepatocellular carcinoma develops against a background of advanced cirrhosis, physical signs of cirrhosis and perhaps hepatic failure may predominate. Spider nevi, palmar erythema, gynecomastia, and testicular atrophy may be present in these patients, especially when the cirrhosis is a consequence of alcohol abuse. For example, these signs were present in half of the patients in a series from Great Britain [4] but in only 16% of Taiwanese patients [12]; they are seldom seen in African patients.

4.10 Budd-Chiari syndrome

Hepatocellular carcinoma has a propensity to invade venous radicles in the liver. This occurs most often with the portal vein radicles, macroscopic evidence of invasion being found in about 70% of patients at necropsy [13, 17]. Invasion of the hepatic veins is less frequent but has equally important consequences. Malignant infiltration of the hepatic veins was found in 14% of Black patients at necropsy [17]. Tumorous obstruction of the hepatic veins produces the clinical picture of the Budd-Chiari syndrome with tense ascites and a uniformly enlarged tender liver. In about two-thirds of patients with hepatic vein infiltration, the tumor plug grows along the hepatic veins and enters the inferior vena cava [17]. The tumor-thrombus plug may completely or partially occlude the lumen of the inferior vena cava, causing the patient to develop severe pitting edema of the lower limbs. The tumor may grow up the inferior vena cava and into the right atrium, where it may be responsible for cardiac failure or cardiac arrythmias [31]. Either the right atrial tumor or a large tumor-embolus from the inferior vena cava may impact in the tricuspid valve, causing sudden death [32].

5 Rare sites for metastases

5.1 Skin

Cutaneous metastases are extremely rare in hepatocellular carcinoma [33]. They present as single or multiple, firm, painless, reddish-blue nodules, which may vary in size from 1 to 2.5 cm; they may enlarge rapidly. Cutaneous deposits of tumor in the surgical scar resulting from previous hepatic surgery have also been described [14].

5.2 Virchow-Troisier glands

Hepatocellular carcinoma rarely spreads to the supraclavicular lymph glands [34].

5.3 Maxillary gingiva

In seven reported patients, hepatocellular carcinoma metastasized to the maxillary gingiva [35].

5.4 Rectus abdominis muscle

An umbilical vein which has reopened as a result of prolonged portal hypertension may allow hepatocellular carcinoma to spread to the rectus abdominis muscle. One such case has been reported [36] and I have seen one additional patient.

5.5 Paranasal sinuses and parasellar region

Two patients have been described in whom hepatocellular carcinoma metastasized, presumably via Batson's vertebral venous plexus, to the sphenoid sinus [37]. The patients presented with orbital pain and ophthalmoplegia. Metastasis to the parasellar region has been reported in one patient with hepatocellular carcinoma [38]. The patient complained of pain and hyperesthesia of the side of the face.

6 Differential diagnosis

In low-risk populations, hepatocellular carcinoma must be distinguished mainly from cirrhosis and hepatic metastases. These two conditions are also important in the differential diagnosis in high-risk populations, although hepatic metastases are relatively less common. In addition, major diagnostic difficulties are posed by amebic hepatic abscesses, parasitic hepatic disease, and tuberculous hepatitis.

7 Paraneoplastic syndromes

Hepatocellular carcinoma is capable of producing a large number and a great diversity of paraneoplastic phenomena [39]. Most of these result in characteristic biochemical changes rather than clinically recognizable syndromes. However, the latter are important because they may precede the local manifestations of the tumor and may direct the clinician's attention to the presence of hepatocellular carcinoma. The clinically important paraneoplastic syndromes associated with hepatocellular carcinoma are hypoglycemia, erythrocytosis, hypercalcemia, and hypercholesterolemia. Rare syndromes are porphyria cutanea tarda, feminization, carcinoid syndrome, hypertrophic osteoarthropathy, hypertension, and hyperthyroidism.

8   Hypoglycemia

The frequency with which hypoglycemia complicates hepatocellular carcinoma is uncertain. The reason for the confusion is the discrepancy between the high prevalence reported in Hong Kong Chinese (27%) [40] and in South America (24%) [40] and the much lower figures recorded in southern African Blacks (6.7%) [17] and in North America (4.6%) [14].

McFadzean and Yeung [40] described two forms of hypoglycemia in Chinese patients with hepatocellular carcinoma. The first occurred during the last few weeks of life in patients with a rapidly growing and poorly differentiated tumor accompanied by rapid wasting and severe muscular weakness (type A). This form of hypoglycemia was characterized by moderate decreases in fasting blood sugar levels, which were readily controlled. Patients with type A hypoglycemia are usually not obviously symptomatic from the glycopenia, although they have severe symptoms attributable to the advanced tumor, and a low blood sugar level may easily be overlooked unless specifically sought. This may offer a partial explanation for the discrepancies in the recorded prevalence of hypoglycemia in different series. The second form of this complication (type B) was characterized by severe hypoglycemia, which manifested early in the course of the disease in patients with a slowly growing and well-differentiated tumor and was difficult to control. These patients present to the doctor with acute neuropsychiatric syndromes, convulsions, stupor, or coma, and the underlying hepatocellular carcinoma may easily be missed. They have a poor prognosis because of the severity of the glycopenia, which is unresponsive to corticosteroids, glucagon, thiazides, and diazoxide.

While there are unquestionably two forms of hypoglycemia in southern African Blacks with hepatocellular carcinoma (corresponding to types A and B) and some of the patients fit readily into one or other category, this is not always so [17]. Analysis of the degree of histological differentiation of the tumor does not reveal a clear separation between poorly differentiated tumors with mild, late hypoglycemia and well-differentiated tumors with severe, early hypoglycemia. Furthermore, late hypoglycemia is not always easy to control. Therefore, when Black patients, who usually seek medical attention late in the course of the disease, present with glycopenia, it may be impossible to decide in which category of hypoglycemia they belong.

Recent reports have suggested an association between the clear-cell variant of hepatocellular carcinoma and hypoglycemia [41, 42].

The pathogenesis of hypoglycemia in patients with hepatocellular carcinoma is not fully understood. Different pathogenetic mechanisms are almost certainly operative in the two types of the disorder. Hypoglycemia may occur during the terminal stages of any malignant disease [43], as well as in patients with malnutrition or inanition [44]. The mechanism of this metabolic disturbance is not known. In the case of hepatocellular carcinoma, an important factor might be that replacement of liver tissue by the tumor may have become so extensive by this stage that there is insufficient unaffected hepatic tissue to meet the combined demands for glucose by the large and perhaps rapidly growing tumor and the other tissues of the body.

This mechanism per se would not account for type B hypoglycemia. Nor is there evidence of production of insulin or an insulinotropic substance by the tumor [17]. Although two of four patients studied by Gorden et al. [45] had raised levels of insulinlike growth factors I and II— substances with insulinlike activity (ILA)—this was not confirmed in a larger series of Black patients with hypoglycemia [46].

Glycolysis is accelerated in many rapidly growing experimental hepatomas [47]. This results mainly from a reversion in the malignant cells to a fetal glycolytic mechanism which is no longer subject to host regulation. However, although human tumors are frequently rapidly growing, there is as yet no proof that enhanced glycolysis and glucose utilization are themselves responsible for hypoglycemia. Moreover, hepatic tissue is capable of an enormous increase in glucose output, which should normally compensate for increased glucose utilization by the tumor. It has also been suggested that glucose may be able to enter malignant cells in the absence of insulin, and this may contribute to a large hepatocellular carcinoma acting as a "sponge" for glucose [47].

Some patients with hepatocellular carcinoma have impaired glycogenolysis, as shown by a subnormal response to glucagon and a substantially reduced phosphorylase activity [48]. In addition, gluconeogenesis may be impaired [48]. These disturbances affect both the normal hepatic tissue and the tumor and offer a possible explanation for type B hypoglycemia.

9 Erythrocytosis

Erythrocytosis occurs in 3%–12% of patients with hepatocellular carcinoma and is one of the better known paraneoplastic syndromes which complicate this tumor [39]. In spite of this, the pathogenesis of the increased red cell mass is poorly understood. Using a relatively insensitive biological assay, raised serum erythropoietic activity has been demonstrated in some but not all of the few patients investigated in detail, suggesting that the increased red cell mass may result from production and secretion of erythropoietin or an erythropoietinlike substance by the tumor. Assay of tumor tissue has more often than not failed to show such activity. However, malignant hepatocytes from a patient with erythrocytosis and hepatocellular carcinoma grown in tissue culture have recently been shown to produce a substance with erythropoietinlike activity [49].

Erythropoietin is produced by the fetal liver [50], and although the kidney is the main source of erythropoietin in man, the liver has been shown to produce this hormone in the presence of uremia (especially in anephric subjects), in response to hypoxia or hemolysis, or when hepatocytes are regenerating [50]. Using a recently introduced radioimmunoassay with a limit of sensitivity for erythropoietin of 5 μg/ml, raised erythropoietin values were demonstrated in one-quarter of southern African Blacks with hepatocellular carcinoma having normal or increased hemoglobin and packed cell volume [51]; 58% of these patients are anemic when they are first seen [52]. However, only one of the patients had erythrocytosis as judged by hemoglobin and hematocrit values. Possible explanations for this apparent anomaly include an expanded plasma volume attributable to cirrhosis (present in 60% of southern African Blacks with hepatocellular carcinoma) [4], counteraction of the effect of increased serum erythropoietin concentrations by the inhibition of erythropoiesis (occurs in advanced malignant disease), or the possibility that the ectopically produced erythropoietin is not always biologically active [51].

The appearance of erythrocytosis in a patient known to have cirrhosis is highly suggestive of the development of hepatocellular carcinoma developed.

10 Hypercalcemia

Although symptomatic hypercalcemia does occur in patients with hepatocellular carcinoma, the prevalence of this paraneoplastic syndrome has not been defined [39]. The symptoms resulting from hypercalcemia (confusion, weakness, malaise, depression, coma, anorexia, nausea, and vomiting) may easily mask those of the underlying tumor, causing the latter to be overlooked.

Hypercalcemia in malignant disease is most often associated with the presence of osteolytic metastases, and it is presumed that the increased serum calcium concentrations result from the release of calcium from bone [53]. Under normal circumstances, an increased mobilization of bone calcium—unless extremely rapid and widespread—should not cause severe hypercalcemia because of the normal homeostatic mechanisms and the renal clearance of calcium. Probably, therefore, some tumors produce not only factors responsible for bone resorption but also humoral factors which prevent renal clearance of calcium. The latter effect may be achieved by increasing tubular reabsorption of calcium, i.e., it acts like parathyroid hormone. True ectopic production of parathyroid hormone by tumors is extremely rare. It has not been proven to occur in patients with hepatocellular carcinoma, although convincing evidence for ectopic production of this hormone is available in one patient with a cholangiocarcinoma [54].

Many malignant tumors secrete factors which may resorb bone by enhancing osteoclastic activity [53]. Included among these are osteoclast-activating factor, prostaglandins, interleukin 1, and several growth factors derived from tumors (some similar to epidermal growth factor). However, up until the present time, there is no evidence that any of these factors are produced by hepatocellular carcinomas.

11 Hypercholesterolemia

A raised serum cholesterol concentration has been reported to occur in as many as 38% of patients with hepatocellular carcinoma [5, 39]. In the absence of cholestasis, this finding may point to the diagnosis of the tumor, particularly in Blacks.

The pathogenesis of the hypercholesterolemia has not been fully elucidated. However, there is evidence in both human and animal hepatomas that cholesterol biosynthesis in the tumor is autonomous [55–57]. Studies on experimental hepatomas in animals have shown that malignant hepatocytes lack receptors for chylomicron remnants (in spite of having coated pits on the cell surfaces) [58]. Chylomicron remnants and hence cholesterol do not, therefore, enter the malignant hepatocytes and exert an inhibitory effect on β-hydroxy-β-methylglutaryl-CoA (HMG CoA) reductase, the rate-limiting enzyme in cholesterol biosynthesis.

12   Porphyria cutanea tarda

Porphyria cutanea tarda is a rare paraneoplastic syndrome associated with hepatocellular carcinoma [39]. Originally, Tio and his colleagues [59] reported an elderly woman who presented with acquired porphyria. Her urine contained excessive quantities of uro- and coproporphyrin and her stools had large amounts of proto- and coproporphyrin. Her symptoms and the increased porphyrin excretion disappeared after a hepatic tumor, initially described as a liver cell adenoma but subsequently believed to be a hepatocellular carcinoma, was resected. Large quantities of porphyrins were demonstrated in the tumor tissue. Since then, about a dozen similar patients have been reported [60].

One patient with hepatocellular carcinoma has recently been described in whom markedly elevated levels of porphobilinogen were found in the urine and feces but who showed no clinical evidence of porphyria [61].

13   Sexual changes

Three types of sexual change have been described in patients with hepatocellular carcinoma, viz. isosexual precocity, gynecomastia, and feminization [39]. In other patients with this tumor, rised serum concentrations of human chorionic gonadotropin or human placental lactogen are found but they are not accompanied by clinically evident sexual changes [39].

13.1   Isosexual precocity

Although the majority of patients with isosexual precocity complicating hepatic tumors have had hepatoblastomas, hepatocellular carcinoma was responsible in at least six of the reported cases. Sexual precocity is attributed to ectopic production of gonadotropin by the tumor [62]. The children have adult serum testosterone levels.

The apparent limitation of the syndrome to males points to elaboration by the tumor of a substance possessing mainly interstitial cell-stimulating properties capable of stimulating the release of testicular androgens.

13.2   Gynecomastia

A few patients with hepatocellular carcinoma have been noted to have gynecomastia [63]. Elucidation of the pathogenesis of the breast enlargement in these patients is complicated by the frequent coexistence of hepatocellular carcinoma with cirrhosis, which may itself be responsible for gynecomastia. In the one published patient with hepatocellular carcinoma in the absence of cirrhosis, no cause for the gynecomastia was ascertained [63].

13.3   Feminization

Four patients with hepatocellular carcinoma and feminization in the absence of cirrhosis have been described [39]. The pathogenesis of the sexual changes was not determined in the first two. In the third patient, the tumor tissue was shown to behave as trophoblastic tissue, converting circulating dehydroepiandrosterone and dehydroepiandrosterone sulfate to estrone and estradiole [64]. All signs of feminization disappeared and the serum sex hormone changes reverted to normal after successful resection of the tumor.

Raised serum estradiol and urinary estrogen levels were documented in the fourth patient [65]. The responsible mechanism was not elucidated, but the sex hormone values returned to normal and all signs of feminization disappeared after the patient was treated with chemotherapy.

14   Cutaneous signs

Cutaneous signs have rarely been described in association with hepatocellular carcinoma. In fact, some of those reported are so rare that they may well have been coincidental. Vitiligo [66] and thrombophlebitis migrans [67] have been described in one patient each. Cutaneous changes of porphyria and the carcinoid syndrome are occasionally seen.

Pityriasis rotunda (circumscripta) has been reported in Japanese and Black patients with hepatocellular carcinoma [68, 69]. The lesions occur on the trunk, buttocks, and thighs and are round, hyperpigmented, and scaly. They vary in size from 0.5 to 25 cm in diameter and may be solitary or multiple. A preliminary analysis indicates that pityriasis rotunda may occur in 10%–15% of older Black patients with hepatocellular carcinoma.

15 Carcinoid syndrome

One patient with hepatocellular carcinoma presenting with some of the features of the carcinoid syndrome has been described [70]. The patient complained of explosive diarrhoea and fainting, and an abdominal mass was found. Urinary 5-hydroxyindole acetic acid, total 5-hydroxyindoles and serotonin concentrations were increased. Indole derivatives and increased tryptophan hydrolase activity were demonstrated in the tumor, which had the biochemical characteristics of a carcinoid tumor of foregut origin but the histopathological features of hepatocellular carcinoma. The tumor was shown to synthesize albumin and fibrinogen, proving it to be of hepatic origin.

16 Hypertrophic osteoarthropathy

Two patients with hypertrophic osteoarthropathy complicating hepatocellular carcinoma have been reported [71]. Ectopic production of growth hormone has been suggested as the cause of hypertrophic osteoarthropathy in patients with carcinoma of the lung and other tumors [72]. However, similar concentrations of growth hormone have been found in patients with and without this syndrome, and there is as yet no convincing evidence for ectopic growth hormone production by tumors.

Of the two patients with hypertrophic osteoarthropathy complicating hepatocellular carcinoma, pulmonary metastases were present in one but were not commented upon in the other [71]. Immunoreactive growth hormone levels were not measured in either patient.

17 Hypertension

A single patient with hypertension complicating hepatocellular carcinoma has been reported [73]. The plasma angiotensinogen concentration was markedly raised and the tumor tissue, assayed postmortem, contained extremely high levels of angiotensinogen. The authors postulated that the patient's high blood pressure resulted from ectopic production of angiotensinogen by the tumor.

18 Polyneuropathy

The other system, apart from the skin, which seems largely to have escaped from paraneoplastic phenomena in hepatocellular carcinoma is the nervous system. There is, however, a recent report of one patient with a sensorimotor polyneuropathy affecting all four limbs [74]. The authors felt that other possible causes of polyneuritis such as alcohol abuse and cirrhosis could reasonably be excluded and, consequently, that the neuropathy was indeed a nonmetastatic manifestation of hepatocellular carcinoma.

19 Hyperthyroidism

A single patient has been reported in whom hepatocellular carcinoma was accompanied by clinically evident hyperthyroidism [75]. Serum concentrations of thyroid-stimulating hormone, T4, T3, and free T3 were appreciably increased. The authors postulated that the tumor produced a substance which stimulated the synthesis and secretion of thyroid-stimulating hormone, which in turn was responsible for hyperthyroidism.

In other patients without clinically evident hyperthyroidism, increased levels of thyroxine-binding globulin have been demonstrated [76].

References

1. Purves LR (1967) Alpha-fetoprotein and the diagnosis of liver cell cancer. In: Cameron HM, Linsell CA, Warwick GP (eds) Liver cell cancer. Elsevier, Amsterdam, pp 61–80
2. Chlebowski RT, Tong M, Weissman J, Block JB, Ramming KP, Weiner JM, Bateman JR, Chlebowski J (1984) Hepatocellular carcinoma. Diagnostic and prognostic features in North American patients. Cancer 53: 2701–2706
3. Kew MC, Dos Santos HA, Sherlock S (1971) Diagnosis of primary cancer of the liver. Br Med J 4: 408–411
4. Kew MC, Geddes EW (1982) Hepatocellular carcinoma in rural southern African Blacks. Medicine 61: 98–108
5. Alpert ME, Hutt MSR, Davidson CS (1969) Primary hepatoma in Uganda. Am J Med 46: 794–802
6. Epstein S (1964) Primary carcinoma of the liver. Am J Med Sci 48: 137–143

7. Lai CL, Lam KC, Wong KP, Wu PC, Todd D (1981) Clinical features of hepatocellular carcinoma: Review of 211 patients in Hong Kong. Cancer 47: 2746–2755

8. Melia WM, Wilkinson ML, Portmann BC, Johnson PJ, Williams R (1984) Hepatocellular carcinoma in the non-cirrhotic liver: A comparison with that complicating cirrhosis. Quart J Med 53: 391–400

9. Craig JR, Peters RL, Edmondson HA, Omata M (1980) Fibrolamellar carcinoma of the liver: A tumor of adolescents and young adults with distinctive clinicopathologic features. Cancer 46: 372–379

10. Tang Z-Y (1985) Subclinical hepatocellular carcinoma. China Academic Publishers, Beijing

11. Gelfand M, Castle WM, Buchanan WM (1972) Primary carcinoma of the liver (hepatoma) in Rhodesia. S Afr Med J 46: 527–532

12. Sung JL, Wang TH, Yu JY (1976) Clinical study of primary carcinoma of the liver in Taiwan. Am J Dig Dis 12: 1036–1049

13. Okuda K (1976) Clinical aspects of hepatocellular carcinoma—analysis of 134 cases. In: Okuda K, Peters RL (eds) Hepatocellular carcinoma. Wiley, New York, pp 387–436

14. Ihde DC, Sherlock P, Winawer SJ, Fortner JG (1974) Clinical manifestations of hepatoma. Am J Med 56: 83–91

15. Luna G, Florence L, Johansen K (1985) Hepatocellular carcinoma. A 5 year institutional experience. Am J Surg 149: 591–594

16. El-Domeiri AA, Huvos AG, Goldsmith HS, Foote FW (1971) Primary malignant tumors of the liver. Cancer 27: 7–11

17. Kew MC, Paterson AC (1985) Unusual clinical presentations of hepatocellular carcinoma. Trop Gastroenterol 6: 10–22

18. Kojiro M, Kawabata K, Kawano Y, Shirai F, Takemoto N, Nakashima T (1982) Hepatocellular carcinoma presenting as intra-bile duct tumor growth. Cancer 48: 2144–2147

19. Roslyn JJ, Kuchenbecker S, Longmire WP, Thompkins RK (1984) Floating tumor debris. A cause of intermittent biliary obstruction. Arch Surg 119: 1312–1315

20. Brand SN, Brand LJ, Sprayregan S, Brenner S, Bernstein LH (1976) Extra-hepatic biliary tract obstruction secondary to a hepatoma-containing blood clot in the common bile duct. Dig Dis 21: 905–909

21. Chearanai O, Plengvanit U, Asavanich C, Damrongsak D, Sundhvananda K, Boonyapsit S (1983) Spontaneous rupture of primary hepatoma. Cancer 51: 1532–1536

22. Carayon A, Courson B, Virieu R (1967) Compression modulaire par metastase d'un foie cliniquent inapparent. Bull Soc Med Afr Noire Lang Fr 13: 586–593

23. Okazaki H, Yoshimo M, Yoshida T, Hirohashi S, Kishi K, Shimosato Y (1985) Bone metastasis in hepatocellular carcinoma. Cancer 55: 1991–1994

24. Byrne MJ, Scheinberg MA, Mavligit G, Dawkins RL (1972) Hepatocellular carcinoma: presentation with metastases and radicular compression. Cancer 30: 202–205

25. Levy JI, Geddes EW, Kew MC (1976) The chest radiograph in primary liver cancer. S Afr Med J 50: 1323–1326

26. Willett IR, Sutherland RC, O'Rourke MF, Dudley FJ (1984) Pulmonary hypertension complicating hepatocellular carcinoma. Gastroenterology 87: 1180–1184

27. Horie Y, Suou T, Hirayama C, Nagasako N (1982) Spontaneous rupture of the spleen secondary to metastatic hepatocellular carcinoma: A report of a case and review of the literature. Am J Gastroenterol 77: 882–884

28. Stein CM, Gelfand M (1985) Hepatocellular carcinoma presenting as a fever of undetermined origin. Cent Afr J Med 31: 21–22

29. Nakamura T, Nakamura S, Aikawa T (1968) Obstruction of the inferior vena cava in the hepatic portion and hepatic veins. Report of 8 cases and review of the Japanese literature. Angiology 19: 479–498

30. Simson IW (1982) Membranous obstruction of the inferior vena cava and hepatocellular carcinoma in southern Africa. Gastroenterology 82: 171–179

31. Kato R, Tanaka N, Kobayashi K, Ikeda T, Hattori N, Nonamura N (1983) Growth of hepatocellular carcinoma into the right atrium. Ann Intern Med 99: 472–474

32. Dajani YF (1977) Hepatoma causing a massive tumor embolus. Postgrad Med J 53: 405–408

33. Reingold RM, Smith BR (1978) Cutaneous metastases from hepatomas. Arch Dermatol 114: 1045–1046

34. Schwarz KO, Schwartz IJ, Marchervky A (1982) Virchow-Troiier's lymph node as a presenting sign of hepatocellular carcinoma. Mt Sinai J Med 48: 59–62

35. Morishita M, Fukuda J (1984) Hepatocellular carcinoma metastatic to the maxillary nasal gingiva. J Oral Maxillofac Surg 42: 812–815

36. Kim SY, Lim JH (1985) Extension of hepatoma to the rectus abdominis muscle via ligamentum teres hepatis. Gastrointest Radiol 10: 119–121

37. Waxman JS, Seife B, Waxman M (1985) Hepatocellular carcinoma presenting as sphenoid sinus metastasis. Mt Sinai J Med 52: 221–224

38. Bith S, Hasgawa H, Ohtsuki H, Obashi J, Kobayashi Y (1985) Parasellar metastases: Four autopsied cases. Surg Neurol 23: 41–48

39. Kew MC, Dusheiko GM (1981) Paraneoplastic manifestations of hepatocellular carcinoma. In: PD Berk, TC Chalmers (eds) Frontiers in liver disease. Thieme-Stratton, New York, pp 305–319

40. McFadzean AJS, Yeung RTT (1969) Further observations on hypoglycemia in hepatocellular carcinoma. Am J Med 47: 220–235

41. Sasaki K, Okuda S, Takahashi M, Sasaki M (1981) Hepatic clear cell carcinoma associated with hypoglycemia and hypercholesterolemia. Cancer 47: 820–822

42. Ross JS, Kurian S (1985) Clear cell hepatocellular carcinoma: Sudden death from hypoglycemia. Am J Gastroenterol 80: 188–194

43. Wanebo HJ, Schessinger I, Tashima CK (1966) Severe hypoglycemia associated with terminal lymphomas. Cancer 19: 1451–1458

44. Elias AN, Gwinup G (1982) Glucose-resistant hypoglycemia in inanition. Arch Intern Med 142: 743–746

45. Gorden P, Hendricks CM, Kahn CR, Megeyesi K, Ross J (1981) Hypoglycemia associated with non-islet cell tumor and insulin-like growth factors. N Engl J Med 305: 1452–1455

46. Widmer U, Zapf J, Froesch ER, Kew MC (1983) Insulin-like growth factor levels measured by radioimmunoassay and radioreceptor assay in various forms of tumor hypoglycemia. In: Spencer M (ed), Insulin-like growth factors/somatomedins. De Gruyter, Berlin, pp 317–323

47. Horecker BL, Hiatt HH (1958) Pathways of carbohydrate metabolism in normal and neoplastic cells. N Engl J Med 258: 177–184

48. Landon BR, Wills N, Craig RW, Leonard CR, Moriwaki T (1962) The mechanism of hepatoma induced hypoglycemia. Cancer 15: 1188–1196

49. Okabe T, Urabe A, Kato T, Chiba S, Takaku F (1985) Production of erythropoietin-like activity by human renal and hepatic carcinomas in cell culture. Cancer 55: 1918–1923

50. Fried W (1972) The liver as a source of extra-renal erythropoietin production. Blood 40: 671–677

51. Kew MC, Fisher JW (1986) Serum erythropoietin concentrations in patients with hepatocellular carcinoma. Cancer 58: 2485–2488

52. Jacobson RJ, Lowenthal MN, Kew MC (1978) Erythrocytosis in hepatocellular carcinoma. S Afr Med J 53: 658–660

53. Stevenson JG (1985) Malignant hypercalcemia. Br Med J 291: 421–422

54. Knill-Jones RP, Buckle RM, Parsons V, Williams R (1970) Hypercalcemia and increased parathyroid hormone activity in primary hepatoma. N Engl J Med 282: 704–708

55. Goldberg RB, Bersohn I, Kew MC (1975) Hypercholesterolemia in primary cancer of the liver. S Afr Med J 49: 1464–1466

56. Harry DS, Morris HP, McIntyre N (1971) Cholesterol biosynthesis in transplantable hepatomas: Evidence for impairment of uptake and storage of dietary cholesterol. J Lipid Res 72: 313–317

57. Brown MS, Dana SE, Siperstein MD (1974) Properties of 3-hydroxy-3-methyl glutaryl co-enzyme A reductase solubilized from rat liver and hepatoma. J Biol Chem 249: 6586–6589

58. Danilewitz MD, Herrerra GA, Kew MC, Mendelsohn D, Barnes S, Alexander CB, Hirschowitz BI, Spenney JG (11984) Autonomous cholesterol biosynthesis in murine hepatoma. A receptor defect with normal coated pits. Cancer 54: 1562–1568

59. Tio TH, Lejinse B, Jarret A, Rimington C (1957) Acquired porphyria from a liver tumor. Clin Sci 16: 517–527

60. Keczkes K, Barker DJ (1976) Malignant hepatoma associated with acquired hepatic cutaneous porphyria. Arch Dermatol 112: 78–82

61. Pierach CA, Bossenmairer IC, Cardinal RA, Weiner MK (1984) Pseudo-porphyria in a patient with hepatocellular carcinoma. Am J Med 76: 545–548

62. McArthur JW, Toll GD, Russfield AB (1973) Sexual precocity attributable to ectopic gonadotropin secretion by hepatoblastoma. Am J Med 54: 390–403

63. Summerskill WHS, Adson MA (1962) Gynecomastia as a sign of hepatoma. Am J Dig Dis 7: 250–254

64. Kew MC, Kirschner MA, Abrahams GE, Katz M (1977) Mechanism of feminization in primary liver cancer. N Engl J Med 296: 1084–1088

65. Aabo K, Dimitrov NV (1980) Feminization in hepatocellular carcinoma corrected by chemotherapy: A case report. Med Pediat Oncol 8: 275–280

66. Curth W (1969) Hepatoma. Arch Dermatol 99: 374–375

67. Nusbacher J (1964) Migratory venous thrombosis and cancer. New York J Med 64: 2166–2173

68. Ito M, Tanaka T (11960) Pseudo-ichtyose acquise en taches circulaires. Ann Derm Et Syphil 87: 826–837

69. DiBisceglie AM, Hodkinson HJ, Berkowitz I, Kew MC (1986) Pityriasis rotunda—a cutaneous sign of hepatocellular carcinoma in southern African Blacks. Arch Dermatol 122: 802–804

70. Primack A, Wilson J, O'Connor GT, Engelman K, Hull E, Cavellos GP (1971) Hepatocellular carcinoma and the carcinoid syndrome. Cancer 27: 1182–1189

71. Morgan AG, Walker WC, Mason MK (1972) A new syndrome associated with hepatocellular carcinoma. Gastroenterology 63: 340–345

72. Sparagnana N, Philips G, Hoffman C, Kucera L (1971) Ectopic growth hormone syndrome associated with lung cancer. Metabolism 20: 730–736

73. Ueno N, Yoshida K, Hirose S, Yokoyama H (1984) Angiotensinogen-producing hepatocellular carcinoma. Hypertension 6: 931–933

74. Calvey HD, Melia WM, Williams R (1983) Polyneuropathy: An unreported non-metastatic complication of hepatocellular carcinoma. Clin Oncol 9: 199–202

75. Helzeberg JH, McPhee MS, Zarling EJ, Lukert BP (1985) Hepatocellular carcinoma: An unusual course with hyperthyroidism and inappropriate thyroid-stimulating hormone production. Gastroenterology 88: 181–184

76. Kalk JW, Kew MC, Danilewitz MD, Jacks F, van der Walt LA, Levin J (1982) Thyroxine-binding globulin and thyroid function tests in patients with hepatocellular carcinoma. Hepatology 2: 72–76

Part II
Clinical Aspects

Chapter 16
Small Hepatocellular Carcinoma

Kunio Okuda[1] and Masamichi Kojiro[2]

The poor prognosis of hepatocellular carcinoma (HCC) is due in part to the difficulties in early diagnosis. Only after the advent of real-time ultrasonography (US) has early detection become possible. Japanese gastroenterologists soon realized that this modality is most effective in the detection of small HCC [1–3], and a program for early detection has since been established in most gastrointestinal units throughout Japan. In this chapter, the historical background of the early diagnosis of HCC and current experience and understanding of small HCC in Japan and elsewhere will be presented.

1 Mass screening for asymptomatic HCC

In the early 1970s, using a test for alphafetoprotein (AFP), an attempt was made by Masseyeff [4] in Senegal to screen normal persons for early HCC, because this cancer is very common among African Blacks. Masseyeff screened 9000 male workers on three occasions and found HCC in three apparently healthy individuals. However, the tumor could be resected in only one of them. Purves et al. [5] screened gold miners who were sent from Mozambique to work around Johannesburg for elevated serum AFP levels; the miners were known to have a high risk of developing HCC. Radioimmunoassay (RIA) and immunodiffusion methods were used in more than 5000 and 4000 miners, respectively; not a single case of HCC was detected.

The government of the People's Republic of China set out to determine the regional incidence of various cancers as a major health program. This national study, which survived the Cultural Revolution of 1966–1976, utilized the extensive medical network involving barefooted doctors and local hospitals, and 250 000 physicians and their 600 000 assistants were mobilized in a mass survey in 29 provinces, which included 2392 counties with 840 million people as the study population [6]. From this campaign emerged a program for early detection of primary liver cancer. Screening with an AFP test began in China in 1971. First, the Ouchterlony technique and subsequently counter-immunoelectrophoresis and more sensitive semiquantitative methods were employed. For instance, 1 223 912 people were screened during the period of 1974–1979 in Qidong County, where 475 cases of HCC were found. Of these, 35.2% were asymptomatic [7]. Many similar screenings have since been carried out in China; a considerable number of the patients were eventually treated surgically.

2 Clinical follow-up

In 1975, Okuda et al. [8] reported five cases of small HCC detected during routine clinical follow-up. In two of them, a sharp rise in serum AFP aroused suspicion and subsequent scintigraphy and angiography disclosed an HCC. In the other two cases, serum AFP was only slightly but continuously elevated, and the diagnosis was made using imaging studies. Okuda et al. [8] called to attention a group of patients with chronic liver disease in whom serum AFP is continuously elevated, though below the level diagnostic for HCC, and suggested that they were likely to have a small HCC [9]. In 1977, the same group studied 16 autopsied and four resected HCC lesions smaller than 4.5 cm in diameter and concluded that such small HCCs are frequently

[1] First Department of Medicine, Chiba University School of Medicine, Inohana, Chiba, 280 Japan
[2] The First Department of Pathology, Kurume University School of Medicine, Kurume 830 Japan

encapsulated and well-differentiated [10]. Kubo et al. [11] made a diagnosis of HCC in 31 patients with cirrhosis during a clinical follow-up of 1–14 years (average 59 months). These patients comprised 11.2% of the clinical cases of HCC.

In a prospective study, Obata et al. [12] followed a total of 115 patients with cirrhosis in Tokyo and observed the development of HCC in 12 cases. Whereas 7 of 30 Hepatitis B serum antigen (HBsAg)-positive patients developed HCC during this period, the emergence of HCC occurred in only 5 of 85 seronegative cases. Following a continuation of the study, the same group suggested more recently that the proportion of HBsAg-positive cases is decreasing, with a simultaneous increase in seronegative HCC caues. The causes of this change in the relative incidence now seems to be due to increasing chronic non-A non-B hepatitis and cirrhosis in Japan [13].

3   Imaging of small HCC

Before the advent of real-time US, the imaging diagnosis of HCC was not a very sensitive measure, except for celiac angiography [14]. Radiocolloid scintigraphy is relatively insensitive [14, 15] and is only capable of recognizing HCC larger than 3 cm located near the anterior surface. Single-photon emission CT (SPECT) has not drastically improved sensitivity.

The characteristic angiographic features of HCC include arterial tumor vessels, increased arterial supply, vascular lakes and channels, and arterioportal shunts [16]. However, small HCC does not exhibit these angiographic features, and localized stains in the capillary phase are the only findings (see Chap. 21). A special technique called "infusion angiography" is now frequently used for the detection of small HCC [17, 18]. This technique stains not only small HCCs but also some large regenerative nodules, making differentiation difficult.

The role of X-ray computed tomograhy (CT) in the diagnosis of small HCC is rather limited. In our study, only one of seven HCCs smaller than 2 cm were recognized without enhancement, and bolus enhancement failed to improve diagnosis (Table 16.1). However, dynamic enhancement (Fig. 16.1) showed a positive scan in one of five 2- to 3-cm HCCs not recognized on plain CT, and three of four negative 3- to 5-cm HCCs [19]. According to Ebara et al. [20], the detection rate by magnetic resonance imaging was one of three HCCs smaller than 2 cm and eight of nine 2- to 3-cm HCCs. Lipiodol CT is perhaps the most sensitive imaging method [21–24]. In this technique, a catheter is introduced into the common or proper hepatic artery, a small amount of Lipiodol is injected, and a CT scan is made 1–2 weeks later. Lipiodol is quickly cleared from noncancerous tissue whereas it remains in cancer tissue for a long period; a lesion as small as 3 mm may be detected (Fig. 16.2).

With improved imaging diagnosis, small-mass lesions are more frequently found in the liver, creating a problem in differential diagnosis. Benign hemangioma occurs in approximately 1% of the population and is readily detected by US. A very small hemangioma may be mistaken for HCC, although the former is usually hyperechoic. On dynamic CT, a hemangioma is enhanced from its periphery and the contrast medium remains for a long period of time, whereas a typical HCC is rapidly enhanced and the contrast medium leaves it quickly. Several inadvertent resections of small hemangiomas have been carried out in Japan as a result of overdiagnosis by US. It now seems that magnetic resonance imaging is particularly useful in the differential diagnosis of small HCC and hemangioma. According to Itai et al. [25] and our study [20], the majority of hemangiomas appear as a markedly high-intensity area with a spin-spin relaxation (T2) time longer than 80 ms.

Table 16.1. Detection of small HCC by X-ray CT scan

Tumor size (cm)	No. of patients	No. of positive scans	Change from negative to positive scans by bolus enhancement	Overall diagnostic accuracy after enhancement
<2	7	1 (14%)	0	14%
2–3	17	12 (71%)	1	92%
3–5	24	18 (75%)	3	92%

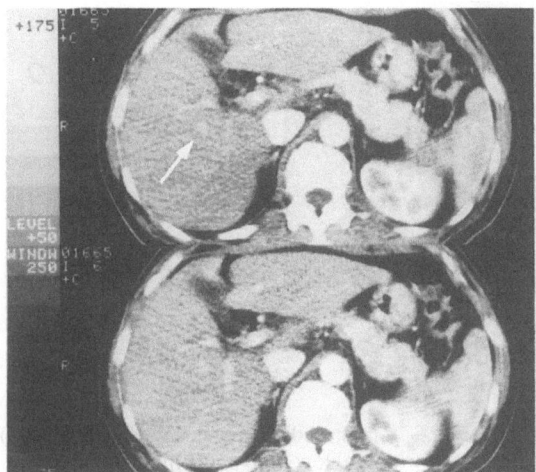

Fig. 16.1. Enhanced CT scan demonstrating a 1-cm lesion (*arrow*)

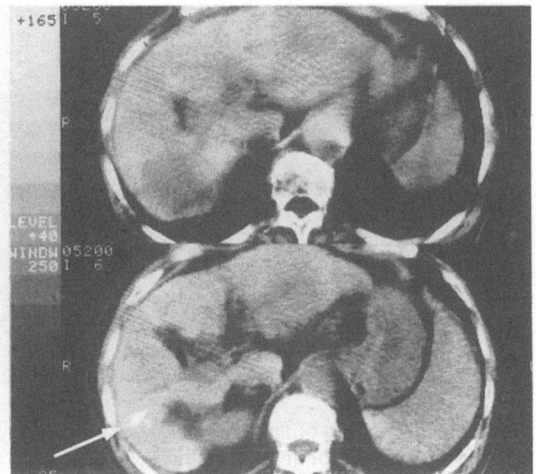

Fig. 16.2. Lipiodol CT demonstrating a 1-cm lesion (*arrow*)

4 Ultrasonography in small HCC and early detection program

With the electronically activated linear-array transducer, the hepatobiliary system may be examined in approximately 20 min. As real-time US became increasingly used, small HCC came to be found both in patients with no symptoms or signs attributable to HCC and in those with symptoms. Subclinical HCC is much more frequently found among patients with chronic liver disease during the clinical follow-up. Thus, gastroenterology units in Japan began a screening program within the hospitals in which patients with established or suspected cirrhosis and chronic active hepatitis were followed regularly by US combined with AFP measurement by RIA [2, 26]. In our experience, the diagnostic signifi-

cance of AFP is rather limited in small HCC, as shown in Fig. 16.3, but some patients with small HCC do show increased levels of AFP. Furthermore, as already discussed, mildly elevated AFP levels which do not fluctuate a great deal also suggest small HCC. Therefore, the determination of serum AFP is essential, unless a more specific and sensitive marker becomes available.

The follow-up interval should vary with the degree of the patient's risk of developing HCC. The minimal interval calculated from the time necessary for detecting a 1-cm increase in a 2-cm HCC by US was 3 months in our study [3], which also showed that the growth speed of small HCC may even be predicted from the echo pattern of the mass. Figure 16.4 represents one example of an intermediate speed of growth with a changing

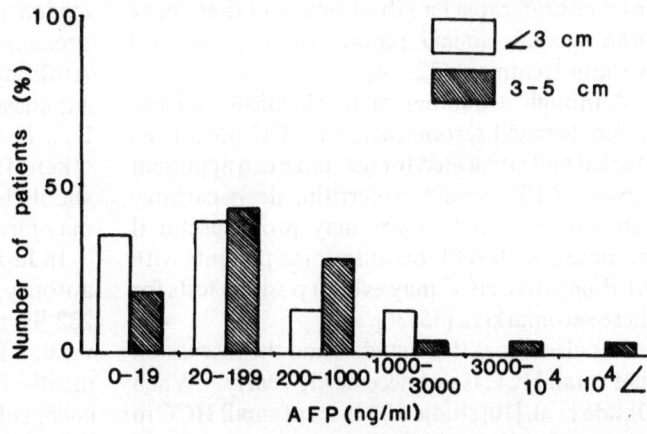

Fig. 16.3. Serum AFP levels in 51 HCCs smaller than 5 cm; 23 were smaller than 3 cm and 28 were between 3 and 4 cm. Note that about 74% of the former and 67% of the latter had AFP levels below 200 ng/ml, suggesting that semiquantitative tests would miss these patients

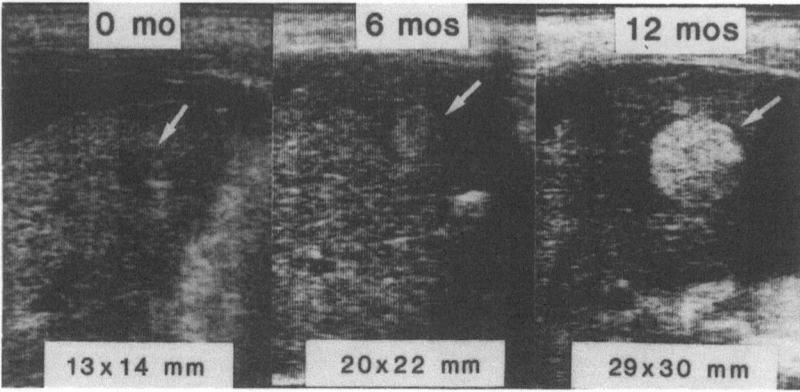

Fig. 16.4. Follow-up of an HCC by ultrasonography. This HCC of an intermediate growth speed (at arrows) had a low echo interior at the beginning. It changed to a pattern of peripheral low echo and a high-echo pattern. The doubling time of this HCC is calculated to be about 6 months

internal echo pattern.

The value of real-time US in the diagnosis of small HCC was soon realized by gastroenterologists in Taiwan, where the incidence of HCC is extremely high and Japanese ultrasonographs are readily available. Several groups in Taipei have been successful in the diagnosis of small HCC and they too adopted the same follow-up program [27–30]. Sheu et al. [29] measured the speed of tumor growth by US and suggested that by extrapolating the growth curve back to the point of size zero it would take 9.8 months to 10.9 years for an HCC to reach a size of 10 cm from the time of emergence. They also reasoned that since it takes 4.6 months for a rapidly growing 1-cm HCC to reach a size of 3 cm, screening at 4- to 5-month intervals should theoretically detect all tumors less than 3 cm. Okazaki et al. were the first to calculate growth speed in terms of the doubling time [31]. These studies, both in Japan and Taiwan, clearly demonstrated that the speed of growth varies tremendously from one HCC to another. Some HCCs remain unchanged in size for a considerable length of time and there have been several clinical reports of long survival without treatment [32–34].

Although a number of biochemical and immunochemical seromarkers of HCC have been studied and advocated for use, none can at present replace AFP. Serum isoferritin, des-γ-carboxy prothrombin, and others may prove useful if combined with AFP because some patients with AFP-negative HCC may exhibit positive tests for these seromarkers [35, 36].

It is clear from these studies and the discussion that small HCC is not necessarily "early." When Okuda et al. [10] studied 20 cases of small HCC in

1977, they defined "mimute" HCC as smaller than 4.5 cm simply because clinical detection of HCC smaller than this was then almost impossible. Within 5 years, as a result of wide use of real-time US, smaller HCCs came to be diagnosed in increasing numbers. In 1983, when the Japan Liver Cancer Study Group published the "General Rules for the Clinical and Pathological Study of Primary Liver Cancer" [37], the definition of "small" HCC was lesions less than 2 cm.

5 Histopathology of small HCC

In the past, many pathologists looked for early lesions of liver cancer in humans and failed to identify unequivocal lesions. Anthony emphasized the presence of dysplastic cells as a putative precursor lesion of HCC [38, 39]. He also demonstrated the close relationship between these and HBsAg-positivity. Although the close relationship between dysplasia and HCC was subsequently confirmed outside Africa [40–42], direct evidence that these dysplastic cells are in fact preneoplastic is lacking. The hypothesis of Anthony has been refuted by several groups of Japanese histopathologists [42–44]. Nevertheless, if dysplasia is seen in a biopsy specimen taken from an HBsAg-positive patient, one should be alerted that the patient may develop or may already have an HCC in the liver.

In Japan, a small HCC is occasionally found at autopsy. In 1984, Nakashima et al. [45] studied 232 livers with HCC autopsied at Kurume University Hospital and found 23 minute HCCs, mostly incidentally; the HCCs were frequently encapsulated [46] and the livers bearing such can-

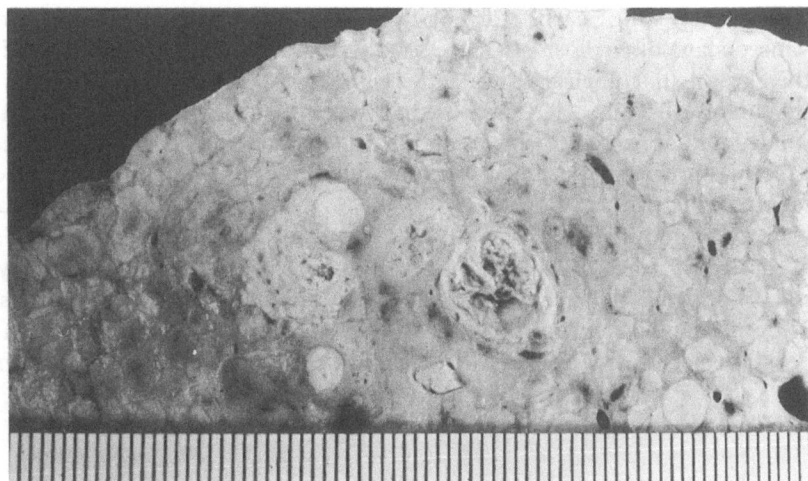

Fig. 16.5. There are five 3- to 10-mm HCCs in an area of about 3 cm square. The largest 1-cm mass shows a necrotizing tendency. A number of portal vessels are invaded in this area. *Scale* in millimeters

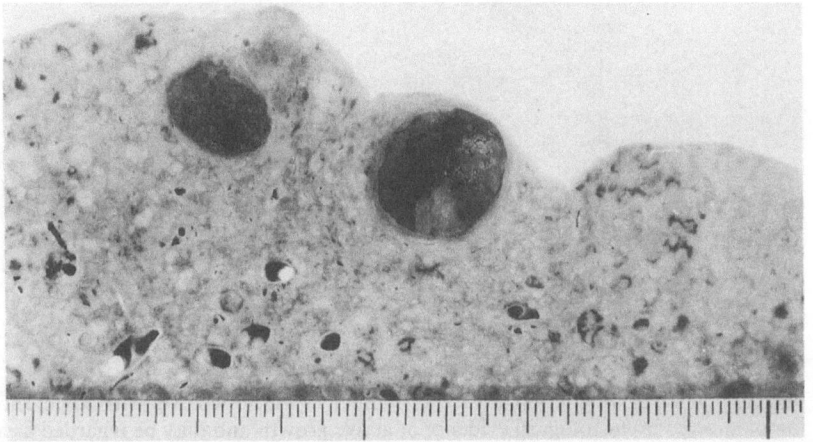

Fig. 16.6. Two green HCCs, 2 cm and 1.5 cm in size, are seen in close approximation. Histologically, both were well-differentiated and produced bile, suggesting the same cancer cell clone or a metastatic origin for the smaller one

cers were small. As more small HCCs came to be clinically detected and resected, it was realized that small HCCs incidentally found at autopsy were not exactly the same as those resected surgically. We studied 27 autopsied small HCC (less than 2 cm) and 25 resected small HCCs with the following results. Only 14 of 27 autopsy cases of small HCC had a solitary HCC; the remaining 13 (48.1%) had more than one lesion. In contrast, all 25 resected small HCCs were solitary. In 11 of 13 cases with multiple HCCs, the tumors were present in the same segment of the liver or close together, as shown in Figs. 16.5 and 16.6. Judging from the similarity of the gross morphology and frequent early intraportal invasion (seen in

5 of 13 cases), it seemed more likely that these lesions in close approximation were due to portal metastases rather than a multicentric emergence of HCC. The difference in the frequency of solitary lesions between the autopsy and surgical material may be due to the selection of patients for resection—multiple lesions are seldom considered for surgery. In other hospitals in Japan, however, resection of multiple lesions is not uncommon, provided that the lesions are not too far apart.

Another observation made was the stage of cirrhosis in which a small HCC was found at autopsy. In one-third of the autopsy cases of small HCC, the weight of the liver was 500–

700 g, suggesting marked atrophy or an advanced stage of cirrhosis. In some small HCCs, there was no histological sign of active growth of the tumor cells. Such HCCs were usually encapsulated and appeared to correspond to "latent" cancers known to occur in the thyroid and prostate (Fig. 16.7).

Grossly, about 90% of small HCCs, whether autopsied or resected, had a fibrous pseudocapsule of varying thickness; some capsules were incomplete. The frequent presence of a capsule does not necessarily exclude the spreading (in-filtrating) growth pattern [47] in small HCC, because small spreading HCC is not readily identified by imaging; expanding HCC is more easily detected. Furthermore, spreading-type HCC occurs more frequently in a noncirrhotic liver and is rarely detected in its early stage. The patient does not succumb to the disease at that stage and hence small spreading HCC is seldom autopsied. Presumably, the incidence of spreading HCC in its early stage (Fig. 16.8) is just as frequent as that in an advanced stage, namely, one of three cases in our autopsy material [48]. It

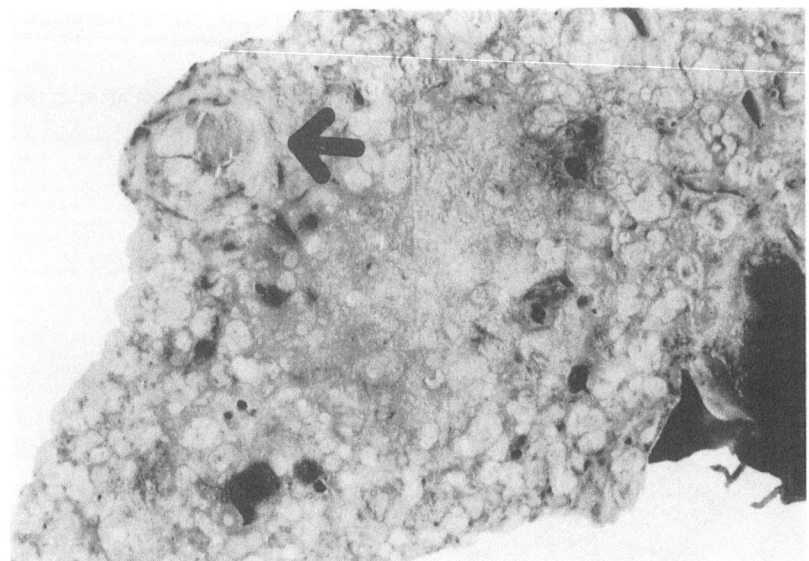

Fig. 16.7. A small HCC lesion (at arrow) found in an autopsied liver with advanced cirrhosis (weight 500 g). This tumor showed no histological evidence of active growth and may be regarded as a latent carcinoma

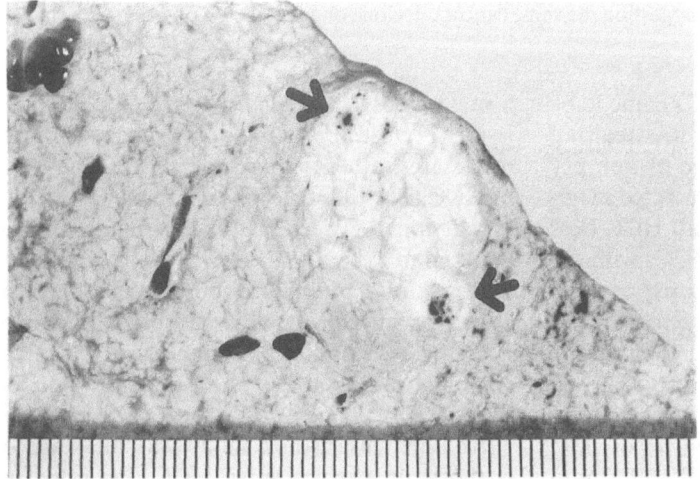

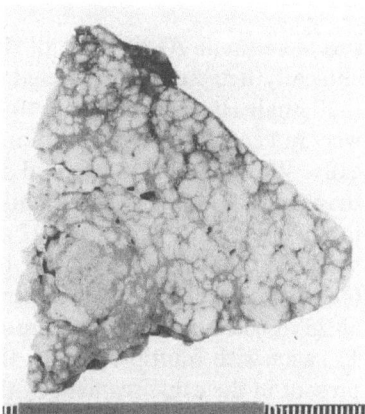

Fig. 16.8. A 2-cm HCC of the spreading-growth type seen in an autopsied liver. Despite the small size of the tumor, two intraportal invasions (*arrows*) are already apparent

Fig. 16.9. A 10 × 12-mm HCC seen in a resected liver. There is no obvious capsule formation

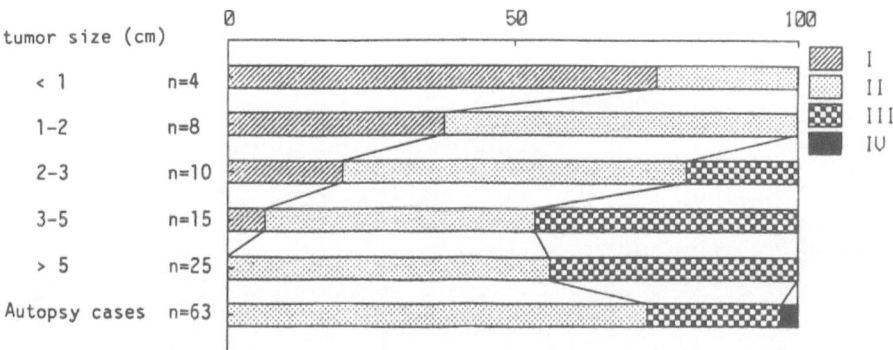

Fig. 16.10. Relative frequency of Edmondson and Steiner's grades in small HCCs in resected and autopsied cases. The grades on this scale of differentiation are I, II, III, and IV. The grade of the predominant cancer cells was used. It is obvious that the smaller the tumor, the more likely was the grade of predominant cancer cells to be I. The suggestion from this study is that the early lesion is more often well-differentiated and that as the tumor grows less-differentiated cancer cells dominate the tumor mass

was also noted that HCC smaller than 1 cm was seldom encapsulated (Fig. 16.9) but that two-thirds of 2-cm HCCs had a recognizable capsule. It was thus suggested that capsule formation often takes place while the tumor gorws to the size of 2 cm. Histological investigation of small HCCs disclosed that they were more frequently well-differentiated than large HCCs and that Edmondson and Steiner's grade I HCC [49] was not uncommon. Whereas only 1 of 33 advanced HCCs having various histological types of HCC cells had Edmondson and Steiner's grade I, seven of eight small HCCs with different tissue types had grade I. It was also found that the smaller the cancer, the more frequent was grade I (Fig. 16.10).

In the clinical setting, surgeons began having problems with more frequent resections. With a clinical diagnosis of HCC or most likely HCC based on imaging findings, resection is carried out, but the pathologist's report of the resected lesion is "nonmalignant." With such experience accumulating at various gastroenterology centers, the serious question was raised as to how to differentiate HCC from such benign lesions and whether or not the seemingly benign lesions were preneoplastic. At the Annual Meeting of the Japanese Society of Hepatology organized by Nakashima in Kurume in 1983, a special session of "Hepatic Lesions Resembling HCC" was held to which the late Prof. Robert L. Peters was invited for comments. A total of 36 papers were presented, which included three cases of HCC with marked fatty changes that made histological diagnosis difficult and ten cases of adenomatous hyperplasia or its equivalent, which was hardly distinguishable from extremely well-differentiated HCC. Although no conclusion was

drawn at this meeting, the problem was clearly defined. These cases were later published in detail in a monograph [50].

Subsequently, Arakawa et al. [51] described 17 small-mass lesions, detected by imaging and resected, from ten patients with cirrhosis. Five of the 17 lesions were unequivocal well-differentiated HCC coexisting with benign-appearing lesions, four were considered to be adenomatous hyperplasia described by Edmondson [52], and eight were equivocal, either an adenomatous hyperplastic nodule undergoing malignant transformation or extremely well-differentiated HCC (Fig. 16.11). In six patients, HCC recurred or occurred *de novo* 11 months to 2 years after operation. Arakawa et al. concluded that these lesions represented an early stage of HCC and that the conventional histological criteria for malignancy were not applicable to such lesions. They further demonstrated [53] in five cases of adenomatous hyperplastic nodules that early malignant foci were seen as small nodules within such lesions (Fig. 16.12)—the so-called nodules-in-nodules, a term coined by Popper [54]. It now seems that in Asia, where HCC is endemic among patients with posthepatitic cirrhosis, and adenomatous hyperplastic nodule or a similar hyperplastic lesion that occurs in cirrhotic livers is preneoplastic and is already committed to malignant transformation [55]. It is likely that many HCCs emerge as extremely well-differentiated (Edmondson and Steiner's grade I lesions) within which less-differentiated HCC lesions develop later (Fig. 16.13). In fact, large expanding HCCs almost invariably contan regions of differing textures. It is yet to be determined whether such a phenomenon is due to the emergence of new clones or to changes in

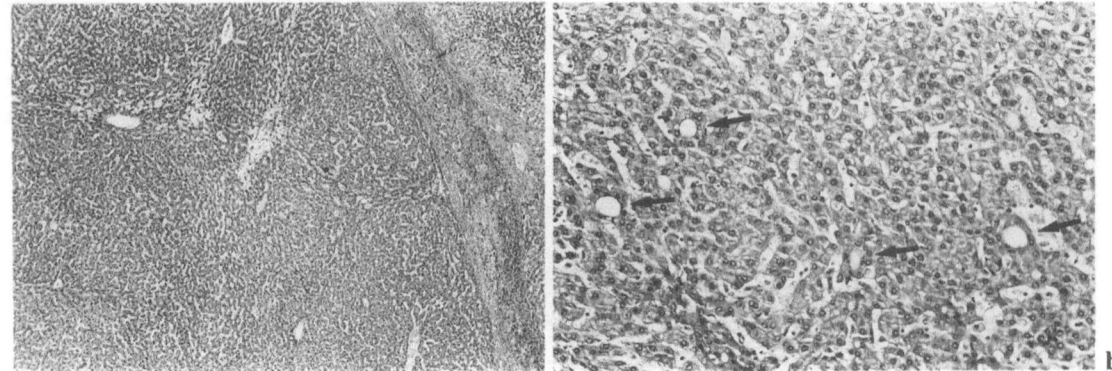

Fig. 16.11. a Low-magnification view of an adenomatous hyperplastic nodule detected by imaging in a cirrhotic liver. The mass was bounded by a pseudocapsule and appears benign with vessels and Kupffer cells; it may be interpreted as an adenoma. H and E, × 40. **b** There are areas where benign-appearing tumor cells are in more than one-cell-thick plates and demonstrate acinar cell arrangements in places (*arrows*). This is perhaps HCC of Edmondson and Steiner's grade I. H and E, × 200

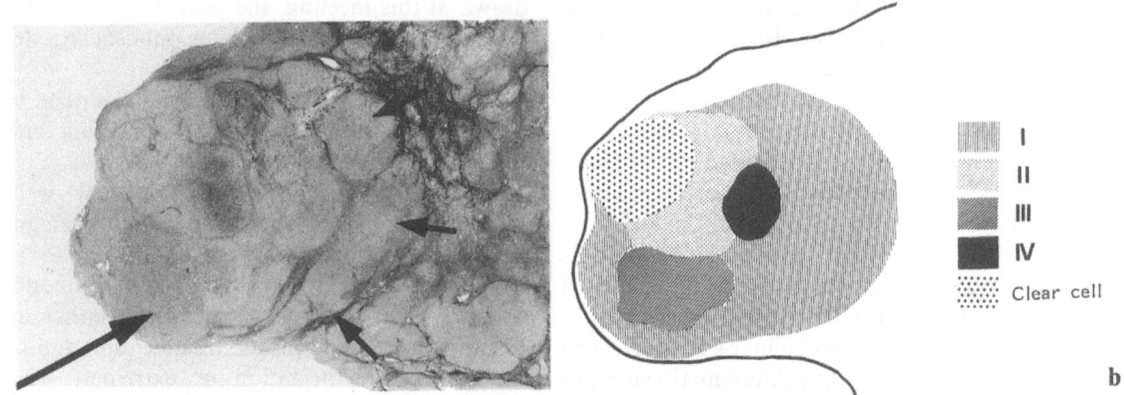

Fig. 16.12. a A 17 × 12-mm HCC lesion resected. Note the irregular texture of the cut surface containing nodules within a nodule. **b** Schematic representation of the tumor histology. There are five different areas of cancer cells that range from Edmondson and Steiner's grade I to IV to clear cells

phenotypic expression occurring within the same clone.

Tumor invasion into the venous system is very common and is even regarded as characteristic of HCC. In our study, it was recognized in 9 of 27 (33.3%) autopsy cases and in 7 of 25 (28%) resected cases of small HCC. In a resected 1-cm HCC, there was a distinct intraportal tumor thrombus at a distance of 1 cm. Figure 16.10 shows a 2-cm spreading-type HCC in which two grossly discernible tumor thrombi are seen in its immediate vicinity. More frequently, however, tumor cells are seen floating in small clusters within the lumen of the portal branches. Such findings call for a sufficient margin to be left from the tumor at the time of resection. Other pathological reports on small HCC made more recently cite similar frequencies of portal invasion [56, 57].

6 Treatment and prognosis of small HCC

When we analyzed the prognosis of 166 patients who had an HCC smaller than 25% of the whole two-dimensional area of the liver, there was a significant difference in survival between those treated surgically (median survival 29 months) and those treated nonsurgically (median survival 13 months). In the resected patients, the survival rate at 2 months was 92%, 84% at 6 months, and 73% at 12 months after surgery [58]. In our separate study of 22 patients with cirrhosis who had an HCC smaller than 3 cm and who did not receive any specific treatment, the 6-month survival rate was 95.5%, 1-year survival 90.9%, 2-years survival 55.0%, and 3-year survival 12.8% (Fig. 16.14). Six of the 12 deaths in this series

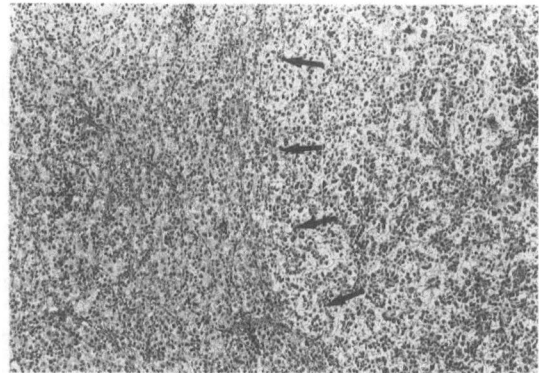

Fig. 16.13. This photomicrograph demonstrates the boundary between grade I and grade II cancer cells within a nodule (*arrows*). Grade II cancer cells are expanding within the grade I cells

were due to hepatic failure, and none was the so-called cancer death or death due to cachexia. Three died from intra-abdominal bleeding due to tumor rupture. The important observations were that whereas 90.7% of patients lived for 1 year, only 12.8% lived as long as 3 years after tumor detection [3]. Therefore, the operative mortality greater than 10% currently observed by some surgeons in patients with small HCCs is inferior to the natural course, but a postoperative survival of greater than 20% after 3 years is better.

Nonsurgical treatment includes transcatheter arterial embolization [59, 60], intra-arterial chemoembolization [61], targeting chemotherapy [62, 63], radiation, and intratumor ethanol injection. Systemic chemotherapy is rarely effective [64], and intra-arterial bolus delivery of a chemotherapeutic agent (such as mitomycin C) is only slightly if at all, better than systemic chemotherapy [58, 65]. If the cancer is of the expanding type [47] and has a fibrous capsule [46] arterial embolization is very effective, provided that the associated cirrhotic changes are not very advanced. Embolization will cause parenchymal damage that could trigger hepatic failure, but our data in patients with stage I disease did not demonstrate a significant effect on survival [58]. Viable cancer cells remain within the capsule because it receives both arterial and portal blood, and these cancer cells cause metastases later. Radiation, using a linear accelerator, may be given following arterial embolization because it will kill cancer cells in the capsule, but the clinical data are inadequate for evaluation at present. Targeting chemotherapy using Lipiodol and polymerized neocarzinostatin (SMANCS) is an effective therapeutic measure [62, 63], but this agent is not commercially available as yet. More recently, we have injected absolute ethanol into small HCCs. Under ultrasonic guidance [66], several milliters of ethanol are injected through a thin Chiba needle into the mass; this is repeated until all cancer tissue is coagulated. Ethanol-treated HCC was subsequently resected in several patients and the tumor was found to be completely necrotic. The size of HCC for which this modality can be used is perhaps no greater than 3 cm. The efficacy of this therapy is currently being assessed.

7 Problems and perspectives for the future

In South Africa, where the incidence of HCC among Blacks is extremely high, early detection and resection have not been described. The frequency of associated cirrhosis is low, the cirrhosis itself is less advanced if present [47] and the cancer is poorly differentiated [67] and generally fast-growing. The difference in the biology of

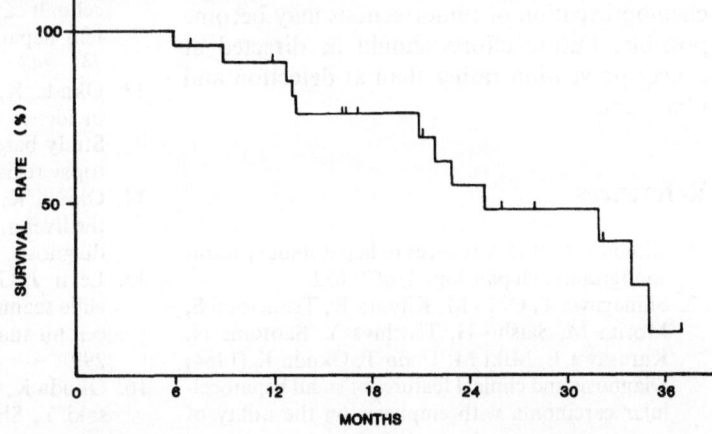

Fig. 16.14. Survival curve for 22 patients with HCC smaller than 3 cm who had no specific treatment as analyzed by the Kaplan-Mjeier method. From Ebara et al. [3], with permission from Elsevier

HCC between South African Blacks and Orientals may be related to etiological factors. It may be that HCC is more often multifocal at the time of detection among African Blacks, whereas it is more often unifocal in livers with posthepatitic cirrhosis in the Far East. The question of multicentric versus unicentric tumorigenesis should also take into account the fact that in chemical carcinogenesis in rodents under experimental conditions [68, 69], numerous preneoplastic foci develop prior to malignant transformation. The early stage of development of HCC is quite different in man, and the diffuse type of HCC, as seen in animal models, is extremely rare. A much longer time-lag between initiation and malignant transformation and different etiological factors, such as integration of viral DNA into hepatocyte chromosomal DNA in humans [70, 71], may account for the difference between chemical carcinogenesis in animals and tumorigenesis in man. Based on recent experience in Japan, it is the opinion of the authors that the question of unicentric versus multicentric emergence may be just a matter of differing intervals between the emergence of the first, second, third tumors, and so on. If the interval is long, the condition is equivalent to a unicentrically emerged HCC, whereas HCCs developing at shorter intervals may appear multicentric.

On the more practical side, there seems to be little room for further refinement and increase in the sensitivity of diagnostic procedures or for prolongation of survival by improved management. Obviously, it is much more desirable to prevent the progression of chronic liver disease to cirrhosis, which, in the opinion of the authors, is itself a preneoplastic state. Molecular biological methodology will provide a measure for predicting the degree of risk of developing HCC in patients with chronic liver disease, and even in patients with fully developed cirrhosis, chemoprevention of tumorigenesis may become possible. Future efforts should be directed at cancer prevention rather than at detection and treatment.

References

1. Okuda K (1981) Advances in hepatobiliary ultrasonography. Hepatology 1: 662–672
2. Shinagawa T, Ohto M, Kimura K, Tsunetomi S, Morita M, Saisho H, Tsuchiya Y, Saotome N, Karasawa E, Miki M, Ueno T, Okuda K (1984) Diagnosis and clinical features of small hepatocellular carcinoma with emphasis on the utility of real-time ultrasonography. A study of 51 patients. Gastroenterology 86: 496–502
3. Ebara M, Ohto M, Shinagawa T, Sugiura N, Kimura K, Matsutani S, Morita M, Saisho H, Tsuchiya Y, Okuda K (1986) Natural history of minute hepatocellular carcinoma smaller than three centimeters complicating cirrhosis. A study in 22 patients. Gastroenterology 90: 289–298
4. Masseyeff RF (1973) Factors influencing α-fetoprotein biosynthesis in patients with primary liver cancer and other diseases. Gann Monogr Cancer Res 14: 3–18
5. Purves LR (1976) Alpha-fetoprotein and the diagnosis of liver cell cancer. In: Cameron HM, Linsell DA, Waruick GP (eds) Liver cell cancer. Elsevier, Amsterdam, pp 61–79
6. Li FP, Shiang EL (1980) Cancer mortality in China. J Natl Cancer Inst 65: 217–221
7. Tang ZY (1985) Subclinical hepatocellular carcinoma—historical aspects and general consideration. In: Tang ZY (ed) Subclinical hepatocellular carcinoma. China Academic Publishers, Beijing, pp 1–11
8. Okuda K, Kotoda K, Obata H, Hayashi N, Hisamitsu T, Tamiya M, Kubo Y, Yakushiji F, Shimokawa Y (1975) Clinical observations during a relatively early stage of hepatocellular carcinoma, with special reference to serum α-fetoprotein levels. Gastroenterology 69: 226–234
9. Okuda K, Suzuki N, Kubo Y, Obata H (1979) Clinical aspects of hepatocellular carcinoma. In: Thatcher N (ed) Advances in medical oncology, research and education, vol. 9. Pergamon, Oxford, pp 133–140
10. Okuda K, Nakashima T, Obata H, Kubo Y (1977) Clinicopathological studies of minute hepatocellular carcinoma. Analysis of 20 cases, including 4 with hepatic resection. Gastroenterology 73: 109–115
11. Kubo Y, Okuda K, Musha H, Nakashima T (1978) Detection of hepatocellular carcinoma during a clinical follow-up of chronic liver disease. Observations in 31 patients. Gastroenterology 74: 578–582
12. Obata H, Hayashi N, Motoike Y, Hisamitus T, Okuda H, Kobayashi S, Nishioka K (1980) A prospective study on the development of hepatocelluralr carcinoma from liver cirrhosis with persistent hepatitis B virus infection. Int J Cancer 25: 741–747
13. Okuda K, Urano Y, Fujimoto I (1976) Rising incidence of hepatocellular carcinoma in Japan. Study based on cancer registry and national autopsy registry. Cancer Res (in press)
14. Okuda K, Iio M (1976) Radiological aspects of the liver and biliary tract. X-ray and radioisotope diagnosis. Year Book Med. Publisher, Chicago
15. Levin J, Geddes EW, Kew MC (1974) Radionuclide scanning of the liver in primary hepatic cancer: an analysis of 202 cases. J Nucl Med 15: 296–299
16. Okuda K, Obata H, Jinnouchi S, Kubo Y, Nagasaki Y, Shimokawa Y, Nakajima Y, Musha H,

Sakamoto K, Kojiro M, Nakashima T (1977) Angiographic assessment of gross anatomy of hepatocellular carcinoma: Comparison of celiac angiograms and liver pathology in 100 cases. Radiology 123: 21–29

17. Kaude J, Jensen R, Wirtanen GW (1973) Slow injection hepatic angiography. A comparison with a high injection rate. Acta Radiol (Diag) 14: 700–712

18. Takashima T, Matsui O (1980) Infusion hepatic angiography in the detection of small hepatocellular carcinoma. Radiology 136: 321–325

19. Tsunetomi S, Ohto M, Iino Y, Shinagawa T, Kimura K, Morita M, Saisho H, Tsuchiya Y, Okuda K, Hirooka N (1984) Diagnosis of small hepatocellular carcinoma by computed tomography. Study in comparison with pathologic findings. Jpn J Gastroenterol 81: 72–81

20. Ebara M, Ohto M, Watanabe Y, Kimura K, Saisho H, Tsuchiya Y, Okuda K, Arimizu N, Konda F, Ikehira H, Fukuda N, Tateno Y (1986) Diagnosis of small hepatocellular carcinoma: correlation of MR imaging and tumor histology studies. Radiology 159: 371–377

21. Yumoto Y, Jinno K, Tojuyama K, Araki Y, Ishimatsu T, Maeda H, Konno T, Iwamoto S, Ohnishi K, Okuda K (1985) Hepatocellular carcinoma detected by iodized oil. Radiology 154: 19–24

22. Nakakuma K, Tashiro S, Hirooka T, Ogata K, Ootsuka K (1985) Hepatocellular carcinoma and metastatic cancer detected by iodized oil. Radiology 154: 15–17

23. Ohnishi H, Uchida H, Yoshimura H, Ohue S, Ueda J, Katsuragi M, Matsuo N, Hosogi Y (1985) Hepatocellular carcinoma detected by iodized oil. Use of anticancer agents. Radiology 154: 25–29

24. Bookstein JJ (1985) Hepatocellular carcinoma: recent advances in diagnosis with iodized oil. Radiology 154: 253–254

25. Itai Y, Ohtomo S, Furui S, Yamauchi T, Minami M, Yashiro N (1985) Noninvasive diagnosis of small cavernous hemangioma of the liver: advantage of MRI. Am J Roentgen 145: 1195–1199

26. Kobayashi K, Sugimoto T, Makino H, Kumagai K, Unoura M, Tanaka N, Kato Y, Hattori N (1985) Screening methods for early detection of hepatocellular carcinoma. Hepatology 5: 1100–1105

27. Chen DS, Sheu JC, Sung JL, Lai MY, Lee CS, Su CT, Tsang YM, How SW, Wang TH, YJY, Yang TH, Wang CY, Hsu CY (1983) Small hepatocellular carcinoma—a clinicopathological study in thirteen patients. Gastroenterology 83: 1109–1119

28. Chen DS, Sung JL, Sheu JH, Lai MY, How SW, Hsu HC, Lee CS, Wei TC (1984) Serum α-fetoprotein in the early stage of human hepatocellular carcinoma. Gastroenterology 86: 14–4–1409

29. Sheu JC, Sung JL, Chen DS, Yang PM, Lai MY, Lee CS, Han HC, Chnang CN, Yang PC, Wang TH, Lin JT, Lee CZ (1985) Growth rate of asymptomatic hepatocellular carcinoma and its clinical implications. Gastroenterology 89: 259–266

30. Liaw YF, Tai DI, Chu CM, Lin DY, Sheen IS, Chen TJ, Pao CC (1986) Early detection of hepatocellular carcinoma in patients with chronic type B hepatitis. A prospective study. Gastroenterology 90: 263–267

31. Okazaki N, Yoshino M, Yoshida T, Okura H, Moriyama N, Matsue H (1981) Growth speed of hepatocellular carcinoma and early diagnosis. Acta Hepatol Jpn 22: 1742 (short communication)

32. Okuda K (1946) Clinical aspects of hepatocellular carcinoma—analysis of 134 cases. In: Okuda K, Peters RL (eds) Wiley, New York, pp 387–436

33. Kan D, Kan M, Fukumoto Y, Noda K, Kodama T, Okita K, Nawata J, Nishioka M, Harada T, Nishimura H, Takemoto T (1979) Long-term survival cases of hepatocellular carcinoma without chemotherapy. Acta Hepatol Jpn 20: 417–422

34. Yoshida T, Okazaki N, Yoshino M, Kitaoka H, Nirohashi S, Shimozato Y (1982) Minute hepatocellular carcinoma without appreciable change in size for seven years: A case report. Cancer 49: 1491–1495

35. Nakano S, Kumada T, Sugiyama K, Watahiki H, Takeda I (1984) Clinical significance of serum ferritin determination for hepatocellular carcinoma. Am J Gastroenterol 79: 623–627

36. Liebman HA, Furie BC, Tong MJ, Blanchard RA, Lo KJ, Lee SD, Caleman MS, Furie B (1984) Des-γ-carboxy (abnormal) prothrombin is a serum marker of primary hepatocellular carcinoma. N Engl J Med 310: 1427–1431

37. Japan Liver Cancer Study Group (1983) The general rules for the clinical and pathological study of primary liver cancer. Kanahara, Tokyo

38. Anthony PP (1973) Primary carcinoma of the liver: a study of 282 cases in Ugandan Africans. J Pathol Bacteriol 110: 37–49

39. Anthon PP (1976) Precursor lesions for liver cancer in humans. Cancer Res 36: 2579–2583

40. Ho JCL, Wu PC, Mak TW (1981) Liver cell dysplasia in association with hepatocellular carcinoma, cirrhosis and hepatitis B surface antigen in Hong Kong. Int J Cancer 28: 571–574

41. Okuda K, Nakashima T, Obata H (1980) Hepatitis B virus and primary liver cell carcinoma. In: Bianchi L, Gerok W, Sickinger K, Stalder GA (eds) Virus and the liver. MTP, Lancaster, pp 209–216

42. Omata M, Mori J, Yokosuka O, Iwama S, Ito Y, Okuda K (1982) Hepatitis B virus antigens in liver tissue in hepatocellular carcinoma and advanced chronic liver disease—relationship to liver cell dysplasia. Liver 2: 125–132

43. Kagawa K, Deguchi T, Okanoue T, Okuno T, Takino T, Kamachi M, Ashihara T (1984) DNA-cytofluorometric analysis for the putative premalignant lesions and the liver cell carcinomas. Hepatology 4: 798 (abstract)

44. Uchida T, Miyata H, Shikata T (1981) Human hepatocellular carcinoma and putative precancerous disorders. Arch Pathol Lab Med 105: 180–186

45. Nakashima T, Okuda K, Kojiro M, Jimi A, Yamaguchi R, Sakamoto K, Ikari T (1983) Pathology of hepatocellular carcinoma in Japan. 232 consecutive cases autopsied in ten years. Cancer 51: 863–877

46. Okuda K, Musha H, Nakajima Y, Kubo Y, Shimokawa Y, Nagasaki Y, Obata H, Okazaki N, Kojiro M, Sakamoto K, Nakashima T (1977) Clinicopathological features of encapsulated hepatocellular carcinoma. A study of 26 cases. 40: 1240–1245

47. Okuda K, Peters RL, Simson IW (1984) Gross anatomical features of hepatocellular carcinoma from three disparate geographic areas. Proposal of new classification. Cancer 54: 2165–2173

48. Nakashima T, Kojiro (1986) Pathology atlas of hepatocellular carcinoma. Springer, Tokyo

49. Edmondson HA, Steiner PE (1954) Primary carcinoma of the liver. A study of 100 cases among 48,900 necropsies. Cancer 7: 462–503

50. Nakashima T, Ohta G, Okudaira M, Arakawa M (1984) Hepatic lesions resembling hepatocellular carcinoma. Chugai, Tokyo

51. Arakawa M, Sugihara S, Kenmochi K, Kage M, Nakashima T, Nakayama T, Tashiro S, Hirooka T, Suenaga M, Okuda K (1986) Small mass lesions in cirrhosis: transition from benign adenmatoud hyperplasis to hepatocellular carcinoma. J Gastroenterol Hepatol 1: 3–14

52. Edmondson HA (1976) Benign epithelial tumors and tumorlike lesions of the liver. In: Okuda K, Peters RL (eds) Hepatocellular carcinoma. Wiley, New York, pp 309–330

53. Arakawa M, Kage M, Sugihara S, Nakashima T, Suenaga M, Okuda K (1986) Emergence of malignant lesions within an adenomatous hyperplastic nodule in a cirrhotic liver. Observations in five cases. Gastroenterology 91: 198–208

54. Popper H (1977) Pathologic aspects of cirrhosis. A review. Am J Pathol 87: 228–264

55. Okuda K (1986) What is the precancerous lesion for hepatocellular carcinoma? J Gastroenterol Hepatol 1: 79–85

56. Hsu HC, Sheu JC, Lin UH, Chen DS, Lee CS, Hnang LY, Beasley RD (1985) Prognostic histologic features of resected small hepatocellular carcinoma. Cancer 56: 672–680

57. Wakasa K, Sakurai M, Okamura J, Kuroda C (1985) Pathological study of small hepatocellular carcinoma: frequency of their invasion. Virchow Arch (Pathol Anat) 407: 259–270

58. Okuda K, Ohtsuki T, Obata H, Tomimatsu M, Okazaki N, Hasegawa H, Nakajima Y, Ohnishi K (1985) Natural history of heptocellular carcinoma and prognosis in relation to treatment. Study of 850 patients. Cancer 56: 918–928

59. Yamada R, Sato M, Kawabata M, Nakatsuka H, Nakamura K, Takashima S (1983) Hepatic artery embolization in 120 patients with unresectable hepatoma. Radiology 148: 397–402

60. Takayasu K, Moriyama N, Nuramatsu Y, Suzuki M, Yamada T, Kishi K, Hasegawa H, Okazaki N (1984) Hepatic arterial embolization for hepatocellular carcinoma. Comparison of CT scans and resected specimens. Radiology 150: 661–665

61. Ohnishi K, Tsuchiya S, Nakayama T, Hiyama Y, Takashi M, Ohtsuki T, Nakajima Y, Okuda K (1984) Arterial chemoembolization of hepatocellular carcinoma with mitomycin C microcapsules. Radiology 152: 51–55

62. Konno T, Maeda H, Iwai K, Tashiro S, Maki S, Morinaga T, Mochinaga M. Hiraoka T, Yokoyama I (1983) Effect of arterial administration of high-molecular-weight anticancer agent SMANCS with lipid lymphographic agent on hepatoma: a preliminary report. Eur J Cancer Clin Oncol 19: 1053–1065

63. Konno T, Maeda H, Iwai K, Maki S, Tashiro S, Uchida M, Miyauchi Y (1984) Selective targeting of anti-cancer drug and simultaneous image enhancement in solid tumors by arterial administered lipid contrast medium. Cancer 54: 2364–2374

64. Okazaki N (1976) Systemic chemotherapy of hepatocellular carcinoma. In: Okuda K, Peters RL (eds) Hepatocellular carcinoma. Wiley, New York, pp 469–476

65. Kubo Y, Shimokawa Y (1976) Arterial injection chemotherapy. In: Okuda K, Peters RL (eds) Hepatocellular carcinoma, Wiely, New York, pp 477–490

66. Ohto M, Karasawa E, Tsuchiya Y, Kimura K, Saisho H, Ono T, Okuda K (1980) Ultrasonically guided percutaneous contrast medium injection and aspiration biopsy using a real-time puncture transducer. Radiology 136: 171–176

67. Steiner PE (1960) Cancer of the liver and cirrhosis in trans-Saharan Africa and the United States of America. Cancer 13: 1085–1166

68. Farber E (1976) Hyperplastic areas, hyperplastic nodules, and hyperbasophilic areas as putative precursor lesions. Cancer Res 36: 2532–2533

69. Bannasch P (1976) Cytology and cytogenesis of neoplastic (hyperplastic) hepatic nodules. Cancer Res 36: 2556–2562

70. Brechot C, Pourcel C, Louise A, Rain B, Tiollais P (1980) Presence of integrated hepatitis B virus DNA sequences in cellular DNA of human hepatocellular carcinoma. Nature 286: 533–535

71. Shafritz DA, Kew MC (1981) Identification of integrated hepatitis B virus DNA sequences in human hepatocellular carcinoma. Hepatology 1: 1–8

Chapter 17

Serological Tumor Markers in Hepatocellular Carcinoma

Norio Sawabu[1] and Nobu Hattori[2]

1 Introduction

A number of substances have been reported to be tumor markers, but many are limited to research use. In the case of hepatocellular carcinoma (HCC), however, several markers are clinically useful, of which α-fetoprotein (AFP) is perhaps one of the best.

The following is a classification of tumor markers, including promising markers for hepatic malignancy. Group Ia includes tumor markers that are highly specific to HCC and hepatoblastomas:

AFP
Novel γ-glutamyl transpeptidase isoenzyme (novel γ-GTP)
Variant alkaline phosphatase
Des-γ-carboxy prothrombin

Group Ib includes markers that are useful for digestive malignancy but have low organ specificity:

Isoferritin
Basic fetoprotein
Aldolase isoenzyme—type A
Glutathione S transferase isoenzyme—type B

In group Ib, false positivity is somewhat frequent in benign hepatic diseases such as hepatitis and liver cirrhosis.

Many group II tumor markers are antigens defined by monoclonal antibodies raised against various adenocarcinoma cell lines by the use of the hybridoma technique:

CA 19-9
CA 125
DU-PAN-2

CA-50
CSLEX-1
ST-4-39
CEA
POA

These are useful mainly as markers for adenocarcinoma of the digestive tract. They are less useful for HCC but may be of diagnostic value in cholangiocellular carcinoma, another histological type of primary liver cancer. In this review, we will mainly discuss group Ia tumor markers, highly specific to HCC, and the problems in the diagnosis of HCC tumor markers.

2 Alpha fetoprotein

2.1 Diagnostic utility of AFP in HCC in recent years

The physiological and pathological properties of AFP have already been reviewed extensively [1, 2] and will not be discussed here. Table 17.1 shows the results of measurement of serum AFP by radioimmunoassay (RIA) in chronic liver diseases. The frequency of positive AFP tests (more than 10 ng/ml) in chronic hepatitis and liver cirrhosis was 22% and 40%, respectively. Even with the dividing value set at 100 ng/ml, there were some positive tests (5% and 11%, respectively). Since levels above 400 ng/ml are rarely encountered in benign hepatic diseases, 400 ng/ml is generally used as the cutoff value to make the test highly specific to HCC [3]. The frequency of HCC with an AFP value of 400 ng/ml or more varies slightly from one report to another. In our studies, it was 58% in 1975–1979 and 49% in 1980–1984 (Table 17.1). Recent progress in diagnostic imaging techiques, including ultrasonography and computed tomography, has made the diagnosis of HCC possible in many cases with a low AFP level, and the diagnostic value of AFP is no longer as important as it was.

[1] Department of Internal Medicine, Cancer Research Institute, Kanazawa University, Kanazawa, 920 Japan
[2] First Department of Internal Medicine, Kanazawa University School of Medicine, Kanazawa, 920 Japan

Table 17.1. Serum AFP levels in various chronic liver diseases

Disease	Total no. of patients	No. of cases			
		Less than 10 ng/ml AFP	11–100 ng/ml AFP	101–400 ng/ml AFP	More than 401 ng/ml AFP
Chronic hepatitis	152	118	27	5	2
			99%[a]		1%[b]
			95%[c]		5%[d]
Liver cirrhosis	116	70	33	9	4
			97%[a]		3%[b]
			89%[c]		11%[d]
Hepatocellular carcinoma 1975–1979	144	13	21	26	84
			42%[a]		58%[b]
			24%[c]		76%[d]
1980–1984	148	27	29	20	72
			51%[a]		49%[b]
			38%[c]		62%[d]

[a] Total percentage less than ∼10, ∼11 to ∼100, and ∼101 to ∼400 ng/ml AFP
[b] Percentage more than ∼401 ng/ml AFP
[c] Total percentage less than ∼10 and ∼11 to ∼100 ng/ml AFP
[d] Total percentage ∼101 to ∼400 and more than ∼400 ng/ml AFP

2.2 Early diagnosis of HCC by AFP measurement

HCC confirmed histologically following surgery or at autopsy or clinically diagnosed from the typical angiographic changes in addition to other findings may be classified according to tumor size into small HCC (a tumor smaller than 3 cm in diameter), medium-size HCC (a main tumor of 3–5 cm in diameter with less than three daughter nodules), and large HCC (a tumor larger than 5 cm in diameter). At diagnosis, the AFP level was 400 ng/ml or more in only 7 (25%) of 28 small-HCC patients (Fig. 17.1). Similar data have been reported in Taiwan where HCC is very prevalent; the frequency of AFP levels above 400 ng/ml was only 18%–21% for small HCC [4, 5]. Thus, determination of AFP alone is not so significant in the early diagnosis of HCC.

As shown in Fig. 17.1, however, the positivity rate for AFP levels above 400 ng/ml in the medium-size HCC groups was 60% (14 of 23 patients), which is about the same as that for large HCC. Furthermore, AFP was above 100 ng/ml in 43% (12 of 28 patients) of patients with small HCC. AFP also has the advantage of being easily measured in repeatable tests, thus facilitating early detection in many patients.

Figure 17.2 illustrates the sequential changes in AFP level in patients with small HCC in whom AFP values could be monitored prior to diagnosis. In 7 of 16 patients (44%), the value remained low and showed no significant changes. In the remaining nine patients, there was a rapid elevation at about the time of detection, after a period of little change or relatively slow increase. In five of these patients, however, the AFP value demonstrated a borderline change only over a range of 92–267 ng/ml (mean 194 ng/ml). It is expedient when a rapid elevation in AFP is detected in patients with chronic liver disease during periodic follow-up that a thorough examination by diagnostic imaging is peformed.

It is important to determine AFP once every few months in patients at high risk to HCC and at least once every 4–5 months even in those at low risk [6]. When the AFP value shows a tendency to increase continuously, even though slightly, diagnostic imaging should be done repeatedly [7].

As illustrated in Fig. 17.1, the AFP test was negative or less than 10 ng/ml in 15 of 154 patients (10%) even with a large HCC. Furthermore, in the small-HCC group a negative AFP test, or a value of less than 10 ng/ml, occurred in 5 of 28 patients (18%), and an AFP level of less than 50 ng/ml was found in 13 of 28 patients (46%). Thus, there are limitations to the diagnosis of HCC by AFP. When AFP is not diagnostic, one should make efforts to improve the diagnostic accuracy by the additional use of other markers, such as novel γ-GTP [8].

2.3 Usefulness as a trace marker

When a patient is obseved clinically, the serum AFP value often increases with the growth of the HCC. The size of the tumor does not always correlate with serum AFP level; even a small tumor can give a high AFP level. This is thought to be due mainly to the varying AFP-producing capacity of HCC. A decreased value or the disappearance of blood AFP is seen after tumor resection or treatment with effective anticancer drugs. When transcatheter arterial embolization is performed, a steady decrease in blood AFP level is observed as the tumor undergoes necrosis. AFP is also useful for monitoring the clinical course in HCC patients, e.g., the recurrence of HCC can be predicted from the postoperative reelevation of blood AFP levels.

2.4 Analysis of AFP by lectin affinity

Recently, the sugar structure of AFP derived from HCC and yolk sac tumor has been identified by Kobata et al. [9, 10]. AFP purified from ascitic fluid from HCC patients has a sugar structure which readily binds to concanavalin A (Con A), as shown in Fig. 17.3a. By contrast, AFP produced by a yolk sac tumor is characterized by glycolinkage with N-acetyl-glucosamine (bisecting GlcNAC) found in the mannose part, as illustrated in Fig. 17.3b. It has been suggested that this residue inhibits the binding with Con A.

The presence or absence of fucose (Fuc) attached to N-acetyl-glucosamine, adjacent to asparagine, is believed to cause the difference in the binding to lentil lectin (LCA). An attempt has been made to quantitate such differences in lectin affinity by affinity chromatography using lectin sepharose, crossed affino-immunoelectro-

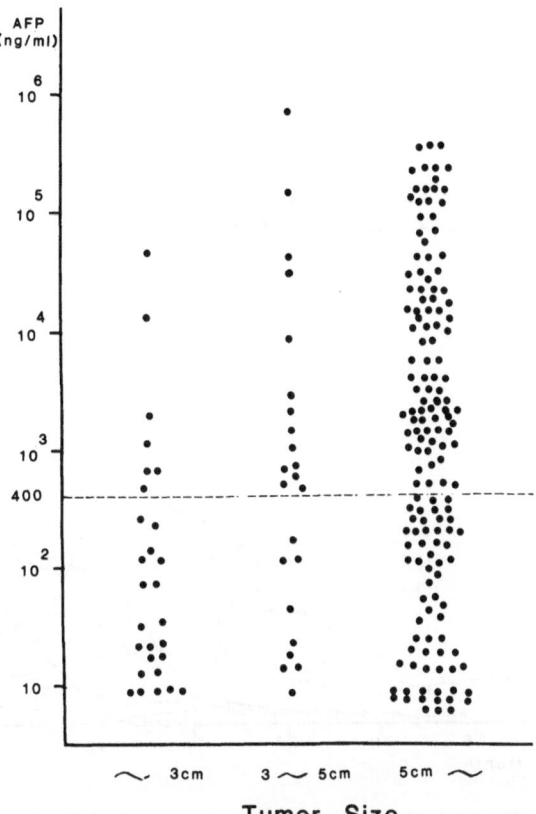

Fig. 17.1. Serum AFP levels at diagnosis and size of HCC

phoresis, or electroaffinity transfer [11–13]. The LCA-unbound fraction accounts for the majority of the AFP molecules found in benign liver diseases, such as liver cirrhosis, or cord serum, whereas in AFP from HCC the proportion of the LCA-unbound fraction is lower and the LCA-bound fraction is increased in varying degrees. In yolk sac tumor and metastatic liver cancer, the LCA-bound fraction is the major component.

The Con A-bound fraction accounts for the large proportion of AFP in cord serum and in the sera of patients with liver cirrhosis or HCC, while the Con A-unbound fraction is considerably greater (often 50% or more) in AFP from patients with yolk sac tumor and metastatic liver cancer. Benign liver diseases can be differentiated from HCC using the test for binding to LCA, and HCC can be distinguished from metastatic liver cancer by the binding to Con A. Such methods are important in differentiating cases with a slight increase of AFP (up to 400 ng/ml), which could be due either to HCC or to other diseases. Efforts have been made to develop a monoclonal antibody that directly recognizes these differences [14].

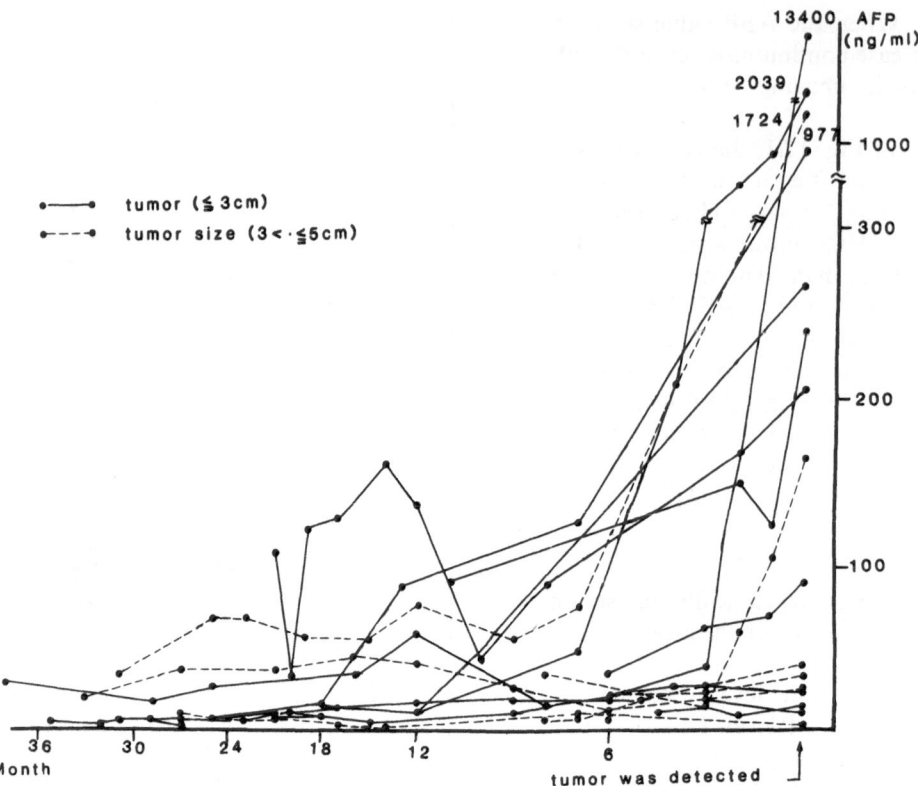

Fig. 17.2. Sequential changes of serum AFP levels in patients with small hepatocellular carcinoma

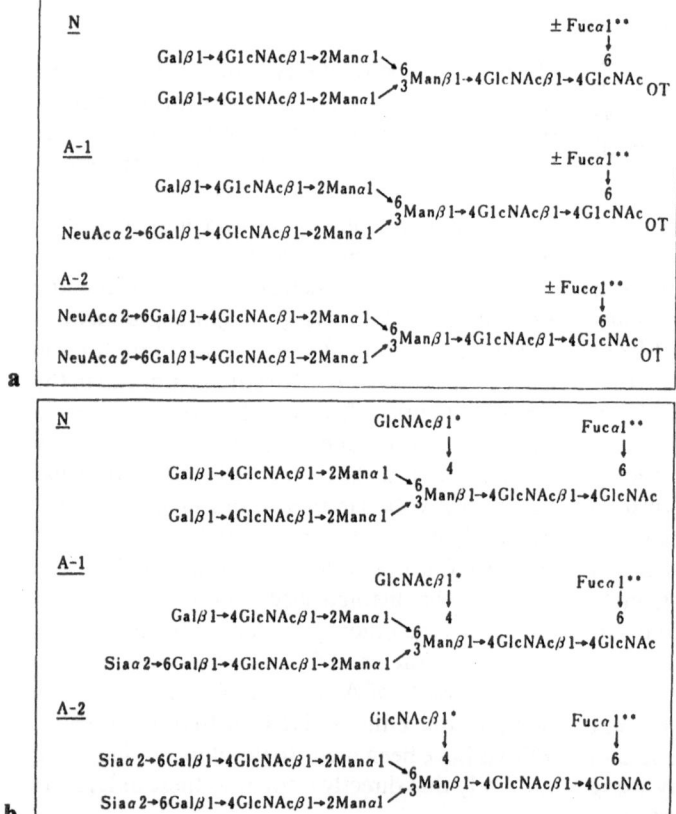

Fig. 17.3a, b. Structures of the asparagine-linked sugar chains of AFP obtained from **a** hepatocellular carcinoma and **b** yolk sac tumor. After Yoshima et al. [9] and Yamashita et al. [10], with permission of Cancer Research

3 Novel γ-GTP isoenzyme

Experimental studies have shown that γ-GTP is strikingly activated during the course of tumorigenesis induced by several hepatocarcinogens in animals and that it is significantly increased in liver cells both during the precancerous stage and when liver cell carcinoma develops [15–19]. As is the case with AFP, γ-GTP activity is quite low in the adult liver but is extremely high in the fetal liver and in HCC [15, 20]. These observations strongly suggest that the fetal activity of γ-GTP resurges in hepatoma cells and that this fetal isoenzyme may be detectable in the sera of patients with HCC. We previously reported the presence of a γ-GTP isoenzyme specifically found in the sera of patients with HCC; this isoenzyme is referred to as novel γ-GTP [21, 22]. The remainder of this chapter will deal with the clinical value and certain properties of this isoenzyme.

3.1 Fractionation of γ-GTP isoenzyme and HCC-specific bands

There are several methods of fractionating γ-GTP isoenzymes. However, to distinguish specific bands in HCC, polyacrylamide gradient gel electrophoresis is the most useful. Figure 17.4 shows γ-GTP zymograms of sera from patients with hepatobiliary diseases. By this method, as already described in detail [21, 22], γ-GTP isoenzymes separate into 13 bands. No bands other than II, II', and I' are characteristic of any group of patients so far studied. On the other hand, bands II, II', and I', which are seen in the region of α-globulin, have a high specificity for HCC. We have referred to these bands as HCC-specific novel γ-GTP isoenzyme (novel γ-GTP). Band I' is not obvious because it overlaps with band I. As will be shown below in detail, band I' does not bind to Con A. this property readily distinguishes band I' from band I.

Bands II, II', and I' have been detected in 97, 93 and 95 of 200 patients with HCC, respectively. Their presence or absence has been documented in diseases othe than HCC, such as cholangiocellular carcinoma (0/8 cases) metastatic cancer to the liver (3/52), biliary carcinoma (0/16), pancreatic carcinoma (0/11), liver cirrhosis (1/57), chronic hepatitis (1/43), acute and subacute hepatitis (0/14), alcoholic liver injury (2/36), intrahepatic cholestasis (0/16), and cholelithiasis (0/16). The concomitant appearance of all three bands was observed in 79 of 109 patients with HCC in whom one or more of these bands were found. The frequency of other combinations is

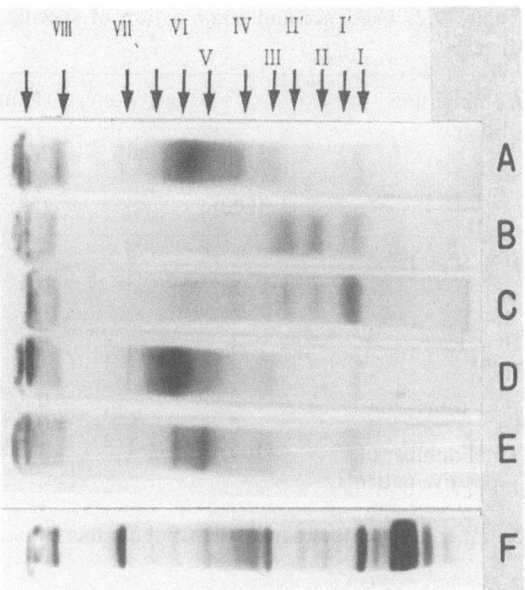

Fig. 17.4. Gamma-GTP isoenzymogram of serum from a patient with alcoholic liver injury (*A*), hepatocellular carcinoma (*B, C*), obstructive jaundice due to choledocholithiasis (*D*), and metastatic liver cancer (*E*). *F* is normal serum protein stained with amido black

shown in Table 17.2. At least one or more of these bands were detectable in 109 of 200 patients with HCC. In contrast, among 279 patients with hepatobiliary diseases other than HCC, they were found in three patients with metastatic liver cancer, two with alcoholic liver damage, one with liver cirrhosis, and one with chronic hepatitis. The prevalence of novel γ-GTP was about 3% among patients with hepatobiliary diseases other than HCC. Kojima et al. [23] and Kew et al. [24], who used the same method for electrophoretic fractionation of γ-GTP in the sera of HCC patients, reported results similar to ours

3.2 Clinical significance of novel γ-GTP

The serum activity of γ-GTP in HCC patients with and without novel γ-GTP is compared in Fig 17.5a. Novel γ-GTP could not be detected in patients whose serum γ-GTP activity was less than 80 mU/ml. By contrast, there were some patients without novel γ-GTP in whom serum γ-GTP activity was remarkably elevated. All of these patients had complications, such as obstructive jaundice, which could have raised the level of serum γ-GTP activity. Although the prevalence of novel γ-GTP was only 55% among all HCC patients, it was 72% in patients whose serum γ-GTP activity was above 100 mU/ml.

Table 17.2. Incidence and combination of specific bands in sera from patients with various hepatobiliary diseases

Combination of bands	Number of patients with specific bands				
	Hepatocelluar carcinoma (200)	Metastatic liver cancer (52)	Liver cirrhosis (57)	Chronic hepatitis (43)	Alcoholic liver injury (36)
II + II' + I'	79	1	0	0	1
II + II'	8	2	1	0	0
II + I'	6	0	0	0	0
II' + I'	4	0	0	0	1
II	4	0	0	0	0
II'	2	0	0	0	0
I'	6	0	0	1	0
Total number of positive patients	109	3	1	1	2

Number in parentheses indicates total number of patients in each group

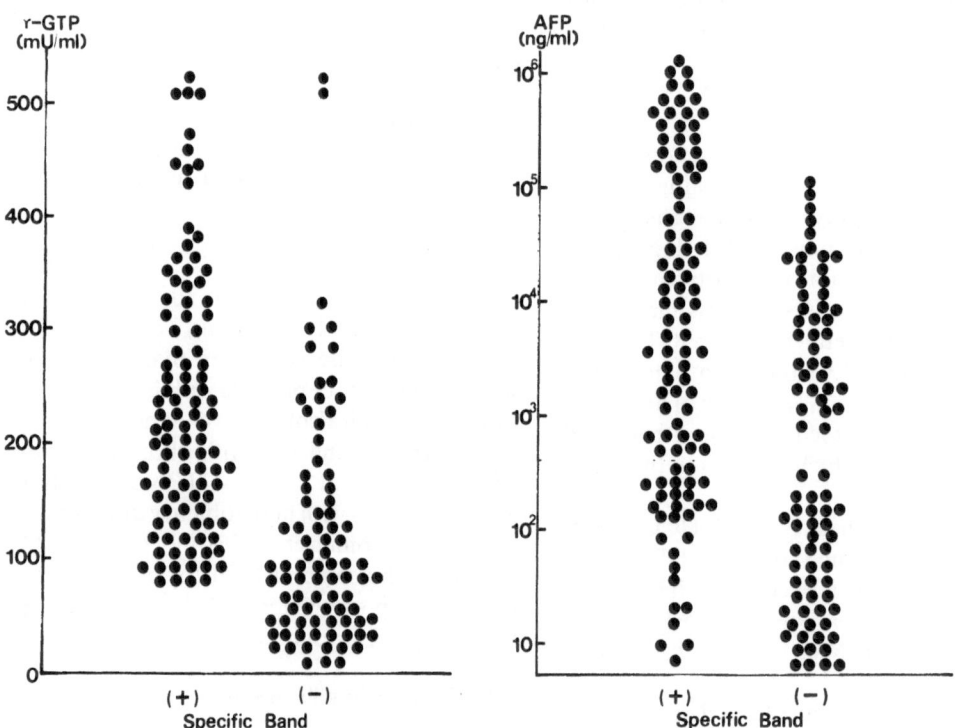

Fig. 17.5a, b. Correlation between positivity for novel γ-GTP isoenzyme and **a** serum activity of γ-GTP or **b** serum levels of AFP. The *dotted line* indicates AFP levels of 400 ng/ml

The same comparison is shown for serum AFP in Fig. 17.5b. Novel γ-GTP occurred more frequently in patients with higher AFP levels. However, it was found in 29 (38%) of 76 patients with AFP levels lower than 400 ng/ml. Furthermore, 11 patients with novel γ-GTP were included among 41 patients with an AFP level below 100 ng/ml. As mentioned in the previous section, about 40%–50% of HCC patients had AFP levels below 400 ng/ml, typical of sera from patients with hepatic diseases other than HCC. Thus, novel γ-GTP may be especially useful in the diagnosis of HCC in patients who have very low serum AFP levels.

The incidence of novel γ-GTP was compared with the stage of HCC, classified by liver scintiscanning, in 132 patients. The results showed that 53% (9/17) of patients were positive in stage

I, 52% (26/50) in stage II, 59% (48/82) in stage III, and 43% (3/7) in stage IV. Thus, the incidence of novel γ-GTP was found to be independent of the stage of the disease. Regarding carcinoembryonic antigens (CEA), now widely used as tumor markers, there is an obvious correlation between tumor mass and CEA blood concentration, whereas the AFP level does not necessarily parallel the size or stage of HCC. Novel γ-GTP in our study did not increase parallel with the advancing stage of HCC as classified by liver scan. Moreover, even in stage I, where the filling defect was undetectable by liver scanning, the incidence of novel γ-GTP was 53%, about the same as the figure of 55% for all HCC patients. In conclusion, novel γ-GTP seems to be a useful marker for the relatively early detection of HCC.

3.3 Characterization of novel γ-GTP isoenzyme

The physicochemical and immunological properties of γ-GTP purified from HCC tissue were compared with those of γ-GTP purified from adult kidney by the same procedure. The enzymes from HCC tissue and kidney were found to be similar or identical with respect to Km value for the substrate, optimum pH, thermostability, effect of various amino acids as acceptors, behavior to cations or ethylenediamine-tetraacetate, and immunological properties. However, the HCC tissue γ-GTP was distinguishable from normal kidney γ-GTP by molecular weight, electrophoretic mobility before and after neuraminidase treatment, Con A affinity, sensitivity to neuraminidase and isoelectrophoretic point, as demonstrated in our previous report [25].

Moreover, in order to elucidate differences in the properties of the band II, II', and I' subfractions of novel γ-GTP [26], they were separated and studied. Table 17.3 summarizes the properties of these subbands. Specific γ-GTP isoenzymes such as bands II, II', and I' in the sera of HCC patients were immunologically indistinguishable not only from each other but also from band I, the nonspecific band, the normal kidney enzyme in the double diffusion and activity inhibition tests. On the other hand, a considerable difference among the subbands was observed by affinity to various lectins and by the effect of neuraminidase, as shown in Table 17.3.

These results suggest that specific γ-GTP in the sera of HCC patients is largely due to structural differences in the carbohydrate moieties. Different carbohydrates reflect altered postribosomal

Table 17.3. Some properties of each band of γ-GTP isoenzyme

	Band			
	I	I'	II	II'
Neuraminidase	+ +	+	±	−
Concanavalin A	+ +	−	+ +	±
Lentil lectin	±	−	+ +	±
Riccimus communis I	+	+ +	+	+ +
Wheat germ lectin	+ +	+ +	+ +	+ +
Bromeline	−	−	+ +	+ +
Cibacron blue	−	−	+ +	±
Anti-HCC γ-GTP	+ +	+ +	+ +	+ +
Anti kidney γ-GTP	+ +	+ +	+ +	+ +

+ + Very sensitive, + sensitive, ± slightly sensitive, − non-sensitive

processing of glycoprotein in HCC cells. However, the structure of the glycolinkage in novel γ-GTP that is specific to HCC and the mechanism that produces this glycolinkage remain to be determined.

In experimental hepatocarcinogenesis, γ-GTP preparations from different organs are immunologically identical for a given mammalian species, but they differ significantly not only in sialic acid content but also in some other carbohydrate moieties [19, 27–29]. Furthermore, Yamashita et al. [30] reported several qualitative and quantitative differences in the sugar chains between γ-GTP purified from rat liver and that from rat ascites AH-66 hepatoma. Among them, the occurrence of a bisecting GlcNAc residue in half of the sugar chains of HCC γ-GTP is the most important because the same residue is not found in the sugar chian of γ-GTP from normal liver. Thus, it may be possible to distinguish human serum γ-GTP associated with HCC from that of non-HCC patients by making use of the structural change in the sugar chains of this enzyme [31].

4 Variant alkaline phosphatase

The isoenzymes of alkaline phosphatase (ALP) have a relatively distinct organ specificity and can be divided into the liver, bone, intestinal, and placental types by electrophoresis, as illustrated in Fig. 17.6. Immunologically, however, the liver type cannot be distinguished from the bone type; isoenzymes of the liver-bone, intestinal, and placental types can be differentiated immunologically.

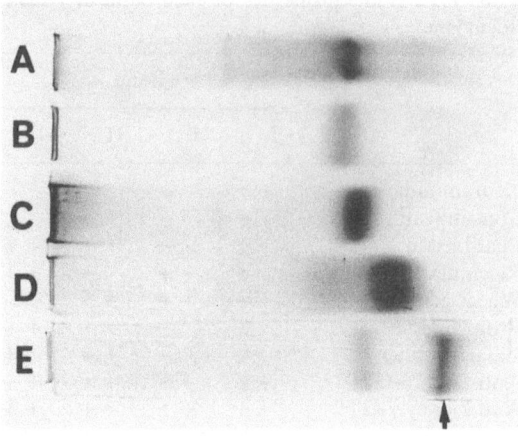

Fig. 17.6. Alkaline phosphatase isoenzymogram on polyacrylamide gradient gel (8%–16%). Extract of bone (*A*), extract of intestine (*B*), serum of patient with benign biliary disease (*C*), extract of placenta (*D*), serum of patient with hepatocellular carcinoma having a variant ALP (*E*). The *arrow* indicates a variant ALP

Table 17.4. Incidence of variant ALP and placental ALP in sera from patients with various disease

Diseases	No. of patients	Variant ALP	Placental ALP
Hepatocellular cancer	94	17	0
Metastatic liver cancer	17	0	1
Pancreatic cancer	7	0	0
Cancer of biliary tract	8	0	0
Cancer of gastro-intestinal tract	33	0	3
Lung cancer	4	0	2
Liver cirrhosis	21	0	1
Acute hepatitis	3	0	0
Intrahepatic choles-tasis	3	0	0
Benign diseases of biliary tract	16	0	0
Others	32	0	0
Total	238	17	7

The Regan isoenzyme discovered by Fishman et al. [32], Nagao isoenzyme by Nakayama et al. [33], and variant ALP (VAALP) by Warnock and Reisman [34] are regarded as ALP isoenzymes that appear with carcinogenesis specifically in the serum or cancerous tissue. The former two are of the placental type but show a slight difference physicochemically. Their prevalence in the sera of cancer patients is given as about 10% in most reports. In our study too, the placental ALP was found in 6 of 69 patients (9%) with digestive cancer, as shown in Table 17.4, but it was not found in HCC nor did it show any organ specificity [35].

VAALP has been studied extensively in Japan; it was called hepatoma ALP by Suzuki et al. [36], because of its high specificity in HCC patients, and Kasahara isoenzyme by Higashino et al. [37]. Opinions are divided as to the origin of this isoenzyme, but it shows a character most akin to the fetal intestine type of ALP. It also resembles the adult intestine type, but its electromobility is far to the anodic side; it is sensitive to sialidase and slightly heat stable and shows a greater affinity to Con A than the adult intestine type of ALP.

The prevalence of VAALP in the sera of HCC patients was reported to be 31% among 51 patients by Suzuki et al. [36], 14% in 56 patients by Higashino et al. [38], and 18% of 94 patients by us [35], as shown in Table 17.4. This isoenzyme was found in the sera of patients other than those with HCC, but its prevalence was very low. We found no positivity in 69 patients with other forms of cancer or in patients with benign hepatobiliary diseases. It thus seems to be a tumor marker that is highly specific to HCC. The frequency of this isoenzyme is low compared with the positivity rate for AFP and novel γ-GTP. As illustrated in Fig. 17.7, however, it was found to be independent of AFP level and of the presence of novel γ-GTP. This isoenzyme was positive in 5 of 36 patients in whom the AFP level was less than 400 ng/ml and novel γ-GTP was negative. In this respect, its clinical significance is complementary to that of AFP or novel γ-GTP. The utility of this method for diagnosis would be increased if a microassay utilizing a monoclonal antibody could be established.

5 Des-γ-carboxy prothrombin

The role of vitamin K in the synthesis of active prothrombin lies in carboxylation of the glutamic acid residue of a prothrombin precursor. The absence of vitamin K or ingestion of a vitamin K antagonist, such as sodium warfarin, inhibits the vitamin K-dependent carboxylase activity of the liver, and des-γ-carboxy prothrombin (abnormal prothrombin) is released into the blood. Blanchard et al. [39] prepared an antibody against des-γ-carboxy prothrombin (DCP) and measured its level in serum by RIA. It was hardly detectable in normal subjects but was increased in some patients with acute hepatitis, liver cirrhosis, and metastatic liver cancer. High

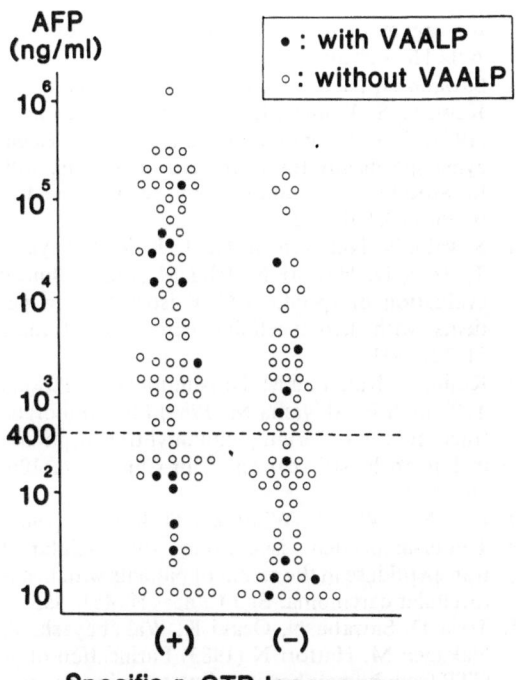

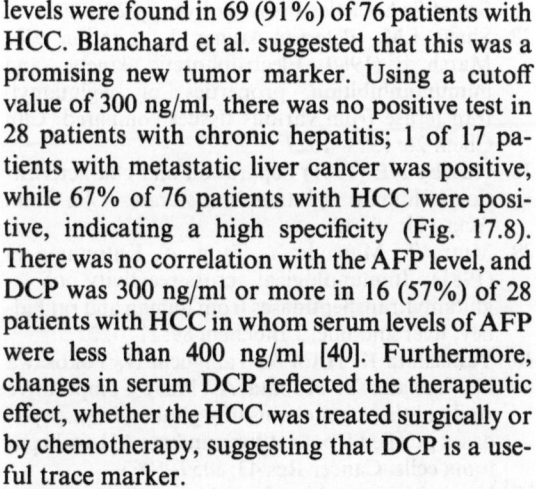

Specific r–GTP Isoenzyme

Fig. 17.7. Correlation between serum levels of AFP and positivity for novel γ-GTP and VAALP

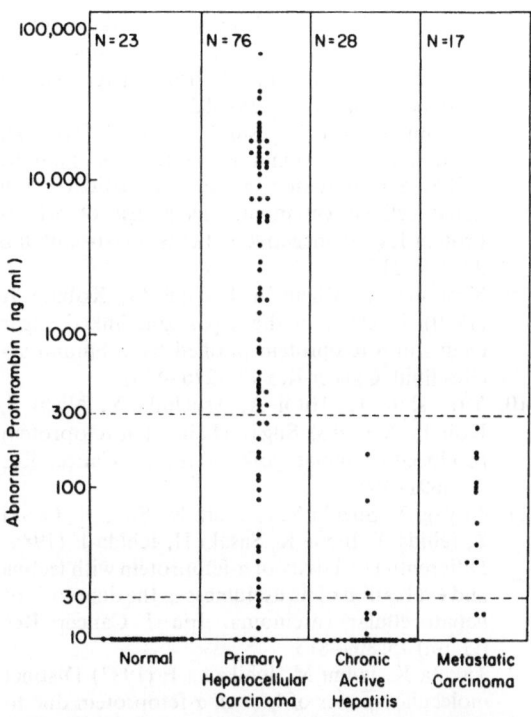

Fig. 17.8. Serum levels of des-γ-carboxy prothrombin in normal subjects and patients with various liver diseases. After Liebman et al. [40], with permission of New England Journal of Medicine

levels were found in 69 (91%) of 76 patients with HCC. Blanchard et al. suggested that this was a promising new tumor marker. Using a cutoff value of 300 ng/ml, there was no positive test in 28 patients with chronic hepatitis; 1 of 17 patients with metastatic liver cancer was positive, while 67% of 76 patients with HCC were positive, indicating a high specificity (Fig. 17.8). There was no correlation with the AFP level, and DCP was 300 ng/ml or more in 16 (57%) of 28 patients with HCC in whom serum levels of AFP were less than 400 ng/ml [40]. Furthermore, changes in serum DCP reflected the therapeutic effect, whether the HCC was treated surgically or by chemotherapy, suggesting that DCP is a useful trace marker.

There have been no reports to indicate that serum DCP levels in HCC patients are affected by administration of vitamin K. Thus, it is speculated that the increase is not due merely to the deficiency of vitamin K and that DCP may be produced directly in HCC by a disorder in the hepatic vitamin K-dependent carboxylation system. Further studies in more patients are needed, but currently this substance appears to be a useful tumor marker in low AFP-producing HCC.

Reference

1. Ruoslahti E, Seppälä M (1979) α-Fetoprotein in cancer and fetal development. Adv Cancer Res 29: 275–346
2. Hirai H, Nishi S, Watanabe H, Tsukada Y (1973) Some clinical, experimental, and clinical investigations of α-fetoprotein. In: Hirai H, Miyaji T (eds) α-Fetoprotein and hepatoma. Gann Monogr Cancer Res 14. Japan Scientific Societies Press, Tokyo, pp 19–34
3. Okuda K (1976) Clinical aspect of hepatocellular carcinoma-analysis of 134 cases. In: Okuda K, Peters RL (eds) Hepatocellular carcinoma. Wiley, New York, pp 387–405
4. Chen DS, Sung JL, Sheu JC, Lai MY, How SW, Hsu HC, Lee CS, Wei TC (1984) Serum α-fetoprotein in the early stage of human hepatocellular carcinoma. Gastroenterology 86: 1404–1409
5. Sheu JC, Sung JL, Chen DS, Yang PM, Lai MY, Lee CS, Hsu HC, Chuang CN, Yang PC, Wang TH, Lin JC, Lee CZ (1985) Growth rate of asymptomatic hepatocellular carcinoma and its clinical implications. Gastroenterology 89: 259–266
6. Kobayashi K, Sugimoto T, Makino H, Kumagai M, Unoura M, Tanaka N, Kato Y, Hattori N (1985) Screening methods for early detection of hepatocellular carcinoma. Hepatology 5: 1100–1105

7. Kubo Y, Okuda K, Musha H, Nakashima T (1978) Detection of hepatocellular crcinoma during a clinical follow-up of chronic liver disease. Gastroenterology 74: 578–582

8. Sawabu N, Wakabayashi T, Ozaki K, Toya D, Yoneshima M, Kidani H, Hattori N, Ishii M (1985) Serum tumor markers in patients with hepatocellular carcinoma: Diagnosis of α-fetoprotein-low or -negative patients. Gastroent Jap 20: 209–215

9. Yoshima H, Mizuochi T, Ishii M, Kobata A (1980) Structure of the asparagine-linked sugar chains of α-fetoprotein purified from human ascites fluid. Cancer Res 40: 4276–4281

10. Yamashita K, Hitoi A, Tsuchida Y, Nishi S, Kobata A (1983) Sugar chain of α-fetoprotein produced in human yolk sac tumor. Cancer Res 43: 4691–4695

11. Aoyagi Y, Suzuki Y, Isemura M, Soga K, Ozaki T, Ichida T, Inoue K, Sasaki H, Ichida F (1984) Differential reactivity of α-fetoprotein with lectins and evaluation of its usefulness in the diagnosis of hepatocellular carcinoma. Jpn J Cancer Res (Gann) 75: 809–815

12. Taketa K, Izumi M, Ichikawa E (1983) Distinct molecular species of human α-fetoprotein due to differential affinities to lectins. Ann NY Acad Sci 417: 61–68

13. Ishiguro T, Sugitachi I, Sakaguchi H, Itani S (1985) Serum α-fetoprotein subfractions in patients with primary hepatoma or hepatic metastasis of gastric cancer. Cancer 55: 156–159

14. Bellet DH, Wands JR, Isselbacher KJ, Bohunon C (1984) Serum α-fetoprotein levels in human disease: perspective from a highly specific monoclonal radioimmunoassay. Proc Natl Acad Sci USA 81: 3869–3873

15. Fiala S, Fiala AE, Dixon B (1972) γ-Glutamyl transpeptidase in transplantable chemically induced rat hepatomas and "spontaneous" mouse hepatomas. J Natl Cancer Inst 48: 1393–1401

16. Kalengayi MMR, Ronchi G, Desmet VJ (1975) Histochemistry of γ-glutamyl transpeptidase in rat liver during aflatoxin B_1-induced carcinogenesis. J Natl Cancer Inst 55: 579–582

17. Taniguchi N, Saito K, Takakuwa E (1975) γ-Glutamyltransferase from azodye induced hepatoma and fetal rat liver, similarities in their kinetic and immunological properties. Biochim Biophys Acta 391: 265–271

18. Sells MA, Katyal SL, Sell S, Shinozuka H, Lombardi B (1979) Induction of foci of altered, γ-glutamyltranspeptidase-positive hepatocytes in carcinogen-treated rats fed a choline-deficient diet. Br J Cancer 40: 274–283

19. Tsuchida S, Hoshino K, Sato T, Ito N, Sato K (1979) Purification of γ-glutamyltranferases from rat hepatomas and hyperplastic hepatic nodules, and comparison with the enzyme from rat kidney. Cancer Res 39: 4200–4205

20. Albert Z, Rzucidlo Z, Starzyk H (1970) Comparative biochemical and histochemical studies on the activity of gamma-glutamyl transpeptidase in the organs of fetuses, newborns and adult rats. Acta Histochem 37: 34–49

21. Sawabu N, Nakagen M, Yoneda M, Makino H, Kameda S, Kobayashi K, Hattori N, Ishii M (1978) Novel γ-glutamyl transpeptidase isoenzyme specifically found in sera of patients with hepatocellular carcinoma Jpn J Cancer Res (Gann) 69: 601–605

22. Sawabu N, Nakagen M, Ozaki K, Wakabayashi T, Toya D, Hattori N, Ishii M (1983) Clinical evaluation of specific γ-GTP isoenzyme in patients with hepatocellular carcinoma. Cancer 51: 327–331

23. Kojima J, Kanatani M, Nakamura N, Kashiwagi T, Tohjoh F, Akiyama M (1980) Electrophoretic fractionation of serum γ-glutamyl transpeptidase in human hepatic cancer. Clin Chim Acta 106: 165–172

24. Kew MC, Wolf P, Whittaker D, Rowe P (1984) Tumor-associated isoenzymes of γ-glutamyl transpeptidase in the serum of patients with hepatocellular carcinoma. Br J Cancer 50: 451–455

25. Toya D, Sawabu N, Ozaki K, Wakabayashi T, Nakagen M, Hattori N (1983) Purification of γ-GTP from human hepatocellular carcinoma, and comparison with enzyme from kidney. Ann NY Acad Sci 417: 89–96

26. Sawabu N, Toya D, Ozaki K, Wakabayashi T, Nakagen M, (1983) Clinical value and some properties of novel γ-GTP isoenzyme specific to sera of hepatocellular carcinoma. In: Makita A, Tsuiki S, Fujii S, Warren L (eds) Membrane alterations in cancer. Gann Monogr Cancer Res 29. Japan Scientific Societies Press, Tokyo, pp 291–298

27. Shaw LM, Petersen-Archer L, London JW, Marsh E (1980) Electrophoretic, kinetic, and immunoinhibition properties of γ-glutamyltransferase from various tissues compared. Clin Chem 26: 1523–1527

28. Huseby NE (1981) Separation and characterization of human γ-glutamyltransferases. Clin Chim Acta 111: 39–45

29. Miura T, Matsuda Y, Tsuji, A, Katunuma N (1981) Immunological cross-reactivity of γ-glutamyltransferases from human and rat kidney, liver and bile. J Biochem 89: 217–222

30. Yamashita K, Hitoi A, Taniguchi N, Yokosawa N, Tsukada Y, Kobata A (1983) Comparative study of the sugar chains of γ-glutamyltranspeptidases purified from rat liver and rat AH-66 hepatoma cells. Cancer Res 43: 5059–5063

31. Hitoi A, Yamashita K, Ohkawa J, Kobata A (1984) Application of a phaseolus vulgaris erythroagglutinating lectin agarose column for the specific detection of human hepatoma γ-glutamyl transpeptidase in serum. Jpn J Cancer Res (Gann) 75: 301–304

32. Fishman WH, Inglis NR, Stolbach LL, Krant MJ (1986) A serum alkaline phosphatase isoenzyme of human neoplastic cell origin. Cancer Res 28: 150–154

33. Nakayama T, Yoshida M, Kitamura M (1970) L-leucine sensitive, heat-stable alkaline-phospha-

tase isoenzyme detected in a patient with pleuritis carcinomatosa. Clin Chim Acta 30: 546–548

34. Warnock ML, Reisman R (1969) Variant alkaline phosphatase in human hepatocellular cancers. Clin Chim Acta 24: 5–11

35. Nakagen M, Sawabu N, Sendai H, Wakabayashi T, Ozaki K, Toya D, Hattori N (1980) Evaluation of alkaline phosphatase isoenzyme separated by polyacrylamide gradient gel electrophoresis: Special reference to variant alkaline phosphatase. Jpn J Gastroent 77: 1940–1937 (in Japanese)

36. Suzuki H, Iino S, Endo Y, Torii M, Miki K, Oda T (1975) Tumor-specific alkaline phosphatase in hepatoma. Ann NY Acad Sci 259: 307–316

37. Higashino K, Kudo S, Ohtani R, Yamamura Y, Honda T, Sakurai J (1975) A hepatoma-associated alkaline phosphatase, the Kasahara isoenzyme, compared with one of the isoenzyme of FL ammion cells. Ann NY Acad Sci 259: 337–346

38. Higashino K, Kudo S, Ohtani R, Yamamura Y (1976) Further observation on Kasahara isoenzyme in patients with malignant diseases. Jpn J Cancer Res (Gann) 67: 909–911

39. Blanchard RA, Furie BC, Jorgensen M, Kruger SF, Furie B (1981) Acquired vitamin K-dependent carboxylation deficiency in liver disease. N Engl J Med 305: 242–248

40. Liebmen HA, Furie BC, Tong MJ, Blanchard RA, Lo KJ, Lee SD, Coleman MS, Furie B (1984) Des-γ-carboxy (abnormal) prothrombin as a serum marker of primary hepatocellular carcinoma. N Engl J Med 310: 1427–1431

Chapter 18

Scintigraphy in the Diagnosis of Hepatocellular Carcinoma

Michael C. Kew[1] and Joseph Levin[2]

1 Introduction

The introduction of hepatic scintigraphy in the late 1950s represented a major advance in the diagnosis of focal hepatic lesions because it became possible for the first time to obtain images of the liver with a noninvasive procedure. Several years were to elapse before alternative and perhaps better hepatic imaging modalities became available, and during this time radiotracer scanning proved to be invaluable, both in the recognition of hepatocellular carcinoma and in the evaluation of patients with this tumor. Scintigraphy was used to confirm (or in some patients to establish) the presence of a "space-occupying lesion" in the liver, to provide a reasonably accurate assessment of the size, position, the extent of the tumor when resectability was being considered, and to determine the optimal site for percutaneous biopsy of the lesion.

There are, however, limitations inherent in this technique of hepatic imaging and these soon became apparent. The most serious is that the images obtained with conventional radiocolloid scanning are not specific for any particular type of "space-occupying lesion" in the liver. Because the colloid is normally phagocytosed by the reticuloendothelial cells in the liver, the presence of disease is recognized by failure to accumulate the radiotracer. Inevitably, therefore, specificity of diagnosis must be limited because detection of disease is based on absence of normal hepatic tissue rather than on presence of abnormal tissue. It is thus not possible, by examining the hepatic images, to differentiate with certainty hepatocellular carcinoma (HCC) from other

malignant or benign hepatic tumors, hepatic metastases, hepatic abscesses, parasitic or congenital cysts of the liver, or intrahepatic or subcapsular hematomata. Even cirrhosis, which often coexists with HCC, may cause difficulties in interpretation: Nodular regeneration, fibrosis, and intrahepatic and extrahepatic shunting of blood reduce the exposure of the radiocolloid to the reticuloendothelial cells, resulting in areas of photon deficiency on the image, which could readily be mistaken for a tumor arising in the cirrhotic liver—so much so, that these defects are referred to as "pseudotumors."

The value of all radiotracers in the diagnosis of HCC is hampered by the fact that their uptake depends among other things upon the circulation through the tumor. Interference with this circulation is not infrequent and may have more than one cause. Large tumors frequently undergo central necrosis, presumably on the basis of ischemia. In addition, HCC has the propensity to invade and occlude portal and hepatic venous radicles. Finally, hemorrhage into the tumor substance may occur.

Further diagnostic difficulties arise because overlying breast tissue, loculated ascitic fluid, or the bowel may produce photopenic areas which simulate mass lesions in the liver. Moreover, extrahepatic masses impinging on the liver may be responsible for images which are indistinguishable from those resulting from intrinsic hepatic lesions. Finally, if hepatic function is poor with a marked shift of radiotracer activity to the spleen, it is difficult to identify focal hepatic lesions.

Although there have been appreciable advances in scintigraphic techniques as regards radionuclides, radiopharmaceuticals, instrumentation, and sophisticated computer programs, the diagnostic accuracy of conventional planar hepatic imaging has not improved materially over the years. The nonspecificity of the images obtained

[1] Department of Medicine, University of the Witwatersrand and Johannesburg and Hillbrow Hospitals, Johannesburg, South Africa
[2] Department of Nuclear Medicine, University of the Witwatersrand, Johannesburg, South Africa

with colloidal scanning has been the stimulus to an ongoing search for other radiotracers possessing properties which might enable HCC to be positively differentiated from other mass lesions in the liver.

Another major limitation of scintigraphic imaging for HCC is its inability to detect very small tumors. The resolution limits of this technique mean that hepatic lesions less than 2.0 cm in diameter are not visualized (although slightly smaller lesions may be seen if they are close to the surface of the liver). Consequently, radiotracer scanning is not useful in detecting the early, so-called minute tumors which are being sought in surveillance programs of individuals considered to be at high risk of developing HCC.

The successive introduction of other imaging modalities—ultrasonography, transmission computed tomography and, very recently, magnetic resonance imaging—has unquestionably enhanced our capability of detecting very small hepatic lesions. The use of these procedures has also increased the amount of information which can be obtained about mass lesions in the liver. Continuing technological advances in scintigraphic techniques as well as in ultrasonography and computed tomography have made comparisons between the three imaging modalities difficult. It is, however, likely that these procedures, as well as magnetic resonance imaging, will prove to be complementary to one another. Nevertheless, the new techniques are not without limitations, and the search for more sensitive and specific imaging modalities therefore continues.

What then is the place of radiotracer imaging of the liver in the diagnosis of HCC at the present time?

2 Colloidal imaging

99m-Technetium sulfur (or tin) colloid is routinely used for hepatic scintigraphy. Colloidal markers are rapidly and almost completely removed from the circulation by the hepatic reticuloendothelial cells. The intensity and uniformity of the hepatic image obtained depend upon the size of the colloidal particles, the rate and distribution of hepatic blood flow, and the functional integrity of the hepatic reticuloendothelial system. "Space-occupying lesions" show as photon-deficient areas on the hepatic image (Fig. 18.1).

Scanning with radiocolloids will almost invariably show the presence of one or more photopenic areas in patients with advanced HCC

(Figs. 18.2, 18.3) [1–4]. This applies equally in populations with a high incidence of the tumor and in those in which HCC occurs rarely and the tumor tends to be smaller. For example, in two studies from Great Britain, photopenic areas were evident in 30 of 34 [1] and in 36 of 38 patients [2]. Seven of the 30 patients in the former series showed, in addition, a patchy loss of uptake of the radiotracer or increased splenic uptake suggestive of cirrhosis, although the former could also have been caused by multiple small neoplastic foci throughout the liver. In two other patients, the defects were less definite, and the remaining two showed only patchy loss of uptake consistent with cirrhosis or diffuse HCC. In an analysis of southern African Blacks only 1 of 202 scans was considered to be normal [4]. A solitary defect was seen in 72% of the patients, two or more defects in 15%, and obviously patchy uptake of the radiotracer in 12%. As was the case with the British patients, in the patients with one or more photopenic areas the remainder of the liver frequently appeared patchy. Photopenic defects was noted in both hepatic lobes in 39% of patients, the right lobe only in 57%, and the left lobe only in 4%.

Anterior, posterior, and right and left lateral images should be recorded when looking for suspected HCC to ensure that smaller lesions are not overlooked. It is also important to mark the palpable edge of the liver so that tumors situated predominantly along the inferior hepatic border are not missed [4].

Analyses of the sensitivity and specificity of radiocolloid imaging are somewhat conflicting, both having been reported as low as 70% and as high as 96% [5–8].

How does scintigraphy compare with other imaging modalities in the diagnosis of focal hepatic lesions? Several such comparisons have been published [8]. To quote the results of one: In a prospective study comparing the accuracy of scintigraphy, ultrasonography, and computed tomography in the recognition of hepatic metastases, no statistically significant differences were found in the sensitivity (93% for computed tomography, 86% for scintigraphy, and 82% for ultrasonography) or specificity (88%, 83%, and 85%, respectively) of the three techniques [9]. For the detection of advanced HCC, hepatic scintigraphy is comparable in sensitivity with

Fig. 18.2. Four examples of the types of hepatic image ▶ (anterior view) which are characteristically seen with radiocolloid scanning in African patients with advanced HCC

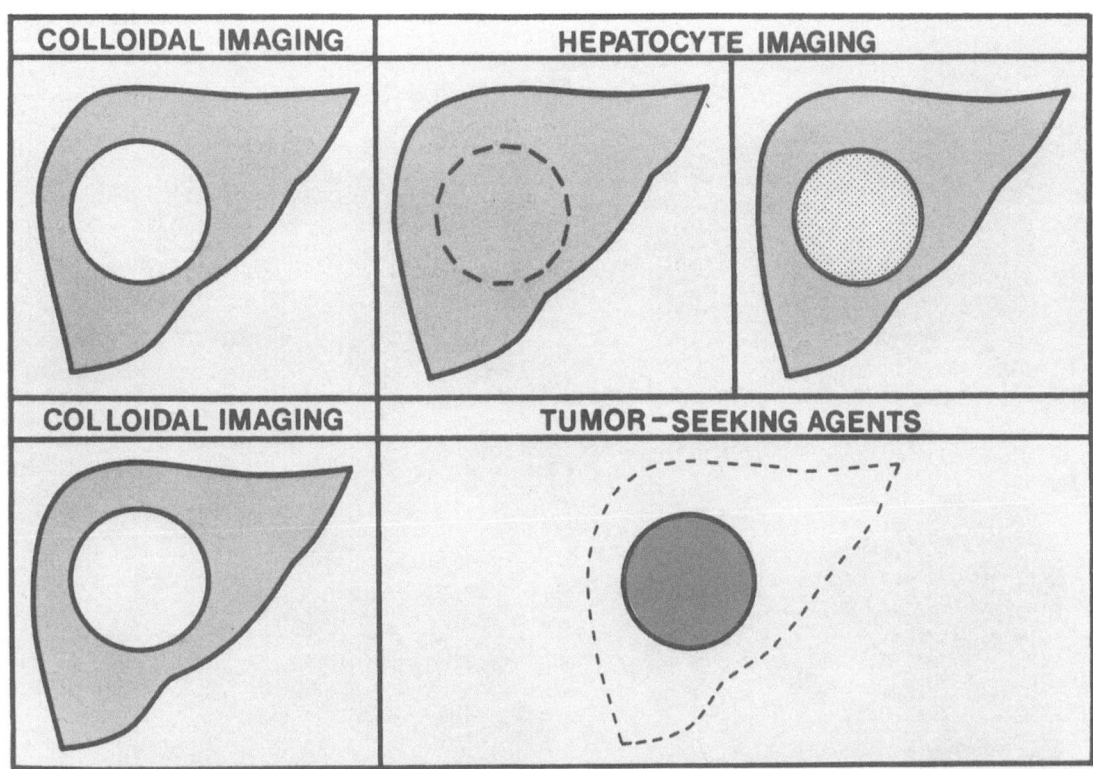

Fig. 18.1. With conventional colloidal imaging, HCC shows as a photon-deficient area on the hepatic image. When radiotracers specifically taken up by hepatocytes are used, the defect seen on the colloidal scan either disappears completely or is partially "filled in" (*upper row of images*). Tumor-seeking radiotracers may be selectively concentrated by the HCC, and the defect seen with colloidal imaging is replaced by a "hot spot" (*lower images*)

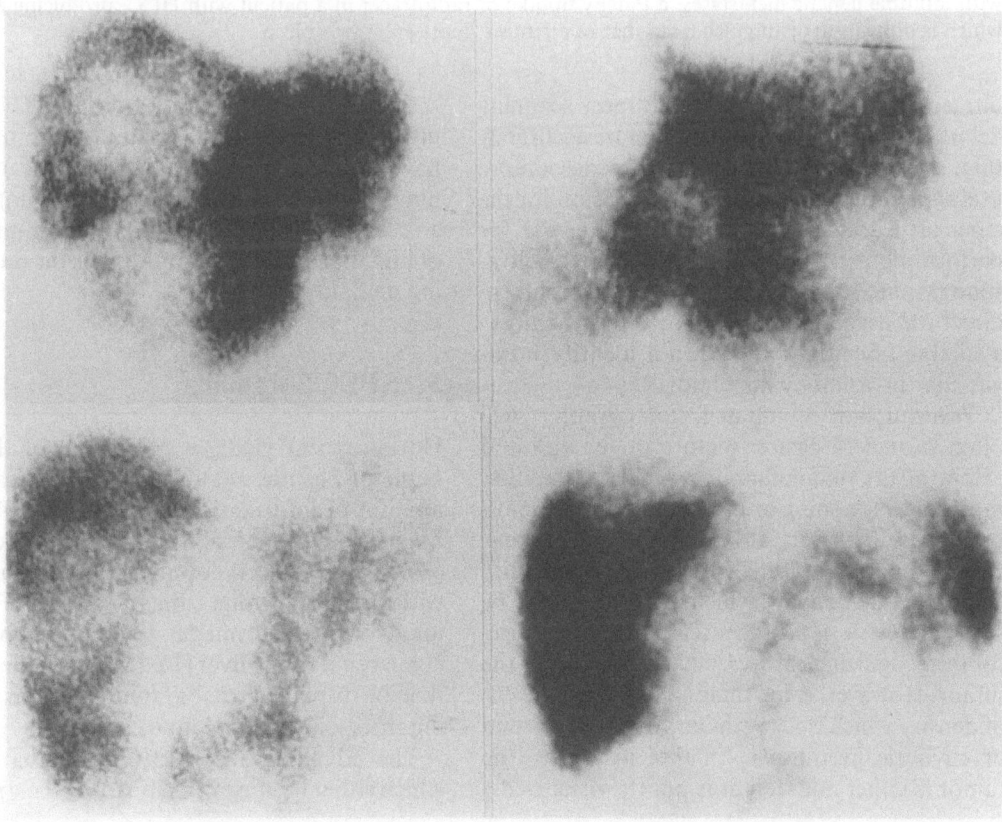

Fig. 18.2

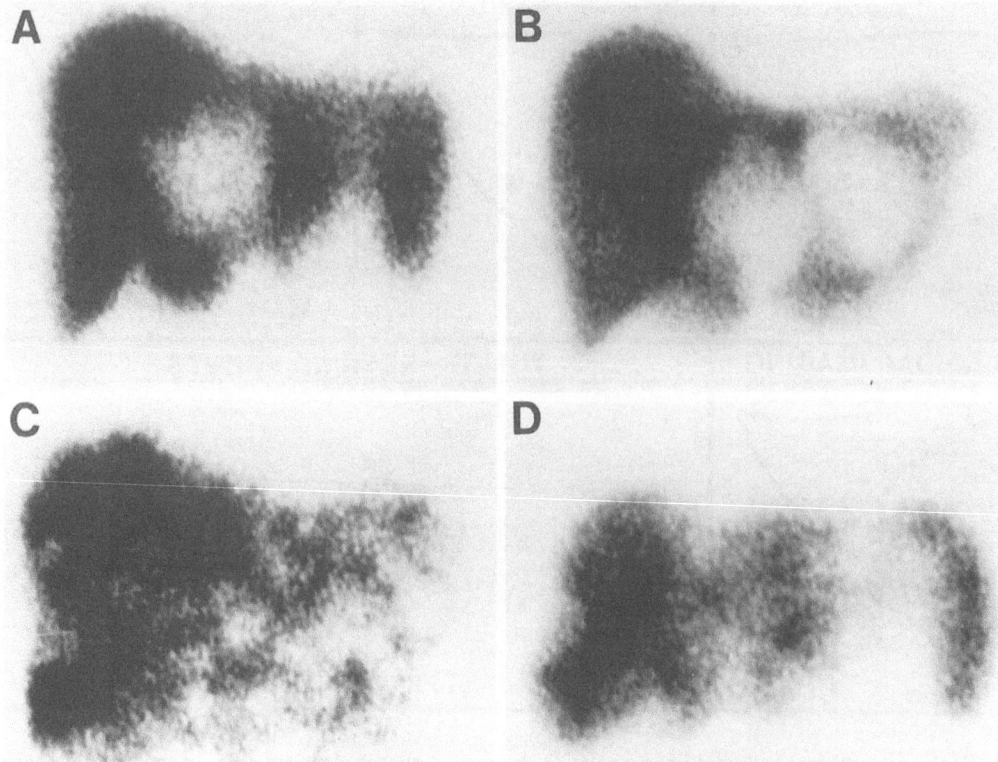

Fig. 18.3. a Smaller and more circumscribed HCC, more typical of those seen in Japanese or Caucasoid patients. **b** Two foci of HCC, each with a well-defined, almost smooth edge, simulating the picture typically seen with hepatic abscesses or cysts. **c** Multinodular HCC producing an image which is indistinguishable from that seen with multiple hepatic metastases. **d** Patchy uptake of radiotracer in a patient with HCC, producing an image which is difficult to distinguish from that of cirrhosis. Note enlarged spleen

ultrasonography. However, radiotracer scanning delineates the extent of the lesion more accurately than does ultrasonography and provides a more useful picture of the position of the lesion for the clinician wanting to know the optimal site for performing a needle biopsy. (Of course, ultrasonographic visualization can be used actually to direct the needle into the tumor if this facility is available.) Scintigraphy will not identify intravascular invasion by the tumor.

Transmission computed tomography will often provide a clearer picture of the size and extent of the tumor than is possible with either radiotracer scanning or ultrasonography. Scintigraphy is, however, an acceptable alternative. Computed tomography will also clearly identify small satellite nodules, which can at best only be suspected with radiotracer scanning, and is useful in recognizing intravascular invasion by the tumor. However, some tumors have a coefficient of density which is very similar to that of normal or cirrhotic liver tissue. In thse instances, the tumor is either not seen or is poorly visualized.

It is in the detection of "minute" HCCs that ultrasonography and computed tomography have a distinct advantage over radiotracer scanning. For this reason, scintigraphy is not used as a screening procedure in surveillance programs of high-risk individuals unless it is the only imaging modality available.

3 SPECT scanning

During recent years, a refinement of the technique of hepatic scintigraphy has increased the amount of information which can be obtained. Single-photon emission computed tomography (SPECT) records computed tomographic scans with a rotating gama camera capable of recording 64 sequential images around the entire circumference of the liver [10, 11]. These images can then be displayed tomographically or as a rotating three-dimensional image.

The advantages of SPECT are that lesions which either because of their size or their position give equivocal pictures on planar scanning can be more clearly seen. At the same time, the number of false-positive results is reduced. In one analysis, it was estimated that SPECT improved sensitivity over conventional planar imaging by 10%–15% [11]. The sensitivity of SPECT was lowest for small lesions in the middle third of the liver. Another advantage of SPECT is that the exact position and extent of "space-occupying lesions" in the liver can be more clearly defined, although, unlike computed tomography, SPECT does not provide information about anatomical landmarks.

Even though SPECT scanning is capable of detecting smaller lesions than is possible with planar scintigraphy, only 52% of hepatic lesions with a diameter of 1.5–2 cm were visualized with this method [11]. For this reason and because of time and financial constraints, SPECT is not a suitable technique for mass screening of "minute" hepatic tumors.

Because the photopenic areas seen in patients with HCC are not diagnostic, attempts have been made over the years to find alternative radiotracers which might make it possible for a specific diagnosis of this tumor to be made. Two approaches have been tried. The first takes advantage of the highly vascular nature of many HCCs by serially recording hepatic images immediately after injection of a radiotracer or by radiolabeling erythrocytes and assessing the pooling of blood in the photopenic area. The other approach involves the search for radio-tracers which are taken up specifically by hepatocytes or by tumor cells (Fig. 18.1). Malignant hepatocytes retain some of the functions of normal hepatocytes, including the ability to secrete bile. The better differentiated the tumor, the more likely this is to occur. By attaching radionuclides to substances known to be taken up and metabolized or secreted by hepatocytes it was hoped that malignant hepatocytes could specifically be imaged. With the exception of hepatocellular adenomas and focal nodular hyperplasia, both of which are rare, and cirrhotic "pseudotumors," the only mass lesions in the liver which contain hepatocytes are HCCs.

4   Scintiangiography and blood pool scanning

Hepatic arteriography has shown that about 85% of HCCs are vascular [12]. Moreover, this tumor derives its blood supply exclusively or predominantly from the hepatic artery [12]. By recording serial images at short intervals starting immediately after injection of the colloidal radiotracer, it is possible to ascertain whether a "space-occupying lesion" in the liver is vascular or avascular; with vascular lesions, including HCC, the photopenic area visible on colloidal imaging "fills in" early during dynamic scintiangiography (perfusion scanning) (Fig. 18.4) [13, 14].

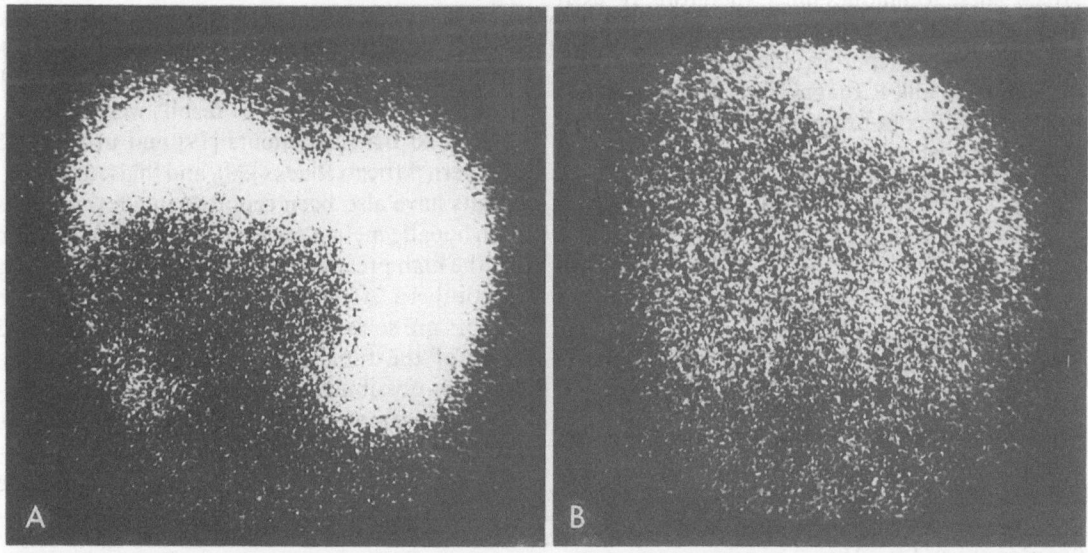

Fig. 18.4A, B. Large photopenic area visible on a 99m-technetium sulfur colloid scan (**A**) is not seen during dynamic scintiangiography (**B**), indicating the presence of a highly vascular HCC

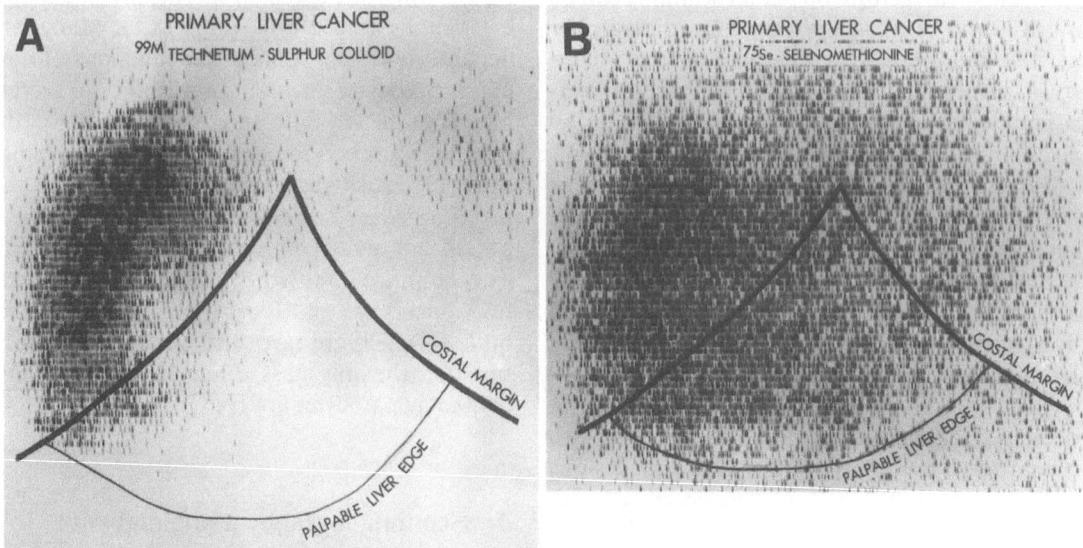

Fig. 18.5A, B. Primary liver cancer. Large photopenic area visible on **A** a 99m-technetium sulfur colloid scan is not seen on **B** a 75-selenium selenomethionine scan

The blood pool scan has been used to provide information similar to that derived from dynamic scintiangiography. This procedure involves labeling erythrocytes with 99m-technetium stannous fluoride. Vascular HCCs show up as "hot spots" during imaging [15].

A major drawback of both of these methods is that cavernous hemangioma, the most common benign hepatic tumor, gives the same picture. Hepatic metastases may also be vascular, and they too will give a false-positive result. Furthermore, a negative study does not exclude HCC. These techniques must, therefore, be used in conjunction, not only with colloidal scanning, but also with a hepatocyte-labeling radiotracer in order to be able to diagnose HCC with any certainty. This has been done by Lee and his colleagues [16], who used a combination of colloidal scanning, scintiangiography and 67-gallium scanning.

5   Specific hepatocyte imaging

The first radiotracer used specifically to label hepatocytes was 131-iodine rose-bengal. This substance is taken up and secreted by hepatocytes in the same way as bilirubin and could, therefore, be used both for hepatic imaging and functional studies. However, there are many technical difficulties associated with the use of 131-iodine rose bengal and it is no longer used to any extent.

5.1   75-Selenium-selenomethionine

This radiotracer is formed by the substitution of 75-selenium (^{75}Se) for the sulfur atom in methionine. The resulting substance follows the same metabolic pathways as the parent molecule and its incorporation into a tissue is, therefore, determined by the tissue's blood supply and its ability to metabolize methionine. In 1967, Ben-Porath et al. [17] showed that the uptake of ^{75}Se selenomethionine by HCC approached that of the surrounding normal liver tissue (Fig. 18.5), a property which should not have been shared by most "space-occupying lesions" in the liver. The diagnostic usefulness of this radiotracer was subsequently confirmed in other studies [18, 19]. However, "false-negative" results were obtained in 4 of 26 British patients [19] and in 22 of 45 southern African Blacks [20], and "false-positive" results have also been reported in a few patients with hepatic metastases [19, 21]. One explanation for the high prevalence of "falsenegative" results in southern African Blacks could be that the tumors are so anaplastic that they have retained none of the functions of normal hepatocytes. Another possibility is that the tumors are necrotic, a not infrequent occurrence in the very large HCCs frequently seen in Black patients. In cirrhosis, hepatic uptake of ^{75}Se selenomethionine is variable, even in the absence of an HCC.

5.2   67-Gallium citrate

In early studies of patients with HCC, selective uptake of 67-gallium citrate by the tumor was found in 11 of 12 [22] and 16 of 18 patients [23]. A review of all published series of patients with HCC indicates that about 90% of these tumors selectively concentrate 67-gallium [24]. However, two studies showed appreciably lower sensitivities for the radionuclide. We recorded "false-positive" results in 29% of southern African Blacks [25], as did Waxman and his colleagues in the same proportion of patients from the United States [26]. Unfortunately, from the diagnostic point of view, 67-gallium citrate is also concentrated in hepatic abscesses, in some hepatic metastases, especially melanomas, and in hepatocellular adenomas [24]. Because hepatic metastases are common in all populations and amebic hepatic abscesses are common in some populations, and because both may mimic HCC clinically, this nonspecificity in the uptake of 67-gallium citrate lessens its usefulness in the diagnosis of HCC. Nevertheless, as already mentioned, Lee et al. have used 67-gallium citrate in conjunction with colloidal imaging and hepatic scintiangiography in the diagnosis of the tumor [16].

67-Gallium may also have a specific use in the recognition of HCC when it occurs in a cirrhotic liver [25]. Because the majority of patients with HCC have coexisting cirrhosis, this problem is not infrequently encountered. Cirrhotic pseudotumors do not take up 67-gallium, whereas the tumor would be expected to concentrate the radionuclide. In an investigation of 18 patients with HCC and coexisting cirrhosis, the defect could be positively identified as a tumor in 12 patients; in the remaining six, however, failure by the tumor to take up 67-gallium could have resulted in the latter being overlooked [25].

The reason for the selective uptake of 67-gallium by HCC is not known. The vascularity of the tumor as well as the extent of necrosis will obviously have an influence on the uptake. Because 67-gallium is taken up by normal hepatocytes, selective concentration by malignant hepatocytes may depend upon their degree of differentiation, and there is some evidence in support of this. Four out of five patients reported by Waxman et al. [26] in whom selective concentration did not occur had anaplastic tumors, whereas 11 of 12 patients with selective concentration had well or moderately differentiated tumors. However, 67-gallium is also concentrated in macrophages and in reticuloendothelial cells.

5.3 Hepatobiliary imaging agents

Three case reports published in 1980 first suggested the possibility that hepatobiliary imaging agents might be useful in the specific diagnosis of HCC. In the first, pulmonary metastases in a patient with HCC concentrated 99m-technetium-p-isopropyliminodiacetic acid [27], and in the other two HCC took up 99m-technetium pyridoxylidene isoleucine and 99m-technetium pyridoxilidene glutamate, respectively [28, 29]. Radiotracers used for hepatobiliary imaging are concentrated by normal hepatocytes and excreted into bile, sharing the same anionic transport pathway as bilirubin. Malignant hepatocytes, especially when well differentiated, may have retained this property. However, when this radiotracer was submitted to formal study in 30 southern African Blacks using 99m-technetium-di-isopropyliminodiacetic acid, nearly two-thirds of the patients showed no uptake of the radiotracer by the tumor (in the remaining patients there was some uptake by the tumor) [30]. Correlation with histological findings failed to show any difference in uptake between well-, moderately, and poorly differentiated tumors. In two patients with multiple pulmonary metastases, the latter did not concentrate the radiotracer. Similar disappointing results were found by Yeh et al. [31]: In only 3 of 80 patients with HCC did selective concentration of 99m-technetium iminodiacetic acid analogues occur.

Recently, Lee et al. [32] have reported uptake of 99m-technetium iminodiacetic acid in four patients in whom delayed scans (after 2.5–4 h) were recorded. They suggested that because the tumor lacks functioning bile ducts, the bile secreted by the malignant hepatocytes accumulates within the tumor, producing a positive delayed scan. Improved results with delayed scanning have also been reported by Hasegawa and colleagues [33].

Other tumors containing hepatocytes might also be expected to concentrate 99m-technetium iminodiacetic acid, and this has been reported to occur with hepatocellular adenomas and focal nodular hyperplasia [34]. Less easy to understand is the uptake by a metastasis from breast carcinoma [35].

5.4 111-Indium Chloride

111-Indium chloride has recently been used in the diagnosis of suspected HCC [36]. In seven of eight patients, the defect present on colloid scintigraphy selectively concentrated the 111-indium chloride. Unfortunately, 6 of 15 patients with defects caused by disease other than HCC did the same. 111-Indium is thought to dissociate from the chloride, forming 111-indium-transferrin. Localization of the complex to HCC suggests that malignant hepatocytes have transferrin receptors, but so do normal hepatocytes, which probably accounts for at least some of the false-positive results obtained.

6 Tumor-seeking agents

6.1 57-Cobalt bleomycin

Bleomycin, a group of polypeptide antibiotics derived from *Streptomyces verticillus*, is an effective cancer chemotherapeutic agent. Labeled with 57-cobalt, bleomycin was tried as a tumor-seeking agent in the early 1970s. The mechanism of localization of bleomycin in tumors is uncertain, but it is known to attach itself to DNA and this may be important in its tumor-seeking properties [37]. In early reports, all three patients with HCC studied showed selective concentration of the radiotracer by the tumor (Fig. 18.6) [38, 39]. However, when this radiopharmaceutical was used in 13 southern African Blacks with HCCs, selective concentration occurred in only four patients (31%) [40]. The parallel between the therapeutic efficacy of bleomycin in squamous cell carcinomas and the diagnostic usefulness of 57-cobalt bleomycin in these tumors suggests the possibility that the uptake of this radiotracer by tumors may be related primarily to the therapeutic efficacy of the antineoplastic agent in those particular tumors. If this is the case, then

the unimpressive findings in the southern African Blacks might have been anticipated because the results of treating HCC with bleomycin in these patients were disappointing.

6.2 99m-Technetium glucoheptonate

99m-Technetium glucoheptonate is selectively concentrated in pulmonary and cerebral tumors and hence has been used in their scintigraphic diagnosis [41, 42]. Pulmonary metastases are less well visualized, and 99m-technetium glucoheptonate scanning is inferior to plain radiography in their detection. However, HCC metastases may be an exception: In one report, these metastases were more readily seen on a 99m-technetium glucoheptonate scan than on chest X-ray [41]. Moreover, the primary tumor concentrated the radiotracer to a greater extent than did the surrounding hepatic tissue. These observations, together with the fact that hepatobiliary excretion of 99m-technetium glucoheptonate has been described, suggest that that this radiotracer might be useful in the scintigraphic recognition of primary and metastatic HCC.

The reason why 99m-technetium glucoheptonate is selectively concentrated by tumor tissue is not known. Glucoheptonate is a saccharide derived from corn syrup, and it has been suggested that 99m-technetium glucoheptonate is taken up like a glucose analogue by an active transport mechanism to be used as a substrate for energy by the metabolically active tumor tissue [42]. If

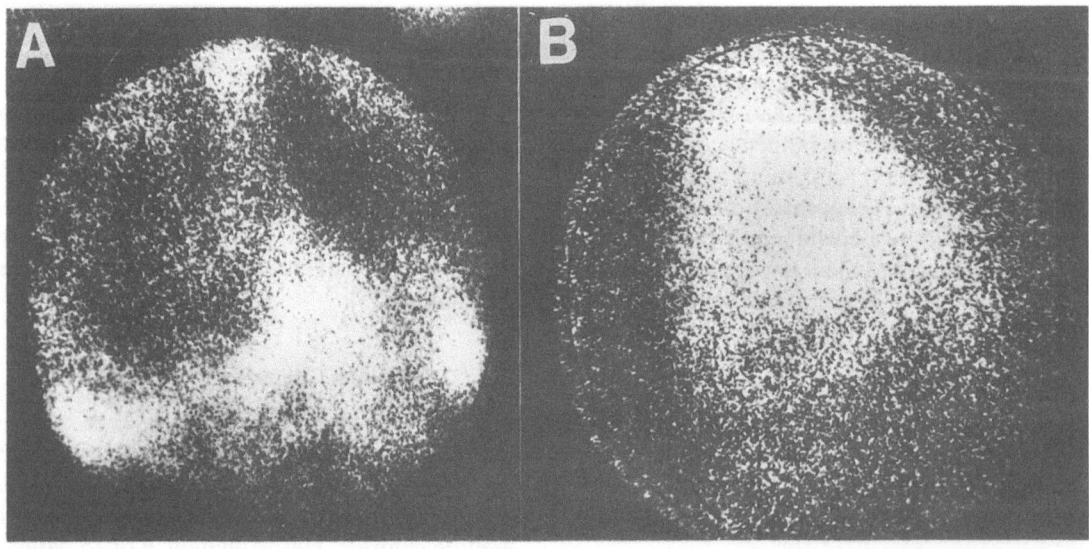

Fig. 18.6A, B. The defect on **A** 99m-technetium sulfur colloid scan and **B** selectively concentrated 57-cobalt-bleomycin in a patient with HCC

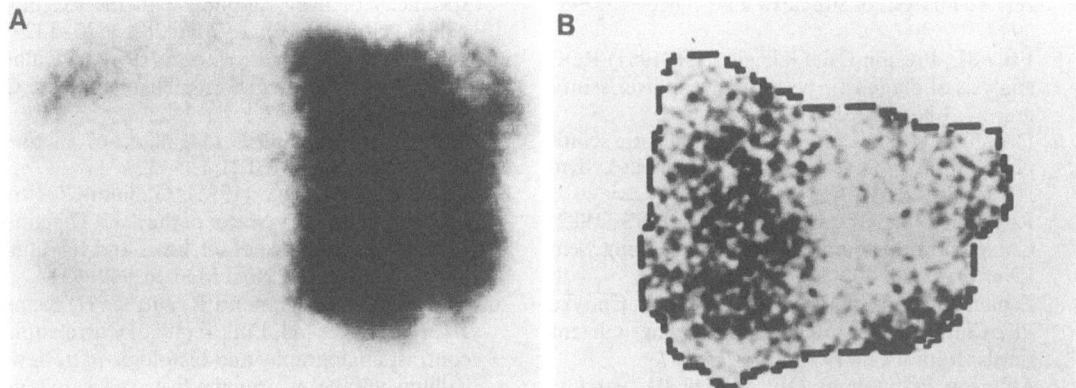

Fig. 18.7A, B. Large defect replacing right hepatic lobe on **A** 99m-technetium sulfur colloid scan in patient with HCC. **B** Subtraction scan showing uptake of monoclonal antibody against alpha fetoprotein by large tumor mass in right lobe and in smaller tumor deposits in left lobe

this were so, one would expect a large amount of the material to be taken up by the liver, a metabolically active tissue. On the contrary, distribution studies in rats show a very low concentration of 99m-technetium glucoheptonate in the liver [43]. If some degree of metabolism of glucoheptonate by the tumor occurred, one would expect a greater uptake by the tumor than the liver. Other possible mechanisms would be nonspecific binding to damaged tissue or a relation to the vascularity and capillary permeability of the tumor.

Of 31 patients studied, uptake in the tumor was greater than that in the nonneoplastic hepatic tissue in two patients, equal in six, lower in ten, and not apparent at all in 13 patients [44]. On the basis of these results, it seems unlikely that imaging with 99m-technetium glucoheptonate will have a major role to play in the diagnosis of HCC.

6.3 Radiolabeled monoclonal antibodies

The recent availability of techniques for producing monoclonal antibodies has opened up exciting new possibilities for the imaging of HCC. Monoclonal antibodies against tumor antigens expressed on the cell membrane of malignant hepatocytes or tumor-specific proteins synthesized by these cells can be labeled with an appropriate radionuclide and used to image the tumor. Preliminary results with a radiolabeled antibody against alpha fetoprotein are encouraging (Fig. 18.7). Antibodies against membrane-expressed antigens have been shown to image hepatomas in experimental animals and are now being used in human HCC.

7 Positron emission tomography

Dynamic positron emission tomography with (^{13}N)-ammonia demonstrates accumulation of this radionuclide in HCC from a very early period, whereas uptake by the rest of the liver progresses more gradually, producing high contrast in the early scans [45]. The mechanism of (^{13}N)-ammonia concentration in HCC is not known. It obviously depends in part on the blood supply to the tumor, but other factors may be responsible for the active uptake by the malignant hepatocytes.

Positron emission tomography with (^{18}F)-fluorodeoxy glucose has been used to assess viability of the tumor in patients with HCC [46]. Fluordeoxy glucose is an analogue of glucose which accumulates in tissues with a high glycolytic demand. Viable tumor tissue has been shown actively to concentrate (^{18}F)-fluorodeoxy glucose, whereas necrotic tissue fails to concentrate the tracer.

References

1. Kew MC, Dos Santos HA, Sherlock S (1971) Diagnosis of primary cancer of the liver. Br Med J 4: 408–411
2. Sharpstone P, Rake MO, Shilkin KB, Williams R (1972) The diagnosis of primary malignant tumors of the liver, Q J Med 41: 99–110
3. Bieler EU, Meyer BJ, Jansen CR (1972) Liver scanning as a method of detecting primary liver cancer. Report on 100 cases (1972) Am J Roentgenol Radium Ther Nucl Med 115: 709–716
4. Levin J, Geddes EW, Kew MC (1974) Radionuclide scanning of the liver in primary hepatic can-

cer. An analysis of 202 cases. J Nucl Med 15: 296–299

5. Fritz SL, Preston DF, Gallagher JH (1981) ROC analysis of diagnostic performance in liver scintigraphy. J Nucl Med 22: 121–128

6. Drum DE (1982) Current status of hepatic scintiphotography for space-occupying disease. Sem Nucl Med 12: 64–74

7. Rothschild MA, Oratz M, Schreiber SS (1982) Comments on radionuclide hepatic scanning. Sem Liver Dis 2: 29–40

8. Zeman RK, Paushter DM, Schiebler ML, Choyke PL, Clark LR (1985) Hepatic imaging: current status. Radiol Clin N Am 23: 473–487

9. Alderson PO, Adams DF, McNeil BJ, Sanders RC, Siegelman SS, Finberg HS, Hessel SJ, Abrams HL (1983) Computed tomography, ultrasound, and scintigraphy of the liver in patients with colon or breast carcinoma: A prospective comparison. Radiology 149: 225–230

10. Strauss L, Bostel F, Clorius JH, Rapton E, Wellman H, Georgi P (1982) Single-photon emission computed tomography (SPECT) for assessment of hepatic lesions. J Nucl Med 23: 1059–1065

11. Brendel AJ, Leccia F, Drouillard J, San Galli F, Eresne J, Wynchank S, Barat JL, Ducassou D (1984) Single photon emission computed tomography (SPECT), planar scintigraphy, and transmission computed tomography: A comparison of accuracy in diagnosing focal hepatic disease. Radiology 153: 527–532

12. Breedis C, Young G (1949) Blood supply of neoplasms of the liver. Am J Pathol 30: 969–985

13. Feeman LM, Mandell CH (1972) Dynamic vascular scintiphotography of the liver. Sem Nucl Med 2: 133–138

14. Stadalnik RC, DeNardo SJ, DeNardo GL, Raventos A (1975) Critical evaluation of hepatic scintiangiography for neoplasms of the liver. J Nucl Med 16: 595–601

15. Lubin E, Lewitus Z (1972) Blood pool scanning in investigating hepatic mass lesions. Sem Nucl Med 2: 128–132

16. Lee VW, Estabaya E, Shapiro JH (1980) Diagnosis of hepatoma by scintigraphy using multiple radionuclides. J Surg Oncol 15: 133–138

17. Ben-Porath M, Clayton G, Kaplan E (1967) Modification of a multi-isotope color scanner for multi-purpose scanning. J Nucl Med 8: 411–425

18. Coakley AJ, Wraight EP (1980) Selenomethionine liver scanning in the diagnosis of hepatoma. Br J Radiol 53: 538–543

19. Eddleston ACWF, Rake MP, Pagaltsos AP, Osborn SB, Williams R (1971) 75-Se-selenomethionine in the scintiscan diagnosis of primary hepatocellular carcinoma. Gut 12: 245–249

20. Kew MC, Geddes EW, Levin J (1974) False-negative 75-Se-selenomethionine scans in primary liver cell cancer. J Nucl Med 15: 234–236

21. Kaplan E, Domingo M (1973) 75-Se-selenomethionine in hepatic focal lesions. Sem Nucl Med 2:139–149

22. Lomas F, Dibos SE, Wager H (1972) Increased specificity of liver scanning with the use of 67-gallium citrate. N Engl J Med 286: 1323–1329

23. James O, Wood EJ, Sherlock S (1974) 67 Gallium scanning in the diagnosis of liver disease. Gut 15: 404–410

24. Hoffer P (1980) Status of gallium-67 in tumor detection. J Nucl Med 21: 394–398

25. Levin J, Kew MC (1975) Gallium-67 citrate scanning in primary cancer of the liver: Diagnostic value in the presence of cirrhosis and relation to alpha-fetoprotein J Nucl Med 16: 949–951

26. Waxman AD, Richmond R, Juttner H, Siemsen JK, Heffelinger MJ, Fink E (1980) Correlation of contrast angiography and histologic pattern with gallium uptake in primary liver cell carcinoma: Non-correlation with alpha-fetoprotein. J Nucl Med 21: 324–327

27. Cannon JR, Long RF, Berens SV (1980) Uptake of 99m-technetium PIPIDA in pulmonary metastases from a hepatoma. Clin Nucl Med 5: 22–24

28. Ueno K, Haseda Y (1980) Concentration and clearance of 99m-technetium-pyridoxyilidene isoleucine by a hepatoma. Clin Nucl Med 5: 196–199

29. Utz JA, Lull RJ, Anderson JH, Lambrecht RW, Brown JM, Henry W (1980) Hepatoma visualization with 99m-technetium pyridoxilidene glutamate. J Nucl Med 21: 747–749

30. Savitch I, Kew MC, Paterson A, Esser JD, Levin J (1983) Uptake of 99m-technetium di-isopropyl iminodiacetic acid by hepatocellular carcinoma. J Nucl Med 24: 1119–1122

31. Yeh SH, Wang SJ, Chu LS (1981) Sensitivity of 99m-technetium HIDA liver scintigraphy for diagnosing hepatoma. J Nucl Med 22: 86

32. Lee VW, O'Brien MJ, Devereux DF, Morris PM, Shapiro JH (1984) Hepatocellular carcinoma: Uptake of 99m-technetium IDA in primary tumor and metastasis. J Nucl Med 25: 57–61

33. Hasegawa Y, Nakano S, Ibuka K, Hashizume T, Sasaki Y, Imaoka S (1984) The importance of delayed imaging in the study of hepatoma with a new hepatobiliary agent. J Nucl Med 25: 1122–1125

34. Vincent LM, Rho TH, McCartney WA, Momro MA (1984) Hepatic adenoma: Demonstration of a discordant uptake of 99m-technetium sulfur colloid and 99m-technetium DISIDA. Clin Nucl Med 9: 415–416

35. Strashun A, Goldsmith SJ (1981) Increased focal uptake of 99m-technetium IDA hapatobiliary agent by a liver metastasis. Clin Nucl Med 6: 295–296

36. Fawcett HD, Sayle BA, Winsett MZ (1985) Indium-III chloride for detecting suspected hepatomas with focal defects on 99m-technetium sulfur colloid liver imaging. Clin Nucl Med 10: 414–412

37. Suzuki Y, Hisada K, Hiraki T (1974) Clinical evaluation of tumor scanning with 57-cobalt bleomycin. Radiology 113: 139–142

38. Maeda T, Tanaka M (1973) Uptake of 57-Co-bleomycin by liver tumor. Radioisotopes 23: 37–38

39. Grove RB, Ribo RC, Eckelman WC, Goodyear M (1974) Clinical evaluation of radio labelled bleomycin for tumor detection. Nuc Med 15: 386–388

40. Kew MC, Allen J, Levin J (1976) 57-cobalt-bleomycin as a tumor scanning agent in primary hepatocellular cancer. Eur J Nucl Med 1: 247–250

41. Vorne M, Sakke S, Jarvi K (1982) TC-99m glucoheptonate in detection of lung tumors. J Nucl Med 23: 250–255

42. Leveille J, Pison C, Karakand Y (1977) 99m-technetium glucoheptonate in brain tumor detection: an important advance in radio-tracer techniques. J Nucl Med 18: 957–967

43. de Kieviet W (1981) Technetium radiopharmaceuticals: chemical characterization and tissue distribution of 99m-technetium glucoheptonate using 99m-technetium and carrier 99m-technetium glucoheptonate. J Nucl Med 22: 703–711

44. Esser JD, Kew MC, Tobias M, Winterton R, Savitch I, Levin J (1985) Technetium 99m glucoheptonate as a scanning agent in hepatocellular carcinoma. Clin Nucl Med 10:586–588

45. Hayashi M, Tamaki N, Yonikura Y, Saida M (1985) Imaging of hepatocellular carcinoma using dynamic positron emission tomography with nitrogen-13 ammonia. J Nucl Med 26: 254–257

46. Paul R, Ahronsen A, Roeda D, Nordman E (1985) Imaging of hepatoma with 18-F-fluoro-dexoxyglucose. Lancet 1: 50–51

Chapter 19
Ultrasonography in the Diagnosis of Hepatic Tumor

MASAO OHTO, MASAAKI EBARA, and KUNIO OKUDA[1]

Great progress has been made in the diagnosis of space-occupying lesions of the liver with the advent of real-time ultrasonography (US) [1, 2]. US is now indispensable in the detection of small lesions such as minute HCC [3–5]. The ultrasonograph has continuously been improved for better resolution and fewer artefacts. The more recent development of the convex-type real-time probe has significantly reduced the dead angle for the linear probe in the right hepatic lobe immediately below the diaphragm. Although large-mass lesions pose no difficulty in US diagnosis, a new problem has arisen with improved resolution of the transducer, namely the differentiation between small HCC and benign hyperplastic nodules [6–8]. In this chapter, we will discuss mainly US diagnosis of hepatic mass lesions and its significance in the clinical setting.

1 Basic US pattern of solid mass lesions

To characterize and determine the common US features of mass-forming diseases, one needs to set several patterns with respect to shape and internal echoes for analysis.

1.1 Shape of mass

This may be divided into the nodular, massive, and diffuse types [9]. (1) Nodular type: The boundary between the mass and parenchyma is discrete and the mass is clearly discerned. The mass may be solitary or multiple, and the gross pathology is closely reflected by the US findings.

(2) Massive type: The mass is usually large, greater than 5 cm in diameter, and the boundary is not clearly defined though the general outline of the mass is recognizable. The gross pathology is usually that of a nonencapsulated expanding tumor. (3) Diffuse type: The mass is not clearly defined and the boundary is indistinct; irregular, coarse, and abnormal echogenic spots are seen diffusely in the parenchyma. The gross pathology is that of the diffuse type of HCC or of widespread multiple small foci of cancer.

1.2 Internal echo pattern

The degree of echogenicity and distribution of echoes are the basis of echo pattern analysis. (1) Low-echo pattern: The echo of the lesion is lower than that of the parenchyma. This is often seen in a mass with a homogeneous tissue structure not accompanied by necrosis and bleeding, and it is common with small HCCs, small metastatic cancers, and large hyperplastic nodules. (2) Low-periphery echo pattern: A round mass is clearly demarcated by a low-echo rim. The internal echo may be about the same as or higher than that of the surrounding parenchyma or mixed low- and hyperechoes. This pattern may be seen in small HCCs and small metastatic cancers. (3) High-echo pattern: The internal echo is generally higher than that of the parenchyma. Histologically, the mass often has extensive necrosis or bleeding. It may be an HCC with fatty changes. A calcified metastatic carcinoma and a hemangioma also demonstrate the high-echo pattern. (4) Mixed-echo pattern: The interior of the mass has an irregular mixture of low- and high-echo areas. Varying histological changes occurring in the same mass may cause this pattern. This is frequently seen in large HCCs and large metastatic cancers.

[1] First Department of Medicine, Chiba University School of Medicine, Inohana, Chiba, 280 Japan

Table 19.1. Ultrasound findings of small HCC

Tumor size (cm)	Number of cases	Echo pattern			
		Low echo	Low periphery		
			Iso	High	Mixed
<2	34	32 (94.1)	2 (5.9)	0 (0)	0 (0)
2–3	41	20 (48.8%)	18 (43.9)	0 (0)	3 (7.3)
3–5	52	5 (9.6)	23 (44.2)	9 (17.3)	15 (28.8)

Numbers in parentheses are percentages

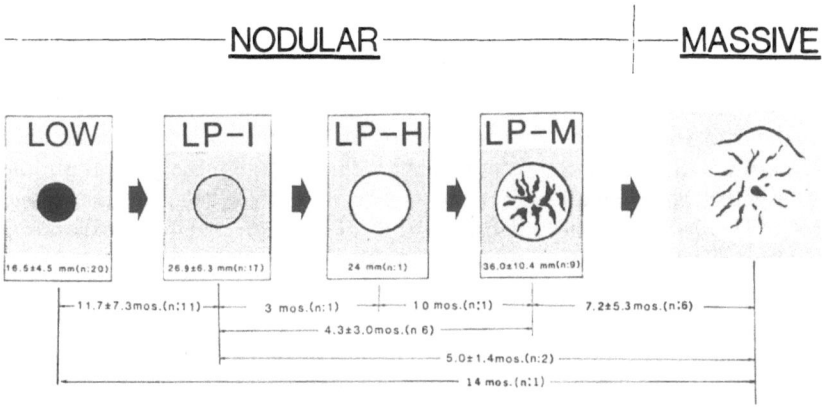

LP : low periphery, I : iso, H : high, M : mixed.

Fig. 19.1. Schematic representation of typical changes in US pattern as a small HCC grows in size. *LP* low-periphery pattern. *Numbers* immediately below *drawings* indicate average size of mass and *lower figures* give the average time required for the pattern to change. After Ebara et al. [4], with permission from Elsevier

2 US features of mass lesions and differential diagnosis

2.1 Hepatocellular carcinoma

2.1.1 Size of mass and US findings

It is important to remember that the echo pattern varies considerably with the tumor size. A lesion smaller than 2 cm more often shows a nodular type with the low-echo pattern [4]. Lesions of 2–3 cm exhibit about equal frequencies of the low-echo and the low-periphery echo patterns. Lesions 3–5 cm in size more often demonstrate the low-periphery pattern and, much less frequently, the low-echo pattern (Table 19.1). With the increasing size of the tumor, the massive type of the high- and mixed-echo patterns becomes more frequent. Most lesions larger than 5 cm in diameter exhibit the high-echo or mixed-echo pattern, and low-echo and low-periphery echo patterns are no longer seen.

2.1.2 Speed of growth and US pattern

Certain changes in the echo pattern occur in HCC as it grows in size. The most common is the transition from the nodular to the massive type, with the concomitant echo pattern change from the low- to low-periphery to high- to mixed-echo patterns, as illustrated in Fig. 19.1. For a small HCC of about 2 cm, there is certain correlation between the echo pattern and growth speed [4]. A slow-growing HCC (doubling time more than 8 months) frequently exhibits the low-echo pattern, a fast-growing HCC (doubling time less than 3 months) the low-periphery echo pattern, and an intermediate growth speed HCC (doubling time 3–8 months) either echo pattern.

2.1.3 Portal invasion and US findings

HCC is known for its tendency to invade the portal vein system. Growth in a major portal vein branch or the portal trunk has serious prognostic implications, particularly with respect to therapy. Thus, US diagnosis and differential diagnosis of a tumor thrombosis are of practical clinical importance.

Tumor thrombosis in a major portal branch is readily recognizable by US as a mass within a

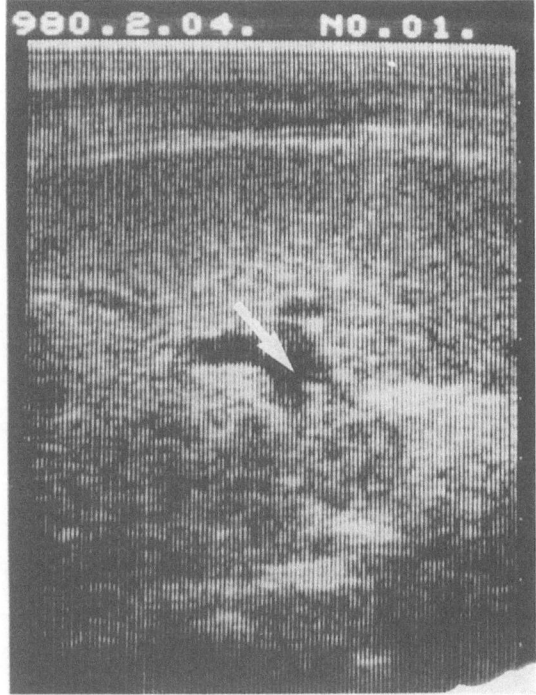

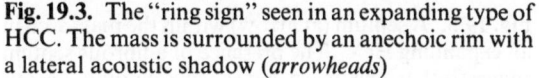

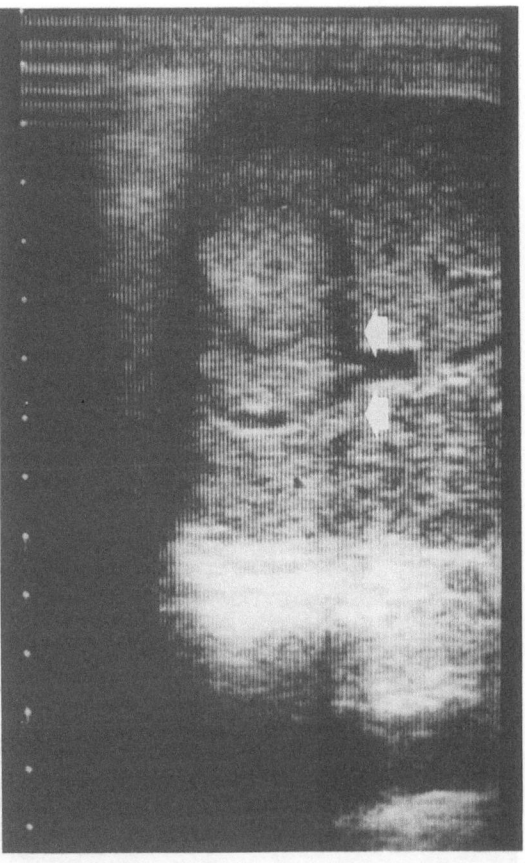

Fig. 19.2. HCC growing in the portal vein as a tumor thrombus (*arrow*)

Fig. 19.3. The "ring sign" seen in an expanding type of ▶ HCC. The mass is surrounded by an anechoic rim with a lateral acoustic shadow (*arrowheads*)

vessel lumen (Fig. 19.2), and the detection rate is greater than that by CT and angiography. Comparison of US, angiography, and CT in our patients demonstrated a detection rate for a tumor thrombus in a third-order portal branch of 71.4%, 28.6%, and 14.5%, respectively [10]. A tumor thrombus grows quite fast: in our experience, it takes 1–6 months (average 2.9 months) for a tumor thrombus in a third-order branch to grow into a first-order branch.

2.1.4 Characteristic US features of HCC
The following US findings are more or less characteristic of HCC.

Ring sign. As it grows to a size greater than about 2 cm, an HCC frequently demonstrates a low-peripheral echo (Fig. 19.3). The HCC is often round and clearly demarcated by a distinct smooth anechoic ring or rim. As the mass enlarges to greater than 3 cm, this ring often demonstrates lateral acoustic shadowing. These changes are closely related to a fibrous capsule typical of the encapsulated HCC [11]. In an in vitro study, we have shown that the lateral

anechoic ring corresponds to a thick fibrous capsule [12].

Nodule in nodule. A nodular mass lesion may occasionally contain another discrete nodule of a differing echo pattern (Fig. 19.4). This is a reflection of the tumor-in-tumor phenomenon, frequently seen in a large expanding HCC in which cancer cell clones form new tumor foci within the preexisting expanding HCC [13].

Septum within mass. Occasionally, a thin anechoic septum or line is seen within an HCC, which corresponds to the phenomenon of septum formation within an encapsulated HCC (Fig. 19.5) [11, 13]. It probably reflects the fibrogenic property of HCC to generate a fibrous septum at the boundary between masses of differing clones of cancer cells.

Small high-echo mass. A small HCC may be seen as a homogeneously high-echo mass. It is due to diffuse fatty changes of the cancer tissue (Fig. 19.6). The difference from hemangioma is in the presence of the low-echo ring at the periphery in HCC.

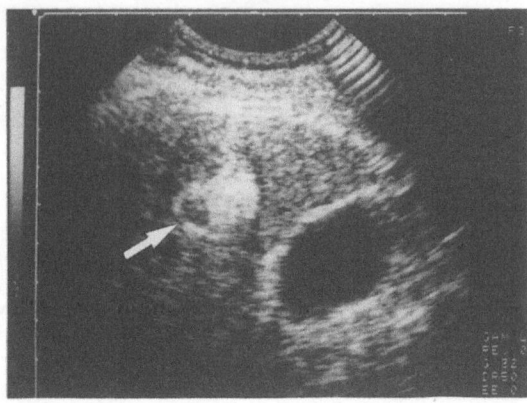

Fig. 19.4. A nodule-in-nodule (*arrow*) seen in an expanding HCC, suggesting growth of a new clone of cancer cells

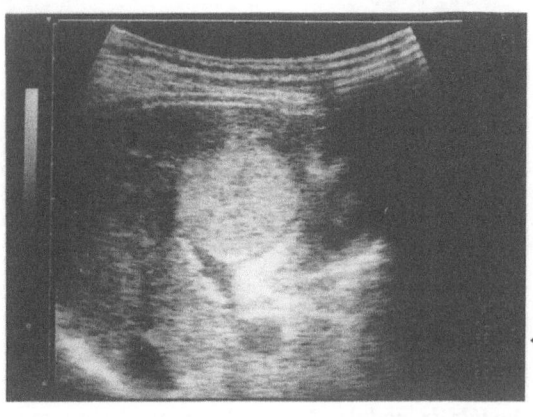

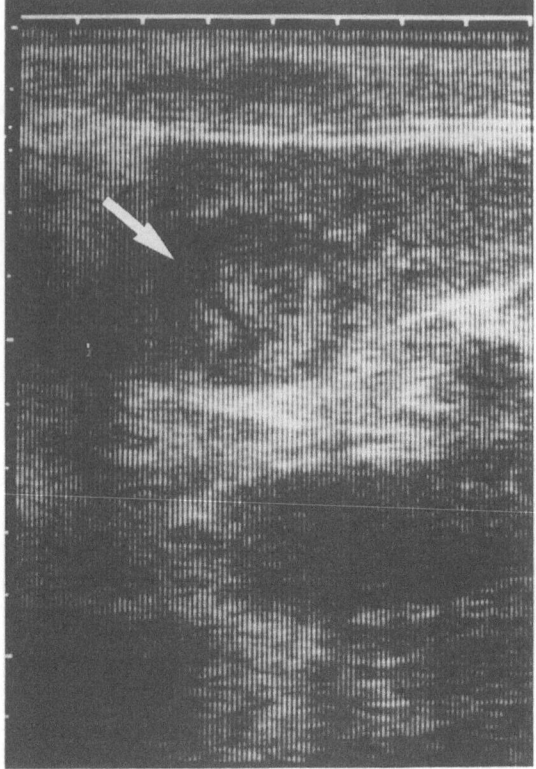

Fig. 19.5. A septum (at arrow) within the mass seen in an expanding HCC. The presence of a fibrous septum suggests that the mass has a surrounding fibrous capsule

Fig. 19.6. A small HCC of the high-echo pattern with a low-periphery rim. A small high-echo HCC usually suggests marked fatty changes

2.2 Metastatic cancer

2.2.1 US findings in relation to tumor size

In the majority (85%) of metastatic cancers, the lesions are multinodular (Table 19.2). In our clinical material, 11.7% of the lesions were solitary and 3.5% diffuse in type. The shape is usually irregular. A small metastatic nodule (< 2 cm) is characterized either by the low-periphery echo or a high-echo pattern (equal in frequency) without additional US changes. Metastatic lesions 2–4 cm in size mostly exhibit the low-periphery echo or a high-echo pattern with frequent additional changes that reflect the histopathology. Large metastatic lesions (> 4 cm) usually show the high- or mixed-echo pattern and additional changes.

2.2.2 Additional US findings

Cluster sign. A cluster of small echogenic nodules may reflect the same gross phenomenon of clustering of small metastatic lesions that form a large mass (Fig. 19.7).

Anechoic center. A round anechoic area is seen in the center of a high-echoic lesion, corresponding to liquefactive necrosis in the center of a metastatic cancer (Fig. 19.8).

Cystic echo within mass. Occasionally, a large cystic anechoic area is seen occupying a large part of a high-echoic mass (Fig. 19.9). It reflects liquefactive necrosis of the interior of a large metastatic lesion.

High echo with acoustic shadow. An irregularly shaped mass demonstrating high echoes and a posterior acoustic shadow, a result of calcification, is usually a metastasis from the colon (Fig. 19.10).

Table 19.2. US findings of metastatic liver cancers in relation to size and primary organ

Tumor size (cm)	Primary	Basic US pattern						Additional US findings					
		Low echo	Low periphery			High echo	Mixed echo	Anechoic	Cystic	Calcification echo	High-echo with acoustic shadow	Cluster sign	Tumor thrombus
			Iso	High	Mixed								
<2 (n = 32)	Stomach	3	2	1									
	Colon			1									
	Pancreas	2	1	2	1	1							
	Biliary tract	1											
	Lung	6	2	2									
	Others	4	2	1									
2–4 (n = 29)	Stomach	1	5	1		1				1	1		
	Colon		1			5		1		1	1		
	Pancreas		1	1		3			1	2	2	1	
	Biliary tract					1						1	
	Lung	1	3			2						1	
	Others					3						1	
>4 (n = 58)	Stomach	1	2	2		7	2	2	2	1	1	2	1
	Colon					17		1	5	10	10	6	
	Pancreas					3		1	1			1	
	Biliary tract					2	2		2				1
	Lung					11	1	1	4			6	
	Others					6	2	1	3				
Total (n = 119)		19	19	11	1	62	7	7	18	15	15	19	2

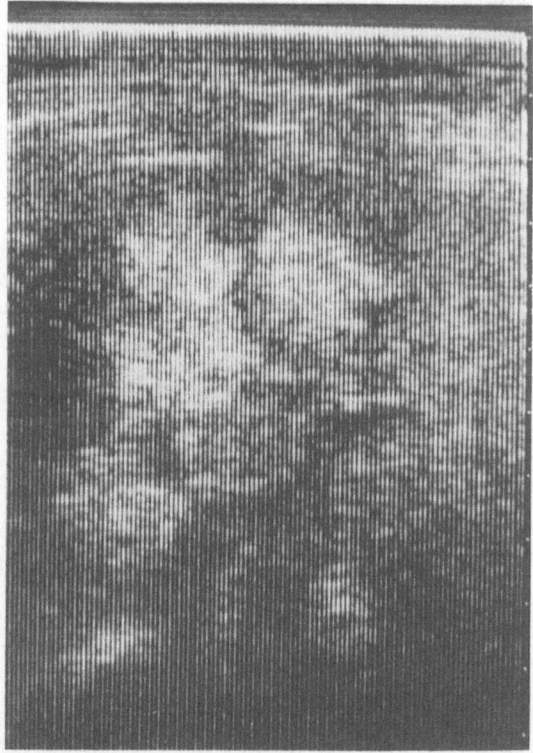

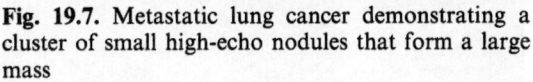

Fig. 19.7. Metastatic lung cancer demonstrating a cluster of small high-echo nodules that form a large mass

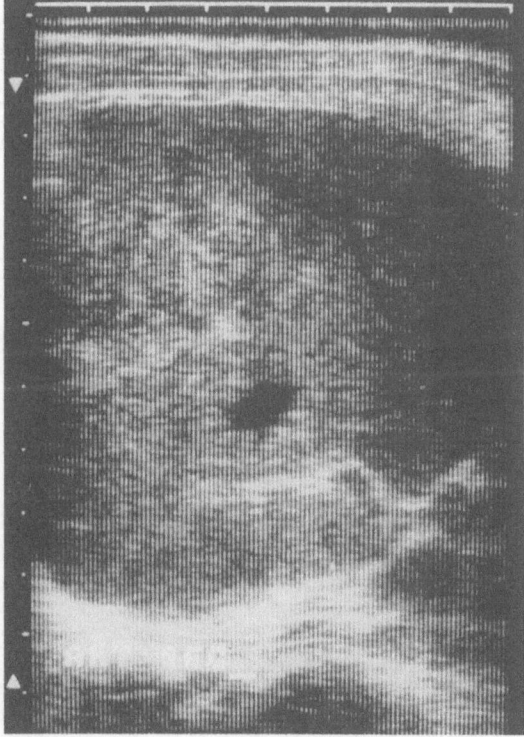

Fig. 19.8. Metastatic colon cancer demonstrating a high-echo pattern with a central anechoic area

2.3 US findings in relation to primary organ

It is generally believed that there are no organ-specific US findings in metastatic cancer. The analysis of our data, however, suggests that there is some, though not an absolute, relationship between the US pattern and the primary site. A mass larger than 4 cm, irregularly nodular or massive in shape and having prominently high echoes with or without an acoustic shadow, is most often (91%) a secondary colon cancer (Fig. 19.10). In our experience, all lesions greater than 4 cm in size that exhibited the low-echo pattern were metastases from the stomach (Fig. 19.11). Small lesions, less than 2 cm, that exhibited the high-echo or low-periphery echo pattern (interior, mixed pattern) were limited to metastases from the pancreas. Thus, consideration of US findings in relation to tumor size may provide information regarding the primary organ.

2.4 Hemangioma

Small hemangiomas do not cause any clinical symptoms. Most autopsy studies have shown an incidence of less than 1%; hemangiomas are now detected frequently by routine US examination. Sometimes, problems arise because a hemangioma has to be distinguished from small HCC. Histologically, cavernous hemangioma may be fibrosed or calcified, and the US findings vary depending on the histological features.

The US findings may be divided into the following three types.

2.4.1 High-echo type

This most common type is characterized by a discrete boundary with parenchyma and diffusely high echoes (Fig. 19.12). It may be confused with a small HCC with fatty changes.

2.4.2 Low-echo type

This rare variety is clearly distinguished by a low-echo interior and a limiting high-echo rim (Fig. 19.13).

2.4.3 Mixed-echo type

High- and low-echo areas are mixed irregularly in the interior, making the boundary indistinct (Fig. 19.14). It may contain small vascular and cystic structures.

3 US-guided biopsy

With the aid of the puncture transducer [14], a lesion as small as 1 cm may be biopsied with accuracy. For aspiration cytology, a 22-gauge Chiba PTC needle is used. For tissue diagnosis, the Silverman or Trucut needle may be used, but to minimize the risk of seeding of cancer cells in

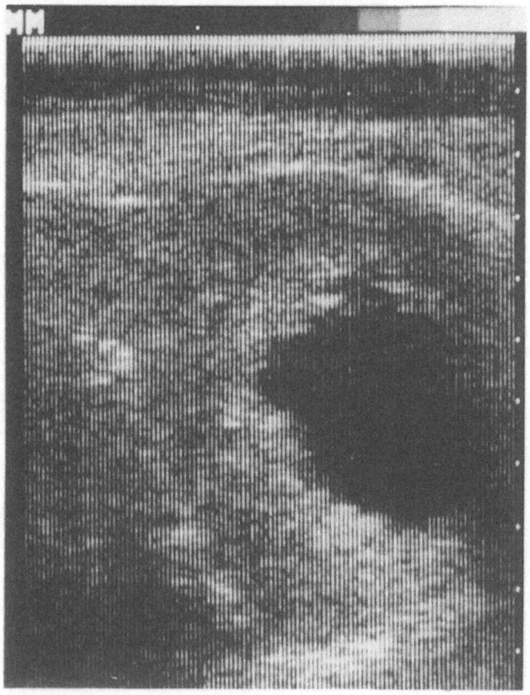

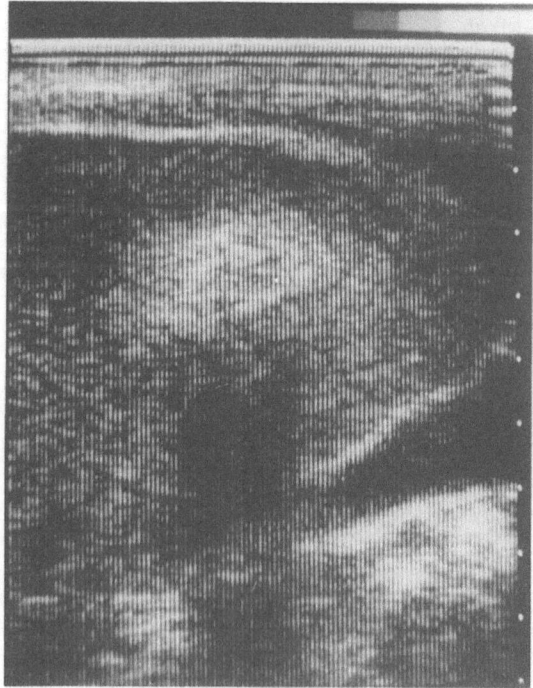

Fig. 19.9. Metastatic colon cancer with a large anechoic (cystic) interior

Fig. 19.10. Metastatic colon cancer demonstrating an irregularly shaped high-echo mass with an acoustic shadow behind. These findings suggests calcification

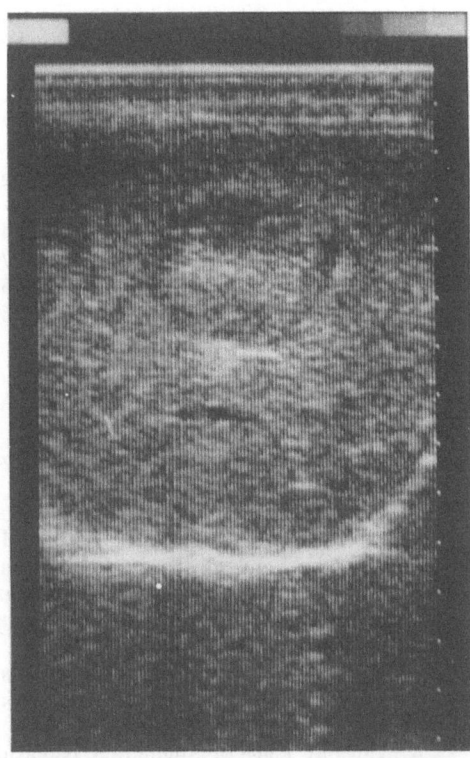

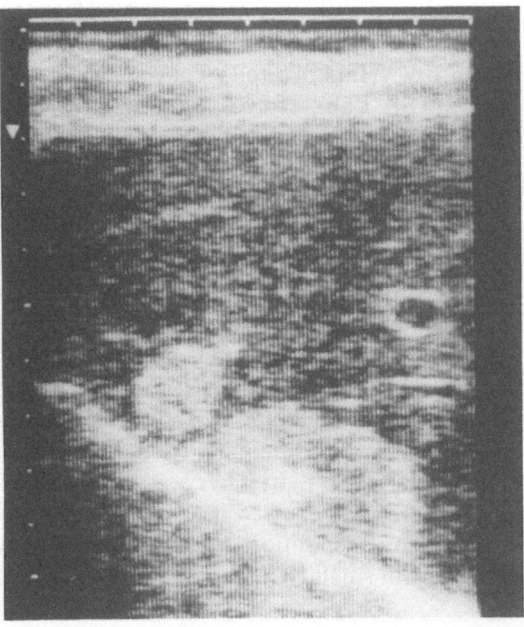

Fig. 19.12. A high-echo hemangioma. Note the direct transition from the parenchymal echo to the high internal echo

Fig. 19.11. Metastatic stomach cancer. Although the mass is larger than 4 cm, it has a low periphery and central isoechoes

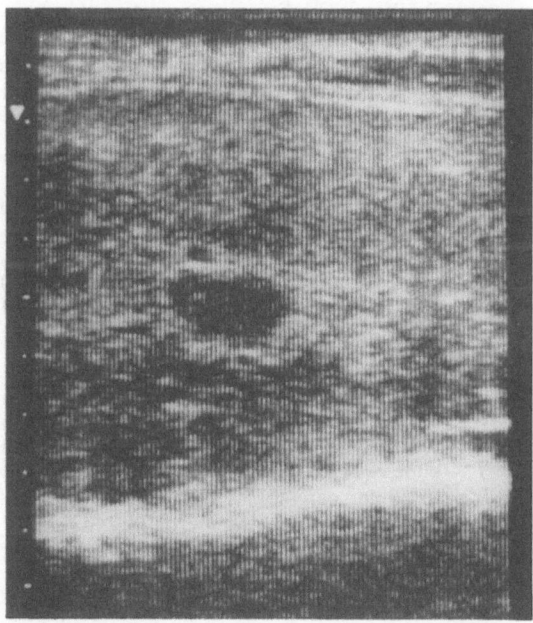

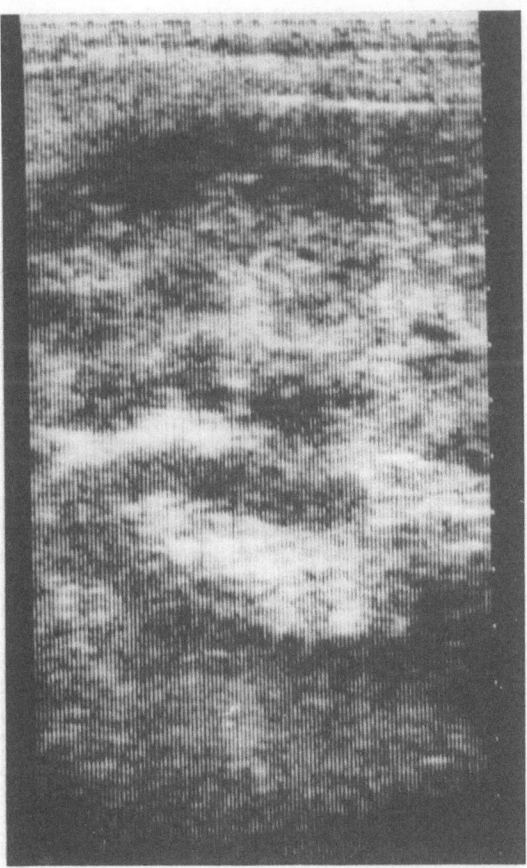

Fig. 19.13. A low-echo hemangioma. The low internal echo is bounded by a high-echo rim

Fig. 19.14. A mixed-echo pattern hemangioma. This mass is poorly demarcated with an irregular boundary, and the interior consists of low and high echoes

the needle track, thinner needles of 21–22 gauge, such as the Sonopsy needle developed in our laboratory (Hakko Shoji, Tokyo) or Surecut needle (TSK Lab., Tokyo), are used. The Sonopsy needle is manipulated with one hand while the other holds the puncture transducer for observation and aiming. For a better aim, a guide needle (thinner than 1 mm) may be inserted up to the peritoneum. The puncture site is chosen according to the size and location of the lesions.

US-guided biopsy is particularly important in the diagnosis of small lesions detected by US, which could be either small HCC or hyperplastic adenomatous nodules [6–8]. The former is usually extremely well-differentiated and difficult to distinguish from the latter by conventional stainings, as already discussed in Chap. 16. For the same reason, aspiration cytology is not very diagnostic in small HCC (Table 19.3).

4 Summary

US imaging alone may distinguish primary from secondary liver cancers, but it is most useful in the detection of small HCC. In the experienced hands of hepatobiliary sonographers, US findings are diagnostic not only for mass lesions but also for the pathology and prediction of the speed of growth of HCC. However, US is not without its drawbacks and there is a limit to its diagnostic accuracy. It should be reinforced by tissue diagnosis made by US-guided puncture whenever possible and by other investigations, particularly in the differential diagnosis of small HCCs and adenomatous hyperplastic nodules— a current problem in the Far East.

Table 19.3. Ultrasonically guided biopsy of small HCC—aspiration cytology versus biopsy histology (November 1979 to October 1985)

Size of tumor	Positive diagnosis	
	Histology	Cytology
<2 cm	13/15 (86.7%)	9/22 (40.9%)
2–3 cm	7/8 (87.5%)	21/30 (70.0%)
3–4 cm	5/5 (100%)	6/8 (75.0%)
Total	25/28 (89.3%)	36/60 (60.0%)

References

1. Cooperberg PL, Burhenne HJ (1980) Real-time ultrasonography. Diagnostic technique of choice in calculous gallbladder disease. N Engl J Med 320:1277–1279
2. Okuda K (1981) Advances in hepatobiliary ultrasonography. Hepatology 1:662–671
3. Shinagawa T, Ohto M, Kimura K, Tsunetomi S, Morita M, Saisho H, Tsuchiya Y, Saotome N, Karasawa E, Miki M, Ueno T, Okuda K (1984) Diagnosis and clinical features of small hepatocellular carcinoma with emphasis on the utility of real-time ultrasonography. Gastroenterology 86: 495–502
4. Ebara M, Ohto M, Shinagawa T, Sugiura N, Kimura K, Matsutani S, Morita M, Saisho H, Tsuchiya Y, Okuda K (1986) Natural history of minute hepatocellular carcinoma smaller than three centimeters complicating cirrhosis. A study in 22 patients. Gastoroenterology 90: 289–298
5. Okuda K (1986) Early recognition of hepatocellular carcinoma. Hepatology 6: 729–738
6. Arakawa M, Sugihara S, Kenmochi K, Kage M, Nakashima T, Nakayama T, Tashiro S, Hiraoka T, Suenaga M, Okuda K (1986) Small mass lesions in cirrhosis: transition from benign adenomatous hyperplasia to hepatocellular carcinoma? J Gastroenterol Hepatol 1: 3–14
7. Okuda K (1986) What is the precancerous lesion for hepatocellular carcinoma? J Gastroenterol Hepatol 1: 79–85
8. Arakawa M, Kage M, Sugihara S, Nakashima T, Suenaga M, Okuda K (1986) Emergence of malignant lesions within an adenomatous hyperplastic nodule in a cirrhotic liver. Observations in five cases. Gastroenterology 91: 198–208
9. Ohto M, Ono T, Tsuchiya Y, Saisho H, Kimura K (1985) Ultrasound diagnosis in gastroenterology. Igaku-shoin, Tokyo
10. Sugiura N, Ohto M, Kimura K, Ebara M, Okuda K (1986) Imaging diagnosis of portal tumor thrombosis and its pathophysiology in hepatocellular carcinoma. Jpn J Gastroenterol 83: 2151–2160
11. Okuda K, Musha H, Nakajima Y, Kubo Y, Shimokawa Y, Nagasaki Y, Sawa Y, Jinnouchi S, Kaneko T, Obata H, Hisamitsu T, Motoike Y, Okazaki M, Sakamoto K, Nakashima T (1977) Clinicopathological features of encapsulated hepatocellular carcinoma. A study of 26 cases. Cancer 40: 1240–1245
12. Shinagawa T, Ohto M, Kimura K, Matsutani S, Kimura M, Unozawa T, Ukaji H, Tsunetomi S, Nakano T, Morita M, Saisho H, Tsuchiya Y, Ono T, Okuda K (1981) Ultrasonographic features of hepatocellular carcinoma. Correlation with histopathology. Jpn J Gastroenterol 78: 2402–2410
13. Nakashima T, Okuda K, Kojiro M, Jimi A, Yamaguchi R, Sakamoto K, Ikari T (1983) Pathology of hepatocellular carcinoma in Japan. 232 consecutive cases autopsied in ten years. Cancer 51: 863–877
14. Ohto M, Karasawa E, Tsuchiya Y, Kimura K, Saisho H, Ono T, Okuda K (1980) Ultrasonically guided percutaneous contrast medium injection and aspiration biopsy using a real-time puncture transducer. Radiology 136: 171–176

Chapter 20

Hepatic Angiography

Vincent P. Chuang[1]

1 Introduction

Despite recent developments in various imaging modalities, including computed tomography (CT), ultrasonography (US), and magnetic resonance (MR), angiography remains an important method for the diagnosis and treatment of hepatic tumors. The mapping of the hepatic artery, portal vein, and hepatic vein anatomy in a single film is only possible with hepatic angiography. Hepatic artery catheterization has become an effective tool for the treatment of liver tumors by embolization and infusion. Although CT and US have greatly improved hepatic mass detection compared with using the nuclear scan alone, with the improved superselective catheterization technique hepatic angiography is still capable of providing the most specific information in tumor diagnosis. The new concepts of hepatic tumor angiography and the changing role of angiography with respect to other imaging modalities will be discussed in this chapter.

2 Vascular anatomy

An aberrant hepatic artery is a hepatic artery arising from a source other than the celiac hepatic artery. In a study of 200 cadavers by Michels, 41.5% had an aberrant artery; 31.5% had only one aberrant hepatic artery, and 10% had two or more [1]. Aberrant hepatic arteries may be either accessory or replaced. An accessory hepatic artery is a supernumerary artery; a replaced hepatic artery is a substitute for a normal hepatic artery that is absent. The aberrant artery may be an aberrant right or left hepatic artery; either may be replaced or be an accessory artery. The incidence of aberrant right hepatic arteries is 26%,

and that of left hepatic arteries 27% [1].

The numerous variations of hepatic blood supply were classified by Michels into ten types with minor variations in each type (Table 20.1). Michels subsequently added a "variant" which was not present in his 200 cases. The "variant" was described as an aberrant right hepatic artery, arising proximal to the celiac bifurcation into the common hepatic and splenic arteries. Harell described the angiographic features of this anomaly in seven additional cases and called it "type X variant" [2]. This is confusing since type X, which is total replacement of the common hepatic artery from the left gastric artery (the gastrohepatic trunk), has no similarity with the "variant," the aberrant right hepatic artery from the celiac trunk. Since this anomaly was more commonly observed than types VII, VIIIa, VIIIb, and X in several thousand cases studied for hepatic tumors in the M.D. Anderson Hospital and Emory University Hospital, Atlanta, GA, USA, it is my opinion that this variation is best termed type XI (Table 20.1). Awareness of this variant can avoid missing a portion of the liver during diagnostic or therapeutic hepatic arteriography.

3 Angiographic technique

3.1 Catheters

A 6.5-F plain polyethylene catheter or a polyethylene catheter with a reinforced shaft for improved torque control (Torcon catheter, Cook Inc.) are frequently used via femoral artery catheterization using Seldinger's technique. If left axillary or brachial artery catheterization is performed, a 5-F catheter is preferable so as to reduce the incidence of arterial spasm and catheterization complications. The basic five catheter configurations are: simple curve, reverse curve, double curve, modified double curve, and hepatic and splenic curves.

---

[1] Department of Radiology, Emory University Hospital, Atlanta, GA, USA

Table 20.1. Hepatic artery variations

Type		Percentage of cases
I	RH, MH, and LH are from CA	55
II	RH and MH from CA; replaced LH from LGA	10
III	MH, LH from CA; replaced RH from SMA	11
IV	MH from CA; replaced RH from SMA, replaced LH from LGA	1
V	RH, MH, LH from CA, and accessory LH from LGA	8
VI	RH, MH, LH from CA, an accessory RH from SMA	7
VII	RH, MH, LH from CA, accessory RH from SMA, accessory LH from LGA	1
VIII	Combination patterns: (a) a replaced RH and an accessory LH (b) an accessory RH and a replaced LH	2
IX	Absent celiac hepatic artery; entire hepatic trunk from SMA	4.5
X	Absent celiac hepatic artery; entire hepatic trunk from LGA	0.5
XI (variant)	Double celiac hepatic arteries (No common hepatic artery); RH from proximal CA, LH from the distal end of CA	

RH right hepatic artery, *MH* midhepatic artery, *LH* left hepatic artery, *CA* celiac artery, *LGA* left gastric artery, *SMA* superior mesentric artery
Modified from Michaels [1]

3.2 Catheterization techniques

There are six superselective catheterization methods: (1) the simple curve method, (2) catheter-exchange methods using a hepatic curve catheter, (3) catheter-guidewire piggyback method, (4) long-reverse catheter with the figure-of-eight method, (5) catheter-deflecting methods, and (6) loop (or triple curve) method [3]. These techniques stress the application of the following principles: tailored catheter configuration to match the arterial anatomy, catheter and guidewire compatibility, and three-dimensional conception of the vascular anatomy. This catheter system and the catheterization techniques have been utilized in the Emory University Hospital and M.D. Anderson Hospital and Tumor Institute to achieve a 95% success rate.

3.3 Angiographic approaches

A celiac arteriogram is routinely performed to reveal the baseline arterial anatomy. With a catheter well seated in the celiac trunk, and injection of 8–12 ml/s contrast medium for a total of 40–50 ml and filming of one film/s for 7 s and one film every 3 s for 15 s provides an adequate arterial phase for the arterial anatomy and a venous phase for portal vein patency. The injection rate is selected so that the contrast medium hardly regurgitates into the aorta, assuring the opacification of the left gastric artery and/or aberrant left hepatic artery. If the portal vein is well seen in the celiac arteriogram, the search for an aberrant right hepatic artery is made only with hand injections of contrast medium into the superior mesenteric artery under fluoroscopy. If the portal vein is poorly visualized or not visualized at all in the celiac arteriogram or if an aberrant right hepatic artery is present in the test injection, a superior mesenteric arteriogram is undertaken with the injection of a vasodilator (25–40 mg Tolazoline) to augment visualization of the portal vein. The injection of contrast medium and the filming rate for superior mesenteric arteriograms are similar to those for celiac arteriograms. In a patient with portal hypertension, a larger contrast medium injection (6 ml/s for 60 ml) and longer filming sequence, such as one film every 2 s for 10 s and one film every 3 s for 24 s (a total of 34 s), frequently assures good visualization of the portal system and portosystemic collaterals.

Following the celiac and/or superior mesenteric arteriograms, a superselective hepatic arteriogram [3] is performed routinely unless multiple tumors are evident in the celiac arteriogram. If no tumor is found, it is essential to proceed with a superselective hepatic arteriogram. In the common hepatic artery, the contrast medium is injected at 4 ml/s for a total of 10 s and the filming rate is similar to that with the celiac arteriogram. If superselective catheterization of the left gastric artery (for aberrant left hepatic artery) or aberrant right hepatic artery (from superior mesenteric artery) is necessary, the injection of contrast medium is 2–3 ml/s for 10 s. The total amount of contrast medium is selected according to the size of the liver and the blood flow of the tumor.

4 Basic concepts in hepatic angiography interpretation

4.1 Hepatic lobulography

The hepatic lobule is the primary functional unit of the liver. Each lobule is a pyramidal hexahedron in shape with a diameter of 0.5–2 mm. In the center of a lobule is the central or intralobular vein; in the periphery, four or five portal spaces are arranged at regular intervals, each containing a branch of the hepatic artery, portal vein, and hepatic duct. Each lobule is composed of anastomosing cords of liver cells, which radiate from the central vein. Between these cell columns, there is a network of sinusoids which receive the mixed blood from the terminal branches of both the hepatic artery and portal vein.

The hepatic lobules have been studied angiographically using wedged hepatic venography. When a small quantity of contrast medium is injected through a catheter wedged in a hepatic vein, the contrast medium floods the hepatic sinusoids, resulting in the angiographic appearance of a homogeneous blush of sinusoids—the so-called sinusoidogram. Close inspection suggests that individual hepatic lobules are visible in the area in which overlapping of sinusoidal densities is not too severe (Fig. 20.1a). Similar nodular densities have been observed in magnification hepatic arteriography. Figure 20.1b illustrates diffuse miliary densities, mostly less than 1 mm in diameter, in the upper portion of the right lobe. These densities probably represent either individual or aggregated lobules, with each lobule either completely or incompletely filled (hepatic lobulogram). The hepatic lobulogram, usually observed in the late arterial or early parenchymal phase of hepatic arteriogram, lasts only for several seconds. These minute uniform-sized hepatic lobules aggregate to form larger, variably sized nodules, 1–3 mm in diameter (Fig. 20.1c), a few seconds later and subsequently fade into a homogeneous hepatogram. The transient formation of these larger nodules is obviously the result of the summation of millions of hepatic lobules. These nodules tend to appear and disappear with the hepatogram, and this is an important feature that helps in differentiating them from small tumor nodules, which usually show prolonged staining.

4.2 Three types of hepatogram

The term "hepatogram" has previously been applied loosely to the homogeneous liver parenchymal stain in the late phase of any visceral arteriogram. Because of the dual blood supply of the liver by the hepatic artery (20%–25%) and portal vein (75%–80%), the hepatogram of a celiac arteriogram is quite different from that of a hepatic arteriogram. The hepatogram can be further divided into the following three types—arterial, portal, and mixed.

Arterial hepatogram refers to the hepatogram resulting from opacification of only the hepatic arterial flow, such as in a selective proper hepatic, right hepatic, or midhepatic arteriogram. The portal vein remains unopacified throughout the study. In the early phase of an arterial hepatogram, thousands of densities of about 1 mm in diameter can frequently be observed; these give a spotted appearance to the hepatogram (Fig. 20.2a). Although definite proof is lacking, these spots probably represent individual or aggregated hepatic lobules, each lobule being completely or incompletely filled.

Portal hepatogram refers to the hepatogram resulting from opacification of only the portal flow, such as in a splenic or superior mesenteric arteriogram and direct splenoportography. Since the portal vein supplies a major portion of the hepatic flow and since the terminal branches of the portal vein freely communicate with hepatic lobules, the portal hepatogram is usually smooth and homogeneous (Fig. 20.2b).

In a celiac arteriogram, the celiac flow is usually divided equally between the common hepatic and splenic arteries, and a mixed hepatogram consists of an initial arterial hepatogram and a subsequent portal hepatogram (Fig. 20.2c). Details of the liver parenchyma in an arterial hepatogram are far superior to those in a mixed hepatogram.

4.3 Hepatogram in hepatic tumors

Unlike the dual blood supply in the normal liver, a hepatic neoplasm receives a single blood supply predominantly from the hepatic artery. This finding was first suggested by Healey and Sheena [4] and Healey [5], using the corrosive technique and injection of dye, particles, and radioactive materials [4, 5]. However, Lin and Lunderquist showed in resected hepatic tumors that the portal vein seemed to contribute to the tumor supply in various degrees [6]. My own evaluation of over 2000 cases of hepatic tumor angiography indicates that the hepatic tumor is always avascular in the portography phase of an arteriogram, thus supporting the concept of a single arterial supply

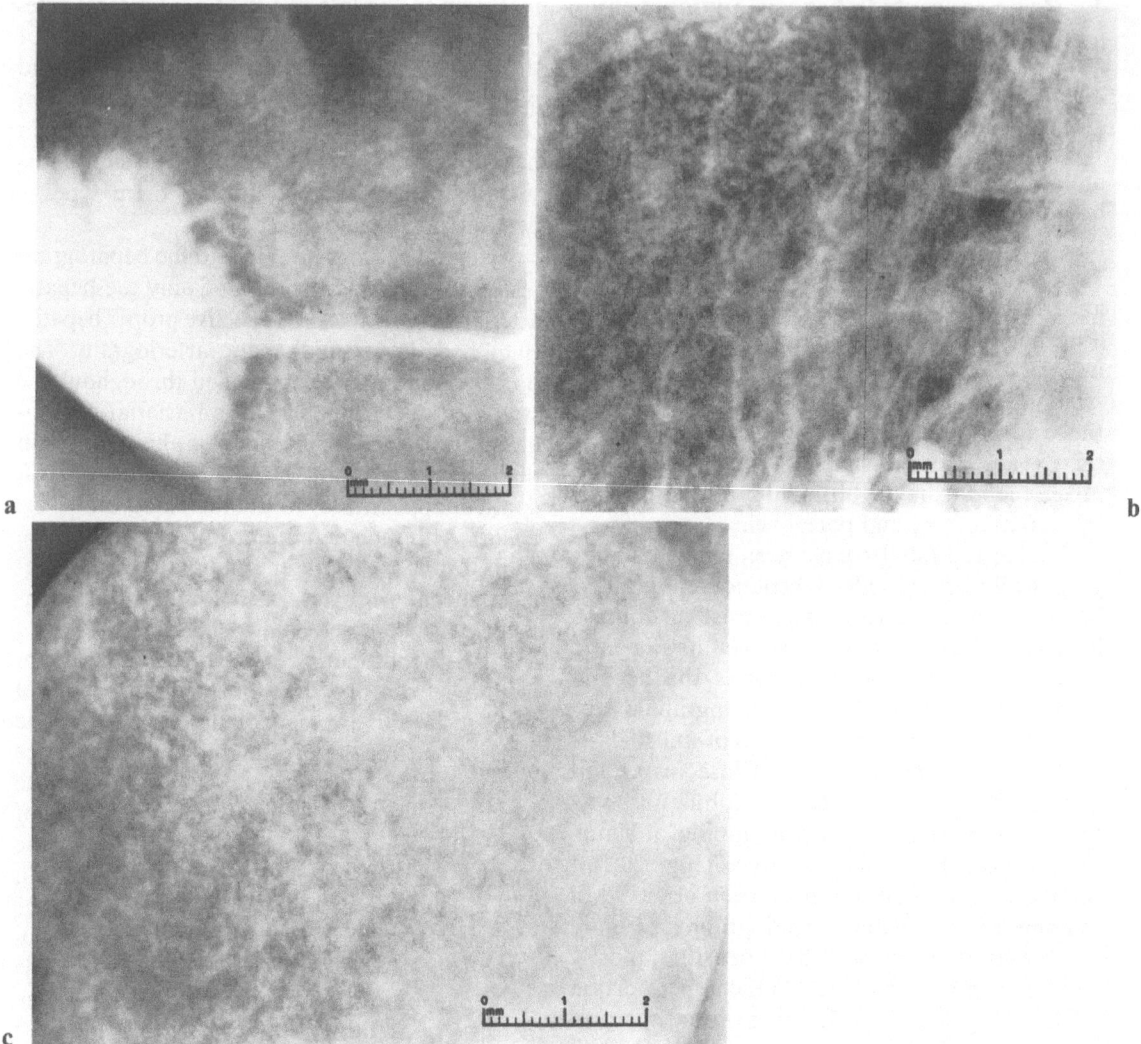

Fig. 20.1a–c. Hepatograms. **a** Wedge hepatic venography. Dense homogeneous hepatogram surrounding the catheter is the result of total opacification of the hepatic sinusoids. In the adjacent area, individual nodules of 1 mm represent "hepatic lobules." **b** In the late arterial phase, individual "hepatic lobules" start to appear, most prominent in the upper portion of the liver. **c** A few second after **b**, the contrast medium has cleared from the hepatic arteries. Aggregation of hepatic lobules results in multiple larger nodules

to liver tumors. If the portal vein does contribute to the tumor blood supply, it is probably hemodynamically insignificant as far as angiography is concerned.

The difference in blood supply between the normal liver parenchyma and the tumor provides an easy and effective means of diagnosis of the tumor. In a hepatic arteriogram, both the normal parenchyma and the neoplasm are initially opacified by the contrast medium; in the normal parenchyma, the contrast medium is subsequently diluted or washed out by the larger amount of

nonopacified portal flow. The tumor, however, stands out as a hypervascular mass due to lack of portal vein washout. This "negative portal vein washout" effect is well illustrated in Fig. 20.3c, d.

In the celiac arteriogram, however, the contrast medium is equally divided between the hepatic and splenic arteries. Since only half the contrast medium arrives at the liver from the common hepatic artery, both the liver parenchyma and tumor are at first not fully opacified. When the second half of the contrast medium arrives through the portal vein, only the normal

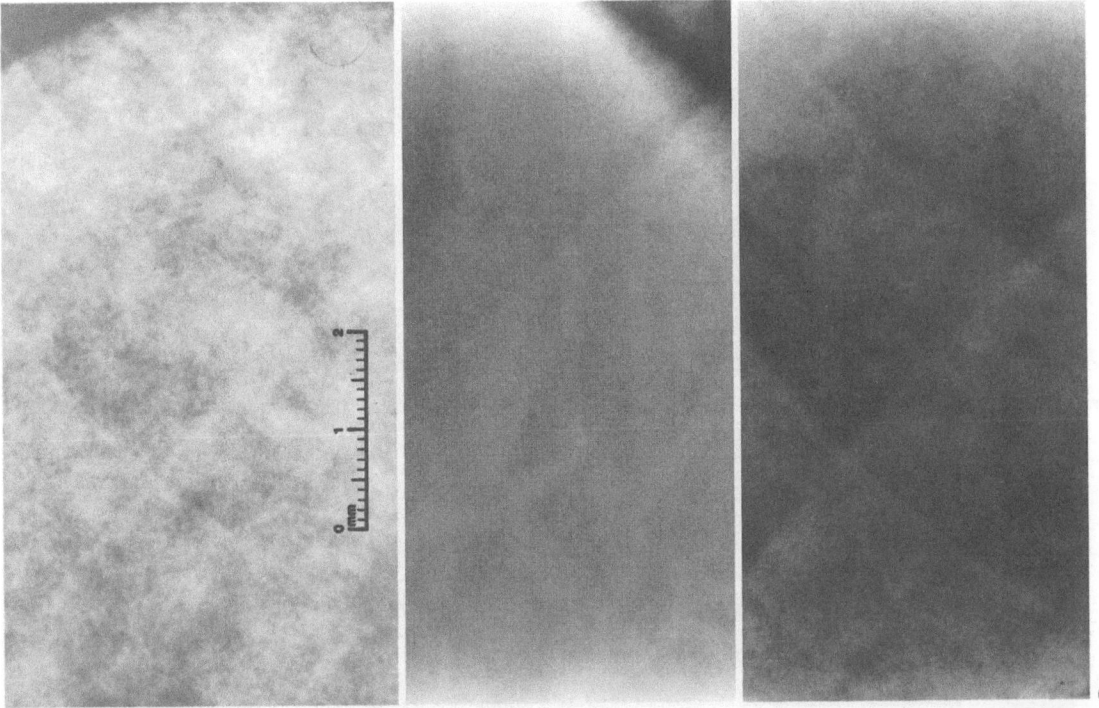

a, b

c

Fig. 20.2. a Arterial hepatogram. The "spotted" appearance of multiple 1-mm fine nodules. **b** Portal hepatogram of the same patient from a superior mesenteric arteriogram. The portal vein branches are still faintly visible. The hepatogram is homogeneous. **c** Mixed hepatogram from celiac arteriogram. The detail of the hepatogram is between **a** and **b**

parenchyma is opacified and its density continues to increase. A hepatic tumor with minimal neovascularity and staining in the arterial phase (Fig. 20.3a) becomes relatively "hypovascular" in the hepatogram phase (Fig. 20.3b) when contrasted with the increased parenchymal stain. This "positive portal vein masking" effect explains why a celiac arteriogram is not as sensitive and reliable in hepatic tumor diagnosis. It also explains why some metastatic tumors have been considered "isovascular" or "hypovascular" in earlier reports [7, 8].

Because the degree of tumor vascularity is a relative comparison with the adjacent liver parenchyma, a tumor with minimal to moderate vascularity, such as in the majority of metastatic neoplasms, appears "hypovascular" in the celiac arteriogram but "hypervascular" in the hepatic arteriogram. Markedly vascular tumors, such as in the majority of primary hepatocellular carcinomas, remain hypervascular in both the celiac and hepatic arteriograms. Because the human eye is more sensitive in detecting increased density than lucency, a small number of tumors with low vascularity can only be diagnosed by infu-

sion hepatic arteriography, where the subtle staining is enhanced by the "negative portal vein washout" effect. This is well illustrated in Fig. 20.4, where a 5 × 6.5-cm metastatic neoplasm beneath the right hemidiaphragm was missed by a conventional celiac arteriogram (Fig. 20.4a, b) as well as by CT scan and US. A selective proper hepatic arteriogram very clearly brings out the tumor vascularity for easy diagnosis (Fig. 20.4c, d).

4.4 Alteration of tumor density in tumor therapy

Since all viable tumors are supplied by branches of the hepatic artery and almost always show tumor staining in the hepatic arteriogram, the stain becomes an important criterion for the evaluation of the tumor response to treatment. A tumor changing from marked "hypervascularity" to "hypovascularity" or "avascularity" after treatment can be considered a significant therapeutic response. This concept is important in the assessment of a nonviable tumor which does not totally disappear. In a sterile metastasis, the necrotic tumor may remain as a mass effect in

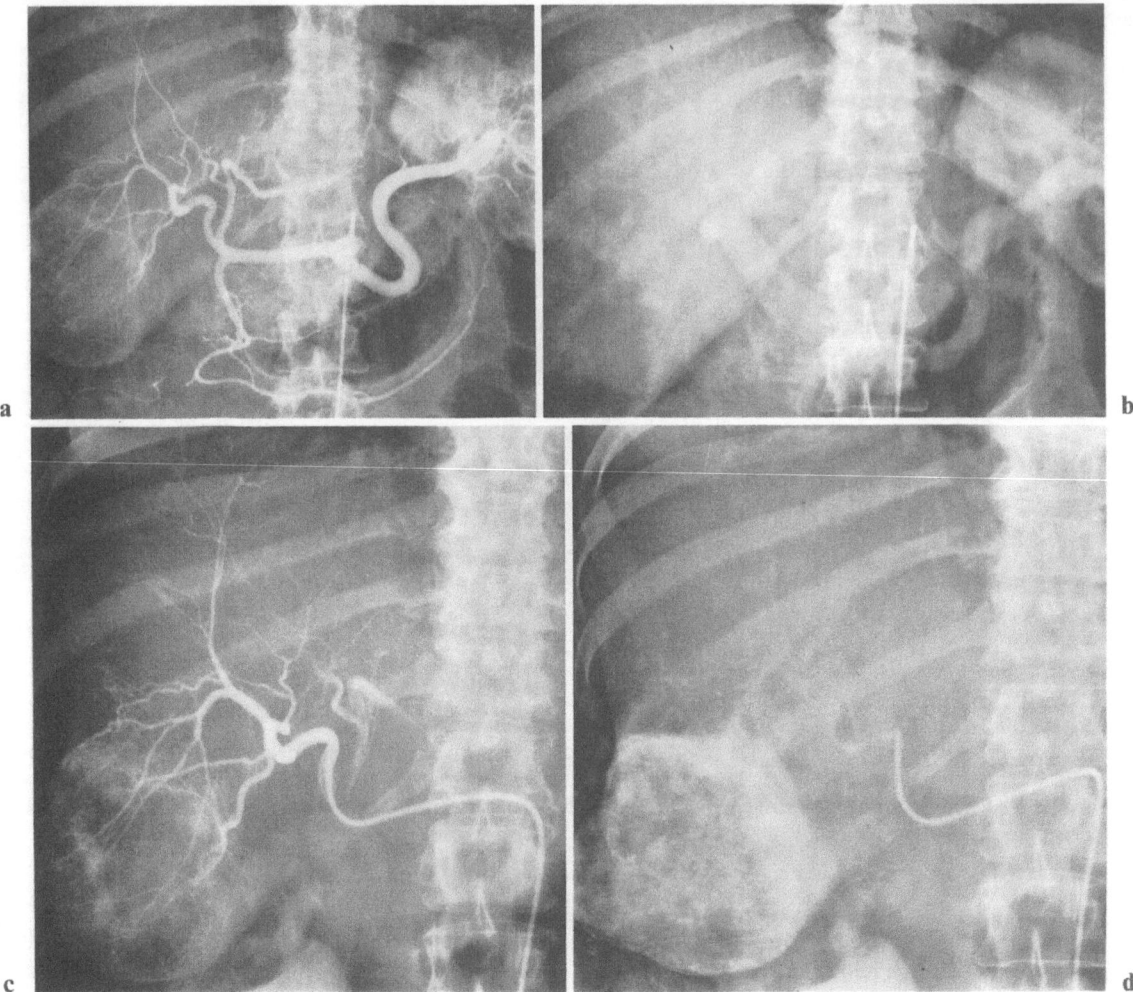

Fig. 20.3a–d. Metastatic colon carcinoma. **a** The arterial phase of the celiac arteriogram. The tumor in right lobe is moderately hypervascular. **b** In the celiac hepatogram, the tumor becomes hypovascular when the density of normal parenchyma increases due to the opacified portal flow. **c** The arterial phase of the right hepatic arteriogram. The tumor is hypervascular. **d** Hepatic hepatogram. The tumor becomes denser when the normal parenchyma has the "washout" from nonopacified portal flow

other diagnostic modalities, such as in an isotopic scan, CT scan, or sonography [9]. Due to its unique ability to demonstrate alterations of the tumor stain, the hepatic arteriogram is the most sensitive and specific diagnostic modality in evaluating tumor response (Fig. 20.5a, b).

5 Patient selection for hepatic angiography

In the diagnosis of a hepatic mass, it is essential to define the presence and nature of single or multiple lesions in order to initiate or alter management. There is little therapeutic significance

in demonstrating ten lesions when five have already been identified. Scintigraphy, US, CT, angiography, and percutaneous biopsy are available for establishing the diagnosis. It is seldom necessary to use all these techniques. Although CT is the most sensitive, accurate, and expensive of the scanning procedures, it also has significant limitations, both in sensitivity and specificity in the detection of small lesions. A mass of low

Fig. 20.5a, b. Metastatic colon carcinoma. **a** A large ▶ hypervascular tumor in the right lobe. **b** One month after hepatic embolization, a marked decrease in the tumor stain suggests tumor response

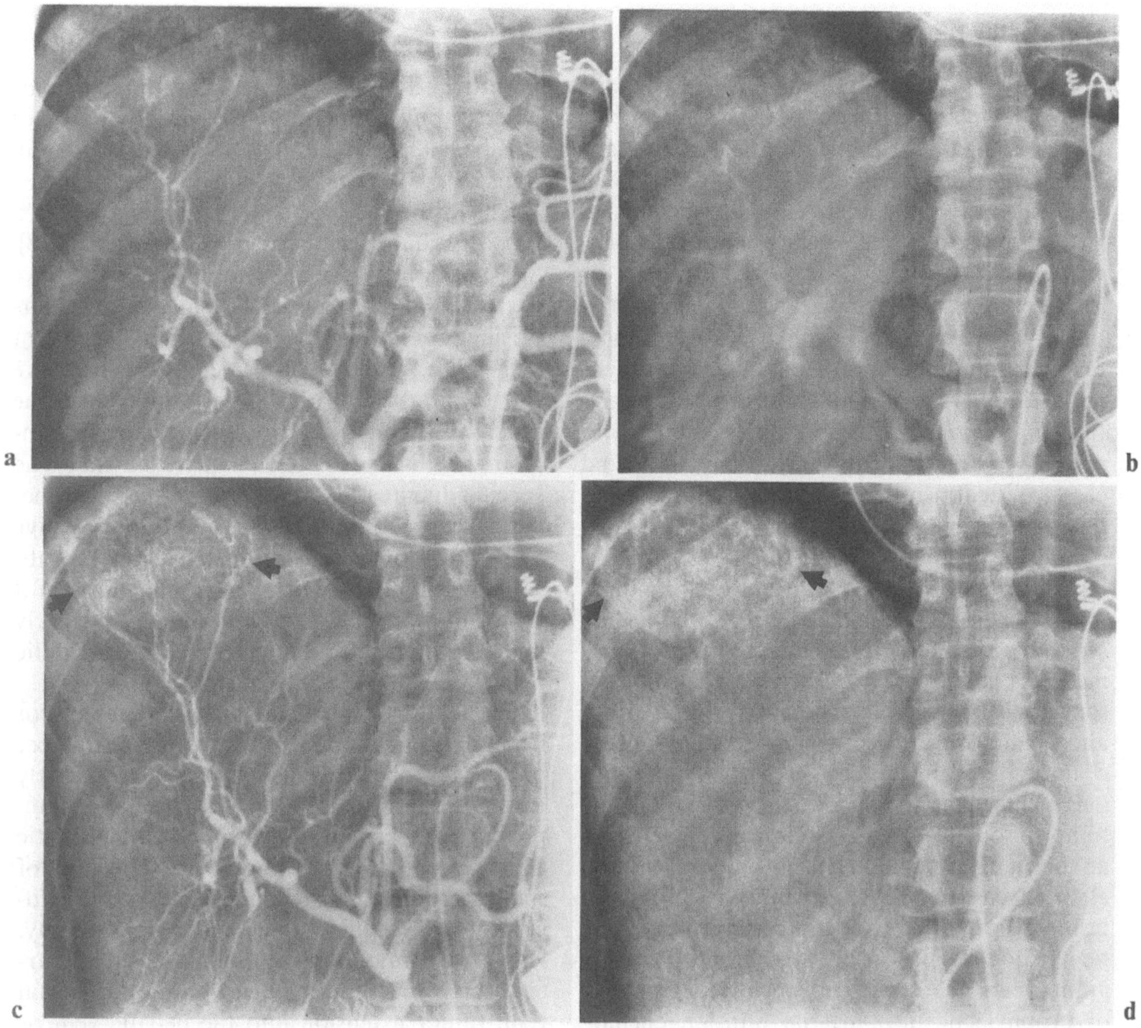

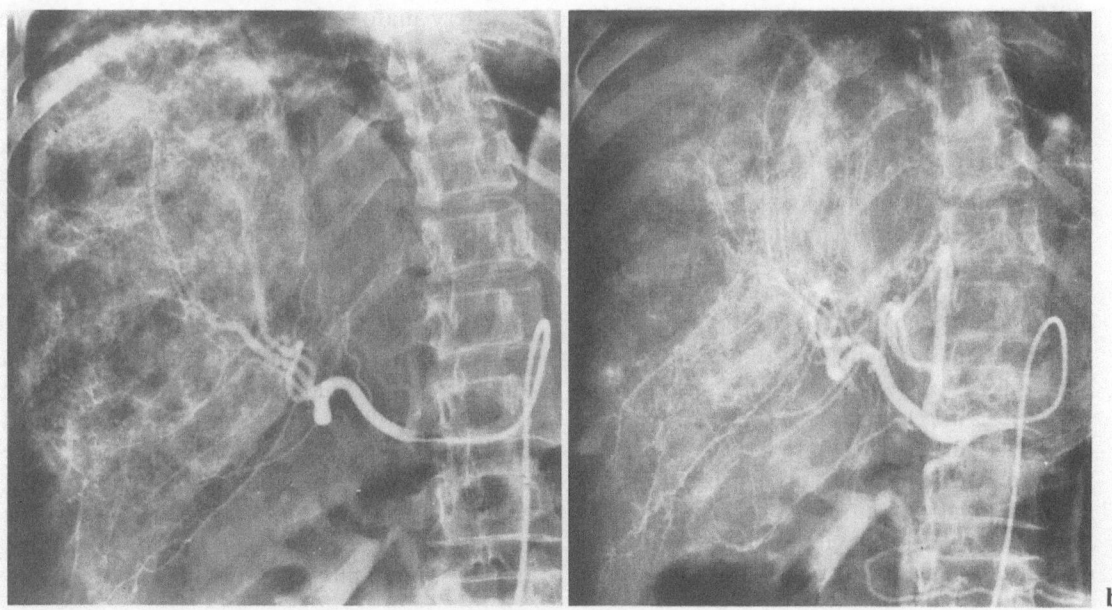

Fig. 20.4a–d. Metastatic colon carcinoma. The isotopic scan reveals an equivocal defect beneath the right hemidiaphragm, but both CT and ultrasonograms are normal. **a, b** The celiac arteriogram; no abnormality. **c, d** Proper hepatic arteriogram. A 5 × 6.5-cm tumor with neovascularity, arterial displacement and tumor stain (*arrows*)

Fig. 20.5a, b

attenuation is a nonspecific finding in CT, and at times a neoplasm is difficult to differentiate from a cyst or a benign hemangioma. Selective hepatic angiography is still necessary for problem solving, especially when there is a discrepancy between the radiological diagnosis and the clinical findings.

Since CT, US, and nuclear scanning are frequently performed initially to detect liver tumors and since routine use of hepatic angiography is impossible, it is important to select patients carefully for angiography. Based on experience with several thousand hepatic tumor diagnoses and cases of treatment, my indications for hepatic angiography include the following: (1) a high clinical suspicion of hepatic tumor, (2) conflicting information among the various scanning imaging procedures—CT, US, radionuclide scintigraphy, and MR, (3) a fatty liver, (4) any mass less than 2 cm on CT or US, (5) evaluation for surgical resectability of any hepatic lesion, and (6) abnormal liver function tests in the face of normal imaging studies.

Patients with a previous history of a malignant tumor in other organs who develop evidence of abnormal liver functions, hepatomegaly, and/or elevated carcinoembryonic antigen (CEA) are prime suspects for liver metastasis. These patients should have an infusion hepatic arteriogram even if CT and US are negative. In a study of prophylactic intra-arterial infusion chemotherapy in 15 patients who had Duke C colon carcinoma but otherwise a normal liver according to CT and/or US, early small metastases were discovered in three patients (20%) by infusion angiography prior to chemotherapy.

When a small mass is detected by CT, it is frequently difficult to differentiate from a benign hemangioma or cyst. The angiographic features of cavernous hemangiomas have been well described and are generally considered to be diagnostic. Recently, it has also been shown that hemangiomas have characteristic CT findings, consisting of gradual contrast enhancement from the periphery toward the center, eventually becoming isodense over a period of time (long delay) [10–12]. This characteristic is best illustrated in larger hemangiomas but is more subtle and, at times, uncertain in smaller ones. Central thrombosis or sclerosis make CT detection more difficult. Hemangiomas have a range of patterns as do some malignancies. When hemangiomas and malignant hepatic tumors coexist (Fig. 20.6), the need for hepatic angiography becomes obvious: Such lesions are extremely difficult to diagnose by CT alone. In our experience, hepatic angiography is superior to CT in the diagnosis of small hemangiomas and is of vital importance in decisions with respect to therapeutic planning.

The problem of detecting a hepatic tumor in a fatty liver has been discussed by Lewis et al. [13]. Since both fatty changes and tumor tissue have decreased attenuation coefficients, it is not surprising that a tumor may be easily hidden by fat (Fig. 20.7). When areas of increased density are present in a liver with diffuse fatty change, the differential diagnosis is between a tumor, hemangioma, or island of normal parenchyma. The specific diagnosis is best accomplished with hepatic angiography or biopsy. Superselective catheterization and infusion technique are absolutely essential for the correct diagnosis of a tumor in patients with a fatty liver, particularly those with a high clinical suspicion of hepatic metastases.

Surgical resection is still the best treatment for hepatic malignant tumors. However, the number of liver tumor resections has decreased recently throughout the world because of the overall improved preoperative diagnosis. Most metastatic liver tumors are multifocal. The detection of small satellite lesions by imaging scans or angiography can avoid unnecessary laparotomy. Hepatic angiography can delineate hepatic artery variations, tumor extension into the portal vein, tumor extension into the hepatic vein or inferior vena cava, and detection of small satellite lesions.

The number and aberrant origin of the hepatic arteries are well known to surgeons. Angiography is the only method to illustrate the hepatic artery anatomy in a single view. The incidence of portal vein tumor involvement is very high in primary hepatocellular carcinoma but is rare, though still possible, in metastatic carcinoma. Portal vein tumors can be detected by CT or US, but angiography best illustrates the extent of the tumor, collateral circulation, and direction of the portal flow. Some surgeons also stress the importance of hepatic vein patency, since tumor involvement of the major right and left hepatic veins is a criterion of nonresectability.

The importance of the selective catheterization and infusion technique in the detection of small liver tumors of less than 1 cm has been discussed earlier in this chapter. It is my experience that the selective infusion hepatic arteriogram and CT angiography are the most sensitive diagnostic modalities in the detection of small liver tumors. If ultrasonography, nuclear scan, and conven-

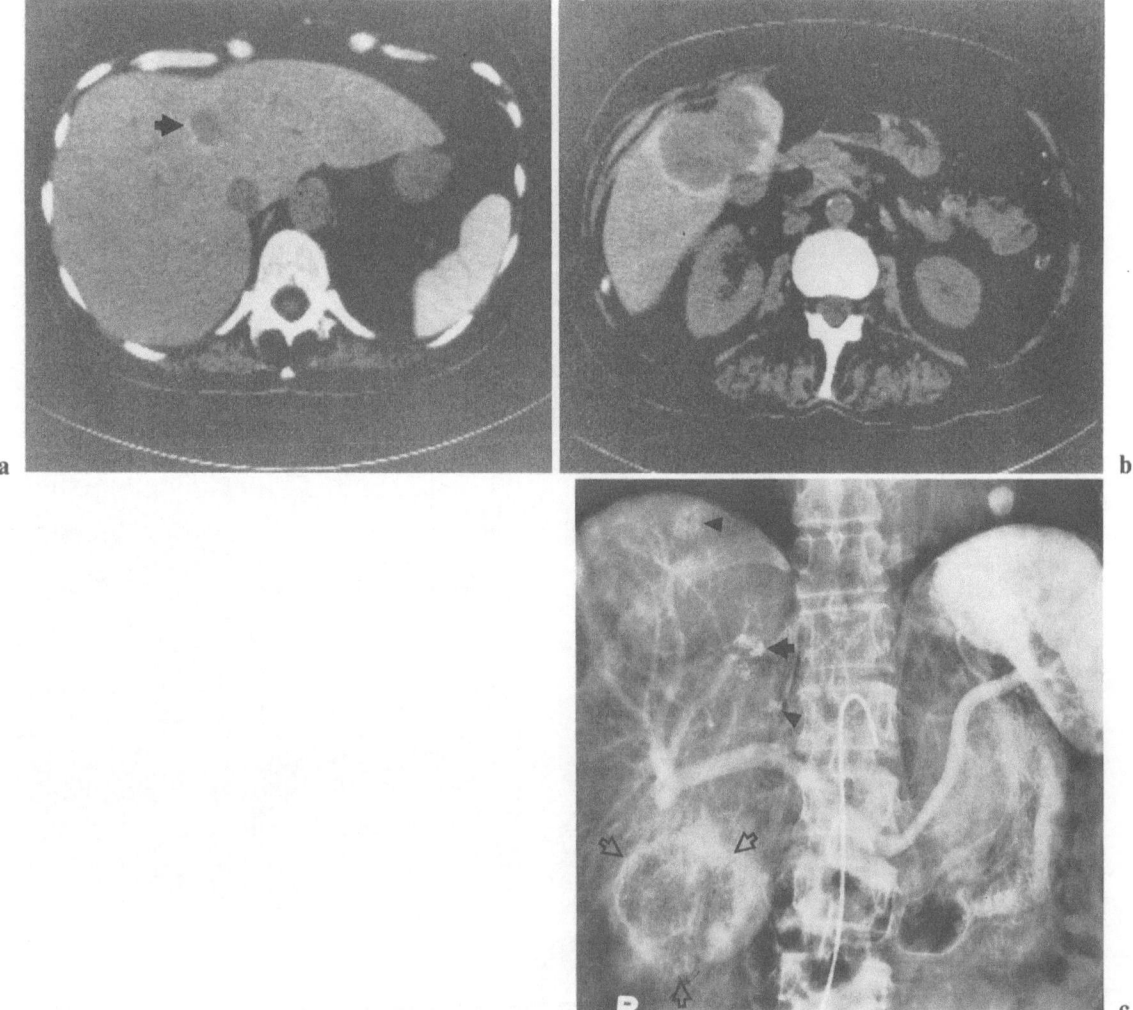

Fig. 20.6a–c. Cholangiocarcinoma and hemangioma. CT with bolus contrast medium shows no liver mass. **a** EOE-13 CT. A low-density lesion arrow. **b** EOE-13 CT, several centimeters lower. Another lesion. **c** Celiac arteriogram reveals that the upper lesion on CT is a hemangioma (*closed arrow*). Two other hemangiomas (*arrowheads*) are seen (not shown by CT). The lower largest lesion (*open arrows*) is a tumor. At surgery, this lower lesion was diagnosed as a cholangiocarcinoma. The smaller hemangiomas were palpated but not resected

tional CT show a resectable liver tumor, hepatic angiography should be routinely performed prior to surgery. After delineation of the vascular anatomy, an infusion hepatic arteriogram should be included to complete the evaluation for tumor resectability. If there is an equivocal lesion in the infusion hepatic arteriogram, then the catheter can be placed in the proper or common hepatic artery and CT angiography performed. If infusion hepatic angiography demonstrates small satellite lesions in the noninvolved segment by conventional CT or US, a CT angiogram can be omitted and save costs.

6 Angiographic features of hepatic tumors

In children, benign tumors are discovered under 2 years of age; they include hemangioendotheliomas and cavernous hemangiomas. The malignant tumor in this age-group is hepatocellular carcinoma or hepatoblastoma. In the adult population, primary carcinoma of the liver displays a remarkable geographical distribution. The incidence of primary carcinoma of the liver among all cancers is 1.4%–2.5% in America, 1.2% in Europe, 16.9% in Singapore, and 50.9%

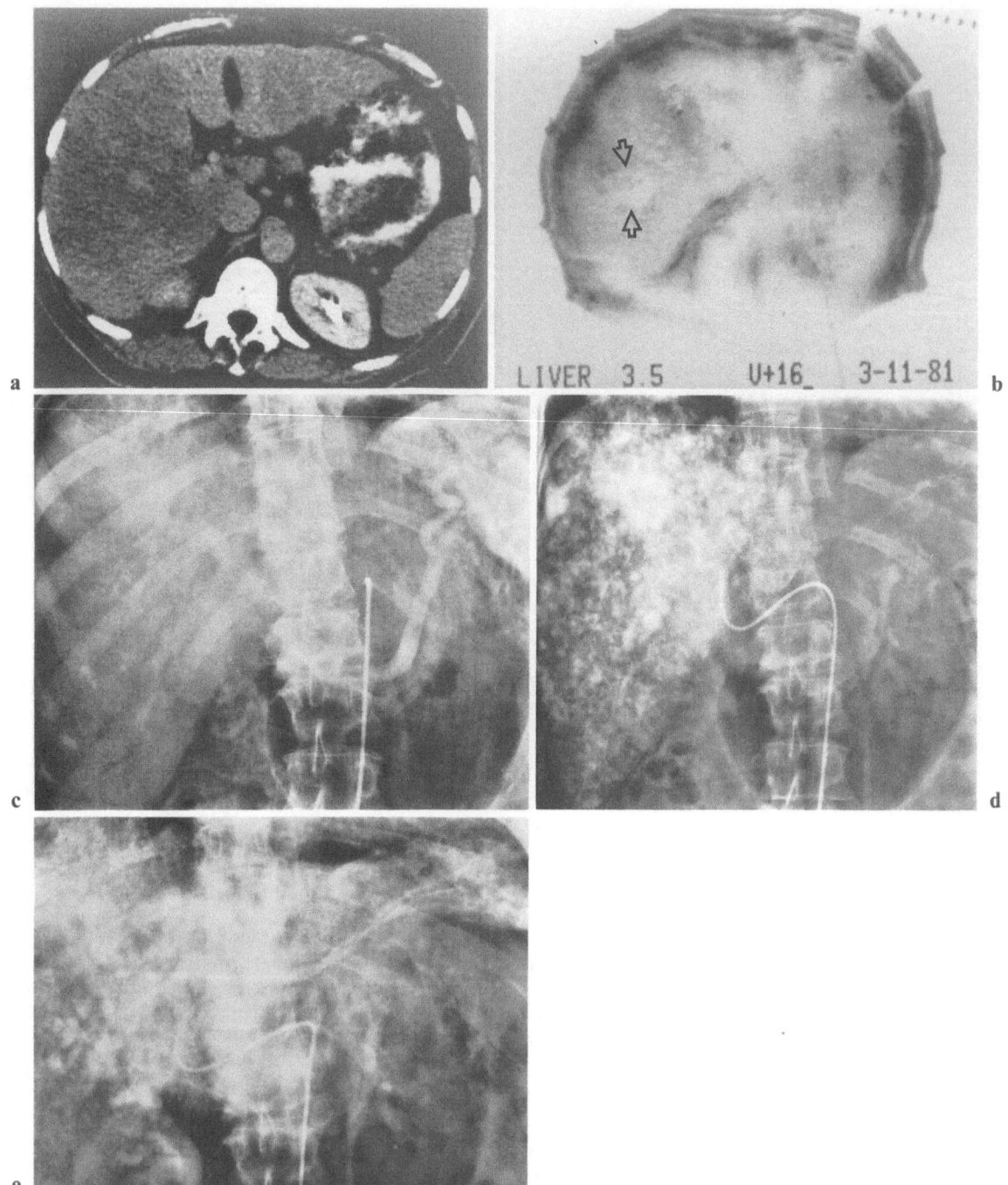

Fig. 20.7a–e. Fatty liver with liver metastasis. **a** CT scan shows fatty degeneration of the liver. **b** US reveals a mass in the right lobe (*arrows*). **c** Celiac arteriogram is grossly normal. **d** Right hepatic arteriogram demonstrates a diffuse tumor. **e** Left hepatic arteriogram shows innumerable small tumors intermingled with the fatty liver. Note also the portal vein filling

in the Bantu in Africa [14]. Benign tumors are approximately one-tenth as frequent [15]. However, the liver is the most common site of metastatic disease. Of all patients who die of cancer, approximately 50%–75% have liver metastases; frequently, the extent of liver disease dictates the length of patient survival [16–19].

The abnormal angiographic findings of the liver tumor include:

1) Distortion, tortuosity, and displacement of the hepatic artery
2) Hypervascularity of the hepatic artery—an increase in the number of opacified vessels
3) Neovascularity—small, abnormal vessels
4) Tumor stain—an increase in capillary blush in the tumor; in small tumors of less than 3 cm, this is frequently the only finding
5) Arteriovenous shunting—more common in the primary carcinoma, but it can also occur in metastatic tumors
6) Arterial encasement—the abrupt and irregular change in the caliber and direction of vessels, more commonly observed in cholangiocarcinoma than other malignancies
7) Pooling or puddling of the contrast medium—usually associated with a hypervascular malignant tumor; the pooling is frequently irregular and is washed out relatively early due to the high flow through the tumor
8) Vascular lakes—usually regular in shape and variable in size, with a delay in washout; they are very typical of a cavernous hemangioma. Pooling of the contrast material, which is more commonly seen in malignancy, should be differentiated from vascular lakes
9) Portal vein tumor—most frequently observed in hepatocellular carcinoma
10) Streak and thread sign—a description of the very small arteries supplying a tumor growing in the portal vein

The classification of hepatic tumors has been described in the other chapters (Chap. 7–12) of this book; many tumors have similar or overlapping angiographic features. Rather than discussing the angiographic findings of each tumor, only tumors with specific angiographic patterns and the key angiographic differential diagnosis will be covered in this chapter.

6.1 Hepatocellular carcinoma

The most common primary malignant neoplasm involving the liver, hepatocellular carcinoma (HCC), has two peak incidences—in children under 2 years old and in adults in the sixth decade of life. HCC presents in the following forms: (1) a solitary mass (usually in noncirrhotic patients), (2) multinodular forms (usually with cirrhosis), and (3) a diffuse infiltrative lesion without a distinct mass. In a typical HCC, all the angiographic features, such as arterial distortion and tortuosity, hypervascularity, neovascularity, tumor stain, and vascular pooling, are present. Kido et al. suggested that these typical features are more commonly observed in well-differentiated hepatomas [20]. If other features such as portal vein tumor extension and arterioportal shunting (thread and streak sign) are also present, the angiographic diagnosis becomes easy (Figs. 20.8, 20.9) [21–23]. Tumor extension to the hepatic vein is rare but can occur (Fig. 20.10). However, some HCC can be of low vascularity especially those 3 cm or smaller. Detection of small satellite lesions is best accomplished with the infusion technique as described above.

6.2 Cholangiocarcinoma

Cholangiocarcinoma commonly originates near the porta hepatis and manifests clinically with obstructive jaundice. Cholangiocarcinoma is an infiltrative tumor but grows more slowly than HCC. Its angiographic feature is typically arterial encasement, a feature rarely seen in HCC and other metastatic tumors. Tumor staining may or may not be present. Arterioportal shunting is rare. Cholangiocarcinoma arising from a peripheral bile duct may resemble a metastatic lesion (Fig. 20.6).

Histological diagnosis is carried out by percutaneous or surgical liver biopsy or by bile cytology and brush biopsy through a cholangiography catheter.

6.3 Metastastic neoplasms

The liver is the organ most commonly involved in metastatic disease. In contrast to some Oriental or African countries, where HCC is the most common liver tumor, metastatic tumors are by far the most common type of tumor in the USA. The median survival for patients with untreated liver metastases is 150 days for colon cancer, 60 days for gastric cancer, and 50 days for pancreatic cancer [19]. Hepatomegaly and nonspecific complaints such as weight loss, anorexia, fever, and right upper quadrant pain are common.

Liver function tests and the serum carcinoembryonic antigen (CEA) values are frequently

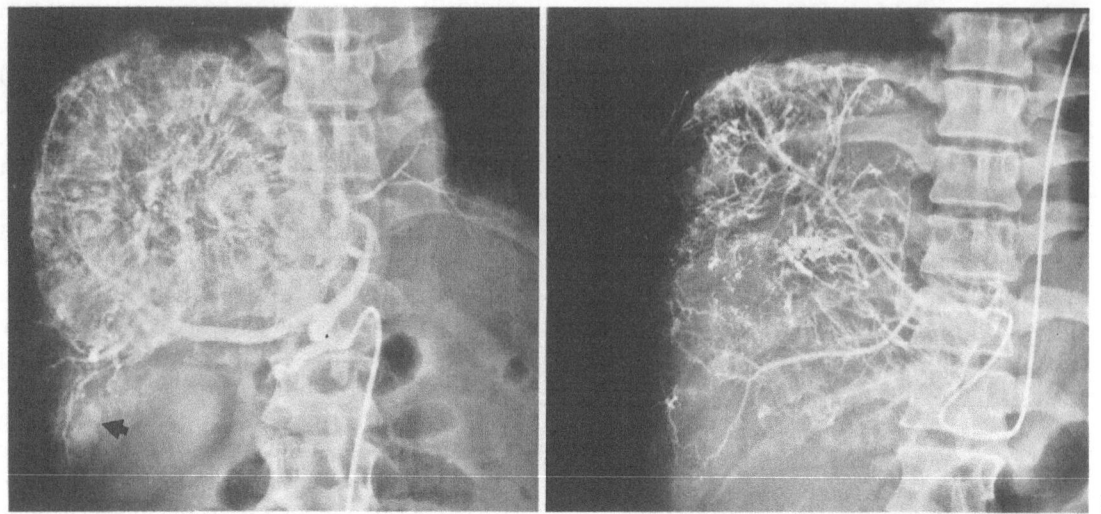

Fig. 20.8a, b. Hepatocellular carcinoma. CT reveals a large solitary mass in the right lobe and the medial segment of the left lobe. **a** Common hepatic arteriogram shows a large hypervascular mass with neovascularity and tumor stain. Another smaller lesion is seen (*arrow*). **b** Superselective midhepatic arteriogram shows significant blood supply to the tumor from the midhepatic artery that was not obvious from the common hepatic artery injection

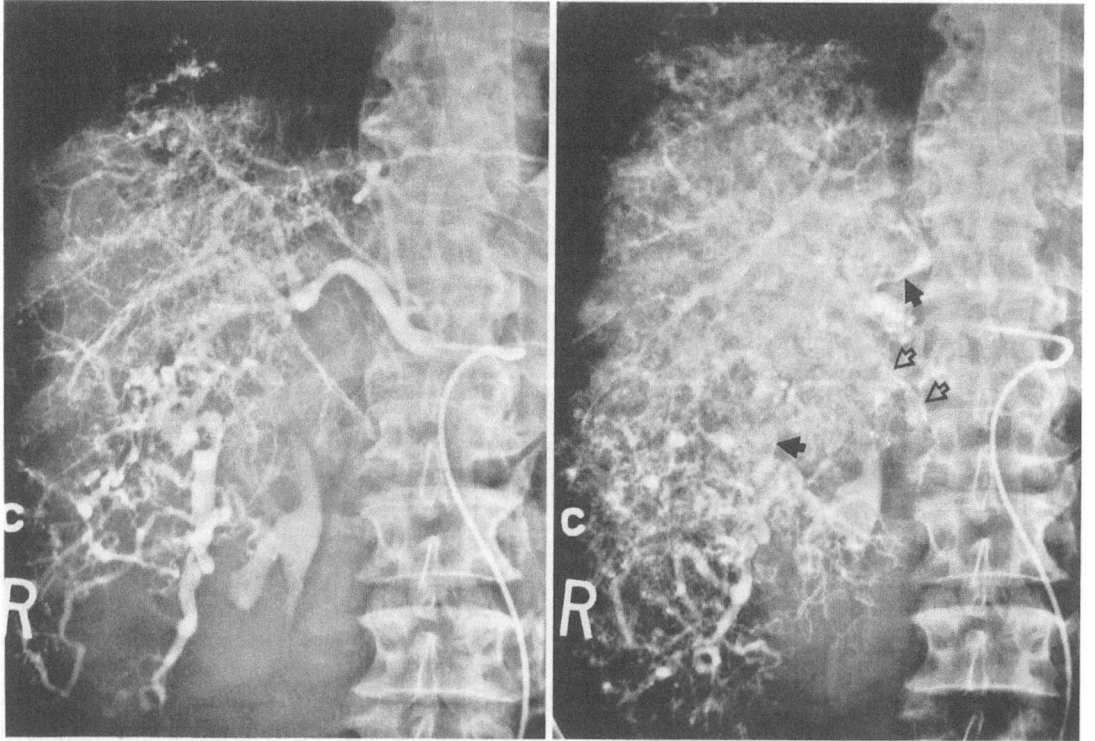

Fig. 20.9a, b. Hepatocellular carcinoma with portal vein tumor extension. **a** Common hepatic arteriogram. The entire right lobe is replaced by tumor. There is arterial distortion, tortuosity, hypervascularity, neovascularity, and vascular pooling. The left lobe is normal. **b** Portal vein tumor (*closed arrows*) and arterioportal shunting (*open arrows*)

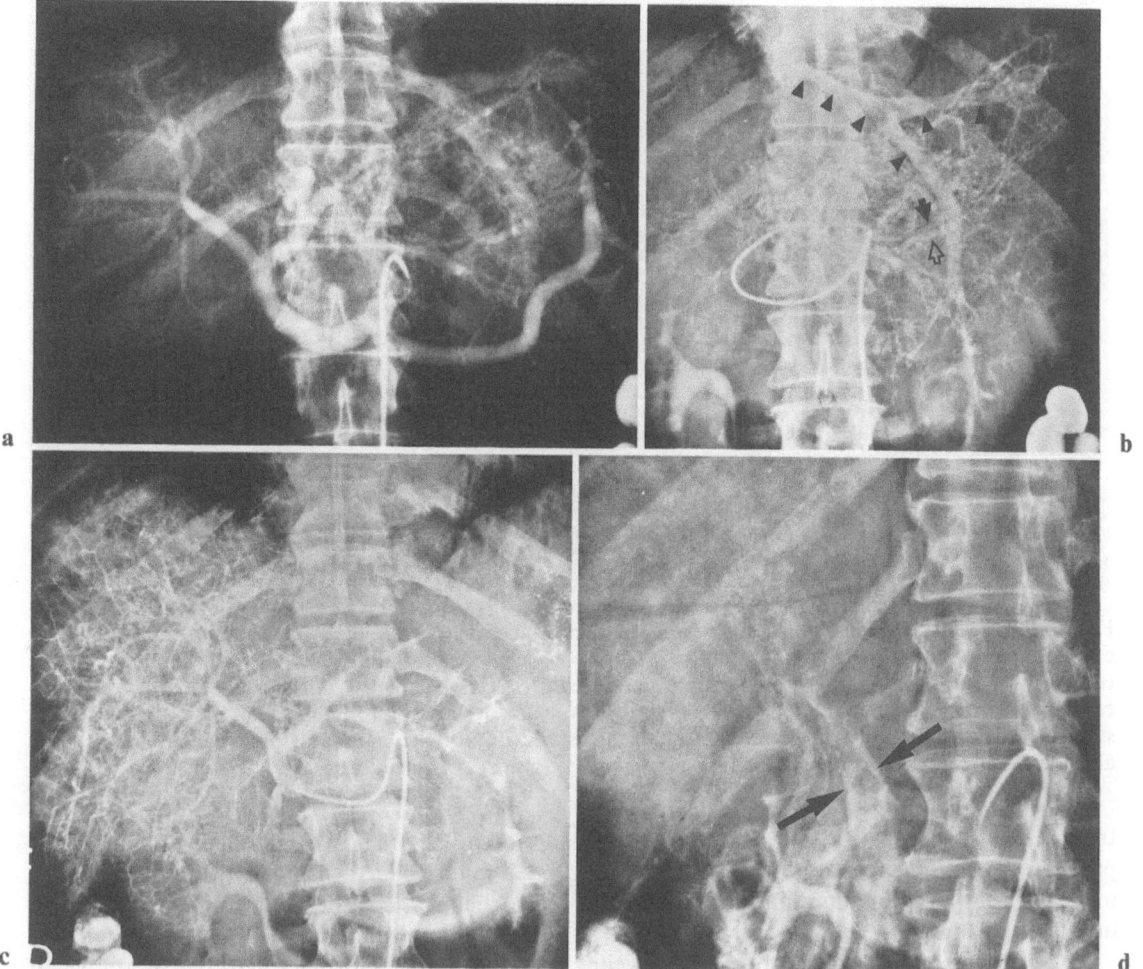

Fig. 20.10a–d. Hepatocellular carcinoma with diffuse bilobar involvement. **a** Celiac arteriogram shows a hypervascular left lobe. Duplication of vessels from arterioportal shunting in the left lobe makes this lobe appear more hypervascular than the right. **b** Superselective left hepatic arteriogram. Arterioportal shunting is seen more clearly (*closed arrow* hepatic artery, *open arrow* portal vein). There is prominent left hepatic vein filling with tumor involvement (*arrowheads*). **c** Right hepatic arteriogram (following left hepatic embolization) reveals hypervascularity and neovascularity indicative of a diffuse right lobe tumor that was poorly appreciated in the celiac arteriogram. **d** The portal vein is occluded by a tumor (*arrows*) in the superior mesenteric arteriogram

abnormal; CEA is particularly useful in monitoring therapy, especially in colon carcinoma.

Although the angiographic features of metastatic tumors range from hypervascular and isovascular to hypovascular in the celiac arteriogram, all such tumors have some degree of "tumor stain" when an infusion hepatic arteriogram is performed. The tumor stain in the infusion hepatic arteriogram is exaggerated by the nonopacified portal flow that results in a "negative portal vein washout" of the normal liver parenchyma with subsequent enhancement of the tumor stain (Fig. 20.3c, d). By contrast, a "hypovascular" metastatic tumor in a celiac arteriogram is the consequence of the opacified portal flow, which enhances the density of the normal liver parenchyma and thus has a "positive portal vein masking" effect (Fig. 20.3a, b). It is essential that a selective infusion hepatic arteriogram be performed in the angiographic diagnosis of all liver masses so as to avoid false-negative results. If the hepatic artery is occluded (due to previous surgery, Infusaid pump chemotherapy, or median arcuate ligament compression), then superselective catheterization of the collateral arteries is frequently possible and should be done for further diagnosis and therapy (Fig. 20.11). Low-vascularity hepatic metastases in the celiac arteriogram are typically from carcinoma of the lung, pancreas, or gastrointestinal

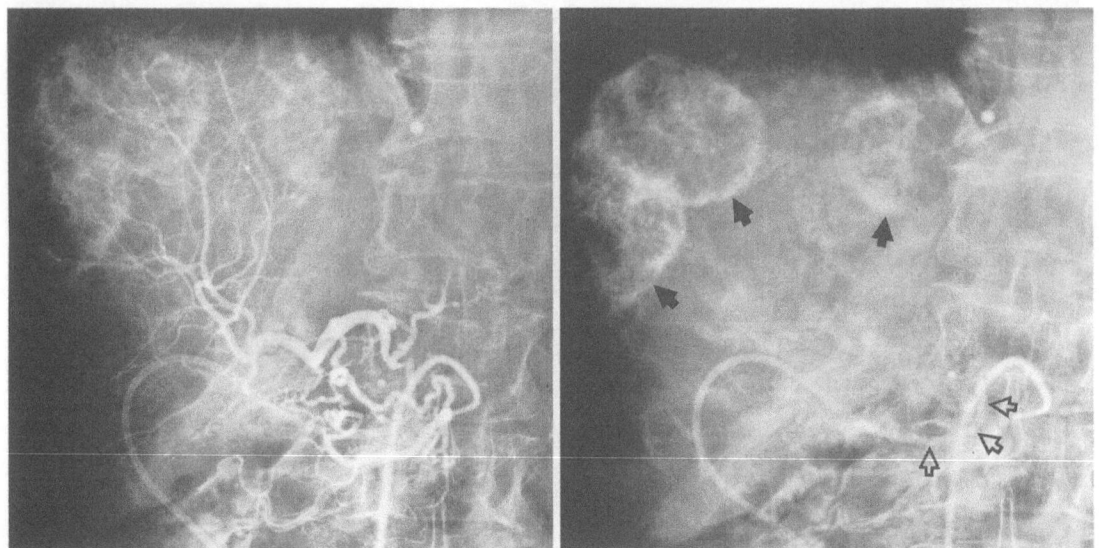

Fig. 20.11a, b. Metastatic colon carcinoma. Despite intra-arterial chemotherapy through a surgically placed catheter for an Infusaid pump. The tumor progressed. Celiac arteriogram revealed total occlusion of the common hepatic artery and gastroduodenal artery. **a** Superselective catheterization of the inferior pancreaticoduodenal artery, the major supply to the liver. Hepatic arteries are not too abnormal, but a tumor stain is starting to show in the upper right lobe. **b** Multiple metastatic tumors with definite staining (*closed arrows*). Note also the catheter (*open arrows*) for the Infusaid pump

tract [7, 8]. Figure 20.12 illustrates a surgically proven pancreatic carcinoma in which the liver metastasis has a tumor stain similar to that seen in other metastases.

For the same reason, a "positive portal vein masking" effect may occur in the conventional CT scan when contrast medium is given intravenously, whether by bolus injection or infusion. A "negative portal vein washout" effect enhances the detection of a liver tumor in CT angiography when the contrast medium is given through a hepatic artery catheter. It is obvious that CT angiography detects small hepatic lesions better than conventional liver CT.

6.4 Metastatic apudoma

The amine precursor uptake and decarboxylation (APUD) cells are diffusely distributed in many organs and systems and include, among others, the cells of the anterior pituitary, parafollicular thyroid cells, chromaffin cells of the adrenal medulla and extra-adrenal paraganglia, enterochromaffin and peptide-secreting cells of the gastrointestinal tract, pancreatic islet cells, and Feyrter's cells of the tracheobronchial tree. APUD derives from their most prominent features, namely, fluorogenic amine content, amine precursor uptake, and the presence of amino acid decarboxylase. The APUD cells and their corre-

sponding neoplasms (apudomas) are closely related in terms of their biosynthetic mechanisms, histochemical and ultrastructural features, and possibly their embryological origin. Apudomas may produce abnormal quantities of amines or peptide hormones, which may or may not be identical to the secretory products of their nonneoplastic counterparts. Apudomas may be benign or malignant; hyperplasias are included among apudomas because of the functional resemblance. Multiple endocrine neoplasia syndromes also comprise these neoplasms. Generally, apudomas grow slowly, and even after metastasizing they are associated with prolonged survival [24].

When an apudoma metastasizes to the liver, the liver tumor frequently becomes the site of excessive hormone secretion. Angiographically, a multifocal tumor with a dense stain is the commonest finding, but it is not dissimilar to other types of metastatic tumor. Partial hepatectomy and hepatic artery ligation have resulted in symptom relief in some patients. Hepatic artery embolization has also achieved significant palliation in these patients [24–26].

6.5 Hemangioma

Cavernous hemangioma is the most common benign tumor in the adult, usually occurring in

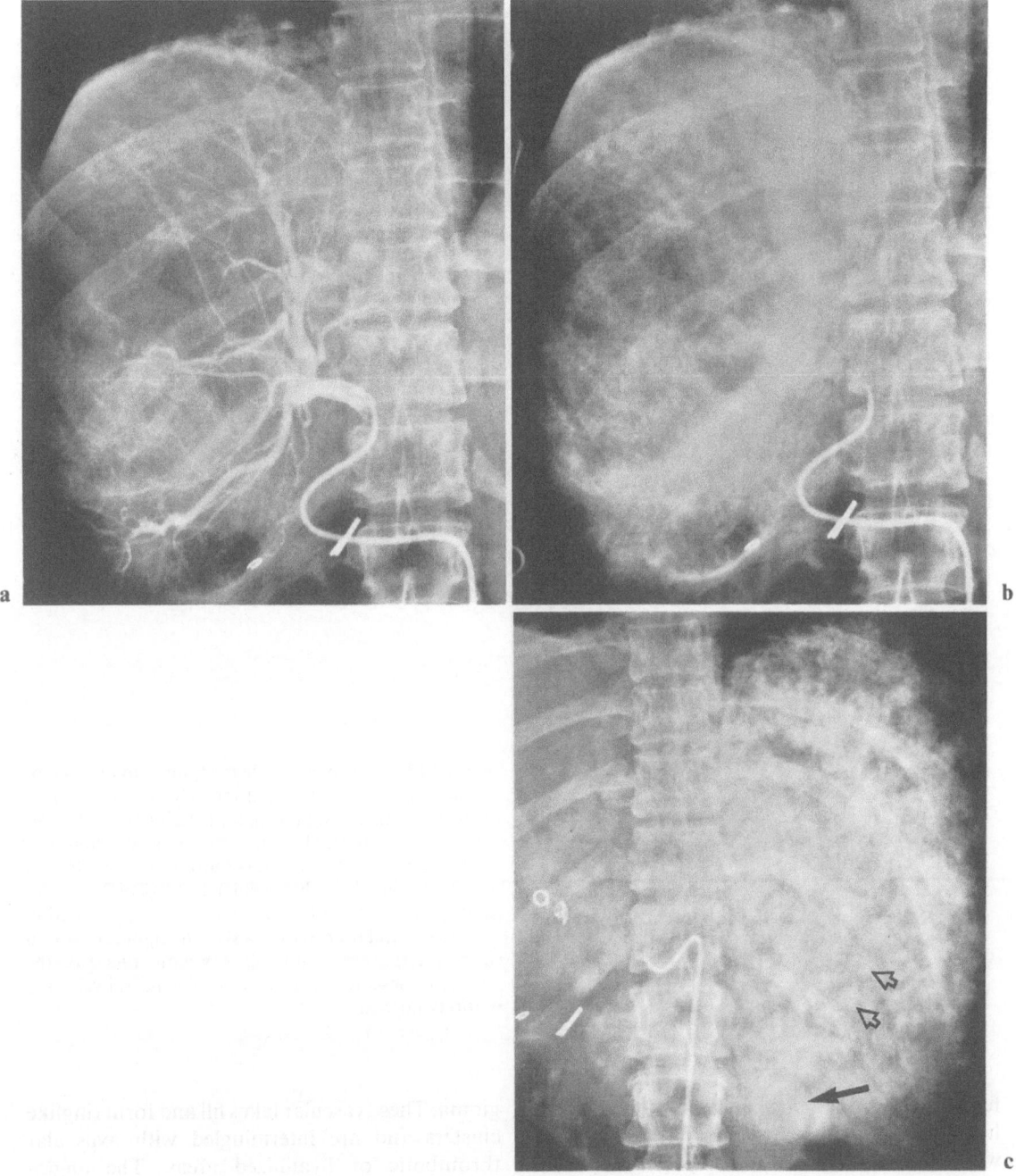

Fig. 20.12a–c. Metastatic pancreatic carcinoma. The primary tumor was previously resected surgically. **a** Right hepatic arteriogram. Displacement of right hepatic segmental arteries is noted around a large mass in the right lobe. Subtle neovascularity and tumor stains are present. **b** Hepatogram phase. There is a hypervascular rim of the large right lobe mass as well as a tumor stain in the center. **c** Hepatogram phase of left hepatic arteriogram. Two coils were placed in the right hepatic artery following Ivalon particle embolization. A 3-cm (*closed arrow*) and several 1-cm tumors (*open arrows*) are present. These metastatic tumors are similar to metastatic tumors from other sites; they were not present in the conventional CT

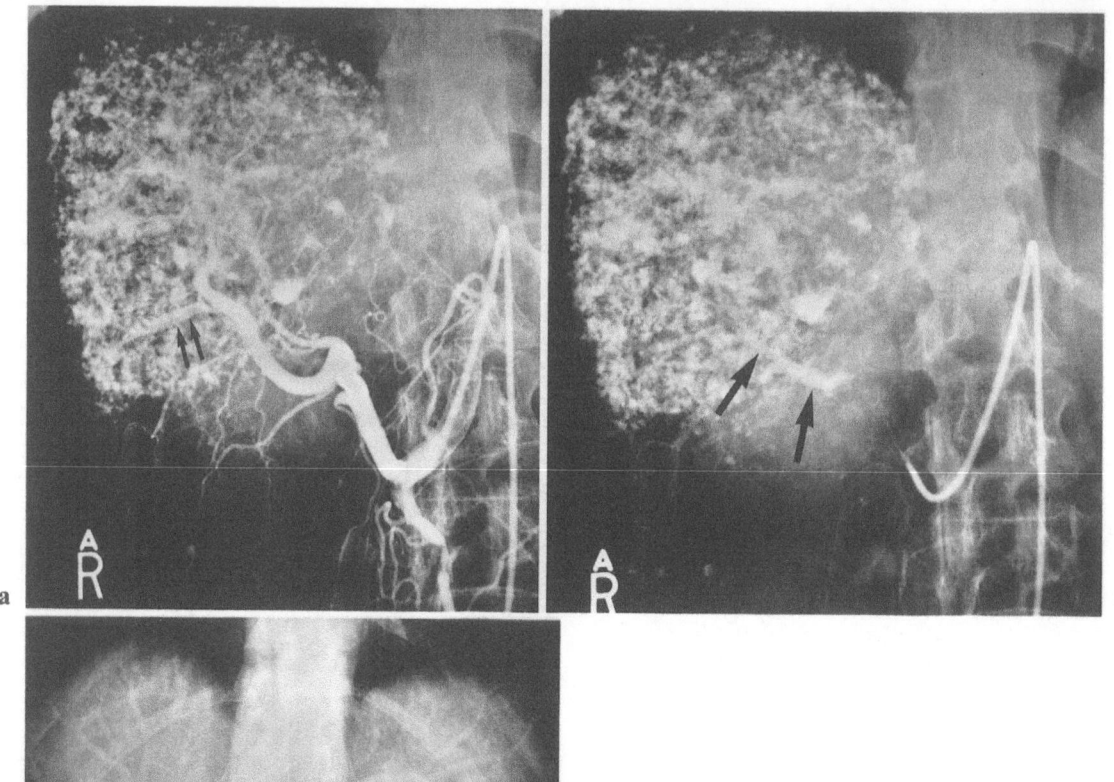

Fig. 20.13a–c. Cavernous hemangioma in an asymptomatic patient with hepatomegaly. Liver enzymes were normal. **a** Right hepatic arteriogram. Hepatic arteries are normal, but arterioportal shuntings (*arrows*) are present. The low third of the right lobe is much less involved. **b** Vascular lakes of various size have persisted for a long time. Note the opacification of a segmental branch (*arrows*) of the right portal vein from arterioportal shunting. **c** Venous phase of the superior mesenteric arteriogram. The portal veins are entirely normal

females. Most patients are asymptomatic, but hepatomegaly may be present. When associated with a primary tumor elsewhere, cavernous hemangioma frequently mimics liver metastasis in imaging modalities such as nuclear scan. Although CT with contrast enhancement may show sequential filling in from the the periphery of the lesion for a histological diagnosis, this is less likely to occur in smaller lesions. Angiography of cavernous hemangioma shows normal, nondilated hepatic arteries and prolonged filling of the dilated vascular lake from the arterial phase to the late hepatogram phase. It has been suggested that a vascular stain of over 18–20 s is very diagnostic of cavernous heman-

gioma. These vascular lakes fill and form ringlike clusters and are intermingled with avascular thrombotic or hyalinized areas. The angiographic features of cavernous hemangioma are so diagnostic (Fig. 20.13) that liver biopsy for histological confirmation is usually unnecessary. Cavernous hemangioma frequently runs a benign clinical course, and malignant transformation is virtually unknown. Very rarely, hemorrhage occurs from either spontaneous rupture or abdominal trauma, and constant abdominal discomfort can develop due to progressive tumor growth. Hepatic artery embolization has proven useful in symptomatic relief without recourse to surgery (Fig. 20.14).

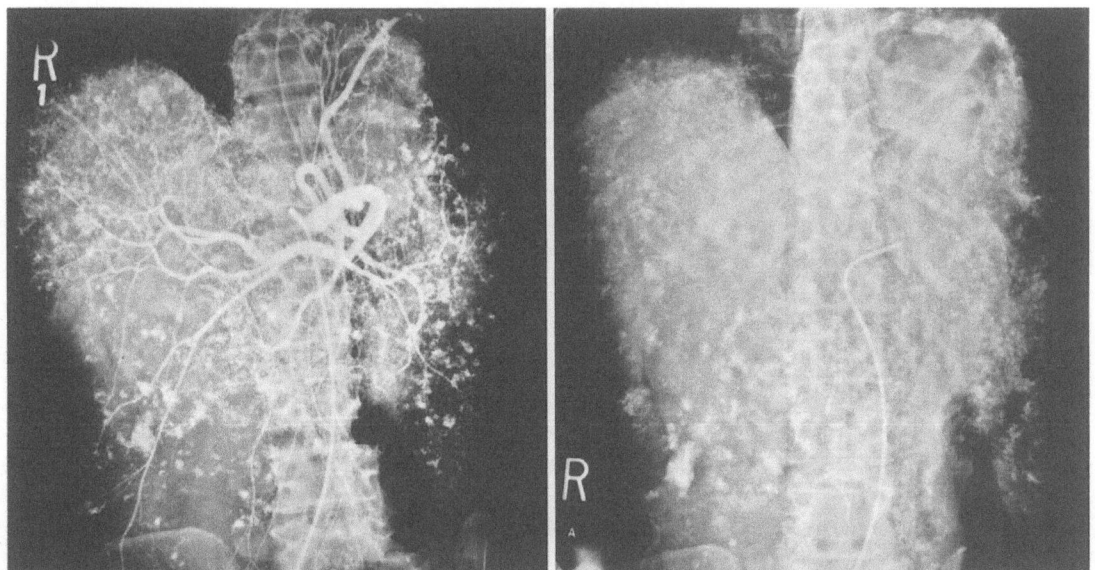

a

b

Fig. 20.14a, b. Cavernous hemangioma in a symptomatic patient who had progressive hepatomegaly with constant abdominal discomfort. **a** Celiac arteriogram. Marked hepatomegaly occupying nearly the entire abdomen. Multiple venous lakes are present throughout both lobes. **b** Hepatogram phase. Persistent venous lake opacification. Eventration of the left hemidiaphragm is present and is thought to be due to hepatomegaly. The patient underwent sequential right and left hepatic artery embolization during a 2-month period and showed significant symptomatic relief

6.6 Infantile hemangioendothelioma

Hemangioendothelioma most frequently occurs in the infant and has a more aggressive clinical course than cavernous hemangioma in adults. A precordial murmur, cough, dyspnea, or congestive heart failure are typical presentations. Spontaneous rupture may occur, resulting in fatal hemorrhage. Angiographic features are similar to those of cavernous hemangioma, but there is a greater degree of arteriovenous shunting, which causes dense filling of the hepatic vein. Arterial embolization has resulted in relief of congestive heart failure and complete remission in some patients.

6.7 Hepatic adenoma

Hepatic adenoma is extremely rare in childhood but common in women of childbearing age. A causal relationship with oral contraceptive agents has been postulated [27, 28]. The patient may have an abdominal mass, pain, and, occasionally, acute abdominal catastrophe from rupture and hemorrhage. There is no evidence that a hepatic adenoma is premalignant. Galloway et al. have suggested the term "minimum deviation hepatoma" for this tumor [29], but this designation has not been universally adopted. The angiographic features of a hepatic adenoma in-

clude a round or ovoid hypervascular mass with hepatic arteries entering from the periphery of the mass. The hypervascularity produces an increased homogeneous stain with a sharply demarcated margin. A fine zone of relative radiolucency, probably representing a liver capsule, may separate the adenoma from the surrounding normal liver.

6.8 Focal nodular hyperplasia

Focal nodular hyperplasia is a hepatic mass with a central area of scar tissue. Multiple fine septa subdivide the nodule into smaller units. Although there is no definite causal relationship with the use of oral contraceptives, focal nodular hyperplasia may grow under the influence of hormones, as has been shown for hemangioma and adenoma [30–34].

Angiographic features show that the hepatic arteries may enter from the periphery of the mass when small or from the center with radiation to the periphery in a larger mass. A fairly homogeneous stain with fine granularity is very typical of the hepatogram phase (Fig. 20.15). Angiographic differentiation between focal nodular hyperplasia and hepatic adenoma is not always easy. It is my belief that the peripheral-entry arterial pattern and central-radiating arterial

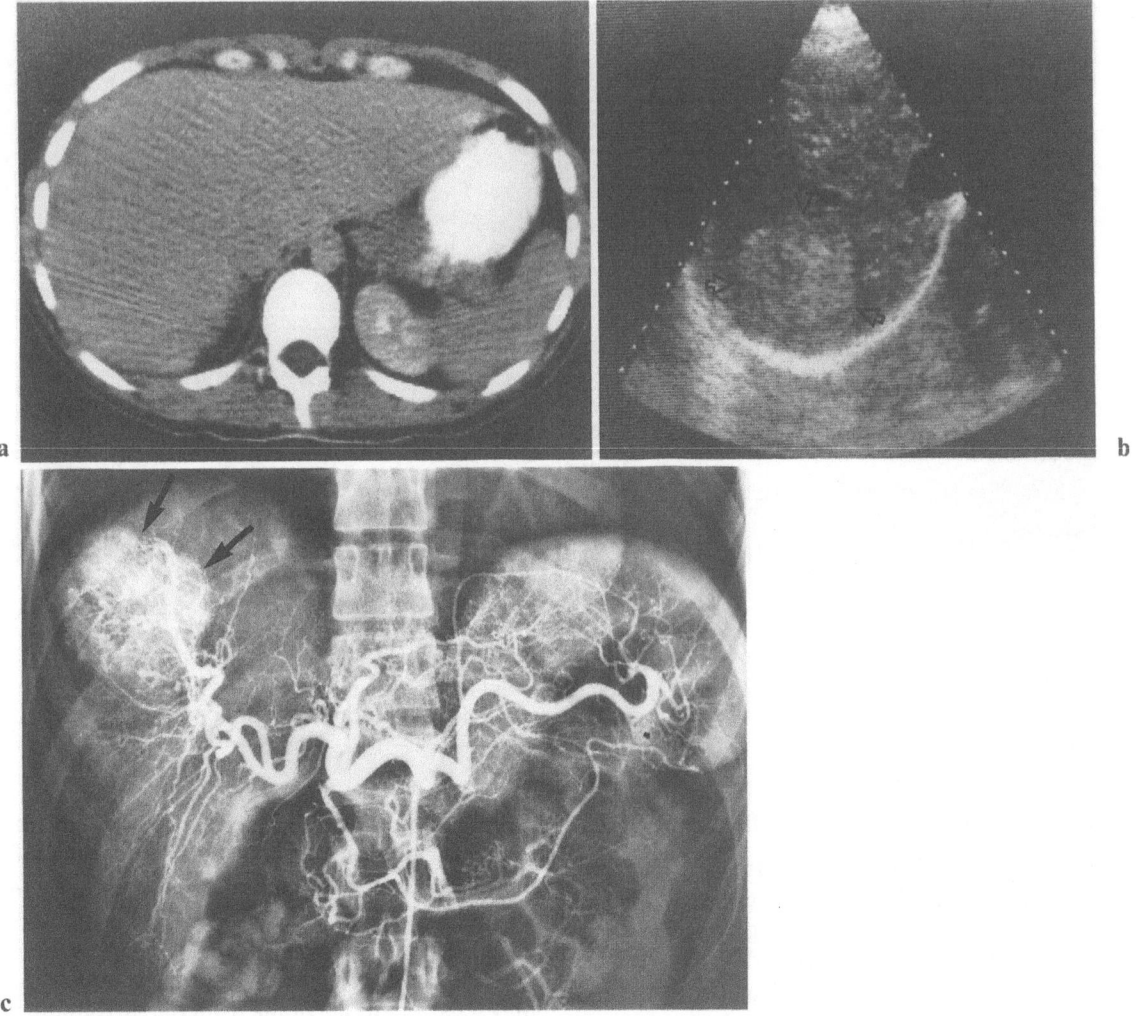

Fig. 20.15a–c. Focal nodular hyperplasia. **a** CT with and without intravenous contrast medium shows no hepatic mass. **b** US shows a hyperechoic mass (*arrows*) in the posterior aspect of the right lobe. **c** Celiac arteriogram. Slightly enlarged segmental hepatic artery supplying a very hypervascular mass (*arrows*). The mass was resected and histologically proven to be focal nodular hyperplasia

pattern could merely be the result of different angles in filming during angiography. By turning a tumor through 90°, a central radiating pattern may turn into a peripheral-entry pattern and vice versa. Rogers et al. suggested that scintigrams are essential for differentiating between focal nodular hyperplasia and adenoma [32]. Casarella et al. reported that a hypovascular mass with a focal defect on liver scan in a young woman taking oral contraceptives would be highly suggestive of adenoma, while a hypervascular mass with a tortuous artery and a septated blush coupled with radioactive colloid uptake was diagnostic of focal nodular hyperplasia [30]. The histological appearance of the two lesions may also be difficult for the pathologist. Thus, further

clinical, angiographic, and pathological evidence of these lesions is required.

6.9 Regenerating nodule

A regenerative nodule is frequently observed in a cirrhotic liver or following partial resection of the liver. A homogeneous stain is frequently the major finding in the hepatogram phase. The arterial phase shows stretched and nondilated arteries entering the lesion. Arterioportal shunting, pooling of contrast medium, or neovascularity are absent. When associated with surgical resection of the liver, the regenerating nodule is frequently in the resected margin of the liver. To differentiate a regenerating nodule from HCC, I have observed in a small number of patients that an epinephrine (2–3 μg) hepatic arteriogram frequently results in disappearance of the stain, whereas the tumor stain frequently persists in HCC.

References

1. Michels NA (1985) Blood supply and anatomy of the upper abdominal organs. Lippincott, Philadelphia
2. Harell G (1974) Ventral portal vein. AJR 121: 369–373
3. Chuang VP, Soo CS, Carrasco CH, Wallace S (1983) Superselective catheterization technique in hepatic angiography. AJR 141: 803–811
4. Healey JE Jr, Sheena KS (1963) Vascular patterns in metastatic liver tumors. Surg Forum 14: 121–122
5. Healey JE Jr (1965) Vascular pattern in human metastatic liver tumors. Surg Gynecol Obstet 120: 1187–1193
6. Lin G, Lunderquist A (1984) Portal blood supply of liver metastasis. AJR 143: 53
7. Baum S (1971) Hepatic angiography. In: Abrams HL, (ed) Angiography, 2nd edn, vol. 2, chap. 61. Little Brown, Boston, pp 983–1002
8. Reuter Sr, Redman HC (1977) Gastrointestinal angiography, 2nd edn, chap. 4. Saunders philadelphia, pp 131–161
9. Lipshitz HI, Jing BS, Wallace S, Logathetis CJ (1983) Sterile metastases: a diagnostic and therapeutic dilemma. AJR 140: 15–20
10. Johnson CM, Sheedy PF, Stanson AW, Stephens DH, Hattery RR Jr, Adson MA (1981) Computed tomography and angiography of cavernous hemangiomas of the liver. Radiology 138: 115–121
11. Itai Y, Furrui S, Araki T, Yashiro N, Tasaka A (1980) Computed tomography of cavernous hemangioma of the liver. Radiology 137: 149–155
12. Barnett DH, Zerhouni EA, White R, Siegelman SS (1980) Computed tomography in the diagnosis of cavernous hemangioma of the liver. AJR 134: 439–447
13. Lewis E, Bernardino ME, Barnes PA, Parvey HR, Soo CS, Chuang VP (1983) The fatty liver: pitfalls in the CT and angiographic evaluation of metastatic disease. J Compt Assist Tomogr 7: 235–241
14. Lin TY (1976) Tumors of the liver: I. Primary malignant tumors. In: Bockus HL (ed) Gastroenterology, 3rd edn, vol. 3. Saunders, Philadelphia, p 522
15. Dehner LP, Ishak KG (1971) Vascular tumors in infants and children. Arch Pathol 92: 101
16. Pack GT, Miller TR (1953) The treatment of hepatic tumors. NY State J Med 134: 59
17. Bloomenthal ED, Spellberg MA (1971) Therapy for carcinoma of the liver. Am J Gastroenterol 92: 101
18. Ariel IM, Pack GT (1961) Intra-arterial chemotherapy for cancer metastasis to liver. Arch Surg 91: 851
19. Jaffe BM, Donegan WL, Watson F, Spratt JS Jr (1968) Factors influencing survival in patients with untreated hepatic metastases. Surg Gynecol Obstet 127: 1
20. Vido C, Sasaki T, Kaneko M (1971) Angiography of primary liver cancer. Am J Roentgenol 113: 70
21. Okuda K, Musha H, Yamasaki T, Jinnouchi S, Nagasaki Y, Kubo Y, Shimokawa Y, Nakayama T, Kojiro M, Sakamoto K, Nakashima T (1977) Angiographic demonstration of intrahepatic arterioportal anastomoses in hepatocellular carcinoma. Radiology 122: 53
22. Okuda K, Musha H, Yoshida T, Kanda Y, Yamazaki T, Jinnouchi S, Kubo Y, Shimokawa Y, Kojiro M, Sakamoto K, Nakashima T (1975) Demonstration of growing casts of hepatocellular carcinoma in the portal vein by celiac angiography: the thread and streaks sign. Radiology 117: 303
23. Okuda K. Obata H, Jinnouchi S, Kubo Y, Nagasaki Y, Shimokawa Y, Nakajima Y, Musha N, Yamazaki T, Sakamoto K, Kojiro M, Nakashima T (1977) Angiographic assessment of gross anatomy of hepatocellular carcinoma: comparison of celiac angiograms and liver pathology in 100 cases. Radiology 123: 21
24. Carrasco CH, Chuang VP, Wallace S (1983) Apudomas metastatic to the liver: treatment by hepatic artery embolization. Radiology 149: 79–83
25. Carrasco CH, Charnsangavej C, Ajani J, Samaan NA, Richli W, Wallace S (1986) The carcinoid syndrome: palliation by hepatic artery embolization. AJR 147: 149–154
26. Mitty HA, Warner RRP, Newman LH, Train JS, Pasnes IH (1985) Control of carcinoid syndrome with hepatic artery embolization. Radiology 155: 623–626
27. Baum JK, Holtz F, Bookstein J, Klein FW (1973) Possible association between benign hepatomas and oral contraceptives. Lancet 2: 926
28. Sherlock S (1976) Hepatic adenomas and oral contraceptives. Gut 16: 753
29. Galloway SJ, Casarella WJ, Lattes R, Seaman WB (1975) Minimal deviation hepatoma: a new entity. Am J Roentgenol 125: 184–195
30. Casarella WJ, Knowles DM, Wolff M, Johnson PM (1978) Focal nodular hyperplasia and liver cell adenoma: radiologic and pathologic differentiation. Am J Roentgenol 131: 393
31. McLoughlin MK, Colapinto RT, Gilday DL, Hobbs BS, Korobkin MT, McDonald P, Phillips MJ (1973) Focal nodular hyperplasia of the liver. Radiology 107: 257
32. Rogers JV, Mack LA, Freeny PC, Johnson ML, Sones PJ (1981) Hepatic nodular hyperplasia: angiography, CT, sonography and scintigraphy. Am J Roentgenol 137: 983
33. Whelan TJ, Baugh JH, Chandor S (1973) Focal nodular hyperplasia of the liver. Ann Surg 177: 150
34. Stauffer JQ, Lopenski MW, Harold DJ, Myers JK (1975) Focal nodular hyperplasia of the liver and intrahepatic hemorrhage in young women on oral contraceptives. Ann Intern Med 83: 301

Chapter 21
Celiac Angiography in the Diagnosis of Small Hepatocellular Carcinoma

KENICHI TAKAYASU[1] and KUNIO OKUDA[2]

Celiac angiography is indispensable in the diagnosis of hepatic tumors, particularly hepatocellular carcinoma (HCC). The characteristic, if not pathognomonic, angiographic findings of HCC include tumor vessels, bizarre vascular lakes or conduits, hypervascularity, arterioportal shunts, and intraportal tumor invasion [1–5], identified as the thread and streaks sign [6]. However, these findings are derived from studies of advanced cases of HCC. With the advent of various newer imaging techniques, the diagnostic significance of angiography is changing. Currently, small HCCs are mostly detected by ultrasonography (US) in Japan and Taiwan and perhaps in some regions of China and Southeast Asia. The established diagnostic policy for early detection of HCC in these areas has been to follow patients with chronic liver disease by regularly scheduled checkups using abdominal US and serum alpha-fetoportein (AFP) measurements [7–9]. Small lesions are often detected among such patients and the lesions mostly prove to be HCC. The usual sequence of diagnostic investigations that follow the detection of a small-mass lesion by US involves CT scan followed by angiography and, finally, perhaps by US-guided biopsy [10]. Although CT scan and angiography are not sufficiently sensitive for the demonstration of lesions smaller than 2 cm, both modalities are necessary, particularly the latter, in patients under consideration for an operation or hepatic resection. The following discussion summarizes our experience with angiography in the diagnosis of HCC smaller than 5 cm in diameter.

1 Patients and methods

A total of 126 patients having an HCC smaller than 5 cm as the main mass were studied by celiac angiography with adequate angiograms for interpretation along with other diagnostic modalities, which included US, CT, AFP measurement, and, in some, US-guided aspiration/biopsy. The studies were conducted at the National Cancer Center Hospital and the First Department of Medicine, Chiba University Hospital over the past several years. The final diagnosis was a combined one based on these diagnostic procedures and histological examination. There were 109 males and 17 females in the study and their ages ranged from 30 to 70 years. Hepatic resection was performed in 126 patients, and a total of 156 small HCC lesions were eventually identified; 19 patients had two lesions, four had three lesions, and one had four lesions.

Superselective angiography of the common hepatic artery or a more peripheral arterial branch was carried out according to the method of Seldinger except for four patients in whom only the celiac angiography was done. Using 25–40 ml of 76% methylglucamine diatrizoate or amidotrizoate at a speed of 4–7 ml/s, films were made at a rate of 2/s for the first 4 s and at a slower rate thereafter. When deemed necessary, further examination with CT combined with angiography (angio-CT) was carried out [11].

2 Angiographic findings

The arteriograms in the arterial phase were analyzed for tumor vessels, hypervascularity, displacement, encasement, arterioportal shunts, and dilated feeding arteries. In this context, a vessel of irregular caliber that runs an irregular course is taken as a "tumor vessel" and much finer, newly formed vessels resembling a brush

[1] Department of Diagnostic Radiology, National Cancer Center Hospital, Tsukiji, Tokyo, 104 Japan
[2] First Department of Medicine, Chiba University School of Medicine, Inohana, Chiba, 280 Japan

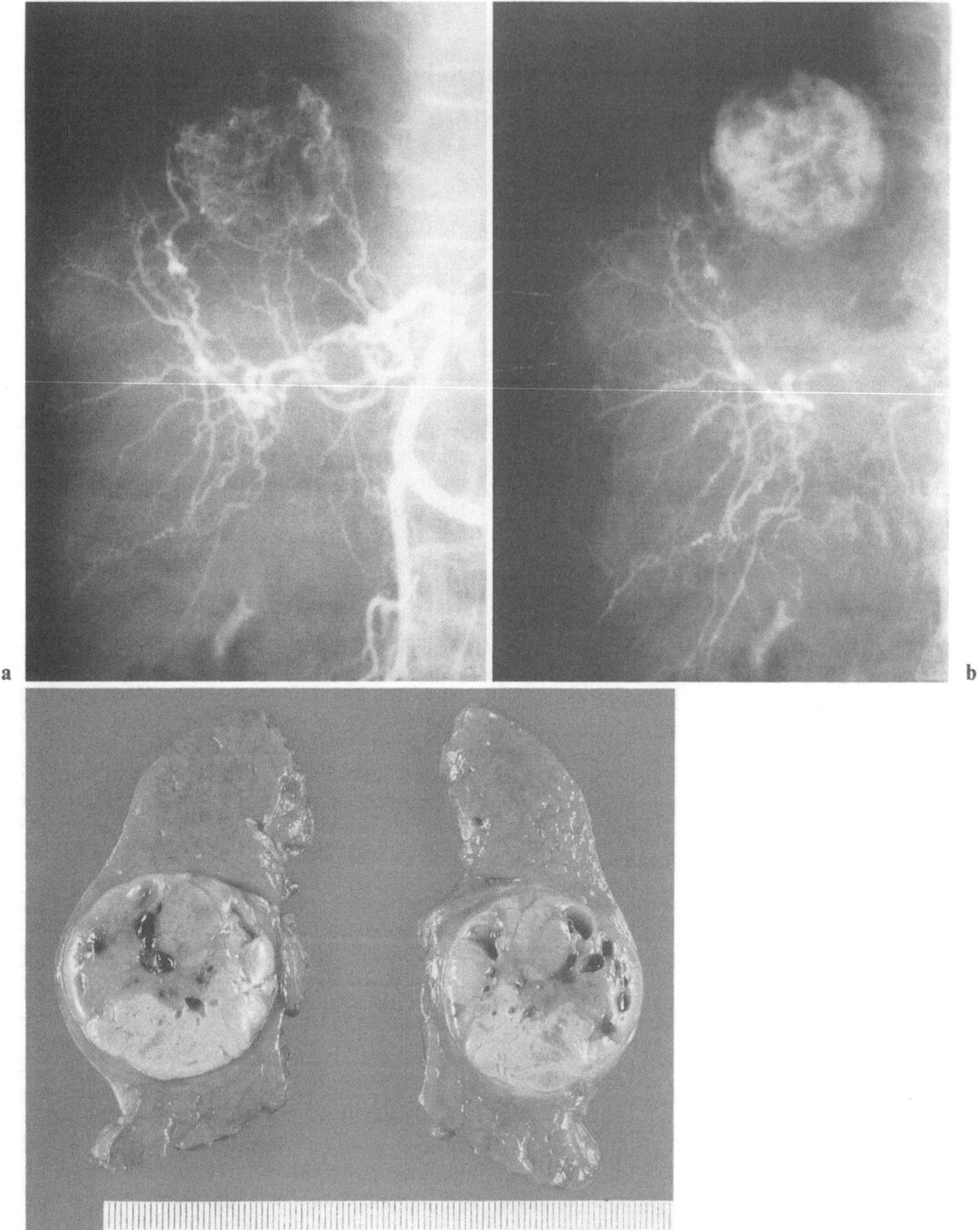

Fig. 21.1a–c. This 69-year-old man with cirrhosis was followed regularly with US and AFP measurement. When US detected a lesion in the anterior superior region, celiac angiography was carried out. **a** In the arterial phase, a large amount of tortuous neovasculature or tumor vessels were seen within the mass; curvilinearly displaced vessels were most likely present on the tumor surface, and there were dilated feeding arteries. **b** In the late arterial phase, there was a stain with a nodular interior containing poorly opacified or nonopacified areas. **c** Cut surface of the resected specimen demonstrating different tissue components of the cancer, large blood spaces or lakes, scattered necrotic areas, and a thick fibrous capsule. The histological diagnosis was Edmondson and Steiner mixed grade II–I. *Scale* in millimeters

are termed "hypervascularity" (Fig. 21.1). An arterial branch that is feeding a mass and is larger than comparable normal arteries is called a "dilated feeding artery." In the venous phase, staining and a translucent rim are discerned. The former is either nodular, nonhomogeneous, or homogeneous. A nonhomogeneous stain is mostly due to necrotic areas within the mass (Fig. 21.1c) [12]. The translucent rim (Fig. 21.2b) has been shown to represent a fibrous capsule or pseudocapsule in advanced HCC by Okuda et al. [13].

Our results were analyzed with respect to tumor size, angiographic findings, and the frequency of undetectability. As shown in Table 21.1, there were 11 lesions smaller than 1 cm, 31 lesions between 1 and 2 cm, 53 lesions 2–3 cm, 35 lesions 3–4 cm, and 26 lesions 4–5 cm in size. Of the 11 lesions smaller than 1 cm, tumor vessels/hypervascularity was seen in only one and tumor stain in five (including the former case). Thus, 6 of 11 cases or lesions (54.5%) showed no angiographic abnormality and were hence undetectable. As tumor size increased, various findings seen in large HCC were also discerned, but staining and tumor vessel/hypervascularity were the most frequent positive findings. Features commonly seen in advanced HCC such as encasement, arterioportal shunt, a translucent rim, and portal tumor thrombosis were only occasionally noted. Displacement and a dilated feeding artery were somewhat intermediate in frequency. The overall frequency of undetectability was 27 of 156 (or 17.3%). Detection failure increased with decreasing tumor size;

there was a singificant correlation between tumor size and detectability by ridit analysis ($p < 0.01$) [14].

3 Grade of cancer cell differentiation and rate of detection

Edmondson and Steiner proposed a four-grade classification [15] that has been used widely in Japan and elsewhere. It has recently been demonstrated in resected specimens that in the early stage of HCC evolution in a cirrhotic liver, cancer cells are generally very well-differentiated and are difficult to distinguish from normal hepatocytes; the lesion looks like a hyperplastic or adenomatous nodule (see Chaps. 13, 16) [16,17]. Therefore, the 19 lesions that were not detected by angiography were compared with 83 lesions detected by angiography among the 102 lesions that could be histologically evaluated [18]; other lesions were not adequate for complete histological assessment. As shown in Table 21.2, more undetected lesions were well-differentiated than detectable ones ($p < 0.01$ by ridit analysis) [14].

Table 21.3 gives the relationship between tumor size and Edmondson and Steiner's grade of cancer cells. Again, there was a definite correlation between the two as analyzed by Kendall's rank correlation method ($p < 0.05$) [19]; 14 of 19 (74%) angiographically undetectable lesions were smaller than 2 cm and were histologically very well-differentiated (Edmondson and Steiner's grade I to II or a mixture of the two grades).

Table 21.1. Relationship between tumor size, angiographic findings, and detection rate in HCC smaller than 5 cm in diameter

Angiographic findings	Tumor size (cm)					Total
	<1	1–2	2–3	3–4	4–5	
Tumor vessel and hypervascularity	1	11	27	26	22	87
	(9.1)	(35.5)	(50.9)	(74.3)	(84.6)	(55.8)
Displacement	0	2	8	20	17	47
Encasement	0	1	2	0	3	6
Arterioportal shunt	0	0	2	3	3	8
Dilated feeding artery	0	2	7	18	22	49
Staining	5	21	46	32	25	129
	(45.5)	(67.7)	(86.8)	(91.4)	(96.2)	(82.7)
Translucent rim	0	0	2	11	7	20
Portal thrombi	0	0	0	0	0	0
Undetected	6	10	7	3	1	27
	(54.5)	(32.3)	(13.2)	(8.6)	(3.8)	(17.3)
Total	11	31	53	35	26	156

Figures in parentheses are percentages

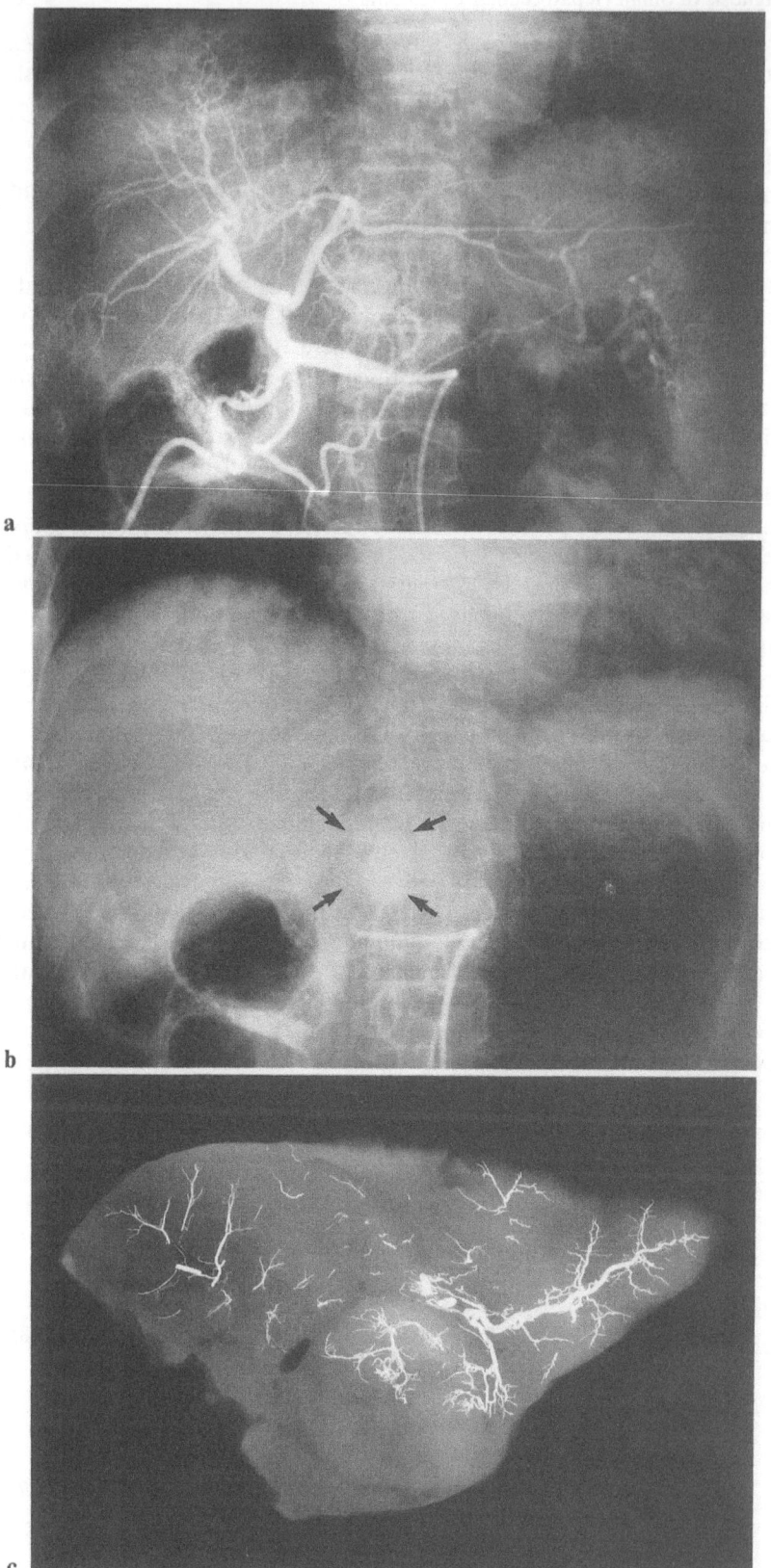

Fig. 21.2a–c. In this 69-year-old female with cirrhosis, a 2.5-cm lesion was found by US. **a, b** Celiac angiography demonstrated a tumor stain with a thin radiolucent rim (*arrows*). **c** The resected specimen had a fibrous capsule, and micro angiography carried out from a feeding artery showed tumor vessels within the mass. It was assumed that the tumor vessels were too thin to be recognized

Table 21.2. Relationship between angiographic detectability of small HCC and grade of cancer cell differentiation according to Edmondson and Steiner

Detectability	Grade of cancer cell differentiation						Total
	I	I–II	II	II–III	III	IV	
Yes	2	4	44	7	26	0	83
No	10	3	5	0	1	0	19
Total	12	7	49	7	27	0	102

Table 21.3. Relationship between tumor size and grade of cancer cell differentiation

Tumor size (cm)	Cancer cell differentiation[a]						Total
	I	I–II	II	II–III	III	IV	
<1	5(4)	1(1)	3(1)	2	0	0	11
1–2	4(3)	3(1)	10(4)	0	5	0	22
2–3	2(2)	1	13(1)	2	9(1)	0	27
3–4	1(1)	1	14	3	8	0	27
4–5	0	0	10	0	5	0	15
Total	12(10)	6(2)	50(6)	7	27(1)	0	102(19)

The predominant grade was used. Figures in parentheses signify HCCs not detected by angiography
[a] According to the classification of Edmondson and Steiner

4 Analysis of angiographically undetectable lesions

There were 19 resected lesions that had not been detected by angiography but were found by other modalities or were found intraoperatively and resected (along with the preoperatively detected lesions). These were analyzed with respect to the cause of failure of detection and the small size of the mass compared with the CT and angio-CT findings. Figure 21.3 shows a case of a 48-year-old man who was suspected of having HCC because of increasing serum AFP levels (from 860 to 1440 ng/ml). Superselective left hepatic arteriography (Fig. 21.3a) failed to show any recognizable changes, yet angio-CT (Fig. 21.3b) in which the catheter tip was placed in the left hepatic artery showed a round nonenhanced mass. The resected specimen demonstrated extensive necrosis affecting about 90% of the cancer tissue (Fig. 21.3c). Altogether, there were four similar lesions.

Figure 21.4 illustrates one patient in whom two lesions were detected by a late-phase dynamic CT [20] but not by angiography, perhaps because of the small difference in the uptake of contrast medium between the cancerous and normal tissues in the early phase of arteriography. In this patient, angio-CT did demonstrate both lesions (Fig. 21.4b). Altogether, there were five such lesions. In 8 of 19 lesions, the cause of failure could not be clearly determined. In two patients, there were two small lesions superimposed in the anterior-posterior projection, producing only one lesion; the smaller lesion was hidden behind the larger one.

5 Small tumor stains

As shown in Table 21.1 and discussed above, tumor stains were the only angiographic changes in most small HCC lesions. It has been our experience that advanced posthepatitic cirrhosis, the commonest variety of cirrhosis in this part of the world, frequently exhibits nodular or reticular stains in late-phase angiograms, particularly following infusion arteriography (see Chap. 16). Such stains create difficulty in differential diagnosis [12]. Some of the stainable cirrhotic nodules may be preneoplastic in view of the difficulty in histological distinction from HCC, and absolute differentiation by imaging alone may be impossible without follow-up studies. For this reason, we analyzed retrospectively the angiograms made in 11 patients with cirrhosis alone who did not develop HCC for at least 1 year after angiography and found stains in nine (72.7%) of

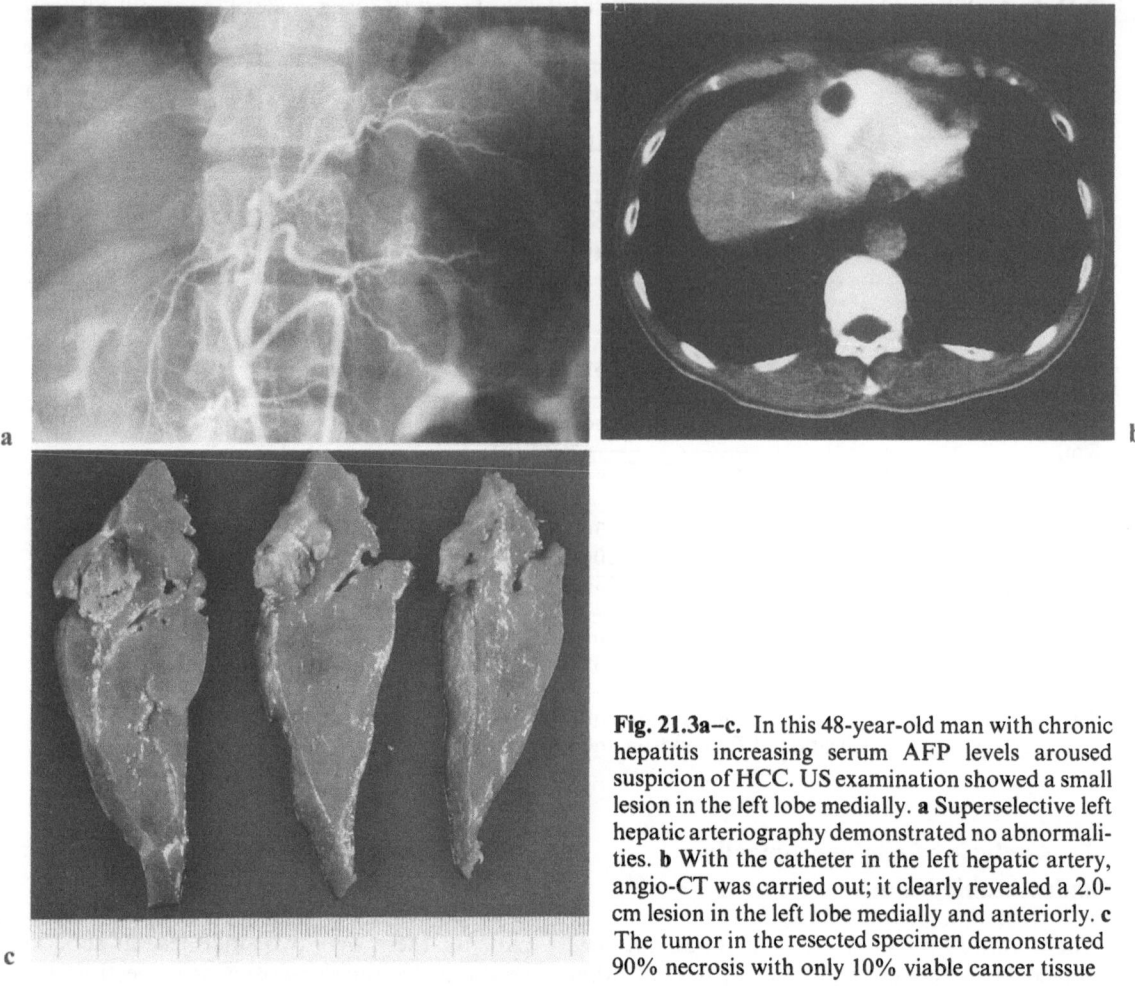

Fig. 21.3a–c. In this 48-year-old man with chronic hepatitis increasing serum AFP levels aroused suspicion of HCC. US examination showed a small lesion in the left lobe medially. **a** Superselective left hepatic arteriography demonstrated no abnormalities. **b** With the catheter in the left hepatic artery, angio-CT was carried out; it clearly revealed a 2.0-cm lesion in the left lobe medially and anteriorly. **c** The tumor in the resected specimen demonstrated 90% necrosis with only 10% viable cancer tissue

Fig. 21.4a–c. This 48-year-old man was followed up with a diagnosis of chronic liver disease and scintigraphy ▶ disclosed a space occupying lesion. Dynamic CT demonstrated two lesions in the late phase. **a** Proper hepatic arteriography failed to detect these lesions. **b** Angio-CT, which followed angiograhy, demonstrated the two lesions as enhanced foci in the same slice. The posterior lesion had a ringlike configuration. **c** The two lesions are seen in the resected specimen after formalin fixation. The posteriorly located lesion showed colloidal degeneration of the interior (*arrow*), the contour of which is almost the same as that in **b**

them. A similar analysis in nine patients with metastatic lesions smaller than 5 cm showed stains in eight (88.9%), and stains were seen in 11 of 12 (91.7%) patients with small benign hemangioma.

Late arteriographic or capillary-phase angiograms made in cirrhotic patients may or may not demonstrate nodular stains, depending upon the amount of contrast medium used, speed of injection, and degree of cirrhotic changes. Figures 21.5–21.7 illustrate the diagnostic features of stains in late-phase angiograms. Figure 21.5 shows several nodular and reticular stains in the late arterial phase in a patient with advanced cirrhosis. Of these stains, the most distinct round one was eventually shown to be HCC; the other stains were regarded as not being due to HCC. However, there was no proof that some of these stains were not preneoplastic or an already well-differentiated HCC. If a round stain is seen in a cirrhotic liver without other nodular stains (Fig. 21.6), the likelihood of this being HCC is high. The stain is usually round in advanced cirrhosis, but it may not be round in a liver without established cirrhosis as in Fig. 21.7.

If the diagnosis is equivocal in such stains, all available imaging modalities should be mobilized, and ultrasound-guided biopsy may become

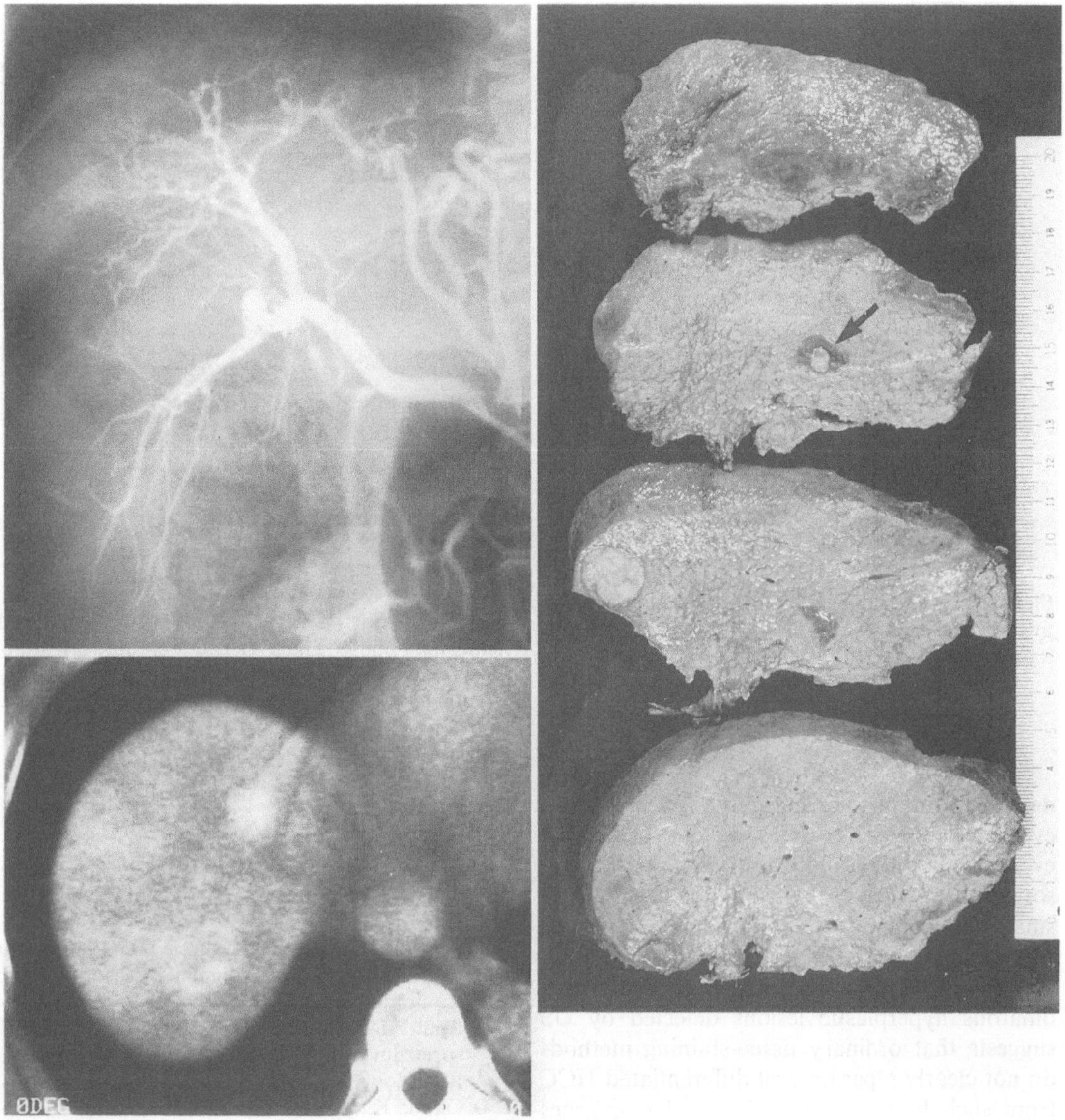

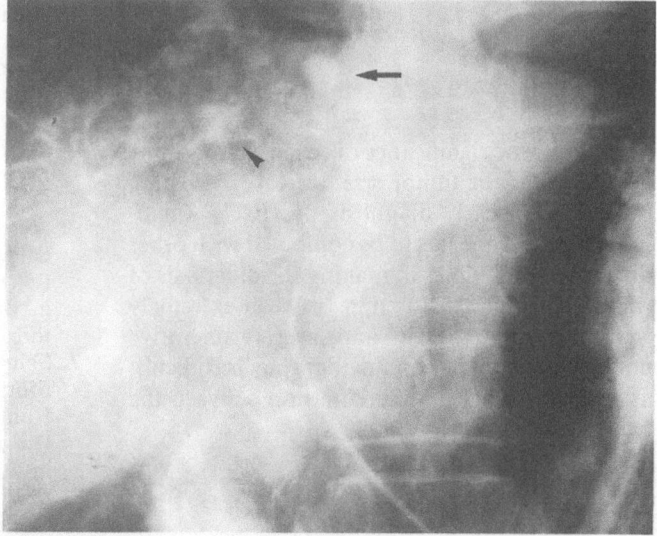

Fig. 21.4a–c

Fig. 21.5. Stains seen in the late arterial phase in a cirrhotic liver. The most distinct stain (*arrow*) is better demarcated from the surrounding tissues than the other ill-defined stain (*arrowhead*) and the smaller nodular and reticular stains. The most clearly demarcated one was subsequently shown to be HCC

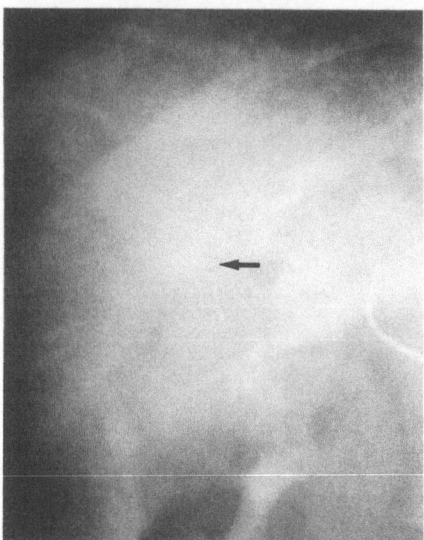

Fig. 21.6. In the sinusoidal phase, a round but indistinct 1.5-cm stain was seen. This was subsequently found to be HCC

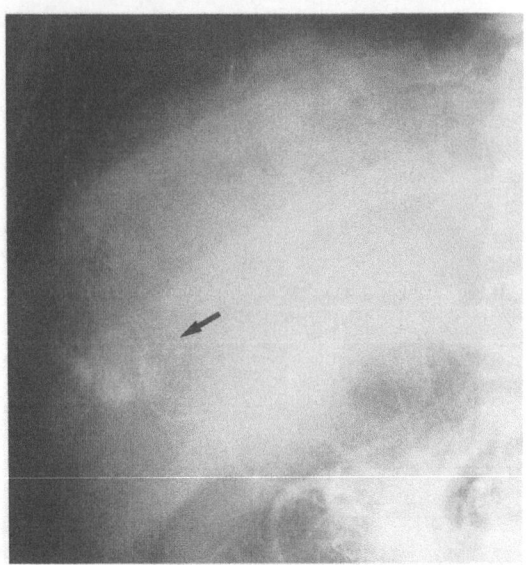

Fig. 21.7. Poorly demarcated but distinct stains in the sinusoidal phase. The liver had a chronic disease but was not cirrhotic. A tumor of this kind of ill-defined stain may grow fast with early intravascular invasion

necessary for histological diagnosis. However, even biopsy may not prove diagnostic. In that event, the lesion should be followed up by ultrasound to see whether it will enlarge or not. Very small hemangiomas are occasionally mistaken for HCC and several such lesions have been resected in Japan. Our recent experience with adenomatous hyperplastic lesions detected by US suggests that ordinary tissue-staining methods do not clearly separate well-differentiated HCC from such lesions. The staining of oncogenes may prove diagnostic in equivocal lesions in the future.

6 Summary

The diagnostic significance of celiac angiography is reduced as the tumor size decreases, creating difficulties in early diagnosis of HCC. Angiography, therefore, has to be combined with other diagnostic modalities in making the diagnosis of small HCC. The distinction between extremely well-differentiated HCC and large regenerative nodules that stain upon angiography is difficult, as is the histological differentiation between the two.

References

1. Boijsen E, Abrams HL (1965) Roentgenologic diagnosis of primary carcinoma of the liver. Acta Radiol (Diag) 3: 257–277
2. Nebesar RA, Pollard JJ, Stone DL (1966) Angiographic diagnosis of malignant disease of the liver. Radiology 86: 284–292
3. Reuter ST, Redman HC, Siders DB (1970) The spectrum of angiographic findings in hepatoma. Radiology 94: 89–94
4. Okuda K, Obata H, Jinnouchi S, Kubo Y, Nagasaki Y, Shimokawa Y, Nakajima Y, Musha H, Sakamoto K, Kojiro M, Nakashima T (1977) Angiographic assessment of gross anatomy of hepatocellular carcinoma: comparison of celiac angiograms and liver pathology in 100 cases. Radiology 123: 21–29
5. Okuda K, Iio M (1976) Radiological aspects of the liver and biliary tract. X-ray and radioisotope diagnosis. Year Book, Chicago
6. Okuda K, Musha H, Yoshida T, Kanda Y, Jinnouchi S, Kubo Y, Shimokawa Y, Kojiro M, Sakamoto K, Nakashima T (1975) Demonstration of growing casts of hepatocellular carcinoma in the portal vein by celiac angiography: the thread and streaks sign. Radiology 117: 303–309
7. Shinagawa T, Ohto M, Kimura K, Tsunetomi S, Morita M, Saisho H, Tsuchiya Y, Saotome N, Karasawa E, Miki M, Ueno T, Okuda K (1984) Diagnosis and clinical features of small hepatocellular carcinoma with emphasis on the utility of real-time ultrasonography. A study in 51 patients. Gastroenterology 86: 495–502

8. Chen DS, Shen JC, Sung JL, Sheu JC, Lai MY, How SW, Hsu HC, Lee CS, Wei TC (1983) Small hepatocellular carcinoma—a clinicopathological study in thirteen patients. Gastroenterology 83: 1109–1119

9. Okazaki N, Yosida T, Yoshino M, Matue H (1984) Screening of patients with chronic liver disease for hepatocellular carcinoma by ultrasonography. Clin Oncol 10: 241–246

10. Ohto M, Karasawa E, Tsuchiya Y, Kimura K, Saisho H, Ono T, Okuda K (1980) Ultrasonically guided percutaneous contrast medium injection and aspiration biopsy using a real-time puncture transducer. Radiology 136: 171–176

11. Prando A, Wallace S, Bernardino ME, Lindell MM Jr (1979) Computed tomographic arteriography of the liver. Radiology 130: 697–689

12. Sumida M, Ohto M, Ebara M, Kimura K, Okuda K, Hirooka N (1986) Accuracy of angiography in the diagnosis of small hepatocellular carcinoma. Am J Roentgenol 147: 531–536

13. Okuda K, Musha H, Nakajima Y, Kubo Y, Shimokawa Y, Nagasaki Y, Jinnouchi S, Obata H, Hisamitsu T, Okazaki N, Kojiro M, Sakamoto K, Nakashima T (1977) Clinicopathologic features of encapsulated hepatocellular carcinoma. A study of 26 cases. Cancer 40:1240–1245

14. Bross IDJ (1958) How to use ridit analysis. Biometrics 14: 18–38

15. Edmondson HA, Steiner PE (1954) Primary carcinoma of the liver. A study of 100 cases among 48,900 necropsies. Cancer 7: 462–503

16. Arakawa M, Sugihara S, Kenmochi K, Kage M, Nakashima T, Nakayama T, Tashiro S, Hiraoka H, Suenaga M, Okuda K (1986) Small mass lesions in cirrhosis: transition from benign adenomatous hyperplasia to hepatocellular carcinoma? J Gastroenterol Hepatol 1: 3–14

17. Arakawa M, Kage M, Sugihara S, Nakashima T, Suenaga M, Okuda K (1986) Emergence of malignant lesions within an adenomatous hyperplastic nodule in a cirrhotic liver. Observations in five cases. Gastroenterology 91: 198–208

18. Takayasu K, Shima Y, Muramatsu Y, Goto H, Moriyama N, Yamada T, Makuuchi M, Yamasaki S, Hasegawa H, Okazaki N, Hirohasi S, Kishi K (1986) Angiography of small hepatocellular carcinoma: analysis of 105 resected tumors. Am J Roentgenol 147: 525–529

19. Kendall MG (1962) Rank correlation methods, 3rd edn. Griffin, London

20. Young SW, Turner RJ, Castellino RA (1980) A strategy for the contrast enhancement of malignant tumors using dynamic computed tomography and intravascular pharmacokinetics. Radiology 137: 137–147

Chapter 22
Imaging Diagnosis with Computed Tomography

Yuji Itai[1]

1 General considerations

The image obtained by X-ray computed tomography (CT) is a computer-assisted reconstruction of averaged X-ray attenuation in the individual pixel of the matrix. Therefore, CT reflects essentially the same information as the conventional X-ray photograph. The advantage and characteristics of CT are seen in better contrast resolution in a true tomogram. With the conventional film-screen system, a normal organ and its neoplasm show a similar X-ray attenuation and cannot be distinguished without the aid of contrast material. CT is capable of distinguishing a 0.5% difference in contrast expressed in Hounsfield units or numbers (which are set at 0 for water and −1000 for air), whereas the conventional film-screen system can barely distinguish ascites from the liver (about 6% contrast).

CT is represented as a true tomogram of a given breadth (i.e., slice thickness, 1.5–10 mm) and its cut plane is usually vertical to the body axis because of a limited diameter of the gantry and X-ray power. The matrix size of CT ranges from 256 to 512 and the spatial resolution becomes 1–2 mm. The scanning time takes 1–10 s with current instruments.

The CT image is displayed by setting an arbitrary gray scale (window width and window level) to the calculated attenuation number (Hounsfield unit). When subtle contrasts between two objects are to be distinguished, a narrow window width is selected. However, any objects having densities scaled out from both ends of the window width are shown as the same black or white shadow. The window level is set at an intermediate value between those of the objects being studied.

The interpretation of a CT scan depends on the recognition of different areas of gray-scale density or the change in absolute Hounsfield number. However, strictly speaking, the Hounsfield number itself is not an absolute value but is rather a relative one that varies with the instrument and the location of the area being scanned.

Many kinds of artifacts cause abnormal density areas; for example, the motion of a markedly high- or low-attenuation subject during scanning gives rise to a radiating high- and low-density zone (streaking artifact), and areas adjacent to a high-density zone occasionally appear as a false hypodense area (undershooting). The types and frequency of artifacts are different from one instrument to another.

2 Plain CT

On plain CT (i.e., without use of contrast material), the normal liver is homogeneous, except for large vessels which are shown as hypodense, round, zonal, or arborescent areas. The density of the liver is almost the same as that of the spleen unless the former has fatty infiltration or iron deposition.

A hepatic neoplasm almost always appears as a hypodense mass, occasionally as an isodense mass, and rarely as a hyperdense mass on plain CT (Fig. 22.1) [1, 2]. Tumors having attenuation values very similar to those of the surrounding liver cannot be recognized, irrespective of their size (limitation of contrast resolution). Even though the contrast of a mass is high, it may not be detected if it is small, since the calculated attenuation number based on the relative volumes of the neoplasm and liver in the individual voxel is below the contrast resolution of the instrument (partial volume phenomenon). For the detection of such an isodense mass, contrast material is given in various ways as described below.

[1] Department of Radiology, University of Tokyo Hospital, Hongo, Bunkyo-bu, Tokyo, 113 Japan

Most hepatic neoplasms appear as hypodense masses whose density is usually between that of the blood and liver. Some tumors have a density as low as but rarely below that of water [3]. Liquefaction necrosis or fatty metamorphosis is the main reason for marked hypodensity in some tumors. Hepatic tumors containing a fat component (lipoma, angiolipoma, hamartoma, etc.) also show hypodensity depending upon the content of fat. A liver abscess occasionally shows air in the mass, but air in a neoplasm is extremely rare except after aggressive anticancer treatment, such as transcatheter arterial embolization and ligation of the hepatic artery [4].

Diffuse hyperdensity is noted in bleeding tumors (adenoma and HCC), HCC, calcified masses (metastatic tumor), and tumors in a fatty liver. A localized hyperdensity in a tumor is associated with calcification and is mainly seen in metastatic tumors (especially colorectal cancer) that have been successfully treated or in long-standing tumors of any kind (Fig. 22.1).

3 Contrast enhancement

A contrast agent is administered for the following purposes: (1) better visualization of a hepatic mass, (2) detection of an isodense mass, and (3) characterization of the mass. The contrast agent (water-soluble iodine compound used for urography), when intravenously administered, is first located in the vascular space and then diffuses into the interstitial space until an equilibrium between the two spaces is attained (around 5 min) [5]. The contrast agent is excreted from the kidney and after equilibrium it comes back from the interstitial space in accordance with the decrease in concentration in the vascular space. The interstitial space in the entire human body is four times as large as the vascular space.

Two additional factors should be taken into consideration in contrast enhancement in the liver—the dual blood supply to the liver and hepatic excretion of the contrast agent [6, 7]. The blood supply to the liver is from both the hepatic artery and the portal vein; the ratio of portal to arterial blood is about 4. This ratio is most important in dynamic studies of hepatic tumors. As much as 1% of the urographic contrast agent is also excreted from the liver in patients with normal renal function and this phenomenon has to be considered in the interpretation of late postcontrast scans using a large volume of contrast agent [8].

A number of methods for contrast enhancement have been reported. The important methods are discussed briefly below.

3.1 Drip infusion

This method is simple; however, the long time necessary for administration results in the contrast agent being supplied through both the artery and vein; thus, the low concentration of contrast agent in the vascular space results in failure to demonstrate the vascularity of the tumor or to evaluate the dynamics of the contrast agent, and it does not impart sufficient contrast to the tumor. Rapid drip infusion may delineate small intrahepatic vessels when combined with a bolus injection [9].

3.2 Bolus enhancement and dynamic study

With a single administration of the contrast agent (bolus enhancement), CT can detect the vascularity of a hepatic tumor, as is clearly demonstrated in angiography. With current instruments, it is possible to scan several to 30 slices in sequence, even in a breath-holding period (single slice dynamic study). Early scans mainly reflect the arterial phase while later ones demonstrate the portal phase of angiography. However, considering the time required for injection and the long circulation pathway, terms such as "arterial-dominant" and "portal-dominant" phases are more appropriate (Fig. 22.2) [7].

Hypervascular tumors become hyperdense in the arterial-dominant phase but usually become iso- or hypodense after the portal-dominant phase because of the massive blood supply by the portal vein to the normal liver; it is worth remembering that hepatic tumors are almost always supplied by the hepatic artery alone and that the portal supply is four times that of the arterial supply in a normal liver. Some hypervascular tumors remain hyperdense after the portal-dominant phase (prolonged enhancement). Hypovascular tumors show negative enhancement and some tumors disclose an enhancement similar to that of the liver [10]. Consideration of both the time-density curve and the location of a highly enhanced area in the mass is useful in differential diagnosis [7]. Recently, the mechanisms of enhancement after the arterial-dominant phase (delayed enhancement) have been clarified. One mechanism is caused by blood draining the tumor (capsule, septa) while the other is induced by the accumulation of contrast agent in a large interstitial space (mainly fibrotic area).

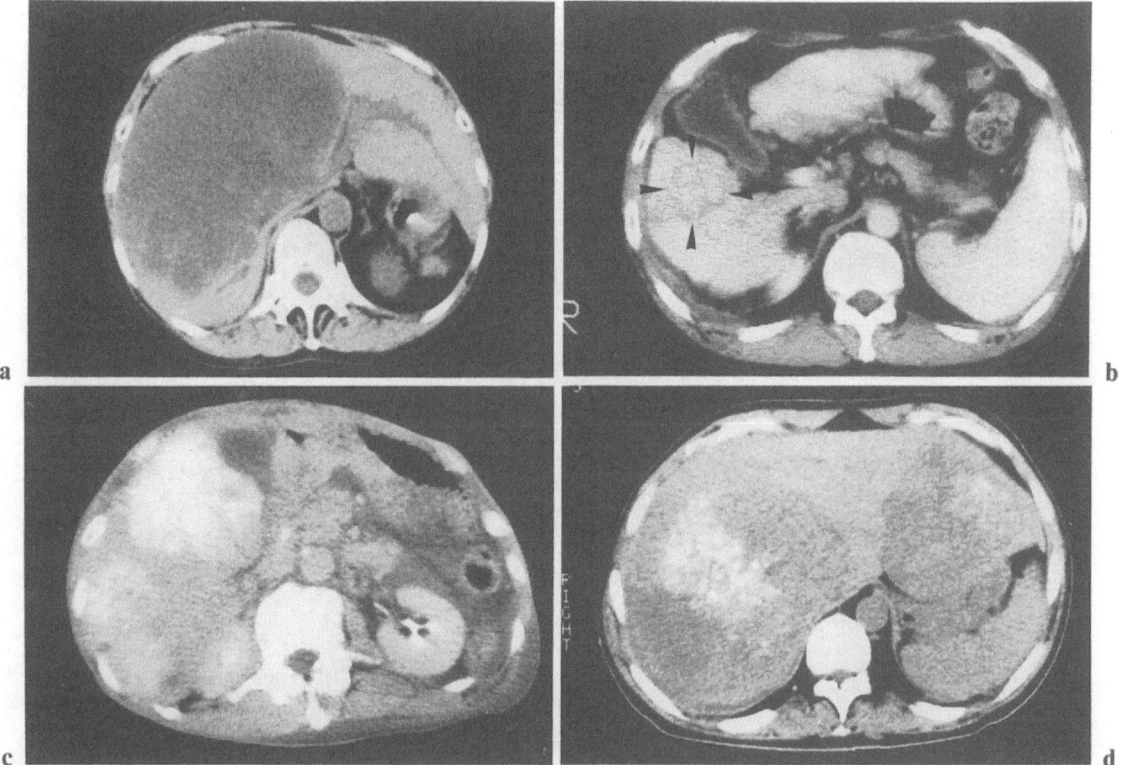

Fig. 22.1a–d. Density of tumor. **a** Markedly low (colonic cancer). **b** Isodense (HCC with a capsule, *arrowheads*). **c** Hyperdense (colonic cancer, due to calcification). **d** Mixed low and high densities (colonic cancer, due to calcification). See also Fig. 22.7a

3.3 CT arteriography

The arterial route is ideal for administration of contrast agent into a short path in high concentrations (per dose) [11]. The combination of CT and an angiographic technique is called CT arteriography. There are two kinds of CT arteriography depending upon the vessel through which the contrast agent enters the liver—arterial, through the hepatic artery (the catheter being inserted in the celiac artery or closer to the liver), and portal, through the portal vein (the catheter being introduced into the superior mesenteric artery) [12].

3.3.1 Arterial CT angiography

Arterial CT angiography provides better contrast resolution and a better tomogram than angiography (Fig. 22.3); a hypervascular tumor as small as 5 mm in diameter may be detected. When the catheter is introduced up to the hepatic artery or further toward the liver, Ethiodol (ethylester of poppy seed oil fatty acid, 38% iodine by weight) can be injected as an embolus that is trapped mainly in a hypervascular hepatic tumor

(Ethiodol CT, Fig. 22.4) [13]. On a scan made 1–4 weeks later, a hypervascular tumor that is a few millimeters in diameter can be demonstrated.

3.3.2 Portal CT angiography

With portal CT angiography, any hepatic tumor is demonstrated as a hypodense mass irrespective of vascularity, and areas of occluded vein (organic or functional) are also shown as wedge-shaped hypodense areas. This method can reveal lesions as small as 5 mm and is useful in detecting hypovascular tumors.

3.4 Miscellaneous

Contrast agent taken up by the reticuloendothelial system or excreted into normal liver tissue (cholangiographic agent or urographic agent at a very late phase, e.g., after 4 h) is useful for demonstrating hepatic tumors as hypodense areas [8]. Thus far, only EOE-13 has been clinically used as a reticuloendothelial contrast agent; 1-cm lesions can be detected by this technique irrespective of tumor vascularity [14].

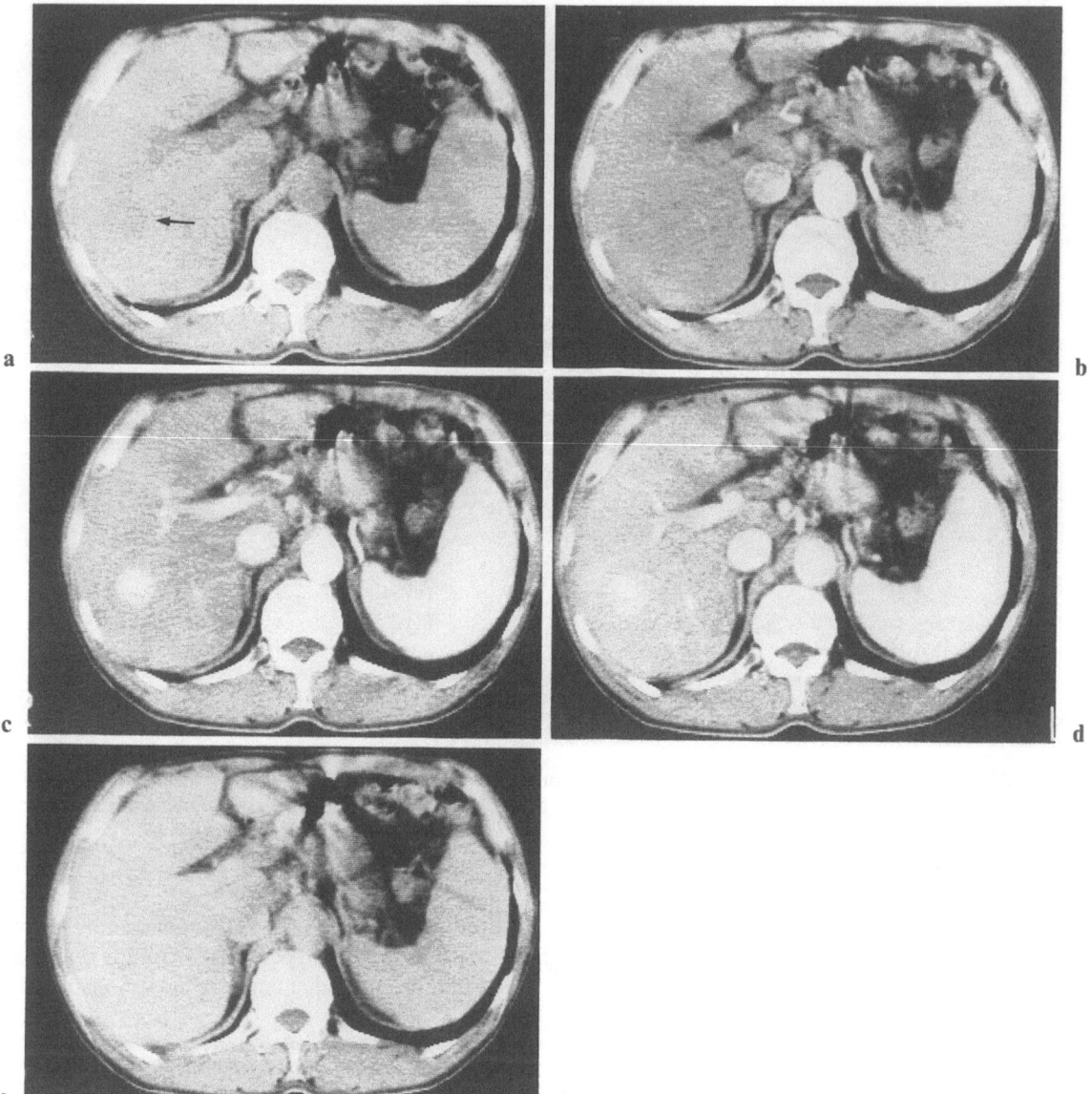

Fig. 22.2a–e. Dynamic study (HCC). **a** Plain; **b–e** 10, 25, 40 s and 3 min, respectively, after bolus injection of contrast enhancement. **a** A hypodense mass (*arrow*) is noted on plain CT. **b** After bolus enhancement, it disappears in an early phase (b) and **c** shows a homogeneous, markedly high density, **d** which rapidly decreases. **e** Three minutes later, the tumor becomes isodense. Note the changes in the densities of the aorta, hepatic artery, portal vein, and inferior vena cava

4 Primary liver cancer

4.1 Hepatocellular carcinoma

Hepatocellular carcinoma (HCC) is divided into localized (nodular and massive) and diffuse types on CT. Localized HCC usually appears as a slightly tŏ moderately hypodense mass and occasionally as an isodense mass on plain CT [1, 2]. It rarely shows hyperdensity in comparison with the surrounding liver or even the spleen. In addi-

tion, findings of liver cirrhosis are often noted, such as disproportionate sizes of individual segments (frequently an enlarged lateral segment and caudate lobe as well as an atrophic right lobe), a generally small size of the liver, prominent fissures and hilus, nodularity of the hepatic surface or even in the parenchyma, splenomegaly, and collateral veins caused by portal hypertension (thickening of the esophagocardiac wall, splenoretroperitoneal or splenorenal shunt, para-

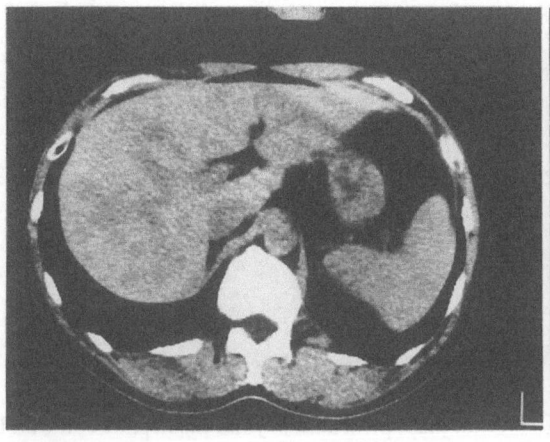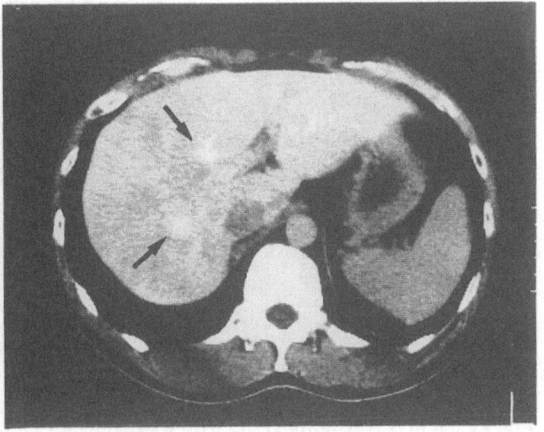

Fig. 22.3a, b. Arterial CT angiography (HCC). **a** Plain. Several hypodense areas are noted on precontrast CT. **b** Fifteen seconds after bolus injection of contrast agent through the catheter inserted into the proper hepatic artery, two masses (*arrow*) show marked enhancement. There is no enhancement in the spleen

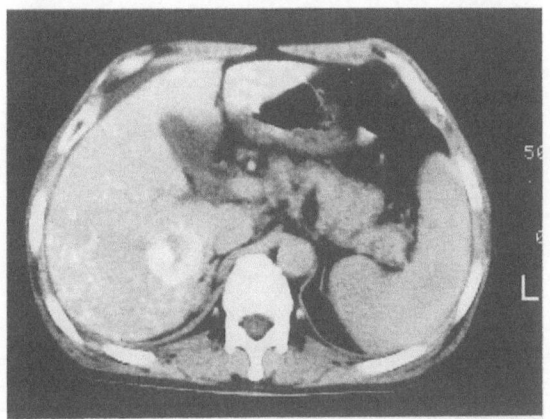

Fig. 22.4. Ethiodol CT (HCC). A well-defined high-density mass as well as innumerable tiny hyperdense nodules are seen. The smallest one is about 3 mm in diameter

umbilical vein, engorged coronary, azygos and hemiazygos veins, etc.). Protrusion from the hepatic contour, a mosaic internal pattern (tumor-in-tumor appearance), and a thin hypodense ring (capsule) are quite characteristic of HCC (Fig. 22.5, 22.6) [2, 7].

On dynamic CT, transient high attenuation occurs in about three-fourths of the patients. It may be diffuse, irregular (mosaic pattern), or dotted (Fig. 22.2, 22.7). An arterioportal shunt and a tumor thrombus in the portal vein or the inferior vena cava are not infrequently noted [15]. An arterioportal shunt appears as early enhancement of the portal vein, showing the same time-density curve as that of the aorta, prolonged enhancement of the portal vein, an abnormally dilated portal vein often surrounded by irregularly enhanced areas (if the shunt is in a large vessel), and as a wedge-shaped area of enhancement distal to the tumor (if it is in a small vessel)

(Fig. 22.7) [16, 17]. Involvement of a main or lobar portal vein is suggested by its hypodensity and enlargement, increased periportal arterial vascularization surrounding the hypodense intraluminal region, nonvisualization of the lobar portal vein, arterioportal shunting, and/or differences in lobar attenuation [15].

A fibrous capsule of HCC appears as a thin hypodense ring surrounding an isodense or subtle hypodense mass and it changes to a hyperdense rim in the portal-dominant phase in dynamic CT following diffuse enhancement of the tumor in the arterial-dominant phase. The capsule may remain hyperdense for up to several minutes (Figs. 22.5, 22.7). According to Otsuji et al. [18], a capsule can be detected in 7% of patients on plain CT alone, 58% on postcontrast CT alone, and 35% on both plain and postcontrast scan [18].

On postcontrast CT, HCC of a localized type almost always becomes hypodense (except for the

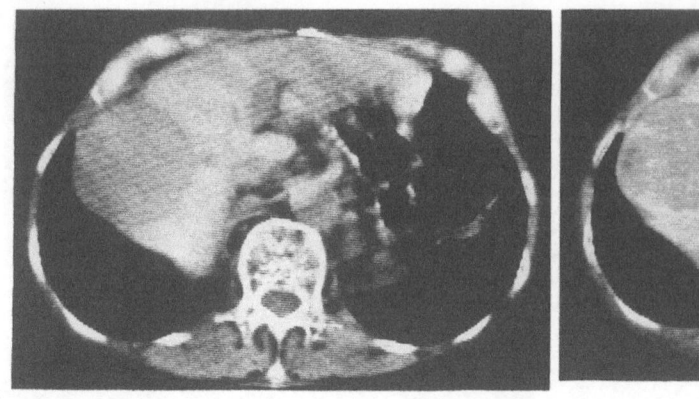
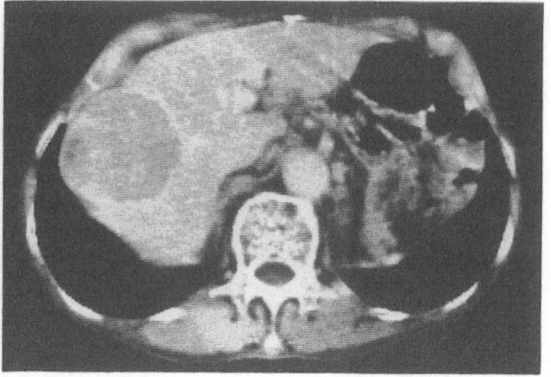

Fig. 22.5a, b. Protruding HCC with a capsule. **a** Plain. A round mass protrudes beyond the hepatic contour. **b** Postcontrast. A hypodense ring surrounding the mass changes to a hyperdense ring on postcontrast CT. This ring corresponds to the capsule of HCC

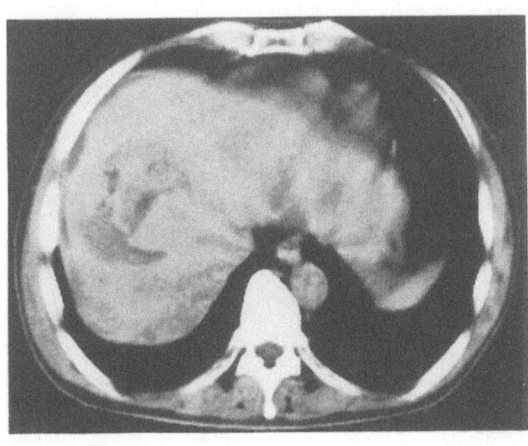

Fig. 22.6. Mosaic pattern. A round mass consists of complex components of varying densities

capsule and/or septa). Large lesions are accompanied by internal lower density areas, which are either solitary and asteroid or multiple and rounded (Fig. 22.7).

HCC of the diffuse type is difficult to diagnose with certainty. Often, diffuse vague hypodense areas are difficult to distinguish from other states such as chronic liver damage with irregular fatty infiltration and artifacts unless an arterioportal shunt and/or tumor thrombus is present.

4.2 Cholangiocellular cancinoma

Cholangiocellular carcinoma (CCC) is far less frequent than HCC in the Far East, and only a small number of cases have thus far been reported in the CT literature. The CT findings are usually nonspecific and variable. Our experience includes a well-defined cystic mass with internal papillary projections, a markedly hypodense mass, localized intrahepatic biliary dilatation without a definite mass lesion, and a nonspecific mass (Fig. 22.8)

[19]. Recently, delayed enhancement in the central fibrotic area has been encountered (Fig. 22.9), which is also difficult to differentiate from a solitary metastatic cancer.

5 Metastatic liver cancer

Metastatic tumors are charcterized by multiple lesions (Fig. 22.10), whereas primary liver cancer is more often solitary or only a few lesions are present. This generalization, however, does not always hold true. There are a number of patients with a solitary metastasis or only a few metastases, while many patients with HCC may have innumerable lesions as a result of intrahepatic metastatic spread. Metastatic tumors tend to have a large, central necrotic area, which results in a "doughnut-shaped" appearance on CT. Some metastases have marked and diffuse necroses and resemble a hepatic cyst (necrotic metastasis; Fig. 22.1a) [2]. Calcifications are

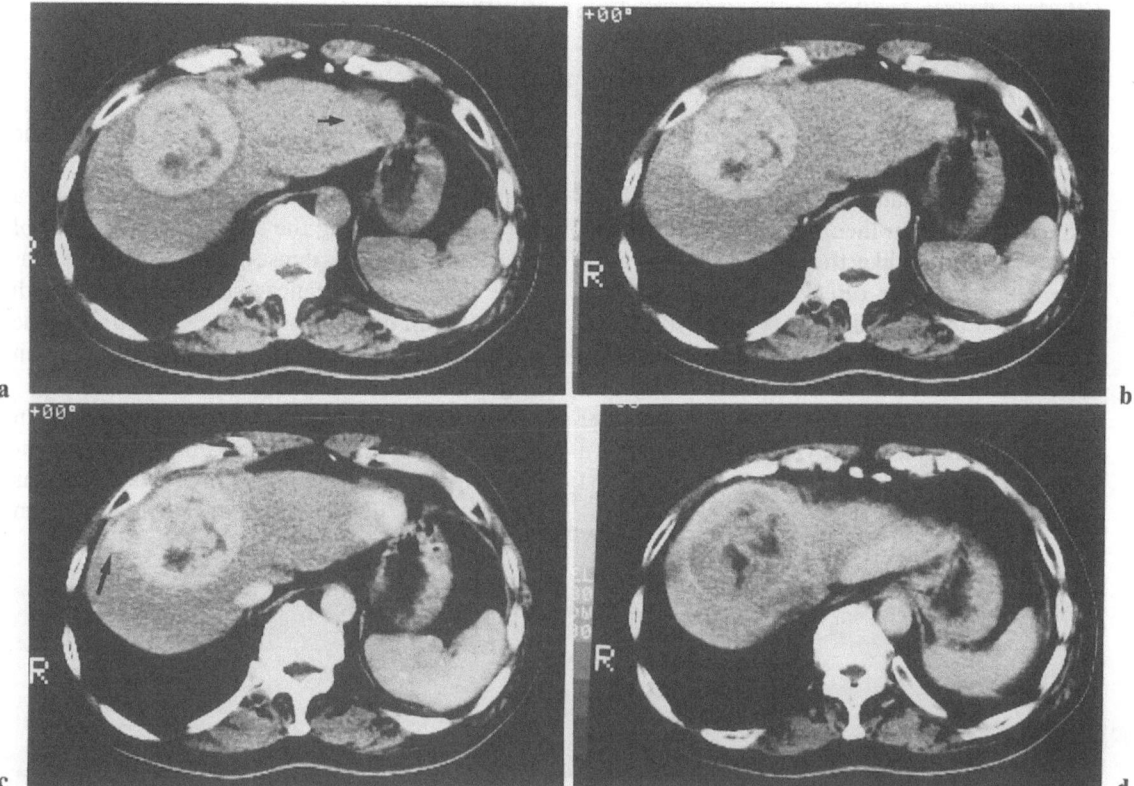

Fig. 22.7a–d. Dynamic study of multiple HCC with an arterioportal shunt. **a** Plain; **b–d** 10, 35 s and 6 min, respectively, after bolus enhancement. **a** There are a round hyperdense mass and a hypodense area (*arrow*). **b, c** After bolus injection, the small mass shows diffuse enhancement, but it is not clear on this display whether the large on has been enhanced. However, a wedge-shaped enhancement (*arrow*) is noted lateral to the hyperdense mass (**b, c** arterioportal shunt). **d** Note also the change in the density of thin ring surrounding the large tumor (capsule)

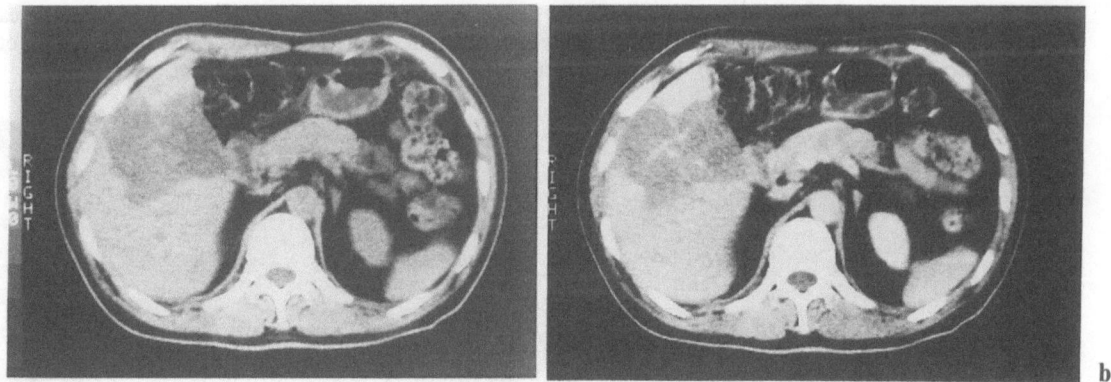

Fig. 22.8a, b. Cholangiocellular carcinoma. **a** Plain. A well-defined, rhomboid hypodense mass is shown. **b** After contrast enhancement, vessel-like structures are clearly demonstrated

occasionally noted within any kind of metastatic tumor (especially colorectal cancer; see Fig. 22.1c, d).

On dynamic CT, the most prevalent pattern of metastatic tumor is a transient, peripheral ring-like enhancement, which is much thicker and more irregular than the capsule of HCC [2]. Some hypervascular metastatic tumors have diffuse enhancement like that of HCC. However, central necroses are often round and large in comparison to those of HCC (Fig. 22.10).

Differentiation of a solitary metastasis from HCC is not difficult if the former is large, since it often has a nodular margin, shows an irregular ringlike enhancement on dynamic CT, and has a delayed central enhancement on postconstrast CT (Fig. 22.11) [2, 6, 7].

6 Benign liver tumor

6.1 Cavernous hemangioma

Cavernous hemangioma has such characteristic findings on dynamic CT that no angiography is required in the diagnosis of the typical case; a hepatic mass having the same density as that of the blood represents dense accumulations of contrast material in or near the periphery which spread in all directions as time elapses [20]. The hyperdensity of the mass lasts more than 3 min in larger lesions (Fig. 22.12).

However, some hemangiomas less than 3 cm in diameter show diffuse enhancement which continues for more than 2 min. Much smaller lesions demonstrate absolute enhancement of even

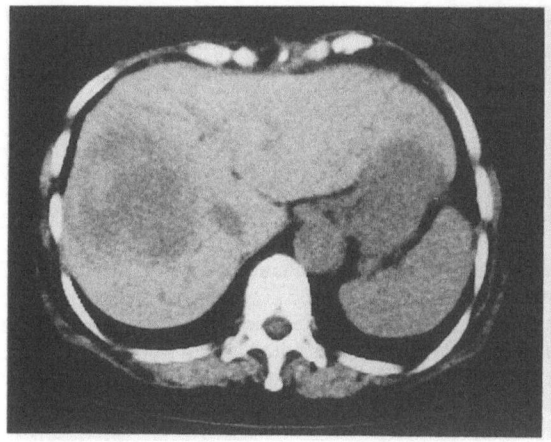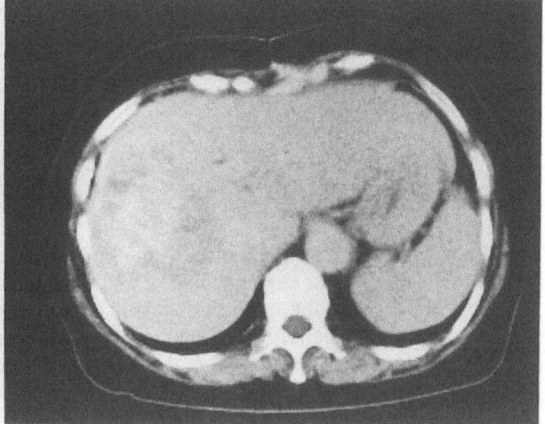

Fig. 22.9a, b. Cholangiocellular carcinoma. **a** Plain. **b** Three minutes after bolus enhancement. The central area of this hypodense mass reveals much delayed but clear enhancement on postcontrast CT. This region did not show hyperdensity in the early phase of the dynamic study

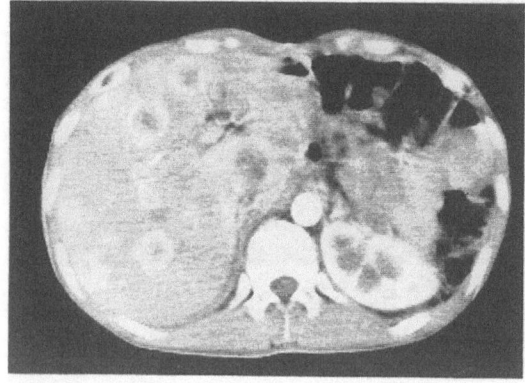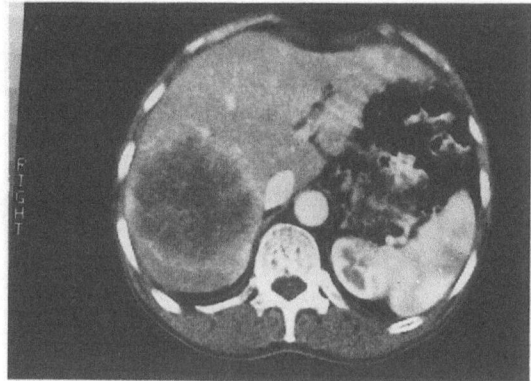

Fig. 22.10. Ring enhancement of metastatic liver cancer (gastric cancer). There are many masses showing prominent rings or diffuse enhancement. Ring enhancement is predominantly noted in patients with metastatic liver cancer

Fig. 22.11. Solitary metastatic tumor (gastric cancer). A solitary mass with a nodular margin shows irregular ring enhancement. Both findings are quite characteristic of metastatic liver cancer

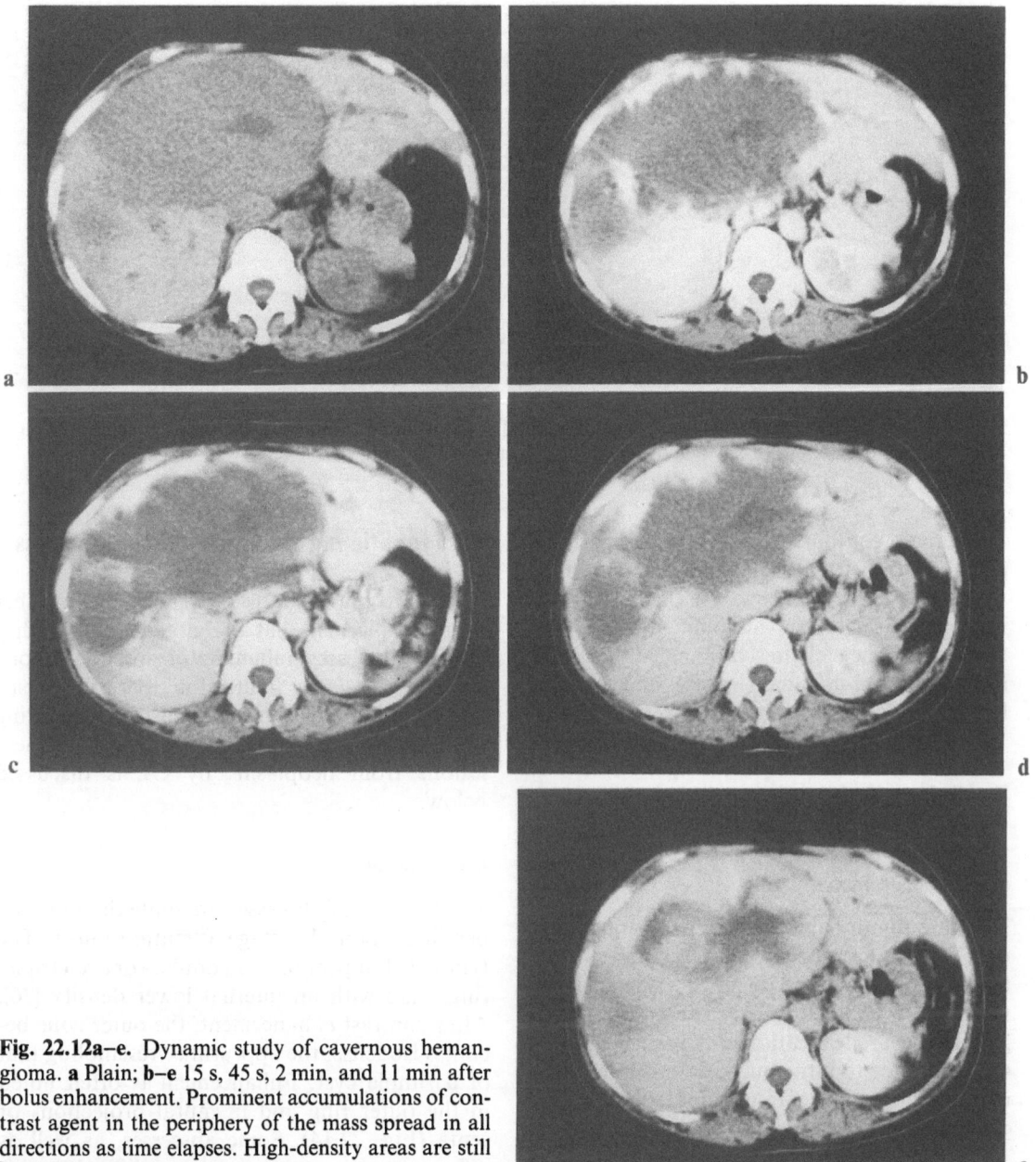

Fig. 22.12a–e. Dynamic study of cavernous hemangioma. **a** Plain; **b–e** 15 s, 45 s, 2 min, and 11 min after bolus enhancement. Prominent accumulations of contrast agent in the periphery of the mass spread in all directions as time elapses. High-density areas are still noted on late postcontrast scans

shorter duration, but this may still be longer than the enhancement of other hypervascular tumors, such as HCC. Almost all cavernous hemangiomas can be correctly diagnosed by dynamic CT as long as the patient can hold his breath repetitively at the same degree of inspiration [21]. Unusually, there are avascular (completely degenerated) or hypovascular hemangiomas which cannot be diagnosed by intravenous dynamic study. Angiosarcoma, hemangioendothelioma, and peliosis hepatis may show the same dynamic pattern; fortunately, they are extremely uncommon.

6.2 Adenoma

Adenoma is difficult to distinguish from well-differentiated HCC, both pathologically and radiologically [22]. Adenoma should be suspected when an HCC-like tumor is seen in a woman who has been taking contraceptive pills and who has no chronic liver disease.

6.3 Focal nodular hyperplasia

Focal nodular hyperplasia (FNH) is also difficult to differentiate from HCC. It may protrude from

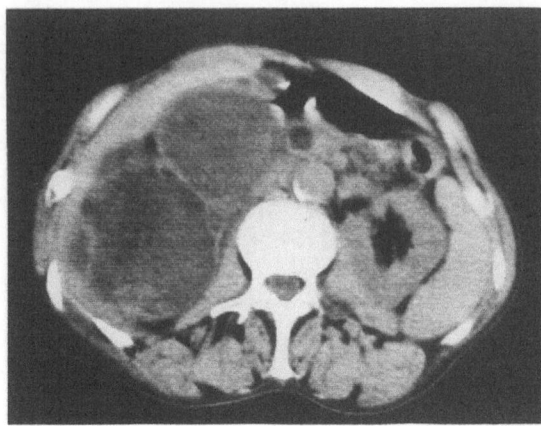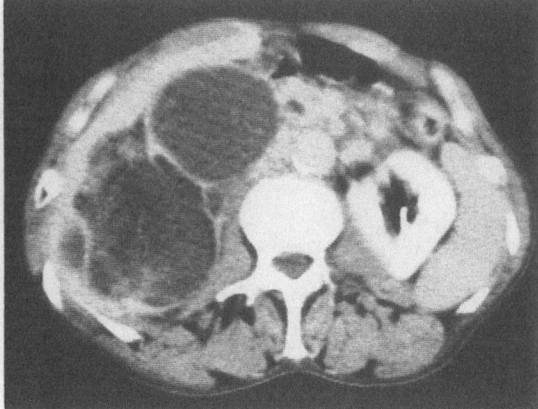

Fig. 22.13a, b. Biliary cystadenocarcinoma. **a** Plain. **b** Postcontrast. A cystic mass shaped like a figure of eight discloses enhancement in its septa and papillary projections

the hepatic contour, be isodense on plain CT, and show transient, diffuse enhancement on dynamic CT [23]. A stellate scar in the center of the mass is characteristic, although it is not seen frequently. The stellate scar remains hypodense in the arterial-dominant phase and becomes hyperdense on later scans.

7 Other tumors

7.1 Biliary cystadenoma and cystadenocarcinoma

This rare tumor has a characteristic appearance on CT. It is a cystic neoplasm associated with mural projections and septa of varying degree which show marked enhancement (Fig. 22.13) [19]. However, delineation of the thin septum by CT is inferior to ultrasound; cystadenoma having radiating, thin septa may look like a simple cyst on plain CT.

7.2 Epithelioid hemangioendothelioma

This rare tumor also shows characteristic CT features; it is a bizarre-shaped hypodense mass localized in the periphery in contact with the hepatic contour over a long distance, has many dense calcification foci throughout the lesion, and becomes isodense on postcontrast scans [24].

7.3 Malignant lymphoma

Primary lymphoma of the liver is rare; secondary involvement occurs in 50%–60% of cases; CT can detect hepatic involvement in only 4% [25]. A liver-specific contrast agent is necessary to raise detectability in this disease.

8 Hepatic masses other than neoplasms

There are many kinds of hepatic mass (other than neoplasms) that are noted on CT; they include abscesses, inflammatory pseudotumors, hematomas, fatty infiltration, parasitic cysts, bilomas, adenomatous hyperplasia, regenerating nodules, etc. The differential diagnosis of these lesions from neoplasms by CT is discussed below.

8.1 Abscess

The features of abscesses are quite different depending upon the stage ("maturation"). The typical CT appearance is a double- or even triple-ring mass with an internal lower density [26]. After contrast enhancement, the outer zone becomes isodense, the appearance resembling that of a simple cyst. Enhancement is often noted in the outer ring and in mural projections or septa (Fig. 22.14). Some abscesses, as well as inflammatory pseudotumors, are difficult to differentiate from neoplasms.

8.2 Fatty infiltration

Fatty infiltration of the liver may be homogeneous and diffuse or may have an anatomical distribution. However, an irregular distribution is not infrequent, and localized, well-defined fatty infiltration together with a fat-free area is also noted (Fig. 22.15) [27]. Areas of relatively dominant fatty infiltration look like a hypodense mass and should be distinguished from a neoplasm, whereas a focally fat-free area appears as a hyperdense mass lesion with the same features as a neoplasm in a fatty liver.

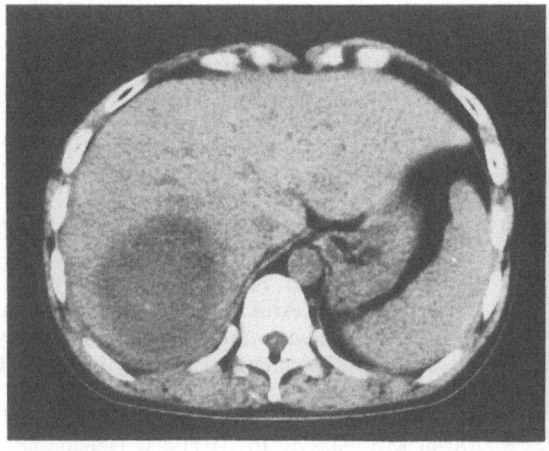 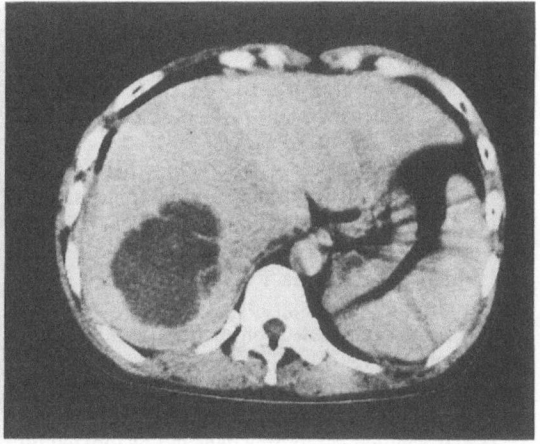

a   b

Fig. 22.14a, b. Liver abscess. **a** Plain. **b** With contrast. Septa appear in a round hypodense mass after contrast enhancement

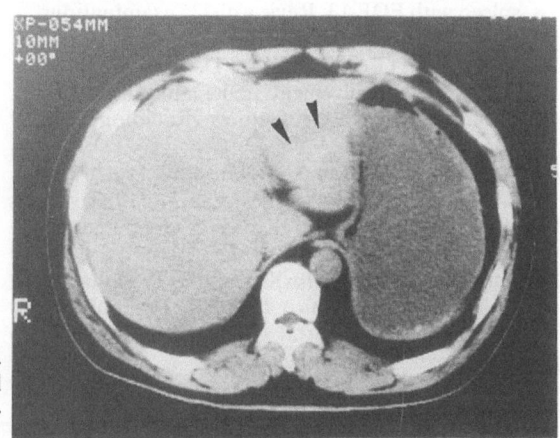

Fig. 22.15. Fatty liver with focally fat-free areas. A protruding hyperdense mass is noted in the lateral segment (*arrowheads*). This density difference had disappeared 1 week later

8.3 Adenomatous hyperplasia and regenerating nodules

Adenomatous hyperplasia and large regenerating nodules are difficult to diagnose on CT. The best way to make a diagnosis is by portal CT angiography, in which these nodules are enhanced to an almost equal extent as in a normal liver, in striking contrast to neoplasms which show no enhancement.

References

1. Itai Y, Nishikawa J, Tasaka A (1979) Computed tomography in the evaluation of hepatocellular carcinoma. Radiology 131: 165–170
2. Itai Y, Araki T, Furui S, Tasaka A (1981) Differential diagnosis of hepatic masses on computed tomography, with particular reference to hepatocellular carcinoma. J Comput Assist Tomogr 5: 834–842
3. Federle MP, Filly RA, Moss AA (1981) Cystic hepatic neoplasms: Complementary roles of CT and sonography. AJR 136: 345–348
4. Furui S, Ohtomo K, Itai Y, Iio M (1984) Hepatocellular carcinoma treated by trascatheter arterial embolization: progress evaluated by computed tomography. Radiology 150: 773–778
5. Kormano MJ, Dean PB (1976) Extravascular contrast material: the major component of contrast enhancement. Radiology 121: 379–382
6. Marchal GY, Baert AL, Wilms GE (1980) CT of noncystic liver lesions: Bolus enhancement. AJR 135: 57–65
7. Itai Y, Ohtomo K, Kokubo T, Yamauchi T, Minami M, Yashiro N, Araki T (1986) CT of hepatic masses: significance of prolonged enhancement and delayed enhancement. AJR 146: 729–733
8. Perkerson RB Jr, Erwin BC, Baumgartner BR, Phillips VM, Torres WE, Clements JL Jr, Gedgaudas-McClees K, Bernardino ME (1985) CT densities in delayed iodine hepatic scanning. Radiology 155: 445–446

9. Pagani JJ (1983) Intrahepatic vascular territories shown by computed tomography (CT). Radiology 147: 173–178

10. Araki T, Itai Y, Furui S, Tasaka A (1980) Dynamic CT densitometry of hepatic tumors. AJR 135: 1037–1043

11. Prando A, Wallace S, Bernardino ME, Lindell MM Jr (1979) Computed tomographic arteriography of the liver. Radiology 130: 697–701

12. Matsui O, Kadoya M, Suzuki M, Inoue K, Itoh H, Ida M, Takashima T (1983) Dynamic sequential computed tomography during arterial portography in the detection of hepatic neoplasms. Radiology 146: 721–727

13. Ohishi H, Uchida H, Yoshimura H, Ohue S, Ueda J, Katsuragi M, Matsuo N, Hosogi Y (1985) Hepatocellular carcinoma detected by iodized oil: Use of anticancer agents. Radiology 154: 25–30

14. Miller DL, Vermers M, Doppman JL, Simon RM, Sugarbaker PH, O'Leary TJ, Grimes G, Chatterji DG, Willis M (1984) CT of the liver and spleen with EOE-13: Review of 225 examinations. AJR 143: 235–243

15. Mathieu D, Grenier P, Larde D, Vasile N (1984) Portal vein involvement in hepatocellular carcinoma: Dynamic CT features. Radiology 152: 127–132

16. Nakashima T, Hiyama Y, Ohnishi K, Tsuchiya S, Kohno K, Nakajima Y, Okuda K (1983) Arterioportal shunts on dynamic computed tomography. AJR 140: 953–957

17. Itai Y, Furui S, Ohtomo K, Kokubo T, Yamauchi T, Minami M, Yashiro N (1986) Dynamic CT features of arterioportal shunt in hepatocellular carcinoma. AJR 146: 723–727

18. Otsuji H, Uchida H, Ohishi H (1983) Dynamic computed tomography of hepatocellular carcinoma with particular reference to capsule. Jpn J Clin Radiol 28: 1465–1471

19. Itai Y, Araki T, Furui S, Yashiro N, Ohtomo K, Iio M (1983) Computed tomography of primary intrahepatic biliary malignancy. Radiology 147: 485–490

20. Itai Y, Furui S, Araki T, Yashiro N, Tasaka A (1980) Computed tomography of cavernous hemangioma of the liver. Radiology 137: 149–155

21. Itai Y, Ohtomo K, Araki T, Furui S, Iio M, Atomi Y (1983) Computed tomography and sonography of cavernous hemangioma of the liver. AJR 141: 315–320

22. Kerlin P, Davis GL, McGill DB, Weiland LH, Adson MA, Sheedy PF II (1983) Hepatic adenoma and focal nodular hyperplasia: Clinical, pathological and radiologic features. Gastroenterology 84: 994–1002

23. Rogers JV, Mack LA, Freeny PC, Johnson ML, Sones PJ (1981) Hepatic focal nodular hyperplasia: Angiography, CT, sonography and scintigraphy. AJR 137: 983–990

24. Furui S, Yamauchi T, Itai Y, Ohtomto K Epithelioid hemangioendothelioma. (in preparation)

25. Zornoza J, Ginaldi S (1981) Computed tomography in hepatic lymphoma. Radiology 138: 405–410

26. Mathieu D, Vasile N. Fagniez PL, Segui S, Grably D, Larde D (1985) Dynamic CT features of hepatic abscesses. Radiology 154: 749–752

27. Halvorsen RA, Korobkin M, Ram PC, Thompson WM (1982) CT appearance of focal fatty infiltration of the liver. AJR 139: 227–281

Chapter 23
Magnetic Resonance Imaging of Liver Tumors

ALBERT A. MOSS and DAVID D. STARK[1]

Magnetic resonance (MR) imaging has been shown to display accurately the normal and pathological anatomy of the abdomen. Pathological conditions of the liver have been detected due to alterations in tissue hydrogen density or tissue relaxation times, T1 and T2 [1–6]. Most MR imaging techniques demonstrate the liver as a homogeneous structure having an intermediate MR signal. The surrounding fat has a very intense signal and abdominal vessels and hepatic vasculature are particularly well demonstrated, as flowing blood has a very low intensity (Fig. 23.1) [1–7].

MR imaging has tremendous flexibility, offering the capacity to tailor examinations to specific clinical questions. Appropriate selection of hepatic MR imaging techniques dramatically improves both anatomical resolution and tissue characterization information [8–11]. As patient throughput and examination cost are directly affected by MR pulse selection, a thorough understanding of the various MR imaging techniques is required to apply MR imaging optimally to the detection and characterization of liver tumors.

1 Technique

The spatial and contrast resolution of a hepatic MR image varies greatly, depending on the MR technique employed. Selection of the optimal MR pulse sequence is both critical and difficult, because an infinite number of techniques are theoretically possible. MR timing parameters TR and TE can be varied independently, and hepatic images can be made using spin-echo, inversion-recovery, phase-contrast, surface-coil, and three-dimensional chemical shift imaging

techniques [8–16]. Direct coronal and sagittal MR images of the liver are obtainable and have proved useful in defining the relationship of the liver to the diaphragm and in evaluating lesions involving the inferior vena cava or right atrium.

The optimal method of MR imaging of the liver has yet to be determined. However, while it is premature to exclude any particular technique, certain trends are evident. Most reported tumors have prolongation of both T1 and T2 values, although the degree of prolongation varies from patient to patient and even amongst various lesions in the same patient [4, 5, 9]. Thus, MR techniques which are either T1 dependent (inversion recovery, spin-echo imaging with short TR intervals) or T2 dependent (spin echo with long TR/TE) best demonstrate hepatic mass lesions [4, 6, 9, 13]. Further improvement in image quality is possible using techniques which reduce motion artifacts, surface-coil techniques, or average multiple-data acquisitions [9, 17–23].

The principle factor degrading hepatic MR images is physiological motion (cardiac, respiratory, and peristaltic). Respiratory and cardiac gating reduce motion artifacts by synchronizing data acquisition to physiological signals [16, 17, 24]. Cardiac gating is simplified by the availability of an electronic trigger (the electrocardiographic R wave) and periodicity of the cardiac cycle [24]. Respiratory gating is more difficult to implement, as a mechanical linkage is required to convert chest wall motion into an electronic signal [17, 18]. While both cardiac- and respiratory-gating techniques improve image quality, both prolong imaging time. For this reason, first-generation gating techniques have not been widely employed. However, newer techniques have been proposed that do not sacrifice imaging time.

Respiratory-ordered phase (ROTE; encoding), centrally ordered phase (COPE; encoding), and EXORCIST differ from conventional respira-

[1] Department of Radiology, SB-05, University Hospital, Seattle, WA 98195, USA

tory gating by acquiring data throughout the respiratory cycle [25–27]. Whereas ungated images and conventional respiratory-gated images proceed in a linear fashion from 0 to 128 steps (phase angles), ordered phase (encoding) selects a desirable phase angle for each phase of the respiratory cycle. Although imaging time is not prolonged, additional set-up time is required and these techniques do not reduce artifacts produced by cardiac motion or intestinal peristalsis.

Adaptation of pulse-sequence timing parameters is another method to improve hepatic image quality. In this technique, motion artifacts are reduced by signal averaging. Using a short TR spin-echo (SE) technique, data from a large number of acquisitions can be averaged without prolonging imaging time. Stark et al. [9] demonstrated that using a TR interval of 260 ms and a TE of 18 ms, 18 data acquisitions could be averaged with a total imaging time of 10 min. This compares with only two data acquisitions being possible within a 9-min scan time when a 2000-ms TR interval is selected.

Hepatic MR images obtained using a short-TR, short-TE, multiple-averaging technique dramatically reduce motion artifacts and image noise (Figs. 23.2, 23.3). This greatly improves image quality, and the imaging time is acceptable. The trade-off for using this technique is that image contrast is restricted to tissue T1 differences. Another pulse sequence must be employed if hepatic T2 differences are to be demonstrated.

2   Multiple slice imaging

Multislice, two-dimensional MR imaging techniques are time efficient and essential for hepatic imaging [4, 8, 9]. Imaging systems that combine contiguous slices with minimal gaps between slices are preferred. The maximum number of slices obtained using a given pulse sequence is limited by the TR and TE times selected. The formula for this relationship is:

$$\text{Maximum number of slices} = \frac{\text{TR}}{\text{TE} + \text{constant}} \text{ [9]}.$$

The constant will vary between different MR imaging systems and is a function of gradient performance. It follows from this equation that more slices can be obtained using long TR intervals and that the number of slices increases as TE is decreased.

This formula has considerable practical importance in hepatic MR imaging. Transverse images of the liver must span a maximum of 15

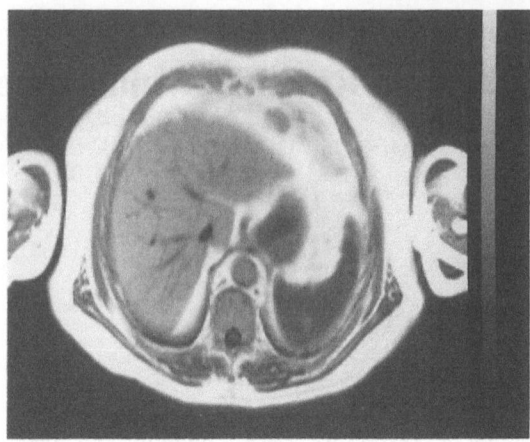

Fig. 23.1. A spin-echo 500/28 image demonstrates subcutaneous fat to be very intense, the liver to be of moderate intensity, and flowing blood in the portal and hepatic veins to have a very low signal intensity

cm if the entire liver is to be included in a single study. If a "constant" of 12 ms is present in a particular MR scanner, selection of a spin echo with a 500/30 pulse sequence will permit a maximum of 11 slices to be obtained and thus require 1.5-cm-thick slices to cover the entire liver. Short TR/TE spin-echo techniques permit simultaneous acquisition of 12 or more contiguous slices and are capable of scanning the entire liver within 10 min (Fig. 23.3).

3   Spatial resolution

Choice of in-plane spatial resolution, i.e., picture element (pixel) size requires a direct trade-off between spatial resolution and imaging time according to the following formula:

Image time
   = number of Y lines · # signal Averages · TR

Where image time equals the number of Y lines resolved multiplied by the number of signal averages multiplied by the pulse-sequence repetition time TR, e.g., 10 mm = 128 × 18 × 0.26 s. The examination time is proportional to the spatial resolution along the in-plane phase encoded dimension (Y), as resolution of each Y line requires a separate pulse repetition. Averaging of multiple data acquisitions to improve the image signal-to-noise level also has a direct time penalty. Slice selection (Z dimension for transverse images) and the in-plane frequency-encoded dimension (X dimension for transverse images) do not have a time penalty. For most hepatic appli-

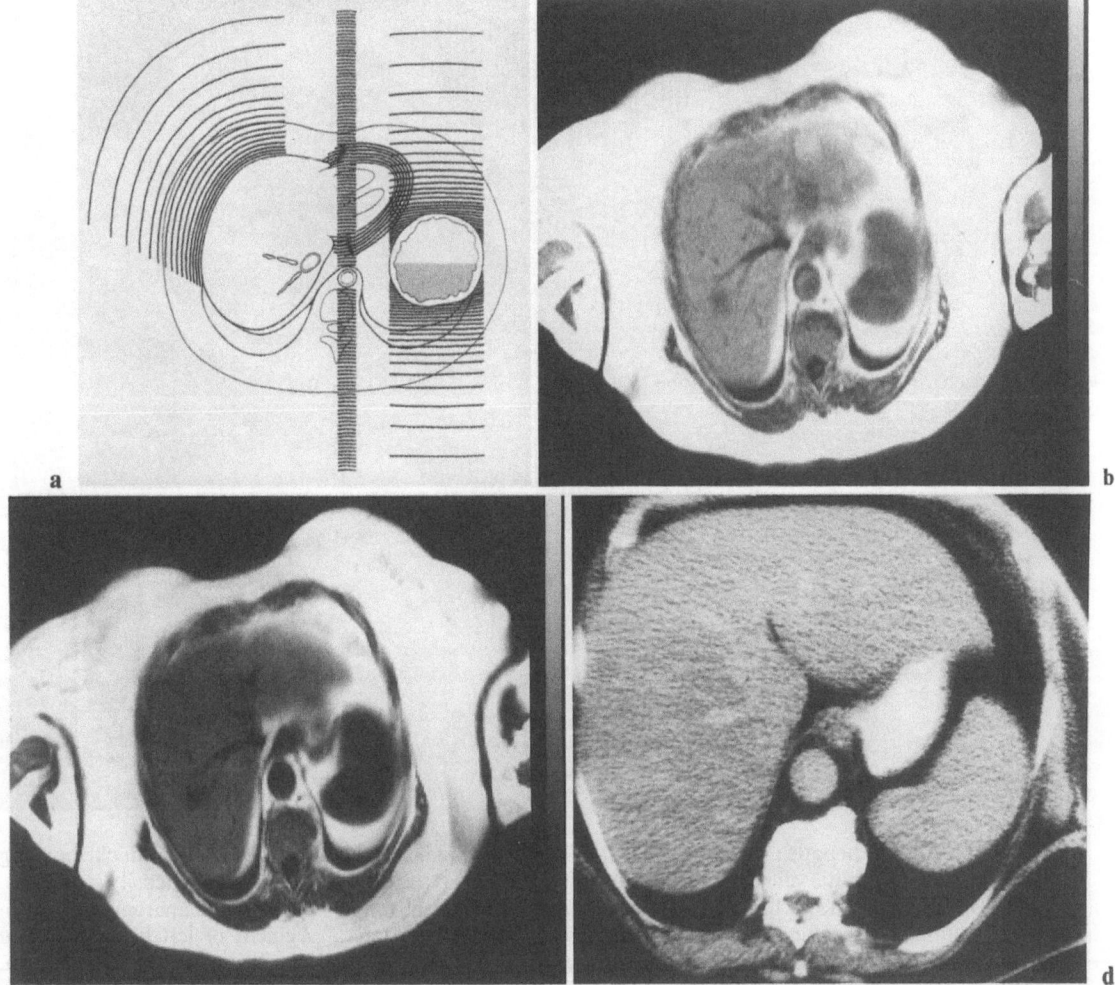

Fig. 23.2. a Motion artifacts. Schematic diagram of the upper abdomen in transverse section. "Ghosts" of moving structures (subcutaneous fat, aorta, heart, stomach) propagate along the phase-encoding axis (vertical). **b** IR 1500/450/15/3 pulse sequence obtained by averaging three data acquisitions required 10 min of imaging time. Ghost artifacts resulting from aortic pulsations are seen overlying the left hepatic lobe. The right lobe lesion now has a low signal intensity due to its long T1. **c** SE 260/15/18 image obtained by averaging 18 data acquisitions required an imaging time of 10 min. The image is less grainy (less noisy); detailed vascular anatomy is well seen. The left heptic lobe is visualized free of motion artifacts, and the single right hepatic lobe lesion is easily identified. **d** CT scan with bolus contrast administration missed the lesion shown by MR imaging

cations, MR images use 128 phase-encoded lines and 256 frequency-encoded points along each line. In a field of view that measures 46 × 46 cm, this typically allows the pixel size to be 3.6 × 1.8 mm.

4 Surface coils

Most abdominal MR imaging is performed using a cirrcumferential "saddle"-type radio frequency coil that serves as an antenna for both transmission and reception. This coil design has a large uniform sensitive volume, permitting the acquisition of images with a large field of view.

Surface coils can be placed adjacent to an anatomical region of interest to replace the receiver functions of the circumferential coil, which usually remains in use as a transmitter only. Surface coils have the advantage of improved radio frequency (RF) signal reception, resulting in greater signal-to-noise levels [19]. The small field of view and nonuniformity of the sensitive volume are disadvantages of surface coils.

Surface-coil examination of superficial structures such as the spine and temporal mandibular

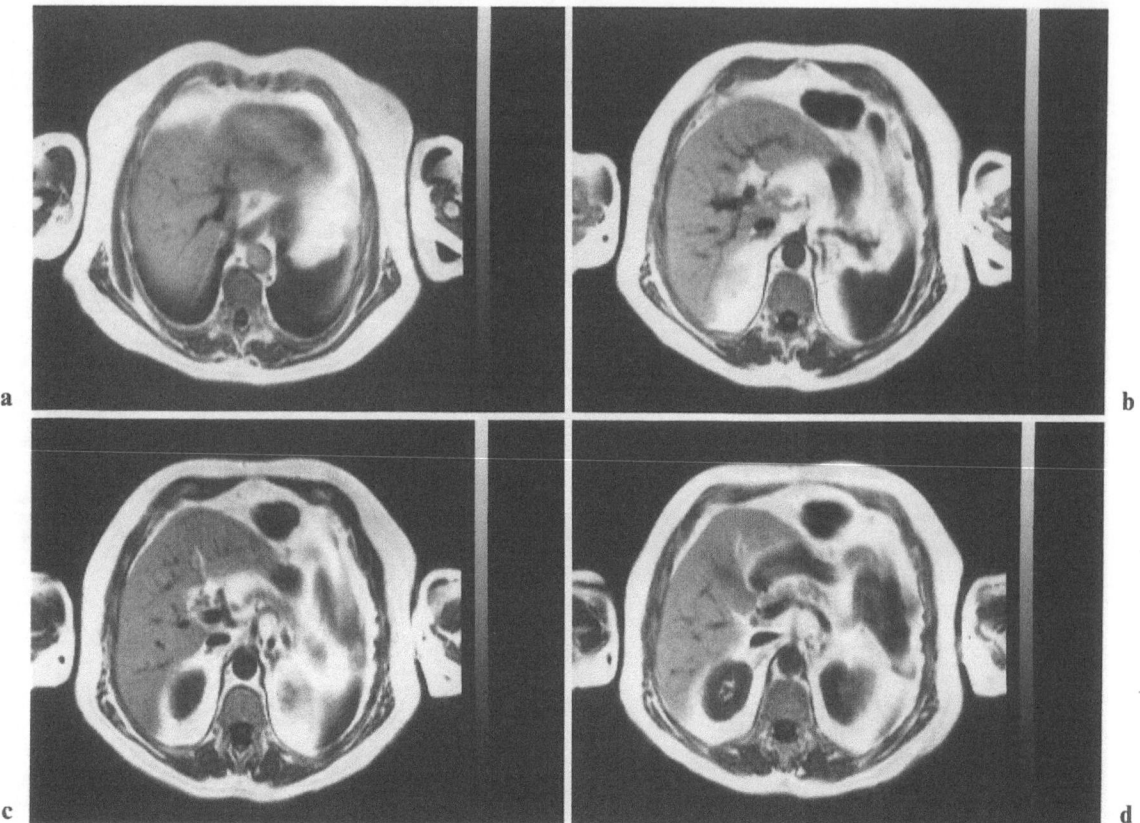

Fig. 23.3a–h. Normal hepatic anatomy (SE 260/15/18 pulse sequence). Each section is 1.5 cm thick. Imaging time 10 min. **a** Right hepatic vein and intrahepatic inferior vena cava are clearly seen as low-intensity structures. **b** Caudate lobe of liver shown between inferior vena cava and portal vein. **c** Porta hepatis anatomy; falciform ligament containing ascending left portal vein is seen demarcating lateral segment of left hepatic lobe. **d** Pancreatic body seen above splenic vein. **e** Gallbladder has low intensity. Renal arteries and veins clearly shown. **f** Right lobe of liver at level of uncinate process of pancreas. **g** Transverse duodenum is seen as low-intensity structure. High signal intensity within inferior vena cava indicates this is bottom slice of multislice imaging technique. **h** A SE 2000/60/3 image. Three data acquisitions; imaging time 15 min. This T2-weighted image corresponds to **d**

joint provide superior images. The development of larger surface coils (15–30 cm in diameter) offers significant gains in signal-to-noise ratio and allows improved visualization of the liver. An additional advantage of hepatic surface coil imaging is reduction of motion artifacts. The signal from moving structures outside the coil's sensitive volume does not cause image artifacts. Surface-coil MR imaging of the liver has shown the potential for improved detection of small surface metastases [19].

5   Tissue characterization

The capacity of MR imaging to characterize normal and abnormal tissues is based on the ability of specific pulse-sequence techniques to detect the difference in one or more MR tissue parameters. Four distinct tissue parameters contribute to the appearance of the hepatic MR image: (1) hydrogen density, (2) motion-physiological (macroscopic) and diffusion (microscopic), (3) chemical shift (spectroscopy), and (4) relaxation times T1 (longitudinal) and T2 (transverse).

Depending on the imaging technique chosen, each parameter has a different degree of influence on image contrast. Hydrogen density usually has the least influence as only fat differs significantly from other tissues. Adipose tissue has approximately 50% greater hydrogen density than liver [15]. Macroscopic motion in the form of blood flow is responsible for the excellent delineation of

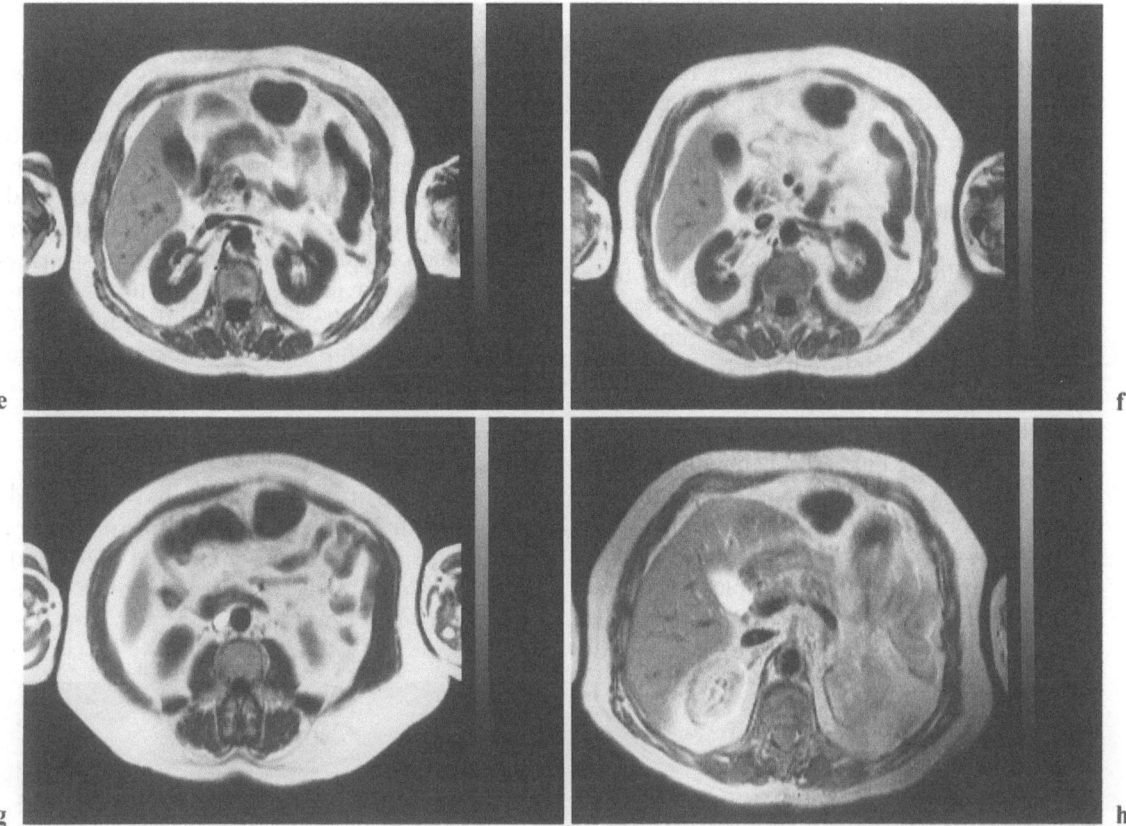

Fig. 23.3e–h

hepatic blood vessels. The contribution of micro-scopic flow (diffusion) to the MR hepatic image appears to be small but requires further study [16].

Chemical shift, which shows differences in resonance frequency between hydrogen nuclei chemically bound to different molecules, can be used in hepatic imaging. Chemical-shift imaging has been employed to separate liver water signal intensity from liver fat signal intensity (Figs. 23.4, 23.5) [12, 14–16].

Dixon developed a method for obtaining pure fat and pure water hepatic images using phase-contrast imaging techniques [12]. In Dixon's opposed phase image, pixel brightness is the net difference between fat and water magnetization [12]. Although detection of a fatty liver itself may be of limited clinical significance, fat-water contrast can be manipulated to improve detection of hepatic metastases in patients with hepatic tumors (Fig. 23.6) [16]. As noncancerous liver tissue contains the predominant amount of ob-servable lipid, the phase-contrast technique can improve cancer/liver contrast, thereby enhanc-ing lesion detectability [14, 16].

Opposed phase images alter cancer/liver con-trast by decreasing the signal intensity of fatty liver tissue, while cancer signal intensity shows little or no change. Though phase-contrast imag-ing has great potential, currently it is not widely employed. The technique is somewhat cumber-some and time consuming, particularly when long TR pulse sequences are employed to obtain T2-weighted phase-contrast images. Opposed phase T1 pulse sequences show loss of cancer/liver contrast due to a decrease in both cancer and liver signal intensity. Furthermore, when conventional T1-weighted images are compared with T2-weighted (conventional or phase con-trast) images they show greater cancer/liver con-trast and better anatomical resolution [16].

Tissue relaxation times, T1 and T2, are by far the most important parameters for selecting the optimal hepatic MR-imaging technique. Although both T1 and T2 times are increased in nearly all pathological hepatic conditions, they have opposite effects on image signal intensity. Long T1 relaxation times lead to decreased signal intensity, while long T2 relaxation times lead to increased signal intensity. It is possible to mask pathological increases in T1 and T2 by allowing both T1 and T2 to influence image contrast (Fig. 23.7). Therefore, imaging techniques should be selected to maximize either T1 or T2 contrast, but not both.

6   Liver tumor detection

Detection of liver tumors by MR imaging is dependent on both anatomical resolution and image display of differential tissue characteristics. Anatomical resolution is a complex function of image geometry (spatial resolution) and signal-to-noise ratios. For example, decreased signal intensity or increased background noise results in a dark or grainy image with poor resolution of normal anatomical structures (Fig. 23.6). Motion artifacts also degrade MR images in a complex manner. For example, respiratory

motion causes blurring (reduced edge sharpness) while aortic pulsations result in "ghost" artifacts which may obscure the left hepatic lobe (Figs. 23.2, 23.6).

MR pulse-sequence performance quantitated by signal difference-to-noise (SD/N) ratio correlates closely with anatomical resolution and conspicuity of hepatic tumors [9]. Quantitative comparison of pulse sequences requires image acquisition using identical imaging time or standardization of noise measurement to reflect the known relationship between background noise levels and hepatic imaging time.

6.1   T2-weighted spin-echo images

Improvements in gradient design have permitted imaging with TE intervals of 180 ms or longer. This results in significantly improved SD/N and improved conspicuity of hepatic tumors com-

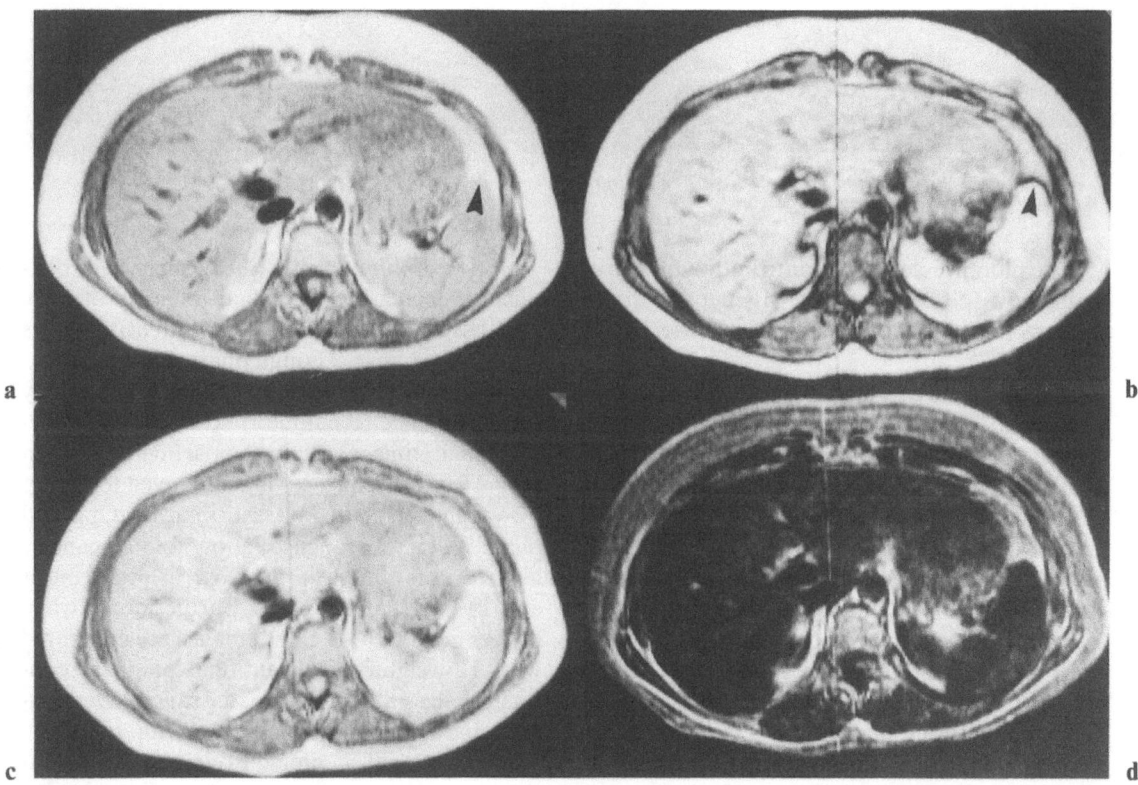

Fig. 23.4a–d. Chemical shift imaging. Normal liver. **a** Conventional in-phase SE 1500/30 image shows spleen to have slightly higher signal intensity than liver. **b** Phase-contrast SE 1500/30 image again shows the nonfatty spleen to have a slightly higher signal intensity than the nonfatty liver. Dark band (*arrowhead*) demarcates interfaces between water-containing viscera and fat-containing adipose tissue. **c** Calculated "water" image is derived by adding the in-phase and opposed-phase images. The obtained image is very similar to the in-phase image, indicating that all liver and spleen signal intensity is from water. **d** Calculated "fat" image is derived by subtracting opposed-phase from in-phase image. Absence of signal from spleen and liver indicates that neither tissue contains fat observable with MR imaging

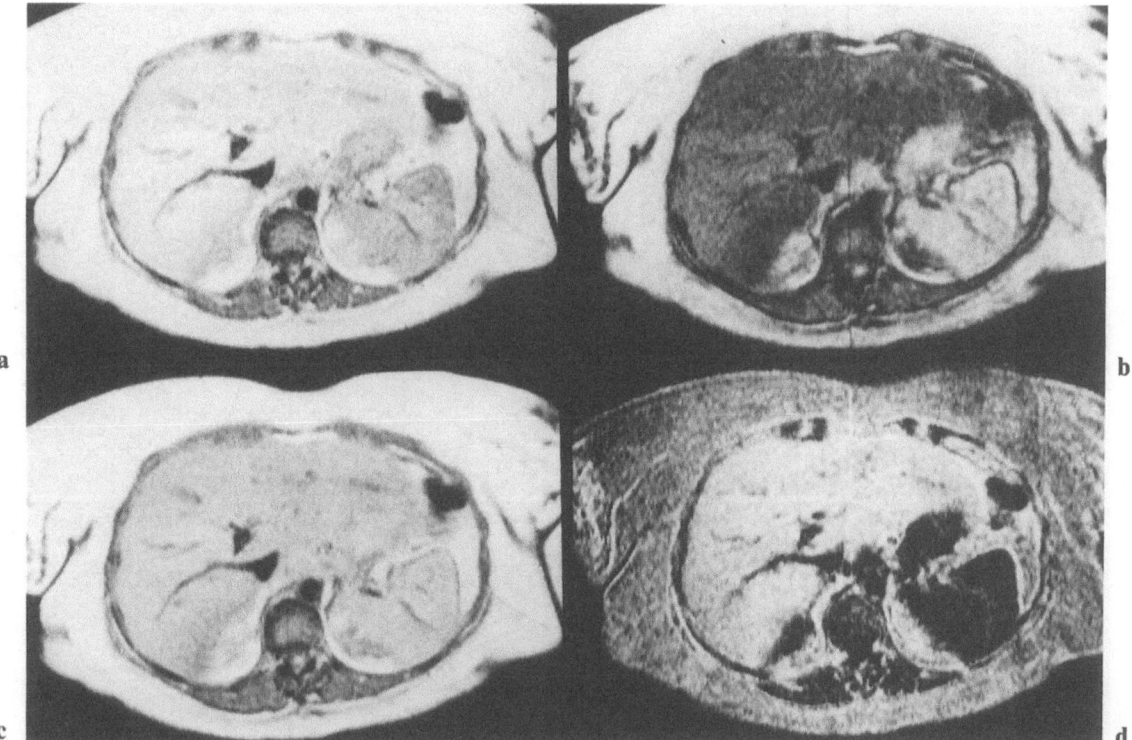

Fig. 23.5a–d. Chemical-shift imaging in patient with diffuse fatty infiltration of the liver. **a** The in-phase SE 1500/30 image reveals the liver to have a higher signal intensity than the spleen. **b** Phase-contrast opposed-phase SE 1500/30 image reveals a dramatic decrease in hepatic signal relative to spleen. **c, d** Calculated "water" and "fat" images show no MR-observable fat in the spleen but considerable fat signal intensity in the liver

pared with imaging using shorter TE intervals. A study of 22 patients with liver metastases demonstrated that an SE 2000/120 sequence was superior to either imaging using a TE of 60 or 180 ms [28]. Hepatic T2-weighted SE pulse sequences obtained using TR intervals of a least 2000 ms appear superior to those using shorter TR intervals. This is due to the long T1 relaxation time of hepatic tumors, which prevents complete recovery of the longitudinal magnetization at TR intervals less than 1500 ms. Unfortunately, increasing TR and TE to improve T2 hepatic contrast requires an unfavorable trade-off of reduced signal averaging, decreased signal-to-noise ratio, increased sensitivity to motion artifacts, and decreased anatomical resolution.

6.2 T1-weighted spin-echo imaging

Hepatic MR imaging using T1-weighted sequences with short TR intervals is time efficient and provides superior tissue discrimination [9]. As the TR interval is reduced to 260 ms or less, there are several beneficial effects. First, T1

weighting of the image is increased, which improves tumor-to-liver contrast. Second, since more data acquisitions can be averaged within a given time, signal-to-noise ratios and anatomical resolution are preserved. Third, signal averaging reduces artifacts due to physiological motion. Reduction in TE complements reductions in TR by further increasing T1-dependent image contrast, increasing signal-to-noise (S/N) ratios, and further reducing motion artifacts (Fig. 23.7) [9].

6.3 T1-weighted inversion-recovery imaging

In vivo studies have shown cancer-liver T1 differences to be substantially greater than T2 differences [9–11] and inversion-recovery (IR) MR-imaging sequences have proven superior to T2-weighted SE sequences with respect to lesion conspiquity [8, 9, 13]. Reducing the TE to 18 ms or less improves the performance of IR sequences. Centering the 90° pulse of the IR sequence near the inversion or "null" point of the magnetization recovery for cancer tissue (at

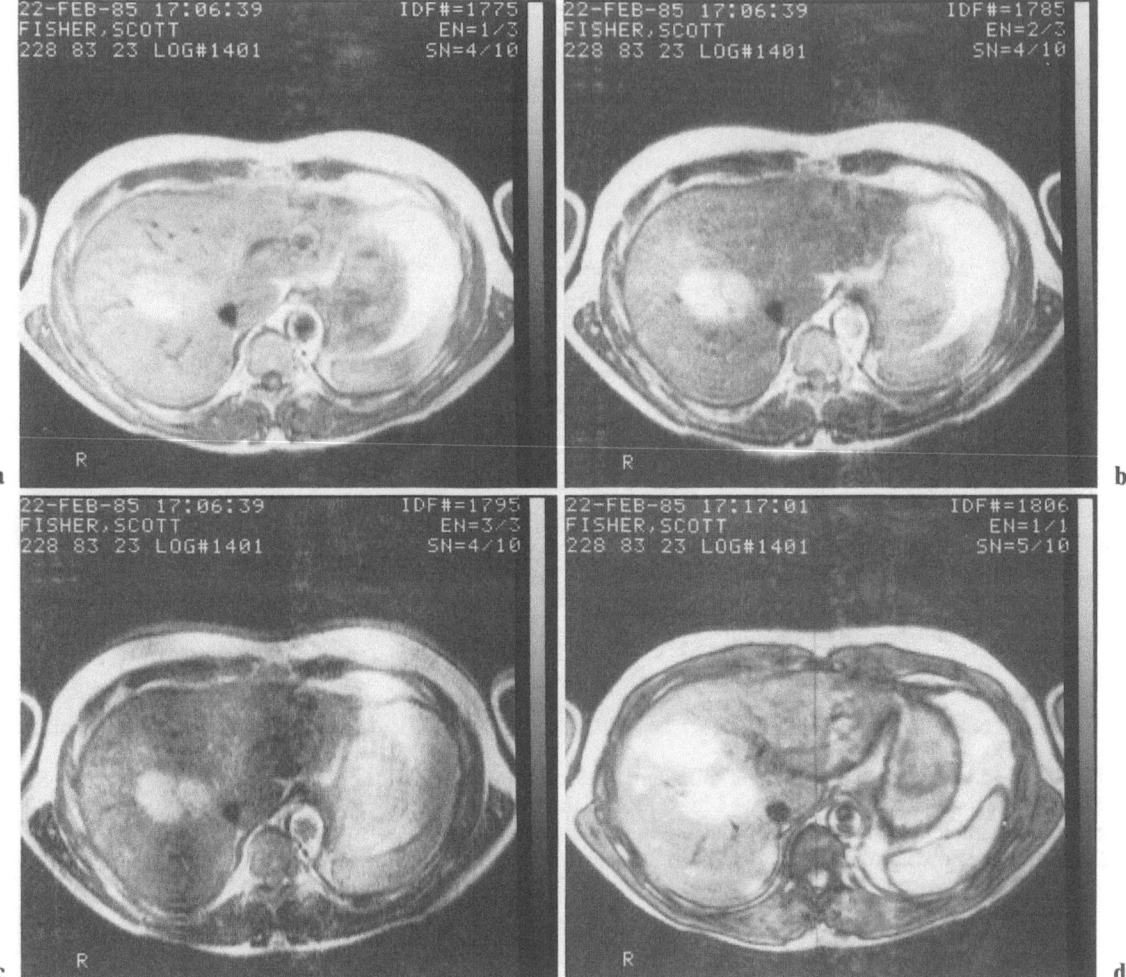

Fig. 23.6a–d. Conventional and chemical shift MR imaging in metabolic liver cancer. **a** Liver metastases, T2-weighted spin-echo images. SE 2000/60/2 acquisition (9 min) image shows a metastasis to the right hepatic lobe as a poorly marginated high-intensity lesion. The left hepatic lobe is partially obscured by motion artifacts ("ghosts") from aortic pulsation. **b** SE 2000/90/2 image. The metastases are better seen due to increased contrast with the surrounding liver. However, the image is grainy and anatomical resolution of structures is decreased due to a decreased signal-to-noise ratio compared with the TE = 30 ms image. Aortic pulsation artifact again obscures part of the left hepatic lobe. **c** Conventional in-phase SE 2000/30 image (T2 weighted) shows only a subtle difference in signal intensity between the left and right hepatic lobes. **d** Chemical shift phase-contrast (opposed-phase) SE 2000/30 image shows a high-intensity mass consistent with metastatic cancer. Overall hepatic signal intensity is decreased due to diffuse fatty infiltration, the metastasis does not contain MR-observable fat and its signal intensity relative to the surrounding liver is increased

TI = 280 ms) decreased the liver S/N ratio but increased cancer-liver contrast (Fig. 23.8).

Due to the frequency dependence of tissue T1 relaxation [29, 30], the optimal pulse sequence for hepatic imaging varies with field strength. As image noise will also vary depending on the imaging sequence employed, specific pulse-sequence recommendations are directly applicable only to individual MR systems. However, methods of pulse-sequence selection and image analysis will apply to all MR systems and should be valuable as general quidelines in selecting optimal hepatic MR-imaging techniques.

7 Hepatic anatomy

The normal liver and its contents are well delineated by MR-imaging techniques. Although the image intensity of tissues varies depending on the pulse sequence used, the normal liver usually

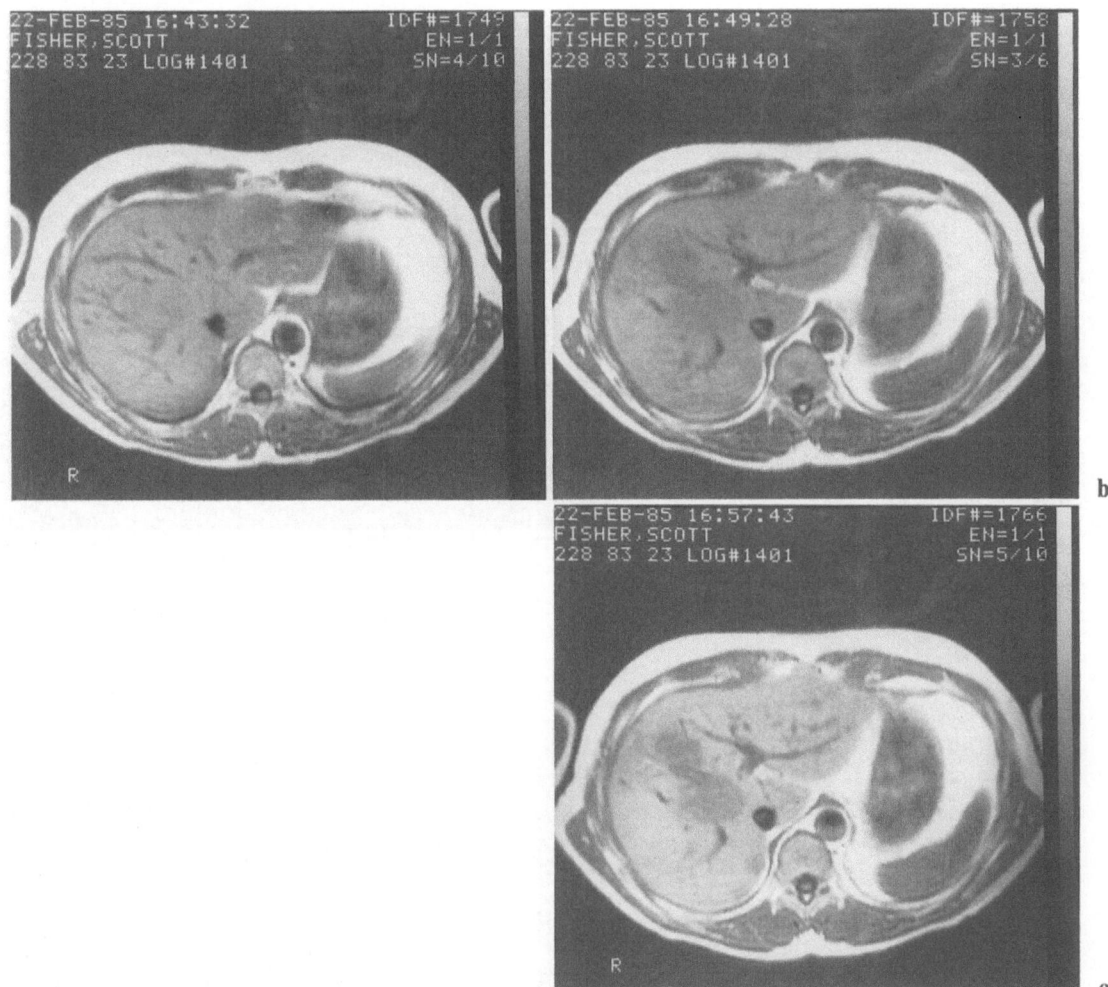

Fig. 23.7a–c. T1-weighted spin-echo images. **a** SE 500/30/4 (4.5-min image). This T1-weighted sequence has poorer tumor–liver contrast than any of the "T2-weighted" or IR pulse sequences. Note that the artifacts due to aortic pulsation persist. **b** SE 260/30/8 (5-min image). Reduction of TR allows increased singal averaging without increased examination time. Compared with the SE 500/30/4 pulse sequence, tumor–liver contrast is increased, anatomical resolution of the left portal vein is imporved, and motion artifacts are decreased. **c** SE 260/18/16 (10-min image). Reduction in TE further increases T1 weighting, increasing tumor–liver contrast. Small metastases in the posterior segment of the right hepatic lobe are now easily seen. Shorter TE also increases the signal-to-noise ratio, improving anatomical resolution of structures such as the left portal vein. Furthermore, artifacts due to aortic pulsation are now eliminated

appears as an organ of moderate intensity (Figs. 23.1–23.3). Due to the rapid flow of blood within the hepatic vascular system, normal hepatic vessels are clearly delineated as low-intensity structures without contrast media administration. The biliary system can be differentiated from the vascular system by varying the pulse sequences used to scan the liver. Periportal fat permits the anatomy of the portahepatis to be displayed without the administration of biliary or vascular contrast media.

Using a 0.35-T imaging system, the T1 and T2 relaxation times of the normal liver have been reported to average 350–533 ms and 46–56 ms, respectively [4, 9]. Currently, most in vivo imaging systems estimate T1 and T2 relaxation times using a two-point nonlinear least square fit while in vitro MR methods use 8–32 points to calculate precisely the relaxation times. Therefore, T1 and T2 relaxation times calculated by various clinical imaging systems should be accepted with caution and never considered "absolute values." Furthermore, because of differences in magnetic field strength, relaxation times obtained on one MR system cannot be quantitatively compared with times calculated on a different system.

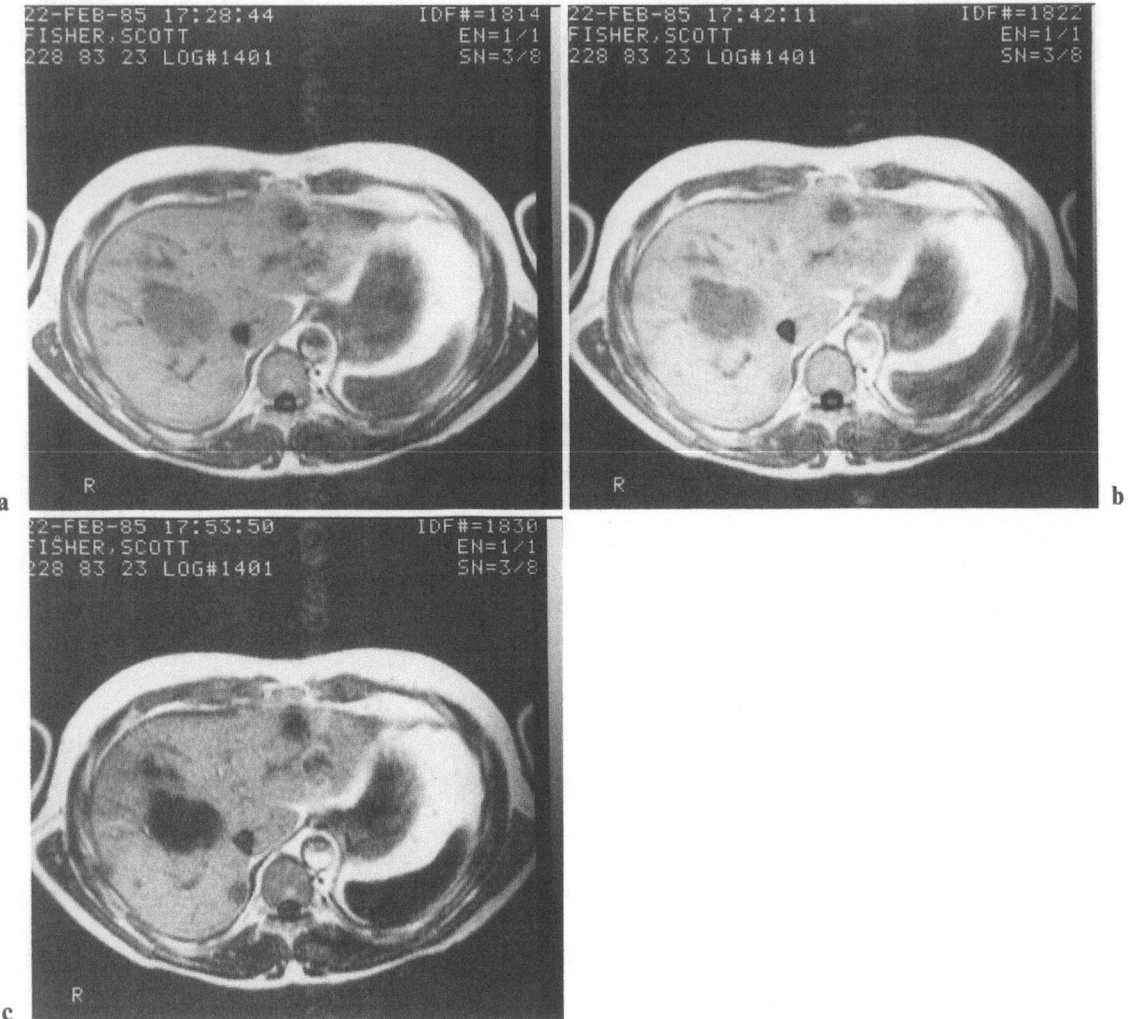

Fig. 23.8a–c. Inversion-recovery (T1-weighted) images. **a** IR 1500/450/30/3 acquisition image. The metastases are now seen as low signal-intensity lesions relative to the surrounding liver as metastases have a longer T1 relaxation time than the surrounding liver. **b** IR 1500/450/18/3 image. Reduction in TE increases the T1 weighting of IR images, increasing tumor–liver contrast. Furthermore, reduction in TE has increased the signal-to-noise ratios, resulting in improved anatomical resolution of left portal vein. **c** IR 1500/280/ 18/3 image. Reduction in T1 decreases the signal intensity of metastases (long T1) more than the surrounding liver, resulting in tumor–liver contrast. Anatomical resolution is slightly reduced due to decreased signal-to-noise ratios

8 Primary hepatic tumors

8.1 Hepatocellular carcinoma

The intensity of hepatocellular carcinoma (HCC) compared with the normal liver varies depending on the MR-imaging sequences employed to obtain the image. HCC has been shown to have prolonged T1 and T2 values and thus is usually best visualized using spin-echo techniques, which are strongly T1 or T2 weighted [3, 4, 6, 9, 31, 32]. HCC are usually of higher intensity than the normal liver when T2-weighted

(long TR/TE) spin-echo techniques are employed (Fig. 23.9). Using T1-dependent (short TR/TE) spin-echo images, HCC usually appear as masses with a lower intensity than the normal liver. When IR techniques are employed, HCC are usually shown to have a lower intensity than the normal liver.

MR-imaging demonstrates the internal structure within HCC, accurately displays the margin of the lesion, and depicts the relationship of malignancy to the hepatic vasculature with great clarity (Fig. 23.9). Both T1 and T2 relaxation times can vary in different regions of a solitary

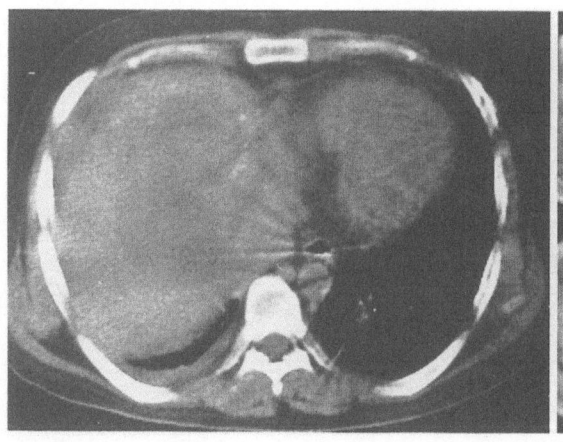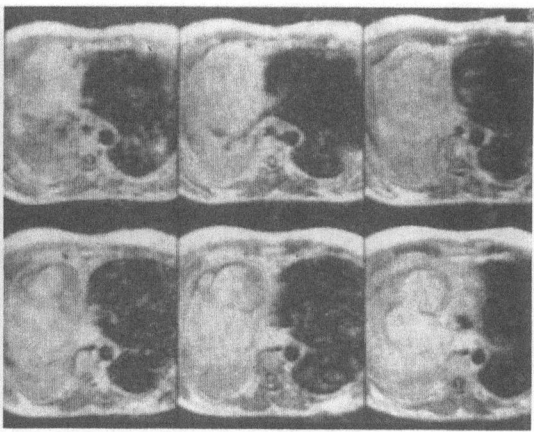

a   b

Fig. 23.9a, b. Hepatoma. **a** CT scan reveals large low-density mass in the central portion of the liver. **b** Six contiguous SE images through the hepatoma reveal the tumor to have a generally higher signal than the normal liver. The tumor margins are well seen. Normal hepatic vascular structures are not seen. The tumor has invaded the inferior vena cava

HCC and among multifocal HCC in individual patients [4].

MR detection of solitary or multifocal HCC is usually easy as significant differences exist in the T1 and T2 relaxation times of HCC and the normal liver [4, 9]. Infiltrating HCC which replace most of the liver are the most difficult to diagnose, as the tumor–liver interface is often ill defined. An accurate diagnosis can be made by noting the loss of normal hepatic vascular structures within the tumor mass and comparing T1 and T2 measurements with those of the normal liver.

8.2 Cholangiocarcinoma

Cholangiocarcinoma is an uncommon but potentially curable primary hepatic malignancy [33, 34]. While the appearance of cholangiocarcinoma has been studied using a variety of imaging techniques, the use of MR to detect and characterize this tumor has only recently been employed [33]. Cholangiocarcinoma is usually detected by MR imaging because it produces a soft tissue mass. Two types of soft tissue mass have been demonstrated. Well-differentiated cholangiocarcinoma produces a mass having a very high signal intensity while the scirrhous subtype of adenocarcinoma demonstrates only a slightly higher signal intensity than the normal liver on T2-weight spin-echo sequences. T2 relaxation time measurement in patients with the scirrhous form of cholangiocarcinoma were shorter than in patients with well-differentiated adenocarcinoma [33].

MR imaging can readily demonstrate encasement or displacement of adjacent vascular structures as well as extension of the tumor into adjacent organs. Associated MR findings in cholangiocarcinoma are demonstration of bile duct obstruction [34], enlargement of hilar lymph nodes, and invasion of the tumor into the gallbladder or portal vascular structures. At present, there is insufficient evidence to assess whether MR imaging can be used to differentiate cholangiocarcinoma from sclerosing cholangitis.

8.3 Hepatic adenoma

There has been limited experience using MR to evaluate benign hepatic adenomas. The reported MR appearance of adenomas did not permit them to be differentiated from HCC (Fig. 23.10) [4]. In addition, the calculated T1 and T2 relaxation times of hepatic adenomas fell within that of HCC and metastatic lesions. As with hepatomas, MR depicted the internal architecture and surrounding capsule of adenomas better than nonenhanced computed tomography. A significant drawback was the inability of MR to demonstrate foci of calcification [4].

8.4 Hemangioma

The MR intensity of hemangiomas is influenced by fibrosis and calcification but appears to be relatively independent of size. Hemangiomas usually appear as masses having a high intensity on spin echo obtained with strong T1 or T2 weighting (Fig. 23.11). Moreover, hemangiomas

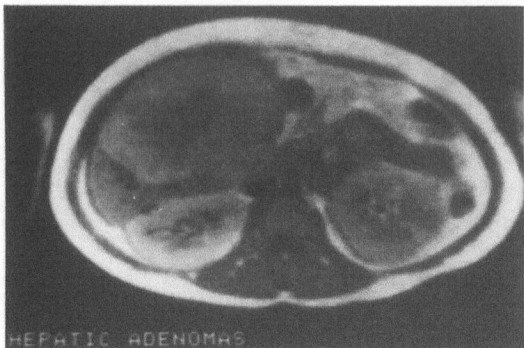

Fig. 23.10. Hepatic adenoma: An SE 1000/28 image shows a large hepatic adenoma to have a signal slightly greater than the normal liver

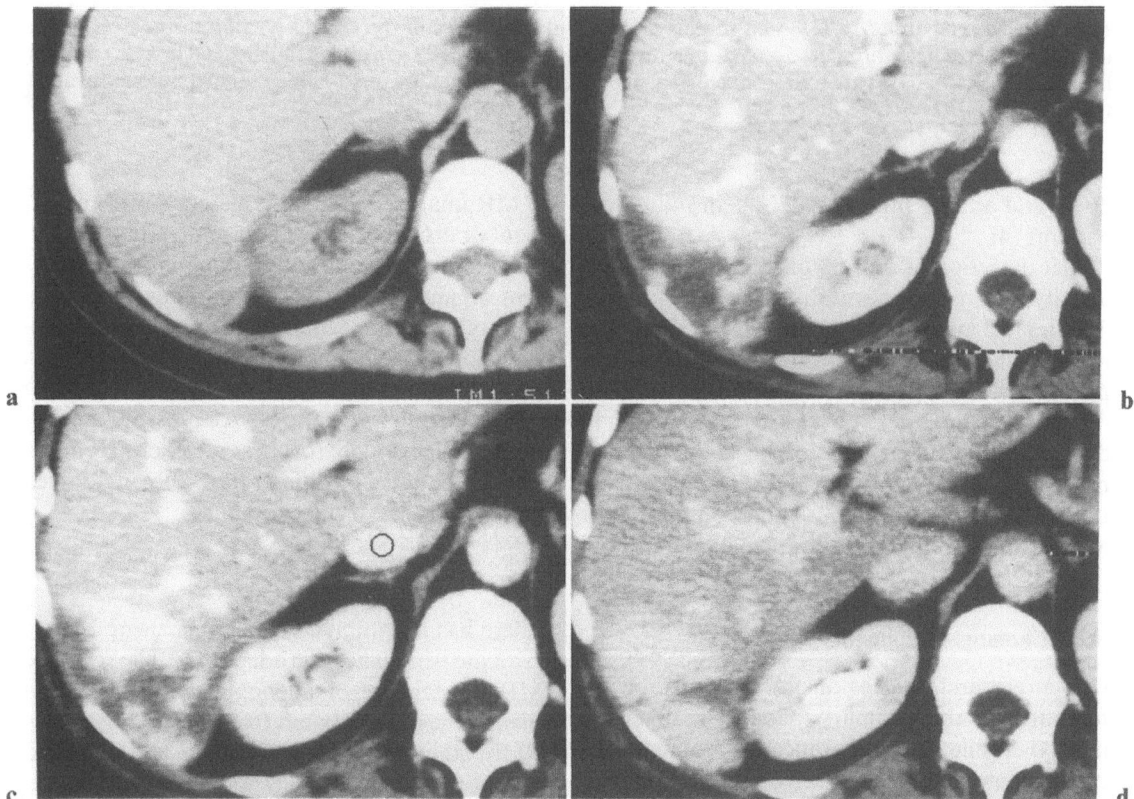

Fig. 23.11a–j. Cavernous hemangioma of the liver. **a** CT scan without contrast reveals an exophytic lesion of the right hepatic lobe. **b** Peripheral enhancement following bolus contrast administration. **c** One minute after contrast bolus, further filling of the lesion is seen. **d** Five minutes after contrast administration, almost complete filling of the lesion is seen. **e** T1-weighted IR 1500/450/30/4 image shows the hemangioma to have a relatively low signal intensity, indicating a long T1 relative to the liver. **f** An SE 500/30/4 image shows reduced contrast between the hemangioma and liver. **g** A T2-weighted SE 2000/30/4 image shows the hemangioma to have increased signal intensity relative to the liver, indicating increased T2. **h** An SE 2000/60 image; signal intensity of the hemangioma has increased relative to liver. **i** Spin-echo 2000/120 image signal intensity of hemangioma equals that of the cerebral spinal fluid in the thoracic spinal canal. **j** An SE 2000/180/4 image shows greatly reduced signal intensity from all solid tissues, hemangioma and cerebral spinal fluid maintain high signal intensity due to extremely long T2 relaxation times

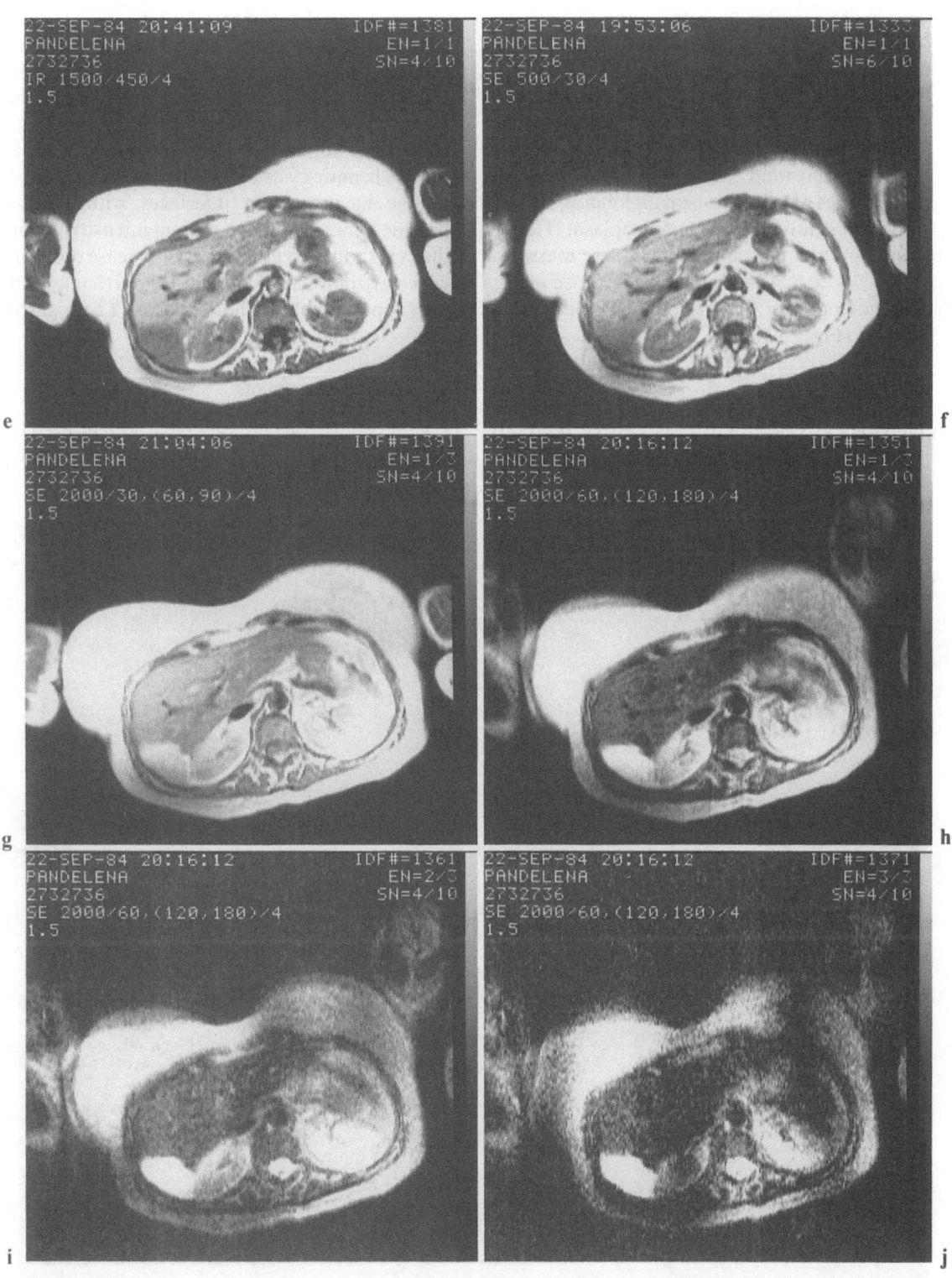

Fig. 23.11e–j

usually have a significantly greater signal intensity than solid neoplasms [28, 35, 36]. The MR appearance of cavernous hemangiomas differs from that of solid hepatic neoplasms because a hemangioma is essentially a fluid, a lake of slowly flowing blood. As fluids have much longer T1 and T2 relaxation times than solids, the MR appearance of a hepatic hemangioma should differ significantly from a solid neoplasm. Hepatic hemangiomas thus appear as intense masses on both T1- and T2-weighted imaging sequences and have greater S/N ratios than solid hepatic tumors (Fig. 23.11) [28, 35, 36].

8.5 Hepatic cysts

Hepatic cysts, like cysts elsewhere in the body, tend to appear as low-intensity masses on IR

images or on T1-weight spin-echo images with short TR intervals [37]. While hepatic cysts contain fluid with relatively long T1 and T2 values, the brightness of the cyst contents relative to the hepatic parenchyma depends upon the exact chemical composition of the hepatic cyst. MR reveals hepatic cysts as clearly delineated, round lesions having sharp interfaces with normal hepatic parenchyma. The signal intensity within the cyst should be uniform and increase on scans which are more T2 weighted. Hemorrhagic cysts may appear bright on both T1- and T2-weighted spin-echo images [37].

8.6 Metastatic tumors

A variety of MR techniques have been utilized to study metastatic tumors. Young et al [8, 38] re-

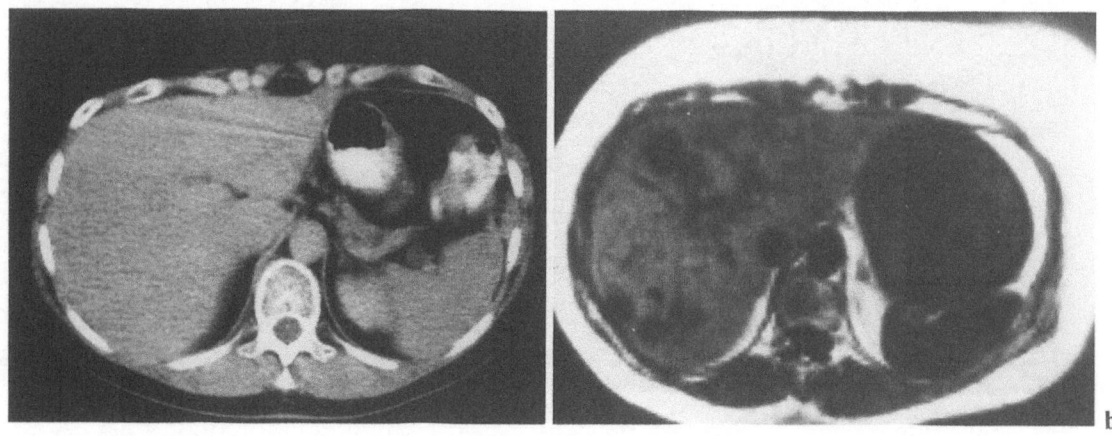

Fig. 23.12a, b. Metastatic colon carcinoma. **a** CT scan following contrast administration is normal. **b** IR scan reveals multiple metastatic deposits as rounded masses of low signal intensity

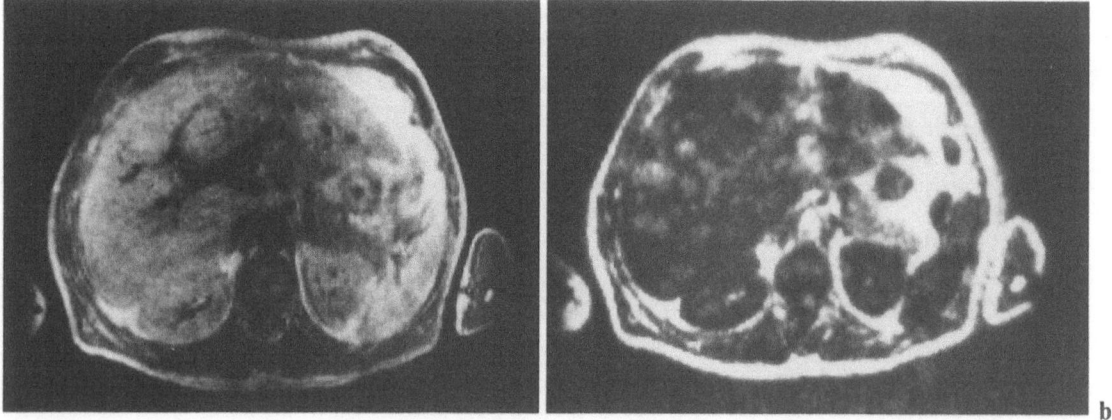

Fig. 23.13a, b. Metastatic colon cancer to liver. **a** SE 2000/28 image shows loss of a right portal vein branch, but it is difficult to detect discrete metastatic foci. **b** IR 1800/420/56 image reveals multiple metastatic foci. Many have low-intensity rims surrounding higher intensity masses. Some tumors have very high signal intensity

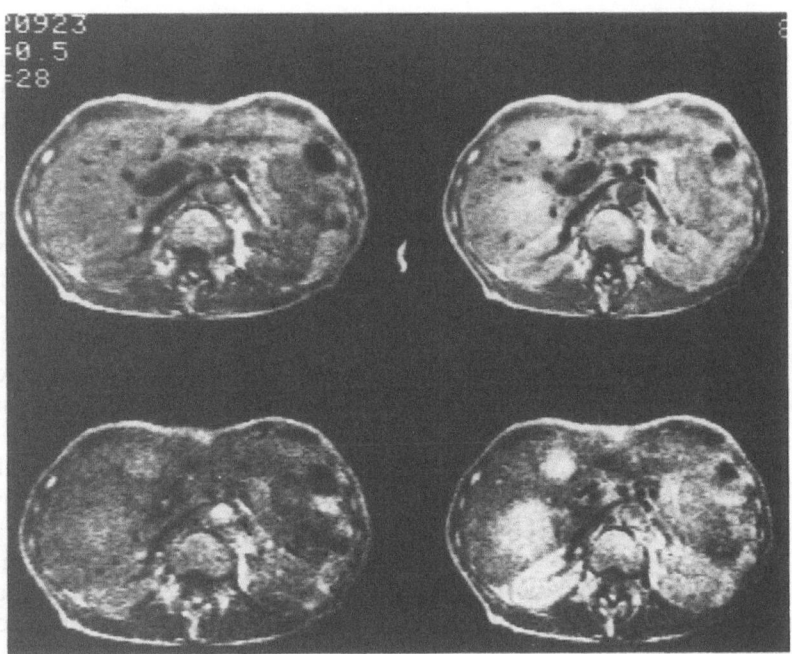

Fig. 23.14a–d. Metastatic carcinoid. **a** SE 500/28 image reveals distortion of the normal right portal vein anatomy but the tumor is isointense with the normal liver. **b** SE 500/56 image reveals two metastatic foci having a higher signal intensity than the liver. **c** SE 1000/28 image is barely able to detect the lesions. There is decreased spatial resolution on this image as compared with **a**. **d** SE 1000/56 image (the most T2 weighted) clearly reveals the metastatic foci although anatomical resolution is further degraded

ported that IR images had greater contrast than images obtained using the technique of partial-saturation recovery and provided the best tumor–liver contrast difference. Haaga et al. [39] comparing saturation-recovery, inversion-recovery, and calculated T1 images also felt that inversion and T1-weighted images were superior to saturation-recovery images. A recent comparison of spin-echo and IR techniques revealed some tumor to be better demonstrated by spin-echo techniques (Figs. 23.12–23.14).

Metastatic tumors are typically shown as masses of low intensity on IR and spin-echo sequences using short TR and TE intervals. IR images using different TR, TI and TE parameters alter the tumor–liver contrast with slightly improved contrast on images obtained using long TR, short TI, and short TE intervals. The center of the metastatic foci often has a longer T1 time than the periphery of the lesion and thus may appear as a mass having a low-intensity peripheral rim surrounding a center of higher intensity.

T1 and T2 relaxation times have been shown to vary between similar tumors in different patients and even among tumors of the same cell type in a single patient [4]. As in primary hepatic neoplasms, both T1 and T2 values of metastatic tumors are usually longer than those of normal hepatic tissue but probably vary slightly more than those found in HCC [4]. Although the average calculated T1 and T2 relaxation times of both primary and metastatic disease differ from those of the normal liver, there is sufficient overlap between the values such that a single T1 or T2 calculation or combination of relaxation time measurements has not yet proved to be specific for a particular hepatic neoplasm. The wide range of T1 and T2 relaxation times in primary and metastatic tumors probably reflects different degrees of tumor cellularity, hemorrhage, blood flow, necrosis, and water content superimposed upon the inaccuracy of many of the current measurements provided by clinical MR instruments. Although improved accuracy and precision of T1 and T2 measurements is anticipated, it appears unlikely that T1 and T2 measurements, either alone or in combination, will provide a specific diagnosis of malignant disease or differentiate between various metastatic lesions.

9 Comparison with computed tomography

There is growing anticipation that MR will become superior to computed tomography (CT) in the detection of primary and metastatic tumors of the liver. Current studies have demonstrated similar detection rates for the two technologies, although early MR imaging was compared with mature CT technology [4, 9, 14, 16, 28, 32, 40]. CT can best demonstrate calcified foci within tumors and assess blood flow after intravenous contrast injection. However, surgical clips produce artifacts on CT and direct coronal and sagittal images are not possible. MR best displays the relationship of the tumor to the hepatic vasculature and permits more precise localization of tumors within the liver. Internal architecture of tumors is more clearly displayed by MR

and in most cases surgical clips do not cause artifacts. Additional advantages of MR are the ability to obtain direct sagittal and coronal images and to distinguish blood vessels from bile ducts without contrast injection. Various paramagnetic contrast materials such as gadolinium-DTPA (diethylenetriamine pentaacetic acid) are undergoing initial evaluation and have the potential for further improving MR detection of hepatic tumors [20–23].

Tissue-specific paramagnetic contrast agents, such as paramagnetic iron complexes, nitroxides, and particulate contrast agents, have recently been described for use within the liver [22]. Iron has been bound to ethylenebis-2-hydroxyphenylglycine (EHPG), a analogue to the class of scintigraphic agents employed for nuclear medicine studies of biliary function and studied experimentally [22]. This prototype tissue-specific hepatobiliary agent has known a

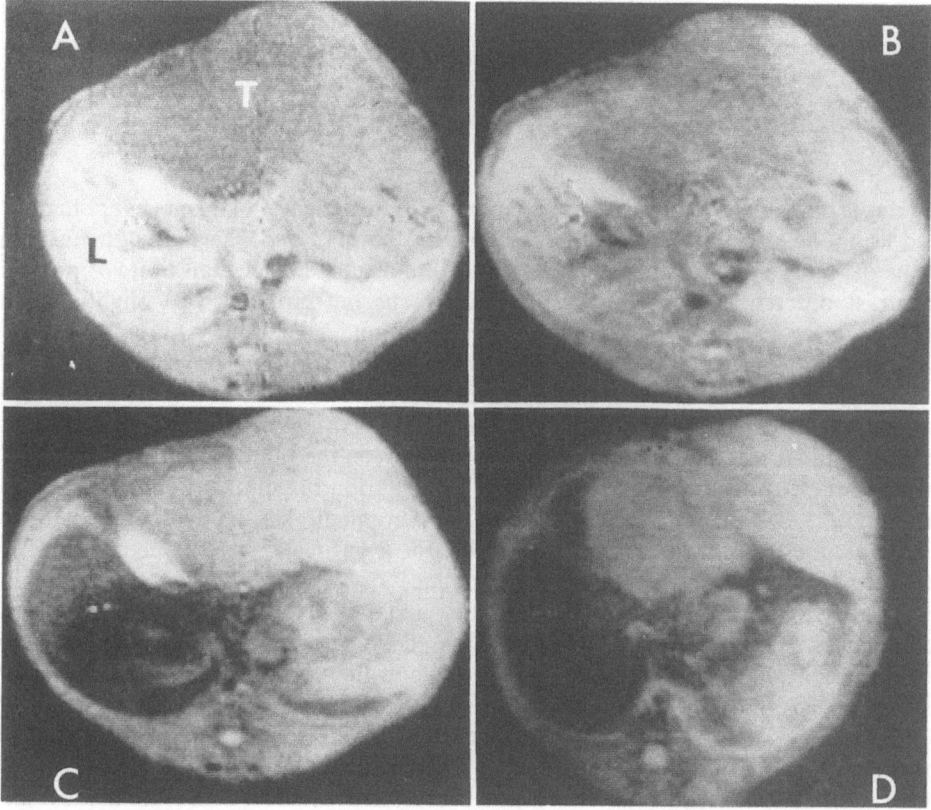

Fig. 23.15A–D. Rabbit model of metastatic liver cancer. V × 2 carcinoma implanted in left hepatic lobe. **A** SE 260/15/16 image shows tumor (*T*) as low signal-intensity mass due to long T1 relative to liver (*L*). **B** SE 500/30/8 image shows reduced tumor–liver contrast and decreased anatomical resolution. **C** SE 500/30/8 image following i.v. administration of magnetite. Particles shows marked decrease in liver signal intensity, no change in tumor signal, and, thus, increased tumor–liver contrast. **D** SE 1600/60/2 T2-weighted image shows complete loss of signal from the magnetite-enhanced normal liver, but a high signal from the tumor. This image has increased noise and motion artifacts due to the use of long TR and TE

Fig. 23.16. Hemochromatosis. An SE 1000/28 image in the axial and sagittal planes shows the marked loss of hepatic signal produced by excessive hepatic iron deposition

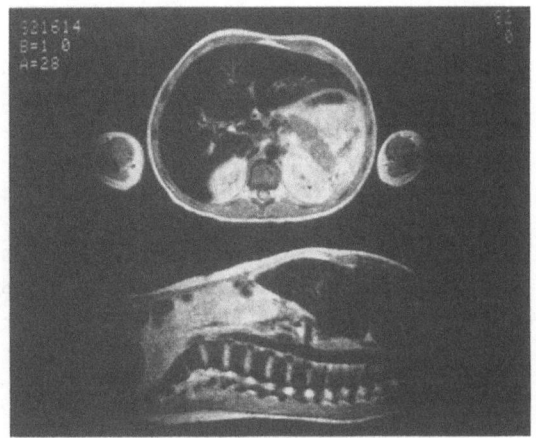

significant (6%) fraction of tissue-specific uptake and excretion by functioning hepatocytes [22]. This class of contrast agent may permit selective enhancement of functioning liver tissue, thereby improving detection of nonfunctioning hepatic tumors.

Investigation of particulate iron oxide MR contrast agents has shown them to have great tissue specificity. Iron oxide particles in the form of magnetite (Fe_3O_4) particles have been demonstrated to be selectively phagocytosed by the reticuloendothelial system of the liver and reduce the relaxation parameters of the liver and spleen. Magnetite particles are not phagocytosed by liver tumors as they lack reticuloendothelial cells; thus, magnetite selectively decreases the T2 of the normal liver, increasing tumor–liver contrast (Fig. 23.15).

10 Differential diagnosis

A variety of metabolic, inflammatory, toxic, and autoimmune disease processes produce hepatic abnormalities which must be differentiated from hepatic tumors. Imaging with MR has proved capable of detecting and characterizing a variety of these hepatic diseases.

10.1 Hepatitis

Prolongation of the T1 and T2 times of patients with proven hepatitis has been demonstrated using MR [41]. With spin-echo techniques, the involved liver appears more intense than the normal liver and histological sampling has shown that the most severe foci of hepatitis appear the most intense. Hepatitis experimentally produced in laboratory animals has been shown to alter markedly the MR signal intensity and

T1 and T2 relaxation times. It thus appear that MR imaging may be capable of detecting, and to some degree quantitating, hepatocellular damage from hepatitis. The degree to which concurrent hepatitis affects MR detection of hepatic tumors is unclear.

10.2 Steatosis

Standard spin-echo and inversion-recovery MR techniques have not proven sensitive to fatty infiltration of the liver [41, 42]. As hepatic T1 and T2 relaxation times are within the normal range for the liver, the MR images usually appear normal. However, recently developed chemical shift-imaging techniques which exploit the shift in resonant frequency (3.7 ppm) between fat and water protons have proven capable of detecting hepatic steatosis [12, 15, 16]. As most hepatic tumors do not contain large amounts of fat, the use of two-dimensional chemical-shift imaging may permit improved detection of hepatic tumors in patients with fatty liver (Figs. 23.4, 23.5).

10.3 Hemochromatosis

Excessive iron deposition in hepatic parenchymal cells produces a dramatic reduction in hepatic MR signal intensity (Fig. 23.16) [43, 44]. The reduced intensity of liver on T2-weighted spin-echo images is due to the reduction in T2 caused by hepatic parenchymal iron. Tissue iron is largely bound to ferritin and hemosiderin as crystalline iron oxyhydroxide [43]. In hydrogen MR imaging, the paramagnetic iron decreases the T2 relaxation time of nearby hydrogen nuclei. Thus, a liver with a very low intensity most likely reflects excessive hepatic iron deposition rather than hepatic malignancy.

10.4 Cirrhosis

Cirrhosis (hepatic fibrosis) has been difficult to detect using conventional spin-echo techniques, as it produces little or no change in hepatic relaxation time or hydrogen density [45]. Morphological changes, such as decreased liver size, surface irregularity, portal vein enlargement, and collateral circulation, have been seen in patients with cirrhosis [46]. The lack of focal mass lesions and intensity differences makes distinction between a cirrhotic nodule and a primary or secondary hepatic tumor relatively easy.

Clinical applications of MR imaging of the liver are in their infancy. As we learn more about the ultimate potential of MR imaging, some applications will become routine, while others will remain research techniques. Due to the complex interations between multiple biological parameters and technical features unique to first-generation MR-imaging instruments, it is too early to determine the ultimate clinical value of MR in hepatic imaging. It is highly probable that hepatic MR imaging will become an important tool in the evaluation of focal hepatic disease. With additional technical developments, MR imaging is likely to have a significant role in the clinical evaluation of many other hepatic diseases.

References

1. Doyle FH, Pennock JM, Banks LM, McDonnell MJ, Bydden GM, Steiner RE, Young IR, Clarke GJ, Pasmore T, Gilderdale DJ (1982) Nuclear magnetic resonance imaging of the liver: initial experience. AJR 138: 193–200
2. Borkowski GP, Buonocore E, George CR, Go RT, O'Donovan PB, Meaney TF (1983) Nuclear magnetic resonance (NMR) imaging in the evaluation of the liver: a preliminary experience. JCAT 7: 768–774
3. Margulis AR, Moss AA, Crooks LE, Kaufman L (1983) Nuclear magnetic resonance in the diagnosis of tumors of the liver. Seminars in Roentgenology 17: 123–126
4. Moss AA, Goldberg HI, Stark DD, Davis PL, Margulis AR, Kaufman L, Crooks LE (1984) Hepatic tumors: magnetic resonance and CT appearance. Radiology 150: 141–147
5. Bernardino ME, Small W, Goldstein J, Sewell CW, Sones PJ, Gedgaudas-McClees K, Galambos JT, Wenger J, Casarella WJ (1983) Multiple NMR T2 relaxation values in human liver tissue. AJR 141: 1203–1208
6. Ohtomo K, Itai Y, Furui S, Yashiro N, Yoshi-kawa K, Iilo M (1985) Hepatic tumors: differentiation by transverse relaxation time (T2) of magnetic resonance imaging. Radiology 155: 421–423
7. Fisher MR, Wall SD, Hricak H, McCarthy S, Kerlan RK (1985) Hepatic vascular anatomy on magnetic resonance imaging. AJR 144: 739–746
8. Young IR, Burl M, Bydder GM (1986) Comparative efficiency of different pulse sequences in MR imaging. JCAT 10: 271–286
9. Stark DD, Wittenberg J, Edelman RR, Middleton MS, Saini S, Butch RJ, Brady TJ, Ferrucci JT Jr (1986) Detection of hepatic metastases: analysis of pulse sequence performance in MR imaging. Radiology 159: 365–370
10. Wehrli FW, MacFall JR, Glover GH, Grigsby N (1984) Dependence of nuclear magnetic resonance imaging contrast on intrinsic and pulse sequence timing parameters. Magnetic Resonance Imaging 2: 3–16
11. Hendrick RE, Nelsen TR, Hendee WR (1984) Optimizing tissue contrast in magnetic resonance imaging. Magnetic Resonance Imaging 2: 193–204
12. Dixon WT (1984) Simple proton spectroscopic imaging. Radiology 153: 189–194
13. Bydder GM, Steiner RE, Blumgart LH, Khenia S, Young IR (1985) MR imaging of the liver using short T1 inversion recovery sequence. JCAT 9: 1084–1089
14. Stark DD, Wittenberg J, Middleton MS, Ferrucci JT Jr (1986) Liver metastases: detection by phase-contrast MR imaging. Radiology 158: 327–332
15. Rosen BR, Carter EA, Pykett IL, Buchbinder BR, Brady TJ (1985) Proton chemical shift imaging: an in vivo fatty liver model. Radiology 154: 469–472
16. Lee JKT, Keiken JP, Dixon WT (1985) Detection of hepatic metastases by proton spectroscopic imaging. Radiology 156: 429–433
17. Ehman RL, McNamara MT, Pallack M, Hricak H, Higgins CB (1984) Magnetic resonance imaging with respiratory gating: technique and advantages. AJR 143: 1175–1182
18. Runge VM, Clanton JA, Partain CL, James EA Jr (1984) Respiratory gating in magnetic resonance imaging at 0.5 Tesla. Radiology 151: 521–523
19. Edelman RR, McFarland E, Stark DD, Ferrucci J Jr, Simeone JF, Wismer G, White EM, Rosen BR, Brady TJ (1985) Surface coil MR imaging of abdominal viscera: I. Theory, technique, and initial results. Radiology 157: 425–430
20. Runge VM, Clanton JA, Lukehart CM, Partain CL, James AE Jr (1983) Paramagnetic agents for contrast-enhanced NMR imaging: a review. AJR 141: 1209–1215
21. Carr DH, Brown J, Bydder GM, Steiner RE, Weinmann H-J, Speck U, Hall AS, Young IR (1984) Gadolinium-DTPA as a contrast agent in MRI: initial clinical experience in 20 patients. AJR 143: 215–224
22. Lauffer RB, Grief WL, Stark DD, Vincent AC, Saini S, Wedeen VJ, Brady TJ (1985) Iron-EHPG as an hepatobiliary MR contrast agent: initial imaging and biodistribution studies. JCAT 9: 431–438

23. Grief WL, Buxton RB, Lauffer RB, Saini S, Stark DD, Wedeen VJ, Rosen BR, Brady TJ (1985) Pulse sequence optimization for MR imaging using a paramagnetic hepatobiliary contrast agent. Radiology 157: 461–466

24. vonSchulthess GK, Fisher M, Crooks LE, Higgins CBG (1985) Gated MR imaging of the heart: intracardiac signals in patients and healthy subjects. Radiology 156: 125–132

25. Bailes DR, Gilderdale DJ, Bydder GM, Collins AG, Firmin DN (1985) Respiratory ordered phase encoding (ROPE): a method for reducing respiratory motion artifacts in MR imaging. JCAT 9: 835–838

26. Vinocur B (1985) Motion-reduction software brightens outlook for body MRI. Diagnostic Imaging, pp 79–84

27. Pelc NJ, Glover GH, Charles HC (1985) Respiration artifacts in MRI. Proceedings Society of Magnetic Resonance in Medicine, August 19–23, 1985, London

28. Stark DD, Felder RC, Wittenberg J, Saini S, Butch RJ, White MR, Edelman RR, Mueller PR, Simeone JF, Cohen AM, Brady TJ, Ferrucci JT Jr (1985) Magnetic resonance imaging of cavernous hemangioma of the liver: tissue-specific characterization. AJR 145: 213–222

29. Fullerton GD, Cameron IL, Ord VA (1984) Frequency dependence of magnetic resonance spin-lattice relaxation of protons in biological materials. Radiology 151: 135–138

30. Johnson GA, Herfkens RJ, Brown MA (1985) Tissue relaxation time: in vivo field dependence. Radiology 156: 805–810

31. Vermess M, Leving AW-L, Bydder GM, Steiner RE, Blumgart LH, Young IR (1985) MR imaging of the liver in primary hepatocellular carcinoma. JCAT 9: 749–754

32. Ebara M, Ohto M, Watanabe Y, Kimurak, Saisho H, Tsuchiya Y, Okuda K, Arimizu N, Kondo F, Ikehira H, Fukuda N, Tateno Y (1986) Diagnosis of small hepatocellular carcinoma: correlation of MR imaging and tumor histologic studies. Radiology 159: 371–377

33. Dooms GC, Kerlan RK Jr, Hricak H, Wall SD, Margulis AR (1986) Cholangiocarcinoma: imaging by MR. Radiology 159: 89–94

34. Doons GC, Fisher MR, Higgins CB, Hricak H, Goldberg HI, Margulis AR (1986) MR imaging of the dilated biliary tract. Radiology 158: 337–341

35. Glazer GM, Aisen AM, Francis IR, Gyves JW (1985) Hepatic cavernous hemangioma: magnetic resonance imaging. Radiology 155: 417–420

36. Itai Y, Ohtomo K, Furui S, Yamauchi T, Minami M, Yashiro N (1985) Noninvasive diagnosis of small cavernous hemangioma of the liver: advantage of MRI. AJR 145: 1195–1199

37. Wilcox DM, Weinreb JC, Lesh P (1985) MR imaging of a hemorrhagic hepatic cyst in a patient with polycystic liver disease. JCAT 9: 183–185

38. Young IR, Bailes DR, Burl M, Collins AG, Smith DT, McDonnell MJ, Orr JS, Banks LM, Bydder BM, Greenspan RH, Steiner RE (1982) Initial clinical evaluation of a whole body nuclear magnetic resonance (NMR) tomograph. JCAT 6: 1

39. Haaga JR, Alfidi RJ, LiPuma JP, Bryan PJ, Yousef SJ (1982) NMR imaging of the liver. Presented at 68th Meeting of the Radiologic Society of North America, Chicago, 12 Jan, 1982

40. Heiken JP, Lee JK, Glazer HS, Ling D (1985) Hepatic metastases studied with MR and CT. Radiology 156: 423–427

41. Stark DD, Bass NM, Moss AA, Bacon BR, McKerrow JH, Cann CE, Brito A, Goldberg HI (1983) Nuclear magnetic resonance imaging of experimentally induced liver disease. Radiology 148: 743–751

42. Wenker JC, Baker MK, Ellis JH, Glant MD (1984) Focal fatty infiltration of the liver: demonstration by magnetic resonance imaging. AJR 143: 573–574

43. Stark DD, Moseley ME, Bacon BR, Moss AA, Goldberg HI, Bass NM, James TL (1985) Magnetic resonance imaging and spectroscopy of hepatic iron overload. Radiology 154: 137–142

44. Brasch RC, Wesbey GE, Gooding CA, Koerper MA (1984) Magnetic resonance imaging of transfusional hemosiderosis complicating thalassemia major. Radiology 150: 767–771

45. Goldberg HI, Moss AA, Stark DD, McKerrow J, Engelstad B, Brito A (1984) Hepatic cirrhosis: magnetic resonance imaging. Radiology 153: 737–739

46. Williams DM, Cho KJ, Aisen AM, Eckhauser FE (1985) Portal hypertension evaluated by MR imaging. Radiology 157: 703–706

Chapter 24

Chemotherapy of Primary Liver Cancer*

GEOFFREY FALKSON and BUKS COETZER[1]

1 Introduction

Despite the large number of patients throughout the world who die of primary liver cancer, the number of patients entered on carefully planned clinical trials from which valid conclusions can be drawn remains limited. Uncontrolled clinical trials conducted during the last 30 years have led to a degree of optimism about results that can be obtained with drugs as diverse as alloxan, 5-fluorouracil, and doxorubicin. Prospectively randomized stratified trials continue to show some activity for various agents (or agent combinations) but none of these give a predictable response rate of > 20%, and survival continues to be a function of the patient discriminants rather than be attributable to a specific drug regimen. Response can, however, occasionally be obtained without necessarily causing severe treatment morbidity. It can, therefore, be stated that the disease is not absolutely resistant to treatment by cancer chemotherapy. The response that can be achieved for a group of patients with standard available cancer chemotherapeutic agents or regimens is not, however, good enough. New treatment approaches and new drug trials should be the frontline approach for patients with advanced disease wherever possible.

In evaluating treatment regimens for patients with primary liver cancer, the response rate is of some value but survival time is a more accurate measure. Of particular importance in the past has been the now unacceptable technique of reporting the median duration of survival of responders compared with nonresponders [1]. Of

*In receipt of a grant from the National Cancer Association of South Africa
[1] Department of Medical Oncology, HF Verwoerd Hospital and University of Pretoria, Private Bag X169, Pretoria, 0001, Republic of South Africa

equal importance has been the exclusion from analysis of patients dying within the first weeks after being placed on treatment. To evaluate a treatment regimen, all patients entered on the regimen should be evaluated for determination of the median survival.

Although there is hope that the incidence of primary liver cancer could be significantly decreased by widespread immunization against the hepatitis-B virus, public health programs of immunization are unlikely to make significant inroads in the foreseeable future, and so clinical trials remain important. In Japan, and more rarely in other areas of the world, surgical resection with the hope of cure is performed for patients whose disease is diagnosed early. For the vast majority of patients with primary liver cancer, the hope for disease control (and possible eradication) must lie with oncolytic chemotherapy.

2 Discriminants

The chemotherapy of primary liver cancer must be seen in the light of known prognostic discriminants. The median survival time of patients with advanced primary liver cancer is usually about 2 months.

2.1 Performance status

Performance status (PS) remains one of the most consistent prognostically predictive discriminants. PS is defined as follows: O, normal activity; 1, symptoms, but the patient is ambulatory; 2, the patient is in bed < 50% of the time; 3, the patient is in bed > 50% of the time; and 4, the patient is 100% bedridden. The median survival time for patients with a PS of 0–1 is 22 weeks, whereas for patients with a PS of 2–3 the median survival time is 8 weeks. When bedridden patients are not included, the median overall survival time is about 10 weeks from the time of histological confirmation of the diagnosis. Among placebo-treated patients, decrease of liver volume has been observed and a survival time of longer than a year occasionally occurs in untreated patients [2]. Patients with a PS of 4 have a median life expectancy of less than 4 weeks. Any analysis of survival relative to treatment must take cognizance of the PS. Similarly, response rates on a treatment will be poorer if moribund patients are entered on that treatment.

2.2 Jaundice

Jaundice remains of prognostic significance. Anicteric patients have a median survival time that is two to four times longer than that of patients with an elevated serum bilirubin. Among South African patients, those with even a mild increase in serum bilirubin have a median survival time of 58 days, compared with 115 days for patients with a normal serum bilirubin level.

2.3 Sex

Sex has prognostic significance, with females having a median survival time about twice as long as that of males.

2.4 Age

The effect of age on prognosis is not consistent except when young children are included in the series and this may be due to some of them having hepatoblastomas.

2.5 Other clinical symptoms

Other clinical symptoms and findings are usually only of prognostic significance when they relate to hepatic failure. Apart from bilirubin, biochemical measurements are not of consistent prognostic significance. Increased alkaline phosphatase, decreased serum albumin, and increased serum globulin are associated with suggestively, but not significantly, shorter survival in our series of treated patients. Among African patients elevated alpha fetoprotein tends to be associated with a longer survival time. Hepatitis-B positivity has been associated with shorter survival in one series [3] and longer survival in another [4].

2.6 Histological type

Histological type is of prognostic significance with a high frequency of cases of liver invasion, portal vein involvement, and satellite formation having a poor prognosis [5]. Patients wih fibro-lamellar carcinoma have a significantly better prognosis. Among patients with primary liver cancer the degree of histological differentiation also plays a prognostic role. Of particular importance has been the review of the histological findings by a pathology panel as secondary carcinoma, misdiagnosed as primary liver cancer, is not a rare occurrence in low-incidence areas. Differentiation between cholangiocellular carcinoma and primary liver cancer can occasionally be difficult.

2.7 Spread within liver

The extent of spread within the liver and the volume and site of metastases are of obvious prognostic importance. The extent of spread within the liver is difficult to assess except in very early and very late stages of the disease and is dealt with elsewhere in this book. The prognostic and therapeutic implications of the new classification by gross anatomic features as proposed by Okuda et al. [6], is of great importance. The present chapter excludes, where possible, data from patients with encapsulated carcinomas (relatively common in Japan, rare in North America and South Africa), as well as the fibrosing varieties of expanding types of hepatocellular carcinoma.

2.8 Distal metastases

Distal metastases are of prognostic significance only if the anatomical location of the metastases affects the prognosis, and patients rarely die as a result of distal metastases.

2.9 Race

Race remains one of the contentious factors in prognosis. In prospective trials, the median survival time for South African patients has been poorer than that of North American patients in some series [7] but not in others [8]. The spectrum of disease in Japan further allows for therapeutic and prognostic implications to be drawn by a staging system not readily applicable in Africa and North America. In Japan, the median survival time for untreated patients with primary liver cancer was 1.6 months [9]. The median survival time of Malaysian patients with primary liver cancer was 18 weeks [10].

3 Chemotherapy

As the response to treatment is strongly influenced by the factors discussed above, prospective randomized studies give a more reliable impression of the value of a particular treatment than do uncontrolled studies.

3.1 Single agents

3.1.1 Alkylating agents

In controlled studies, no alkylating agent has been found to be of value in the treatment of patients with primary liver cancer. The alkylating agents include cyclophosphamide (CTX), triethyleneglycol diglycidylether, alanine mustard, DL-serine bis (2-chloropropyl) carbamate ester, bischlorethyl nitrosourea (BCNU), chloroethyl-cyclohexylnitrosourea (CCNU), and chloroethyl-methyl-cyclohexyl-nitrosourea (MeCCNU). Response rates with these drugs are <10% and the median survival time is comparable to that achieved with placebo.

3.1.2 Antimetabolites

Various antimetabolites have been tested and none have proved to be of value as single agents in the treatment of patients with primary liver cancer. The antimetabolites include methotrexate, 6-mercaptopurine, 5-fluorouracil, hydroxyurea, cytosine-arabinoside (Ara-C) and dichloromethotrexate. Although optimistic responses have been claimed in uncontrolled studies, in the large Eastern Cooperative Oncology Group (ECOG) study EST2273, none of 45 patients receiving oral 5-fluorouracil responded; median survival times were as follow: North American White patients—7.3 weeks; North American Black patients—14.7 weeks; and South African Black patients—3.1 weeks [7]. These results are similar to those with placebos; results from smaller uncontrolled trials are best ignored.

3.1.3 Plant alkaloids

Vincristine, vinblastine, and SPG 827, a podophyllin derivative, were found to be of no value in patients with primary liver cancer. Of 26 patients treated with VP-16-213, three achieved a partial remission, respectively, for 12, 16, and 35 weeks [11].

3.1.4 Other single agents

Diverse single agents that have been tested and found to be inadequate include dehydroemetine, procarbazine, cobalti-protoporhyrin complex, and butyryloxyethylglyoxal and dithiosemicarbazone. Table 24.1 shows response rates obtained

Table 24.1. Primary liver cancer—results in patients treated with m-AMSA

Number of patients	Response	Median survival (weeks)	Reference
35	1/35	11	12
26	0/26	11.6	8
33	3/33	NS	13
16	0/16	NS	14

NS not stated

with 4'-(9-acridinylamino)-methanesulfon-m-anisidide (m-Amsa). The response rates reported by Falkson et al. [8, 12], Bukowski et al. [13], and Cheng et al. [14] and the documented median survival times make it clear that this drug had no therapeutic value in primary liver cancer. Acivicin is at present undergoing clinical trial in patients with primary liver cancer.

3.1.5 Cis-diamino-dichloroplatinum

Cis-diamino-dichloroplatinum showed no therapeutic effect in patients with primary liver cancer in a study by Melia et al. [15], and in a subsequent ECOG study it showed a response in only 1 of 30 patients treated with this cytostatic drug.

3.1.6 Antibiotics and related substances

In this group of drugs, no therapeutic value was shown with mitomycin-C, actinomycin-D, carzinophyllin, and chromomycin-A3. Neocarzinostatin showed some promise in a phase II ECOG trial and was further investigated in a randomized clinical trial. Among 31 South African patients treated in these two studies, the median survival time was 12 weeks and the response rate was less than 20% [8].

The anthracyclines and their derivatices have been investigated extensively in patients with primary liver cancer and the results obtained with doxorubicin (ADM) are shown in Table 24.2. In the ECOG study EST 2273, the median survival time for North American/European patients was 12 weeks, while for Black South African patients it was 16 weeks [7]. In total, 146 patients were treated with doxorubicin in ECOG trials, with 16 responding to treatment [8]. Other trials using doxorubicin in the USA have shown response rates of 17% [16], 15% [17], and 11% [18]. Olweny et al. [19], however, reported response in 22 of 74 patients treated with doxorubicin in Uganda.

These and other reports confirm some activity for doxorubicin, but with too low a response rate

Table 24.2. Primary liver cancer—results in patients treated with doxorubicin (ADM)

Number of patients	Response	Median survival (weeks)	Reference
31	3/31	15	7
43[a]	5/43	—	8
46[b]	2/46	—	8
Uncontrolled trials			
41	7/41	NS	16
13	2/13	NS	17
52	6/52	NS	18
74	22/74	NS	19

NS not stated
[a] Previously untreated
[b] Pretreated

Table 24.3. Primary liver cancer—combination chemotherapy response

Cytostatic combination	Response (%)
Oral 5-FU + STZ	12
Oral 5-FU + MeCCNU	5
IV 5-FU + MeCCNU	
North American/European	13
South African Black	0
IV 5-FU + STZ	
North American/European	10
South African Black	0
IV 5-FU + MeCCNU + ADM	19

5-FU 5-fluorouracil, STZ streptozotocin, MeCCNU chloroethyl-methyl-cyclohexyl-nitrosourea, IV intravenous, ADM doxorubicin

and too poor a median survival time to justify its use as a single agent in this disease. Histological grading and other patient discriminants at the start of treatment further explain much of the response claimed in central Africa.

Mitoxantrone, an anthracenedione, was included in a trial by ECOG but showed no response in 34 patents, although a better median survival time was documented.

A doxorubicin analogue, 4'-epidoxorubicin, showed response in 3 of 18 patients, with a median survival time of 12.5 weeks [20]. It is too early to comment on the ongoing ECOG trial of esorubicin (4'-deoxydoxorubicin), though this seems promising.

3.2 Combination chemotherapy

There are no exceptions to the rule that nothing is gained by adding cytostatics that do not have single-agent activity to a drug combination regimen. This procedure leads to increased toxicity and necessitates a decrease of the amount of the therapeutically active agent that could be given at the same time. Various small series of uncontrolled trials of drug combinations in patients with primary liver cancer are reported in the literature; patient discriminants are ignored and the results claimed are best explained by variations in the natural history of the disease.

Among chemotherapy combinations tested and found to be ineffective are: (1) vincristine (VCR), methotrexate (MTX), 6-mercaptopurine (6MP), plus prednisone (Pred); (2) BCNU plus cytosine-arabinoside (Ara-C); (3) 5-fluorouracil (5-FU) plus thiotepa; (4) 5-FU plus mitomycin-C; (5) 5-FU, cyclophosphamide MTX, plus VCR [21–23]. In a randomized double-blind trial of

5-FU plus placebo versus 5-FU plus Ara-C, Gailani et al. [24] documented response in 1 of 22 patients with primary liver cancer treated with 5-FU plus Ara-C compared with a response in 1 of 16 patients treated with 5-FU plus placebo.

In the largest prospectively randomized controlled studies performed [2, 7, 22], the response rates shown in Table 24.3 were documented. These response rates vary from 0% to 19%, the latter being for the most toxic combination. Particularly significant was the severe toxicity encountered in patients treated with intravenous 5-FU + MeCCNU + ADM. The most finite measurement is median survival time and those for the ECOG studies are shown in Table 24.4. The median survival time according to these treatment combinations varied from 6.3 to 13 weeks.

After optimistic reports of the therapeutic effect of ADM for patients in Africa, combination chemotherapy incorporating ADM has been tried by various investigators and these results are shown in Table 24.5, the best reported being 5 of 38 patients on ADM plus 5-FU with none of the other combinations showing more than an occasional response.

4 Present status of chemotherapy

Until a more predictable and satisfactory response has been adequately documented for single agents, or adequate motivation can be found for combination chemotherapy in patients with primary liver cancer, it is not justified treating small groups of patients with drug combinations. The recommended approach is well-

Table 24.4. Primary liver cancer—median survival times on combination chemotherapy

Cytostatic combinations	North America/Europe		South Africa	
	No. of patients	Survival (weeks)	No. of patients	Survival (weeks)
Oral 5-FU + STZ	15 (White)	31.1	11	11.5
	5 (Black)	14.2		
Oral 5-FU + MeCCNU	21 (White)	26.1	13	6.3
	9 (Black)	15.1		
IV 5-FU + MeCCNU	45	28.0	10	8.0
IV 5-FU + STZ	40	22.0	9	8.0
5-FU + MeCCNU + ADM	32	17.0	6	13.0

5-FU 5-fluorouracil, *STZ* streptozotocin, *MeCCNU* chloroethyl-methyl-cyclohexyl-nitrosourea, *IV* intravenous, *ADM* doxorubicin

designed phase II trials of new agents.

The expanding knowledge about primary liver cancer as a disease will hopefully promote better clinical trials in the future as the science of medicine is placed on a sounder footing. Clinical trials remain essential in testing hypotheses generated by epidemiological and laboratory observations. Although no cytostatic agent has shown reproducible response rates of $\geq 20\%$ in patients with primary liver cancer, there are some agents with occasional activity and others that are totally inactive, allowing for a more logical choice of new drugs for clinical trials. Taking cognizance of our increasing knowledge of the biology of the disease and with many new agents that theoretically could have value, clinical trials in primary liver cancer can be approached with cautious optimism.

Table 24.5. Doxorubicin—containing cytostatic combinations in primary liver cancer

Combination	Response	Reference
ADM + 5-FU	5/38	25
ADM + *STZ*	2/23	26
ADM + MeCCNU	3/21	27
ADM + dichloromethotrexate	1/9	19
ADM + 5-azacytidine	1/6	19
ADM + ICRF 159	1/6	19
ADM + CTX	1/6	19

ADM doxorubicin, *5-FU* 5-fluorouracil, *STZ* streptozotocin, *MeCCNU* chloroethyl-methyl-cyclohexyl-nitrosourea, *ICRF 159* rauoxane, *CTX* cyclophosphamide

References

1. Anderson JR, Cain KC, Gelber RD, Gelman RS (1985) Analysis and interpretation of the comparison of survival by treatment outcome variables in cancer clinical trials. Cancer Treat Rep 69: 1139–1144
2. Geddes EW Falkson G (1970) Malignant hepatoma in the Bantu. Cancer 25(6): 1271–1278
3. Chlebowski RT, Tong M, Weissman J, Block JB, Ramming KP, Weiner JM, Bateman JR, Chlebowski JS (1984) Hepatocellular carcinoma: Diagnostic and prognostic features in North American patients. Cancer 53: 2701–2706
4. Falkson G, Böhmer RH, Adam M, Coetzer BJ (1985) Hepatitis-B as a prognostic discriminant in patients with primary liver cancer. Cancer (in press)
5. Hsu H, Sheu J, Lin Y, Chen D, Lee C, Hwang L, Beasley RP (1985) Prognostic histologic features of resected small hepatocellular carcinoma (HCC) in Taiwan. A comparison with resected large HCC. Cancer 56: 672–680
6. Okuda K, Peters RL, Simson IW (1984) Gross anatomic features of hepatocellular carcinoma from three disparate geographic areas. Proposal of new classification. Cancer 54: 2165–2173
7. Falkson G, Moertel CG, Lavin P, Pretorius FJ, Carbone PP (1978) Chemotherapy studies in primary liver cancer. Cancer 42(5): 2149–2156
8. Falkson G, MacIntyre J, Coetzer B, Schutt AJ, Engstrom PF, Carbone PP (1984) Phase II–III trial of neocarzinostatin versus m-Amsa or adriamycin in hepatocellular carcinoma. J Clin Oncol 2(6): 581–584
9. Okuda K, Ohtsuki T, Obata H, Tomimatso M, Okazaki M, Hasegawa H, Makajima Y, Ohnishi K (1985) Natural history of hepatocellular carcinoma and prognosis in relation to treatment. Cancer 56: 918–928
10. Joishy SK, Bennett JM, Balasegaram M, MacIntyre JM, Falkson G, Moertel C, Carbone PP (1982) Clinical and chemotherapeutic study of hepatocellular carcinoma in Malaysia: A comparison with African and American patients. Cancer 50(6): 1065–1069

11. Cavalli F, Rozenzweig M, Renard J, Goldhirsch A, Hansen HH (1981) Phase II study of oral VP-16-213 in hepatocellular carcinoma. Eur J Cancer Clin Oncol 17(10): 1079–1082

12. Falkson G, Coetzer B, Klaassen DJ (1981) A phase II study of m-Amsa in patients with primary liver cancer. Cancer Chemother Pharmacol 6: 127–129

13. Bukowski RM, Legha S, Saiki J, Eyre HJ, O'Bryan R (1982) Phase II trial of m-Amsa in hepatocellular carcinoma. A Southwest Oncology Group Study. Cancer Treat Rep 66: 1651–1652

14. Cheng E, Lightdale C, Young C, Yagoda A, Fortner J, Golbey R (1983) Phase II trial of (m-AMSA) 4'-9-(acridinylamino)-methanesulfon-m-anisidide in primary liver cancer. Am J Clin Oncol 6: 211–213

15. Melia WM, Westaby D, Wilhams R (1981) Diammino-dichloride platinum (cis-platinum) in the treatment of hepatocellular Carcinoma. J Clin Oncol 7: 275–280

16. Vogel CL, Bayley AC, Brocker RJ et al. (1977) A phase II study of adriamycin (NSC 123127) in patients with hepatocellular carcinoma from Zambia and the United States. Cancer 39: 1923–1929

17. Ihde DC, Kane RC, Cohen MH, McIntyre KR, Minna JD (1977) Adriamycin therapy in American patients with hepatocellular carcinoma. Cancer Treat Rep 61(7): 1385–1387

18. Chlebowski RT, Brzechwa-Adjukiewicz A, Cowden, Block JB, Tong M, Chan KK (1982) Full dose adriamycin in hepatocellular carcinoma: Clinical and pharmacokinetic results. Proc AACR 23: 110

19. Olweny CL, Katongole-Mbidde E, Bahendeka S, Otim D, Mugerwa J, Kyalwazi S K (1980) Further experience in treating patients with hepatocellular carcinoma in Uganda. Cancer 46: 2717–2722

20. Hochster HS, Green MD, Speyer S, Fazzini E, Blum R, Muggia FM (1985) 4'-Epidoxorubicin (epirubicin): Activity in hepatocellular carcinoma. J Clin Oncol 3(11): 1535–1540

21. Lee Yeu Tsu M (1977) Systemic and regional treatment of primary carcinoma of the liver. Cancer Treat Rev 4: 195–212

22. Falkson G, McIntyre JM, Moertel CG, Johnson LA, Scherman RC (1984) Primary liver cancer— An Eastern Cooperative Oncology Group Trial. Cancer 54: 970–977

23. Cochrane AMG, Murray-Lyon IM, Brinkley DM, Williams R (1977) Quadruple chemotherapy versus radiotherapy in treatment of primary hepatocellular carcinoma. Cancer 40: 609

24. Gailani S, Holland JF, Falkson G, Leone L, Burningham R, Larson V (1972) Comparison of treatment of metastatic gastrointestinal cancer with 5-fluorouracil (5-FU) to a combination of 5-FU with cytosine-arabinoside. Cancer 29: 1308–1313

25. Baker LH, Saiki JH, Jones SE, Hewlett JS, Brownlee RW, Stephens RL, Vartkevicius VK (1977) Adriamycin and 5-fluorouracil in the treatment of advanced hepatoma: A Southwest Oncology Group Study. Cancer Treatment Reports 61(8): 1595–1597

26. Morstyn G, Ihde DC, Eddy JL, Bunn PA, Cohen MH, Minna JD (1982) Combination chemotherapy with doxorubicin and streptozotocin (DXC/STZ) in hepatocellular carcinoma (HC). Proc AACR 23: 133

27. Chlebowski RT, Chan KK, Tong MJ, Weiner JM, Ryden VMJ, Bateman JR (1981) Adriamycin and methyl-CCNU combination therapy in hepatocellular carcinoma. Cancer 48: 1088–1095

Chapter 25

Arterial Embolization in the Treatment of Hepatocellular Carcinoma

Kunio Okuda[1], Kunihiko Ohnishi[1], and Kenichi Takayasu[2]

Transcatheter arterial embolization (TAE) has been used in the management of arterial bleeding [1–3] and abdominal neoplasms [4–6] since 1975. This modality was first introduced by Yamada et al. in Japan for the treatment of inoperable hepatocellular carcinoma (HCC) in 1978 [7]. It has since completely replaced the earlier modality of choice, intra-arterial one-shot (bolus dose) chemotherapy [8], in this country.

After acquiring some experience with TAE, we used microencapsulated (mc) mitomycin C (MMC) [9], which was developed by Kato et al. [10], with the rationale that these capsules would embolize small arteries supplying the cancer and effect a slow release of the chemotherapeutic agent within the tumor. We further modified this so-called chemoembolization in such a way that it is followed by conventional TAE, in which large embolizing particles are used. Thus, MMC released from the microcapsules would not be immediately washed away by the incoming arterial blood. In this chapter, the procedures, results, and complication of these modalities are discussed.

1 Techniques for transcatheter arterial embolization

The procedure is essentially the same as Seldinger's technique for celiac angiograhy. A polyethylene catheter is introduced into the femoral artery via a stab wound under local anesthesia and guided superselectively into either the right or left proper hepatic artery. For TAE, gelatin sponge (Gelfoam, Upjohn) cut into 1 × 1-mm particles is injected until major arterial branches supplying the tumor are occluded and tumor stains disappear (Fig. 25.1a–c). The Gelfoam particles may or may not be permeated with MMC or Adriamycin (20 mg). At the beginning of our experience with this procedure, contrast medium was also added to the particles in order to see whether the tumor would receive more particles than noncancerous areas.

For chemoembolization, mcMMC, the core of which consists of 80% MMC and the shell 20% ethyl cellulose (containing 20 mg MMC), was suspended in 20 ml saline and infused into the feeding arteries (Fig. 25.2). In some patients, mcMMC was first injected and TAE was then carried out additionally.

2 Changes following embolization

As long as the target HCC is supplied by arteries, occlusion of feeding arteries causes an anoxic state of the tumor and leads to tumor necrosis. This effect is particularly evident if the target HCC is of the expanding type, which is usually encapsulated in Japan [11] and in Taiwan, where more than 80% of small HCCs are encapsulated [12]. The interior is completely necrotized (Fig. 25.3) and, in due time, liquefies. However, the capsule is supplied by both arteries and portal branches, and tumor cells in and around the capsule remain viable [13]. Therefore, if the tumor is thought to be encapsulated, eradication of cancer cells in the capsule should be attempted as the second aim, for which other treatment modalities may be used, such as radiation and transcatheter embolization of the feeding portal veins. In most cases, the cancer cells remaining in the capsule resist treatment and cause late spread within the liver.

These histopathological changes may be seen indirectly by imaging. After embolization, the necrotic area of the tumor is no longer enhanced by contrast CT (Fig. 25.4) [14], and gas often

---

[1] First Department of Medicine, Chiba University School of Medicine, Inohana, Chiba, 280 Japan
[2] Department of Diagnostic Radiology, National Cancer Hospital, Tsukiji, Tokyo, 104 Japan

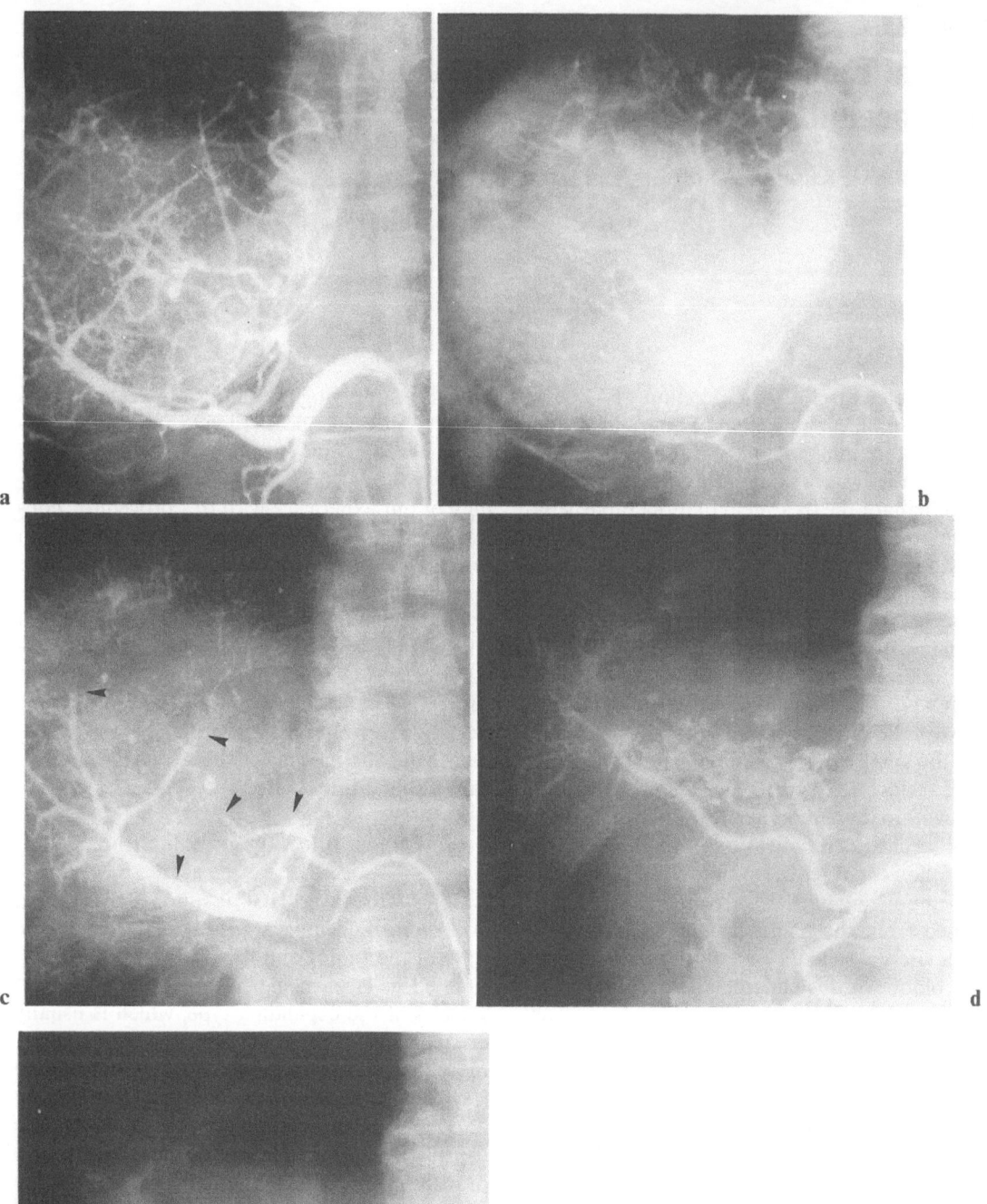

Fig. 25.1. a A large expanding HCC is apparent on this arteriogram. **b** Late-phase arteriogram demonstrating a large tumor stain, with some of the tumor vessels within the mass still containing contrast medium. **c** Immediately after embolization with Gelfoam particles; medium-sized feeding arteries are occluded (*arrowheads*). **d** Nine months after TAE; the previously large mass has regressed with diminution of the size of arteries (arterial phase). **e** Capillary phase film showing a tumor stain, which delineates the exact size of the mass

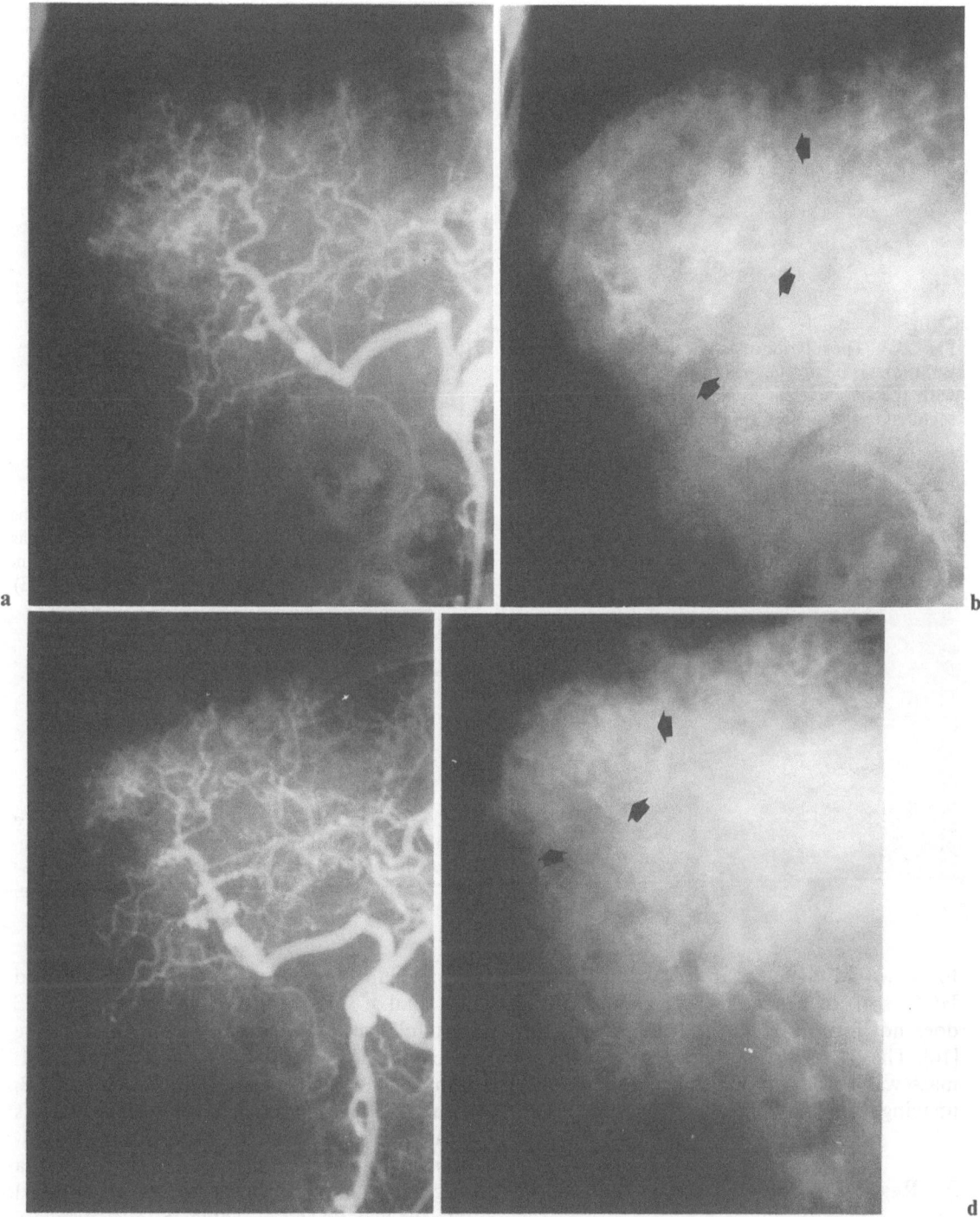

Fig. 25.2. a A hypervascular area is seen in the anterior superior subsegment of the right lobe. **b** A capillary phase film reveals an egg-shaped tumor stain (*arrows*). **c** Five weeks after chemoembolization with MMC microcapsules; note the reduction in the size of the hypervascular area compared with **a**. **d** The capillary phase film corresponding to film **b**. Reduction in the size of the stain is evident (*arrows*)

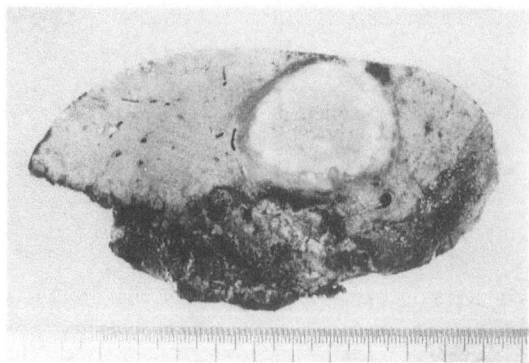

Fig. 25.3. The interior of an encapsulated HCC in the right lobe is completely necrotized, but the boundary with the parenchyma to the *left* is not in this liver segment resected after TAE. *Scale* in millimeters

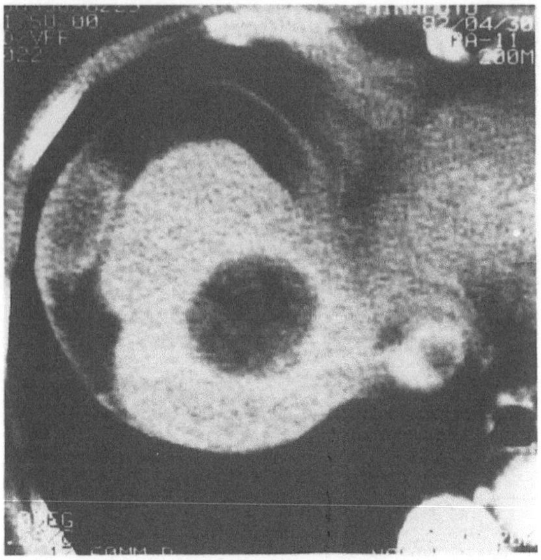

Fig. 25.4. An encapsulated HCC in the right lobe immediately below the diaphragm; it now contains gas on CT scan and no longer receives contrast medium following contrast enhancement (2 weeks after TAE)

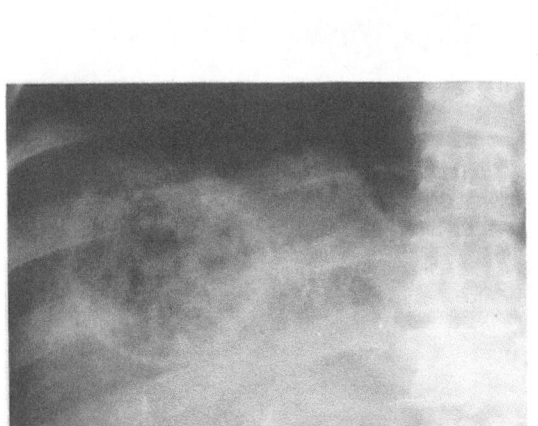

Fig. 25.5. The same HCC as in Fig. 25.4 is seen as a tumor stain following celiac angiography. This encapsulated HCC is clearly outlined and contains gas

forms within the tumor in 1–2 weeks [15] if the HCC is of the expanding type (Fig. 25.5); gas does not form in spreading (infiltrative) HCC [16]. The effect of TAE becomes evident if the mass was reduced in size during follow-up by imaging (Fig. 25.1d, e).

3 Results

TAE alone was carried out in 112 patients with unresectable HCC. Of these, 41 were in stage I, 64 in stage II, and 7 in stage III (for staging of HCC, see Chap. 33 and Okuda et al. [16]). Analysis of the results showed that TAE significantly prolonged survival in patients with stage II HCC, as shown in Fig. 25.6, but not in patients with stage I and III HCC. mcMMC chemoembolization was carried out in 32 patients. TAE

combined with other procedures was performed in a total of 34 patients who were given mcMMC first, followed by TAE. Another 22 patients were given mcMMC first, followed by 20 mg Adriamycin intra-hepatic arterially, and then TAE, Table 25.1 gives the median survivals of patients treated with these three different treatment modalities in comparison with 222 patients in whom a single bolus dose of 20 mg MMC was injected into the hepatic artery. Table 25.1 also provides the survival data published by other investigators for reference [16–22]. Although the staging of these patients was not uniform, making an exact comparison difficult, a marked difference between two modalities, such as mcMMC + TAE versus systemic chemotherapy, and intra-arterial bolus dose chemotherapy and mcMMC alone, may be significant.

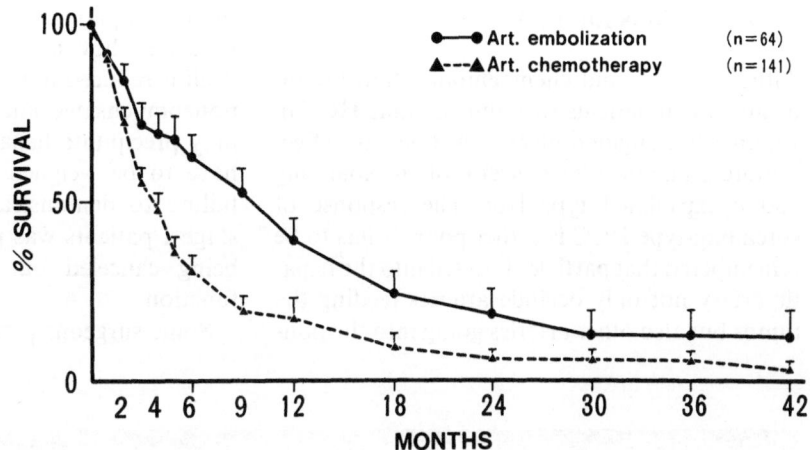

Fig. 25.6. The actuarial survival curves for 64 stage II patients with HCC who were treated by TAE and for 141 state II patients who were given MMC or Adriamycin intra-arterially. The differences are significant for the period from 3 to 18 months

Table 25.1. Survival rates in patients with hepatocellular carcinoma given various types of treatment

Author	No. of cases	Treatment	Median survival (mo.)	Survival 1 year	(%) at 2 year
Okuda, et al [16]	229	None	1.6		
Kew, et al [17]	585	None	1.5		
Sciarrino, et al [18]	107	Systemic ADM		13.0	
Okuda [19]	134	Various modes of chemotherapy	6.4		
Sawa [20]	100	Single intra-arterial bolus of 10–30 mg of MMC or 40–100 mg of ADM alone, or combined with 100 mg of 5-FU	5.5	13.0	
Yamada, et al [21]	120	Embolization of the hepatic artery with gelfoam mixed with 10 mg of MMC or 20 mg of ADM		44	29
Ohishi, et al [22]	97	Intra-arterial bolus of Ethiodol-MMC or ADM followed by embolization of hepatic artery with gelfoam		69	
Current study	52	Single intra-arterial bolus injection of 20 mg of MMC	3.4	8.8	5.9
	32	Single intra-arterial bolus of 20 mg of mcMMC	7.2	16.9	4.3
	34	Single intra-arterial bolus of 20 mg of mcMMC followed by embolization of hepatic artery with gelfoam	12.1	51.2	32.3
	22	Single intra-arterial bolus of 20 mg of mcMMC and 20 mg of ADM followed by embolization of hepatic artery with gelfoam	10.4	46.9	31.2

MMC mitomycin C, *ADM* adriamycin, *FU* fluorouracil

4 Indications for TAE

Although TAE and chemoembolization are indicated in all patients with unresectable HCC in whom celiac angiography can be done, the effect is more dramatic if the cancer is of an expanding and encapsulated type [16]. The response of spreading-type HCC is rather poor. It has to be remembered that particles injected into the hepatic artery not only occlude arteries feeding the tumor but also other arteries going into the non-tumorous parenchyma. Some of the liver function tests show poorer results and liver function itself is reduced to some extent. In patients with noncompensated and advanced cirrhosis, TAE may precipitate hepatic failure, and such risks have to be weighed against the benefits. Our failure to demonstrate a therapeutic effect in stage I patients was perhaps due to the benefit being canceled out by aggravation of liver function.

Some surgeons prefer TAE as a preoperative

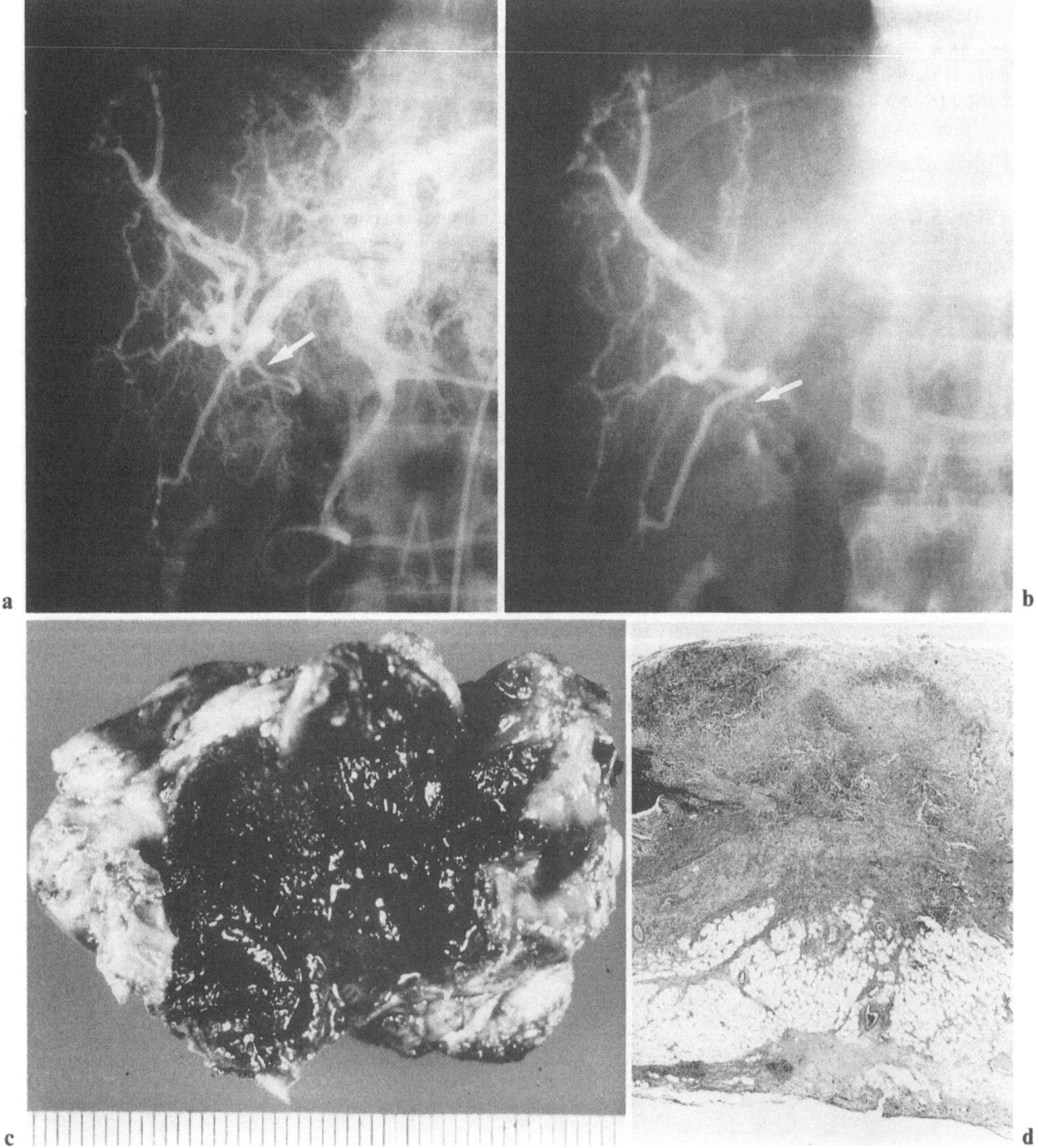

Fig. 25.7a–d

procedure, the rationale being that spread of cancer cells during the operation may be prevented. A national study conducted with the aim of determining an adequate time interval between TAE and surgery suggested that it takes about 3 weeks before the liver recovers from TAE-induced injury.

5 Side effects and complications

Shortly after TAE, high fever almost always develops (96% of cases) and last for a few days. The second common side effect is abdominal pain (68%); other complaints that follow TAE include anorexia (61%), increase of ascites (21%), elevation of serum aminotransferases (18%), and reduction in the formed elements of the blood (10%–21%). The decrease in the counts of red blood cells, white blood cells, and platelets is due to the chemotherapeutic agents rather than to embolization itself. With mcMMC chemoembolization alone, these side effects are less frequent and much milder.

5.1 Embolization of cystic artery

As long as the catheter tip is proximal to the origin of the cystic artery, injected particles can enter and occlude this artery (Fig. 25.7a, b), resulting in necrotizing ulcerative cholecystitis. The patient complains of a right upper quadrant pain of varying degree. It seems that a considerable proportion of abdominal pain following TAE is due to cystic arterial embolism. However, emergency surgery is seldom required. According to Takayasu et al. [23], 10 of 19 TAE procedures caused inadvertent occlusion of the cystic artery, and nine of ten patients in whom the gallbladder was removed during hepatic resection demonstrated necrotizing ulcerative cholecystitis (Fig. 25.7c, d).

◀ **Fig. 25.7. a** Celiac angiogram demonstrating an advanced and unresectable HCC in the left lobe and smaller lesions in the right lobe. The *arrow* points to the origin of the cystic artery. **b** TAE was carried out with Gelfoam particles, and the right and left hepatic arteries were occluded, with some contrast medium still remaining in the right hepatic artery. Note the occlusion of the cystic artery (*arrow*). **c** Resected gallbladder showing a thickened wall and a necrotic and hemorrhagic mucosa. **d** Section of the gallbladder wall, showing bleeding and necrosis across the entire thickness of the wall. H and E, × 10

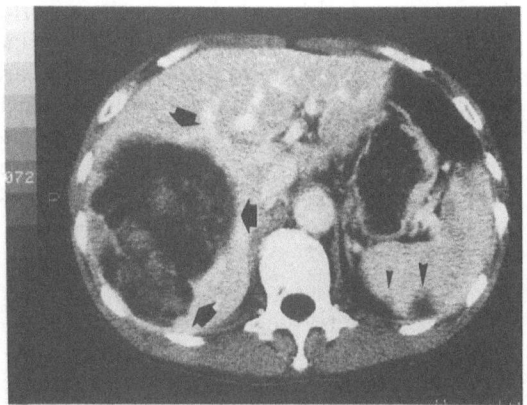

Fig. 25.8. CT scan with enhancement made 8 days after TAE. A large low-density mass (*arrows*) is apparent. Two wedge-shaped low-density lesions are also recognized in the spleen (*arrowheads*), representing infarcts due to embolization resulting from regurgitation of Gelfoam particles that are primarily intended for occlusion of hepatic arteries

5.2 Splenic infarction

After the TAE procedure before withdrawal of the catheter, repeat angiography is carried out to obtain angiograms for comparison with the pre-TAE angiograms. During this procedure, in which contrast medium is injected under pressure, some of the embolizing Gelfoam particles regurgitate and enter the splenic artery. Takayasu et al. [24] described five such cases out of 37 patients who received TAE treatment. Three patients complained of a dull pain in the left upper quadrant shortly after TAE. CT scan of the spleen after the procedure showed wedge-shaped low-density areas (Fig. 25.8), which slowly decreased in size.

6 Summary and discussion

TAE is the current choice in the treatment of unresectable HCC, particularly of the expanding type, in Japan, and it will be so in other Asiatic countries in the near future. The therapeutic efficacy is now well-established in comparison with systemic and intra-arterial bolus dose chemotherapy. mcMMC and iodized oil contrast medium (Lipiodol) containing a chemotherapeutic agent (such as SMANCS, see Chap. 27) are based on the same principle, namely to occlude feeding arteries on which HCC is totally dependent. The fibrous capsule often present at the boundary of an expanding HCC and the parenchyma is supplied by arteries as well as portal veins, and tumor cells remain viable in and around the capsule. Additional measures are needed to kill tumors cells in the capsule, which will cause subsequent spread. Since complete sure of HCC cannot be expected with TAE alone, it has to be combined with other modes of treatment in order to prolong survival further.

References

1. Chuang VP, Reuter SR, Walter J, Foley WD, Bookstein JJ (1975) Control of renal hemorrhage by selective arterial embolization. Am J Roentgenol 125: 300–306
2. Goldstein HM, Medellin H, Ben-Menachem Y, Wallace S (1975) Transcatheter arterial embolization in the management of bleeding in the cancer patinet. Radiology 115: 603–608
3. Jander HP, Laws HL, Kogutt MS, Mihas AA (1977) Emergency embolization in blunt hepatic trauma. Am J Roentgenol 129: 249–252
4. Goldstein HM, Medellin H, Beydoun MT, et al. (1975) Transcatheter embolization of renal cell carcinoma. Am J Roentgenol 123: 577–562
5. Hlava A, Steinhart L, Navratil P (1976) Intraluminal obliteration of the renal arteries in kidney tumors. Radiology 121: 323–329
6. Goldstein HM, Wallace S, Anderson JH, Bree RL, Gianturco C (1976) Transcatheter occlusion of abdominal tumors. Radiology 120: 539–545
7. Yamada R, Nakatsuka H, Nakamura K, Mizuguchi K, Yamaguchi S, Sato M, Miyamoto T, Tamaki M (1978) Transcatheter arterial embolization therapy in 29 patients with various malignancies. J Jpn Coll Angiol (Tokyo) 18: 563–571
8. Kubo Y, Shimokawa Y (1976) Arterial injection chemotherapy. In: Okuda K, Peters RL (eds) Hepatocellular carcinoma. Wiley, New York, pp 477–490
9. Ohnishi K, Tsuchiya S, Nakayama T, et al. (1984) Arterial chemoembolization of hepatocellular carcinoma with mitomycin C microcapsules. Radiology 152: 51–55
10. Kato T, Nemoto R, Mori H, Takahashi M, Tamakawa Y, Harada M (1980) Sustained-release properties of microencapsulated mitomycin C with ethylcellulose infused into the renal artery of the dog. Cancer 46: 14–21
11. Okuda K, Musha H, Nakajuma Y, Kubo Y, Shimokawa Y, Nagasaki Y, Sawa Y, Jinnouchi S, Obata H, Hisamitsu T, Okazaki N, Kojiro M, Sakamoto K, Nakashima T (1977) Clinicopathologic features of encapsulated hepatocellular carcinoma. A study of 26 cases. Cancer 40: 1240–1245
12. Hsu HC, Sheu JC, Lin YH, Chen DS, Lee CS, Hwang LY, Beasley RP (1985) Prognostic histologic features of resected small hepatocellular carcinoma (HCC) in Taiwan. A comparison with resected large HCC. Cancer 56: 672–680
13. Sakurai M, Okamura J, Kuroda C (1984) Transcatheter chemo-embolization effective for treating hepatocellular carcinoma. A histopathologic study. Cancer 54: 387–392
14. Takayasu K, Moriyama N, Muramatsu Y, Suzuki M, Yamada T, Kishi H, Hasegawa H, Okazaki N (1984) Hepatic arterial embolization for hepatocellular carcinoma. Comparison of CT scans and resected specimens. Radiology 150: 661–665
15. Furui S, Otomo K, Itai Y, Iio M (1984) Hepatocellular carcinoma treated by transcatheter arterial embolization: progress evaluated by computer tomography. Radiology 150: 773–778
16. Okuda K, Ohtsuki T, Obata H, Tomimatsu M, Okazaki N, Hasegawa H, Nakajima Y, Ohnishi K (1985) Natural history of hepatocellular carcinoma and prognosis in relation to treatment. Study of 850 patients. Cancer 56: 918–928
17. Kew MC, Geddes EW (1982) Hepatocellular carcinoma in rural southern African blacks. Medicine 61: 98–108
18. Sciarrino E, Sigmonetti RG, Moli S, Gagliaro L (1985) Adriamycin treatment for hepatocellular carcinoma. Experience with 109 patients. Cancer 56: 2751–2755
19. Okuda K (1976) Clinical aspects of hepatocellular carcinoma—analysis of 134 cases. In: Okuda, Peters RL (eds) Hepatocellular carcinoma. Wiley, New York, pp 384–436
20. Sawa Y (1979) Treatment of hepatocellular carcinoma by one shot injection of anticancer agents through the hepatic artery. Acta Hepatol Jpn 20: 852–960
21. Yamada R, Sato M, Kawabata M, Nakatsuka H, Nakamura K, Takashima S (1983) Hepatic artery embolization in 120 patients with hepatocellular carcinoma. Radiology 148: 397–401
22. Ohishi H, Uchida H, Yoshimura H, Ohue S, Ueda J, Katsuragi M, Matsuo N, Hosogi Y (1985) Hepatocellular carcinoma detected by iodized oil: use of anticancer agents. Radiology 154: 25–29
23. Takayasu K, Moriyama N, Muramatsu Y, Shima Y, Ushio T, Kishi K, Hasegawa H (1985) Gallbladder infarction after hepatic artery embolization. Am J Roentgenol 144: 135–138
24. Takayasu K, Moriyama N, Muramatsu Y, Suzuki M, Ishikawa T, Ushio K, Matsue H, Sasagawa M, Yamada T (1984) Splenic infarction, a complication of transcatheter hepatic arterial embolization for liver malignancies. Radiology 151: 371–375

Chapter 26

Radiation Therapy and Percutaneous Ethanol Injection for the Treatment of Hepatocellular Carcinoma

MASAO OHTO, MASAAKI EBARA, MASAHARU YOSHIKAWA and KUNIO OKUDA[1]

Most hepatocellular carcinomas (HCCs) develop in a liver with cirrhosis, which is unfavorable for surgical treatment. In the Far East, particularly in Japan, cirrhosis is often advanced at the time of tumor detection. The current choice of therapeutic modality is transcatheter arterial embolization (TAE), which, if properly executed in patients with moderately advanced HCC, significantly prolongs survival (Chap. 25). It does not afford complete cure, however. TAE necrotizes the arterial blood-dependent HCC, but cancer cells remain viable in the periphery of an expanding HCC, the most common gross type, and later cause intrahepatic spread.

A large-dose irradiation of the liver causes so-called radiation hepatitis [1–3], and radiation therapy was almost abandoned at one time because it was thought to be ineffective [4, 5]. Attempts have been made more recently to deliver radioactive particles [6, 7] and immunoglobulin [8, 9] directly into the hepatic artery, to implant radioactive seeds in the liver [10], and to combine chemotherapy with radiation [11–13]. We recently reevaluated external radiation therapy using the linear accelerator and found it to be effective in a considerable proportion of patients with HCC, though the effects were often unpredictable. It may also serve the purpose of destroying those cancer cells remaining in the capsule of HCC after TAE. Despite the frequent early detection of HCC in recent years [14, 15], these small HCCs are very difficult to treat because of the coexistent advanced cirrhosis. Therefore, we devised a new therapeutic procedure in which absolute ethanol is injected into the tumor percutaneously with the intention of destroying the entire mass by coagulation. In this chapter, we will discuss these two different modalities.

1 Radiation therapy

A total of 39 patients with HCC were treated by irradiation; all had associated cirrhosis. The size of the main mass was less than 3 cm in 11 patients, 3–5 cm in 15, and larger than 5 cm in 13. Tumor thrombi were seen in the major portal vein in four patients. All the patients were given external X-irradiation by the linear accelerator, 200 rads tissue dose/day in two opposing or right-angle fields, as determined by ultrasound (US) and CT imaging, five times a week, or 400 rads/day every other day, for a total dose of 3000–5000 rads.

1.1 Results

Changes in tumor size were assessed by CT or US and calculated as percentages by the equation: $(a \times b - a' \times b'/a \times b) \times 100$ (%), where a and b are the largest longitudinal and transverse axes before irradiation; a' and b' are the same after irradiation. As shown in Fig. 26.1, there occurred a more than 25% tumor regression in 90% of HCCs smaller than 5 cm and a more than 50% regression in 55%. Of the 12 patients with HCC larger than 5 cm, there was a more than 50% regression in seven (58%) of them but four died within 12 months due to metastases. Figure 26.2 illustrates tumor regression in a patient with an expanding HCC slightly larger than 5 cm, following irradiation with 5000 rads. Tumor regression was generally a slow process, as seen in Fig. 26.1. Serum alpha-fetoprotein was quickly reduced in patients with high preirradiation levels. On repeat angiography, the vascularity was reduced, the size of tumor stain was decreased along with the tumor regression, and the tumor stain became unrecognizable in some cases. On CT scanning, the density of the tumor interior was decreased in the majority of cases. In four evaluable cases of portal tumor thrombosis, the tumor thrombi were reduced in size in three; in the

[1] First Department of Medicine, Chiba University School of Medicine, Inohana, Chiba, 280 Japan

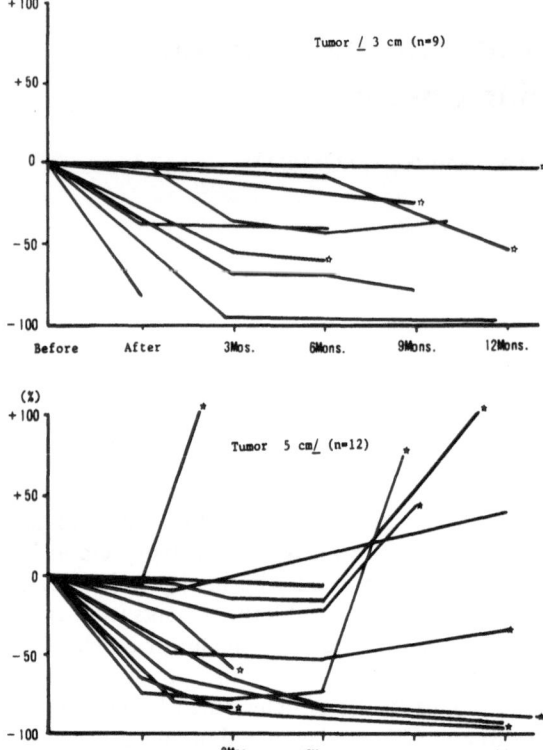

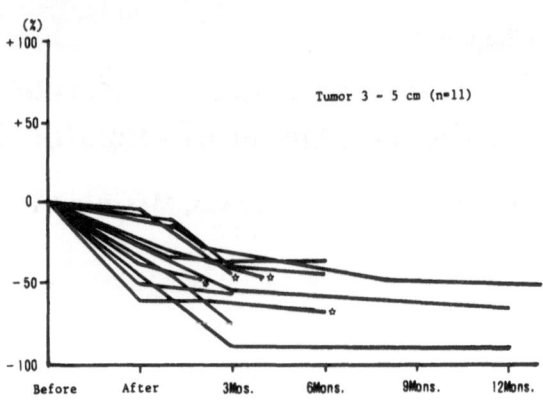

Fig. 26.1. Changes in tumor size following radiation therapy. The *abscissae* give time in months postirradiation and the *ordinates* tumor regression in percentages as assessed by CT or US. The patients were divided into three groups according to the tumor size (> 3 cm, 3–5 cm, and < 5 cm). Tumor regression occurred to varying degrees in the majority of patients

remaining cases, no further growth was seen up to 15 months postirradiation.

The cancer tissue was studied after irradiation in eight patients. It showed extensive coagulative necroses with small numbers of cancer cells. The noncancerous parenchyma showed congestion and bleeding, with increased fibrous tissue along the blood vessels and luminal narrowing. Liver cells also demonstrated degenerative changes with focal necroses.

1.2 Side effects and complications

Complaints of the patient during and shortly after radiation therapy included anorexia, slight fever, abdominal pain, general malaise, and nausea. As shown in Table 26.1, a gastro-duodenal ulcer developed in ten patients, and the white blood cell count dropped on average by more than 1000/mm³, with a slow subsequent recovery. Abdominal pain was usually associated with ulcers. These complaints were more frequent and severe when the irradiated field was greater than 100 cm². Due to leukopenia, irradiation had to be discontinued in two and temporarily suspended in three patients. The ulcer tended to resist treatment, but pain was

relieved within 1 month. In a few patients, intractable ascites developed approximately 3 months after irradiation. Liver function tests showed significant reduction in the values of serum choline esterase and albumin, and the counts of red blood cells and platelets were also reduced. These reductions improved slowly after several months. In two patients with large HCC, the serum aspartate aminsotransferase (AST) level increased by more than 500 milliunits/ml; it could not be determined whether this was due to tumor necrosis or parenchymal damage.

1.3 Prognosis and survival

Table 26.2 gives the prognosis of 37 (excluding two who underwent operation) patients up to 40 months postirradiation. A total of 21 patients died. However, it is noteworthy that 8 (80%) of 10 deaths in patients with an HCC smaller than 5 cm were due to hepatic failure and that no patients died as a result of cancer growth. In contrast 8 (73%) of 11 patients with an HCC larger than 5 cm died from cancer. The prognosis of the patients with an HCC smaller than 3 cm should be compared with that of a comparable group of patients who did not receive any specific treat-

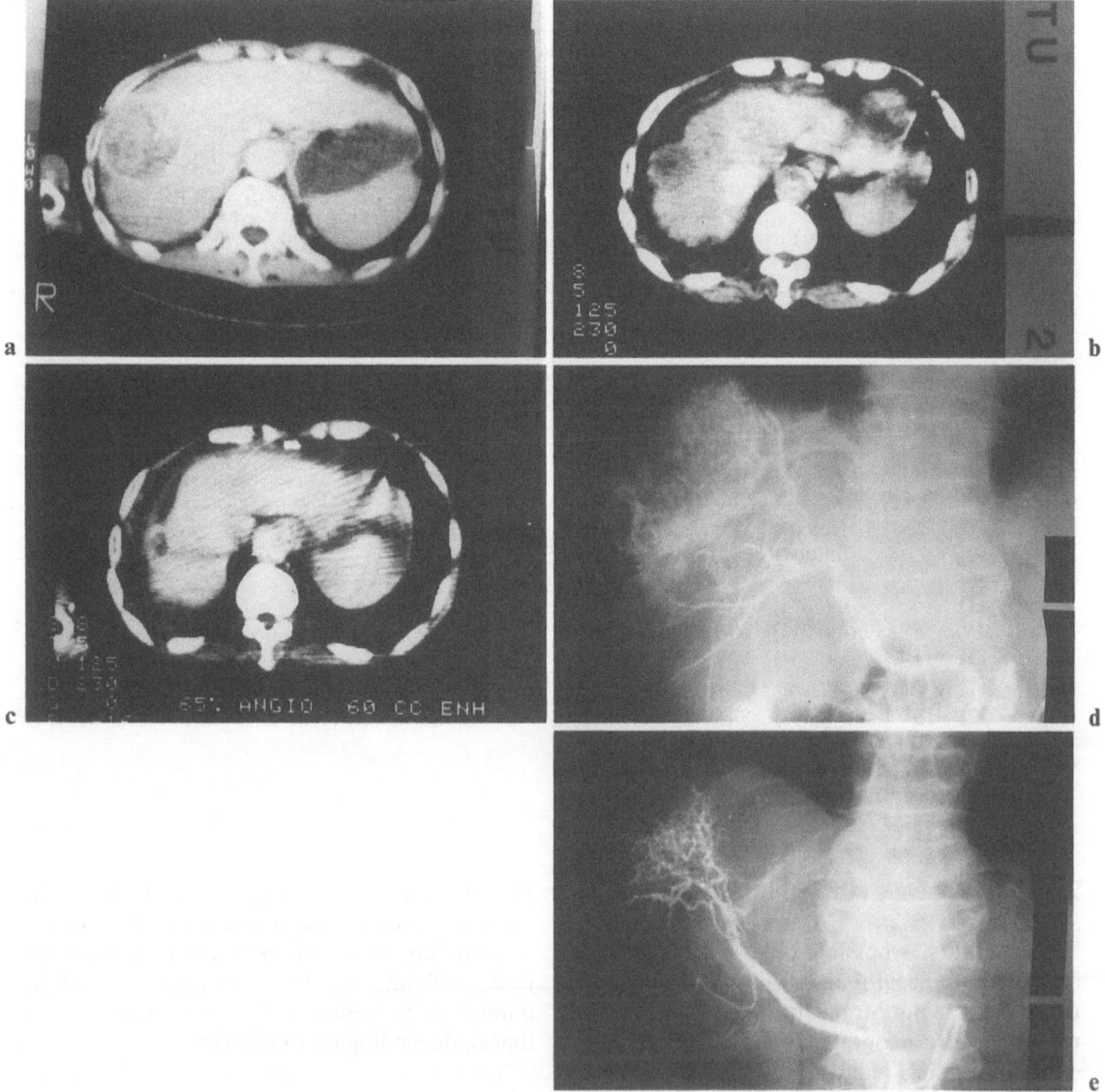

Fig. 26.2a–e. Effects of radiation therapy seen in a 71-year-old male following a total dose of 5000 rads (200 rads five times/week). **a** A typical encapsulated HCC is seen in the anterior superior segement of the right lobe. **b** Two months postirradiations; note the reduced in tumor size as well as density of the mass. Significant atrophy of the liver parenchyma, with reduced density, is also apparent. **c** Twelve months postirradiation; the mass is markedly shrunken and is protruding from the atrophied liver. **d** The angiogram of the mass before radiation therapy; the mass is typically hypervascular with tumor vessels. **e** Postirradiation angiogram with reduced vascularity and diminished size of the mass

ment. In the latter group, shown at the bottom of Table 26.2, 8 (54%) of the 15 patients died from cancer growth.

As shown in Table 26.3, the 2-year survival rate for patients with an HCC smaller than 3 cm was 46%; it was 46% for those with an HCC of 3–5 cm and 17% for those with an HCC larger than 5 cm. The 3-year survival rate was 23% and

46% for those with an HCC smaller than 3 cm and 3–5 cm, respectively. The reason for the lower survival rate in patients with an HCC smaller than 3 cm than in those with an HCC of 3–5 cm was that the former had more advanced cirrhosis (6 of 11 patients were of Child's B or C grade).

Table 26.1. Complications of radiation therapy

Tumor size (cm)	Gastro-duodenal ulcer	Leukopenia		AST[a] increase (> 500 milliunits/ml)
		Treatment temporarily suspended	Treatment abandoned	
<3 (n = 11)	1 (9%)	2 (18%)	1 (9%)	0 (0%)
3–5 (n = 15)	5 (33%)	1 (7%)	0 (0%)	0 (0%)
>5 (n = 13)	4 (31%)	0 (0%)	1 (8%)	2 (15%)

[a] aspartat aminotransferase

Table 26.2. Prognosis of patients treated by radiation therapy

Tumor size (cm)	No. of deaths	Cause of death		
		Hepatic failure	Cancer death	Others
<3 (n = 11)	5	4 (80%)	0 (0%)	1 (20%)
3–5 (n = 15)	5	4 (80%)	0 (0%)	1 (20%)
>5 (n = 13)	11	3 (27%)	8 (73%)	0 (0%)
Untreated control[a]				
<3 (n = 22)	15	5 (33%)	8 (54%)	2 (13%)

[a] For various reasons, these patients did not receive any specific treatment

Table 26.3. Survival of patients with HCC treated by irradiation

Tumor size (cm)	Survival (%)		
	1 year	2 years	3 years
<3 (n = 11)	90	46	23
3–5 (n = 15)	61	46	46
>5[a] (n = 13)	42	17	

[a] Includes cases having portal tumor thrombosis

2 Percutaneous ethanol injection

This modality is possible only in the hands of experienced hepatobiliary ultrasonographers, using the puncture transducer connected to the real-time ultrasonograph [16]. Our preliminary study in animals indicated that the distance of infiltration of absolute ethanol injected from a syringe into liver tissue is limited. Thus, percutaneous intratumor ethanol injection is indicated in HCC smaller than 3 cm, preferably 2 cm in size, provided that the number of lesions is small, perhaps less than three.

2.1 Technique

Under local anesthesia, a percutaneous transhepatic cholangiography (PTC) needle (22 gauge, 20 cm) is introduced into the tumor or its marginal area through a puncture probe of an electronic linear scanning sonograph. Absolute ethanol is slowly injected through the needle while it is being slowly withdrawn in order to produce diffuse necrosis within and around the mass. This procedure is repeated twice a week until the original echo pattern is completely re-placed by a different echo pattern, which persists for some time in the tumor as well as in the surrounding area. The amount of ethanol injected each time is 1–5 ml (average 3 ml), and the number of procedure is two to six (average 3.5 times), depending on tumor size.

2.2 Results

A total of 25 patients with HCC smaller than 3 cm and one patient with a 3.2-cm HCC underwent percutaneous ethanol injection (PEI). The age ranged from 43 to 70 years (mean 59.0) in 24 males; the two female patients were aged 53 and 71 years. Liver cirrhosis coexisted in all these patients. Five of the 26 patients underwent resection within 1 month of PEI. In these surgically treated patients, two tumors smaller than 2 cm (which had been injected with a total of 6 ml ethanol in three procedures) showed complete necrosis as studied histologically. One tumor of 3.2 cm that received a total of 25 ml ethanol in four procedures also showed complete necrosis (Fig. 26.3). The remaining two tumors, 2–3 cm in size, to which 4 ml ethanol was injected in two procedures and 10 ml in three procedures, re-

Fig. 26.3. Resected HCC nodule after PEI. This 32 × 30-mm HCC was treated by PEI with a total of 25 ml ethanol given in four procedures and partial resection was carried out 10 days after the last injection. Histopathologically, the mass was completely necrotic, and some surrounding liver tissue was also coagulated. × 4

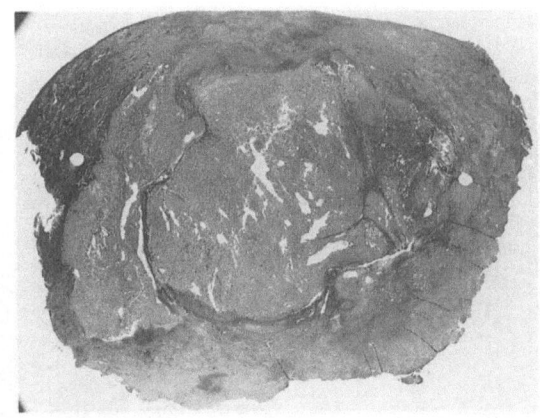

spectively, had nearly complete necrosis with some residual viable cancer cells in the marginal area.

In the 21 patients who were followed without resection, the changes assessed by US and other imaging techniques were as follows. Satisfactory results were obtained in 12 of 13 tumors less than 2 cm to which a total of 3–14 ml ethanol was injected in two to five procedures. Similarly satisfactory results were obtained in eight of nine tumors of 2–3 cm that received 8–25 ml ethanol in three to six procedures. The results were unsatisfactory in a 1.9-cm tumor to which 3 ml ethanol was injected in one procedure and in another 2.7-cm tumor to which 7.5 ml ethanol was injected in three procedures. In the former, the injection was given only once, and in the latter the location of the mass was near the surface of the anterior segment, a location difficult to inject with accuracy.

2.2.1 US findings

All 21 tumors with a long follow-up showed a low or low-periphery echo pattern characteristic of small HCC before treatment (Chap. 19). The echo pattern changed within 1 month to a high-ring echo pattern in nine tumors, low-halo pattern in three, high-ring low-halo pattern in two, mixed pattern in six, low pattern in one, and no recognizable echo in one. All tumors with a high-ring or low-halo echo pattern subsequently showed disappearance of echo or reduction in tumor size. By contrast, one of six tumors with a mixed-echo pattern and one with a low-echo pattern did not disappear or regress. A certain relationship between the echo pattern shortly after PEI and the therapeutic effects was recognized. All 13 tumors that showed a reduction in size demonstrated a high-spot or high-ring echo pattern in the follow-up period 6 months post-PEI

(Fig. 26.4). At that time, the echo pattern had transformed from high ring, low halo, or mixed to high spot in nine of them. Two tumors in which the results were unsatisfactory showed a low-echo pattern during the follow-up period.

2.3 Side effects, complications, and prognosis

2.3.1 Side effects

In 24 of 26 patients, pain occurred locally the instant the needle was withdrawn after the injection. The pain varied from mild to severe and usually lasted a few minutes. A high fever (over 38°C) developed on the day of injection in 13 patients. A slight to moderate rise in serum transaminase occurred transiently in five patients. All these side effects subsided with symptomatic and supportive treatment.

2.3.2 Prognosis and survival curve

One of the 21 patients followed from 6 to 30 months died from HCC, which involved an area of the liver for which no treatment had been given, and two died from variceal bleeding and hepatic coma due to advanced cirrhosis. The remaining 18 are alive without recurrence, with a survival curve (Fig. 26.5) that is better than the survival curve of 22 patients with similarly small HCC who did not receive specific treatment.

3 Discussion and summary

HCC is one of the most malignant neoplasms of man and survival after diagnosis used to be a few months [17, 18]. The chronic liver disease on which HCC develops varies with the geographical region [19, 20]. In South African Blacks, HCC is not associated with advanced cirrhosis and cancer cells are frequently poorly differen-

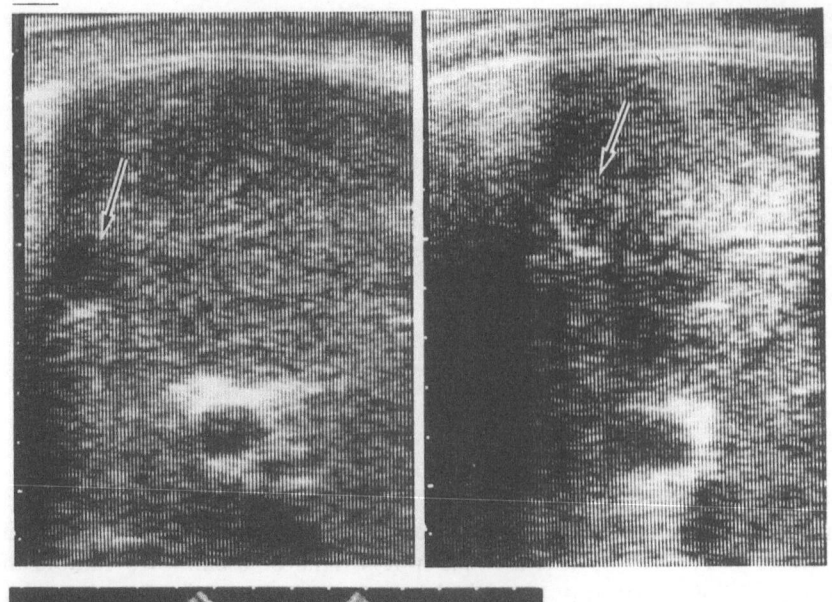

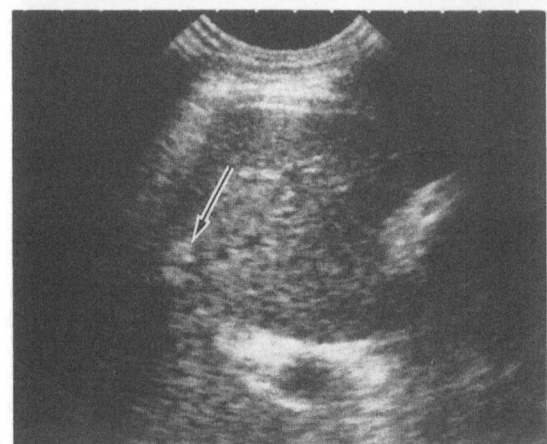

Fig. 26.4a–c. Ultrasonographic changes that followed PEI. **a** A 14 × 12-mm HCC is seen as a low-echo lesion (*arrow*). **b** Immediately after the termination of ethanol injection; the mass (*arrow*) now shows a high-echo rim, a sign suggestive of success. **c** One year post-PEI; the mass is now seen as a high-echo dot with a marked reduction in size (*arrow*). There is no indication of recurrence

tiated [19], whereas in Japan and the far East HCC is often well-differentiated and arises in a liver with advanced cirrhosis [21]. With the current practice in Japan of regular follow-up of patients with chronic liver disease, small HCC is now frequently detected by US [22–24], but treatment is the real problem.

Radiation therapy and PEI have resulted from the difficulties, in treating patients who have very poor liver fuction, preventing surgical intervention. Fortunately, however, tumorigenesis is frequently unicentric or oligocentric in the Orient [21], making these two modalities practicable. Irradiation of the liver unexpectedly caused no serious alimentary tract complications, except for ulcer development. However, radiation damage to the liver parenchyma seemed significant because hepatic failure ensued in some of the patients with Child's C grade. Future adjustment

of radiation dose according to liver function tests may be required. Our earlier attempts to inject anticancer drugs directly into the cancer mass failed because an aqueous solution of anticancer agents immediately entered the circulation rather than remaining in the cancer tissue. Absolute ethanol immediately fixes or coagulates tissue on contact. If ethanol can be injected stereotactically with an automated device into the cancer nodule in such a way that it infiltrates completely into the surrounding noncancerous tissue after fixation of the interior of the mass, then total destruction of cancer cells can be achieved. Ethanol itself is practically harmless and can be injected repeatedly. Although PEI may not prove useful in the Western hemisphere where HCC is uncommon, the majority of HCC patients live in the Far East, and PEI may become one of the treatments of choice.

Fig. 26.5. The survival curve for 21 patients treated by PEI in comparison with that for 22 patients who did not receive specific treatment (Kaplan-Meier method)

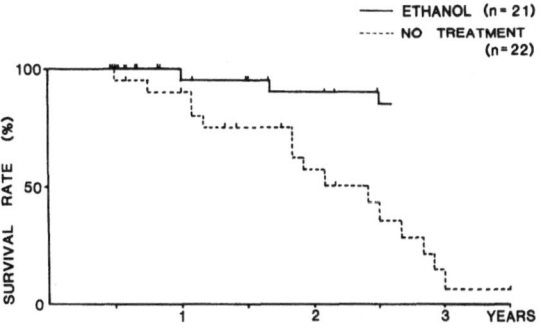

References

1. Ingold JA, Reed GB, Kaplan HS, Bagshaw MA (1965) Radiation hepatitis. Am J Roentgenol Rad Therapy 93: 200–208
2. Johnson PM, Grossman FM, Atkins HL (1967) Radiation induced hepatic injury. Its detection by scintillation scanning. Am J Roentgenol Rad Therapy 99: 435–462
3. Lewin K, Millis RR (1973) Human radiation hepatitis. Arch Pathol 96: 21–26
4. Cochrane AMG, Murray-Lyon IM, Brinkley DM, Williams R (1977) Quadruple chemotherapy versus radiotherapy in treatment of primary hepatocellular carcinoma. Cancer 40: 609–614
5. Bhardwaj S, Bruckner HW, Holland JF (1985) Therapy of malignant tumors of the liver. In: Berk JE (ed) Bockus gastroenterology, 4th edn., vol. 5. Saunders, Philadelphia, pp 3388–3397
6. Grady ED, Nolan TR, Crumbley AJ, Larose JH, Cheek WV (1975) Internal hepatic radiotherapy: II. Intra-arterial radiocolloid therapy for hepatic tumors. Am J Roentgenol Rad Therapy 124: 596–599
7. Grady ED (1979) Internal radiation therapy of hepatic cancer. Dis Col Rect 22: 371–375
8. Order SE, Klein JL, Ettinger D, Alderson P, Siegelman S, Leicher P (1980) Phase I–II study of radiolabeled antibody integrated in the treatment of primary hepatic malignancies. Int J Radiation Oncol Biol Phys 6: 703–710
9. Ettinger DS, Order SE, Wharam MD, Parker MK, Klein JL, Leicher PK (1982) Phase I–II study of isotopic immunoglobulin therapy for primary liver cancer. Cancer Treat Rep 66: 289–297
10. Holm HH, Stryer I, Hansen H, Stadil F (1981) Ultrasonically guided percutaneous interstitial implantation of iodine 125 seeds in cancer therapy. Br J Radiol 54: 665–670
11. Friedman M, Cassidy M, Levine M, Phillips T, Spivack S, Resser KJ (1979) Combined modality therapy of hepatic metastasis. Cancer 44: 906–913
12. Barone RM, Byfield JE, Frankel S (1979) Combination infusional 5-fluorouracil and radiation therapy for the treatment of metastatic carcinoma of the colon to the liver. Dis Col Rect 22: 376–382
13. Lokich J, Kinsella T, Perri J, Malcolm A, Clouse M (1981) Concomitant hepatic radiation and intraarterial fluorinated pyrimidine therapy. Correlation of liver scan, liver function tests, and

plasma CEA with tumor response. Cancer 48: 2569–2574
14. Shinagawa T, Ohto M, Kimura K, Tsunetomi S, Morita M, Saisho H, Tsuchiya Y, Saotome N, Karasawa E, Miki M, Ueno T, Okuda K (1984) Diagnosis and clinical features of small hepatocellular carcinoma with emphasis on the utility of real-time ultrasonography. Gastroenterology 86: 495–502
15. Okuda K (1986) Early recognition of hepatocellular carcinoma. Hepatology 6: 729–738
16. Ohto M, Karasawa E, Tsuchiya Y, Kimura K, Saisho H, Ono T, Okuda K (1980) Ultrasonically guided percutaneous contrast medium injection and aspiration biopsy using a real-time puncture transducer. Radiology 136: 171–176
17. El-Domeiri AL, Huvos AG, Goldsmith HS, Foote FW Jr (1971) Primary malignant tumors of the liver. Cancer 27: 7–11
18. Primack A, Vogel CL, Kyalwazi SK, Ziegler JL, Simon R, Anthony PP (1975) A staging system for hepatocellular carcinoma: Prognostic factors in Ugandan patients. Cancer 35: 1357–1364
19. Steiner PE (1960) Cancer of the liver and cirrhosis in trans-Saharan Africa and the United States of America. Cancer 13: 1085–1166
20. Okuda K, Peters RL, Simson IW (1985) Gross anatomic features of hepatocellular carcinoma from three disparate geographic areas. Proposal of new classification. Cancer 54: 2164–2173
21. Nakashima T, Okuda K, Kojiro M, Jimi A, Yamaguchi R, Sakamoto K, Ikari T (1983) Pathology of hepatocellular carcinoma in Japan. 232 consecutive cases autopsied in ten years. Cancer 51: 863–877
22. Shinagawa T, Ohto M, Kimura K, Tsunetomi S, Norita M, Saisho H, Tsuchiya Y, Saotome N, Karasawa E, Miki M, Ueno T, Okuda K (1984) Diagnosis and clinical features of small hepatocellular carcinoma with emphasis on the utility of real-time ultrasonography. Gastroenterology 86: 495–502
23. Ebara M, Ohto M, Shinagawa T, Sugiura N, Kimura K, Matsutani S, Morita M, Saisho H, Tsuchiya Y, Okuda K (1986) Natural history of minute hepatocellular carcinoma smaller than three centimenters complicating cirrhosis. A study in 22 patients. Gastroenterology 90: 289–298
24. Okuda K (1986) Early recognition of hepatocellular carcinoma. Hepatology 6: 729–738

Chapter 27

Targeting Chemotherapy of Hepatocellular Carcinoma

Arterial Administration of SMANCS/Lipiodol

Toshimitsu Konno[1] and Hiroshi Maeda[2]

1 Introduction

A number of methods utilize the feeding artery of the tumor for the treatment of hepatocellular carcinoma (HCC); such methods include implantation of an infusion pump, placement of a catheter for injection into the artery, and embolization of the artery with gelatin-gel or microspheres containing anticancer agents. However, very few methods have exploited the use of lipid as a carrier and depository of an anticancer agent. Recently, we developed a procedure in which Lipiodol ultrafluid (Lipiodol) is used as a carrier of anticancer agents for injection into the feeding artery, a significant breakthrough in the treatment of solid tumors. The lipid lymphographic agent, Lipiodol, has been found to be selectively retained in HCC when injected into the hepatic artery [1]. In addition, a lipid contrast medium has various diagnostic applications, as described in this chapter. Anticancer agents, such as styrene maleic acid conjugates of neocarzinostatin (SMANCS) [2, 3], mitomycin C (MMC), or aclarubicin (ACR), were dissolved into Lipiodol. As SMANCS/Lipiodol (LPD), MMC/LPD, ACR/LPD, or a mixture of these, these oily anticancer agents were administered by catheterization of the celiac or hepatic artery under X-ray monitor. Anticancer effects and the advantages of this targeting chemotherapy for HCC are described in the succeeding sections of this review.

2 Principle of tumor targeting by LPD

It is now known that tumor cells secrete tumor angiogenesis factor, which is necessary for the

The First Department of Surgery[1] and Department of Microbiology[2], Kumamoto University Medical School, Honjo, Kumanoto, 860 Japan

growth of tumors over 2–3 mm in diameter, and hence an extensive neovasculature develops in the tumor [4].

LPD has been found to be selectively retained in HCC and other malignant solid tumors when injected intra-arterially [1, 5]. The mechanism of the selective accumulation of LPD is not fully understood; LPD that has flowed into normal capillaries is removed within a few days, whereas LPD that has flowed into tumor tissue remains in the neovasculature and extracapillary space for a long period of time. We speculate that the mechanism for selective accumulation of LPD in the nevoasculature is a combination of the nature of the neovasculature (such as vascular structure and mode of blood flow) and the viscosity and surface tension of LPD. Since there is no muscular cell layer in the neovasculature, it cannot constrict; blood flow in the neovasculature is considered to be slow in comparison with that in normal capillaries. It has been speculated that the selective accumulation of LPD in the extracapillary space in a tumor is due to its fairly effective leakage through the neovasculature and the poor development or absence of a recovery mechanism (as exerted by the reticuloendothelial system) in the tumor tissue. This postulated mechanism of vascular permeability and prolonged retention of lipid has been substantiated by separate experiments using various proteins labeled with an isotope or dye [6].

3 Drug preparation

We used SMANCS primarily as a chemotherapeutic agent and LPD as its carrier. SMANCS is a semisynthetic macromolecular compound that consists of an antitumor antibiotic protein—neocarzinostatin (NCS)—and two chains of synthetic copolymers of styrene and maleic acid; the latter two compounds have molecular weights of approximately 12 000 and 1600 per chain, respectively. The detailed structure of SMANCS has been described elsewhere [2, 3, 7]. Briefly, the two amino groups of NCS are attached to two chains of the copolymer by a chemical reaction. Thus, the molecular weight of SMANCS becomes approximately 15 000. Since the styrene-maleic acid copolymer exhibits hydrophobic and anionic characters, the conjugated SMANCS retains these properties and becomes soluble in some organic solvents and lipids, including LPD; this has been designated as SMANCS/LPD. MMC/LPD was prepared by dissolving 2–4 mg MMC in 1 ml LPD; ACR/LPD was prepared by dissolving 6.5–12 mg ACR in 1 ml LPD with the use of appropriate solublizing agents.

LPD is an iodinated fatty acid ester of poppyseed oil containing 38% iodine by weight; it is manufactured by Guerbert Laboratories in France. The viscosity of SMANCS/LPD (1 mg/ml), MMC/LPD (4 mg/ml), ACR/LPD (12.5 mg/ml) and the mixture of these oily anticancer agent were 45.5, 59.5, 38.5, and 49.6 centipoises, respectively. Essential properties of these oily anticancer agents include solubility in LPD, lack of separation into oil and aqueous phases, and slow release of the anticancer drug from LPD. It takes at least 24 h for LPD to be selectively retained in cancer tissue after its removal from the noncancerous parenchyma. SMANCS/LPD was used in this study as a first-choice drug. The other agents or mixtures of these oily anticancer agents were used when the tumor did not respond to SMANCS/LPD.

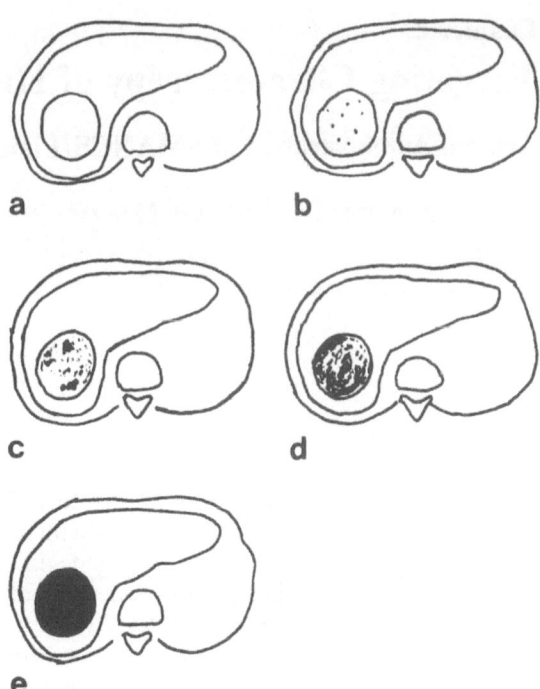

Fig. 27.1a–e. Classification of CT image after administration of SMANCS/LPD. Definition based on the amount of retention of LPD, shown as *black dots*. **a** Grade O; LPD is not recognized. **b** Grade I; LPD is retained in less than 10% of the tumor mass. **c** Grade II; retention in less than 50% of the tumor. **d** Grade III; retention in over 50% of the tumor, but not the entire area. **e** Grade IV LPD retained by the entire tumor. See Maki et al. [8] for details

4 Patients and procedure

We studied 175 patients with HCC, diagnosed either histologically or clinically; 145 patients had unresectable advanced HCC, and 30 patients had resectable tumors. Of the 175 patients, 163 (93.1%) had liver cirrhosis. Of the 145 patients with unresectable HCC (excluding ten patients in whom the disease stage of HCC could not be evaluated on the basis of criteria used by the Japanese Society for Cancer Treatment), there were 13 patients with HCC of stage 1, 35 patients of stage 2, 27 patients of stage 3, and 60 patients of stage 4. These 135 patients were classified according to Child's scheme as 38 patients grade A, 52 patients grade B, and 45 patients grade C.

Selective or superselective catheterization of the celiac artery was performed through the femoral artery under fluoroscopy using Seldinger's method with a Torcon-Blue preshaped-type catheter (Cook Inc., USA). A total of 371 injections of the drug were given to the 175 patients. An average of 4 mg SMANCS/LPD per dose was given by arterial infusion through the celiac (71 times), common hepatic (170 times), proper hepatic (79 times), or other peripheral arteries (51 times). The maximum dose of SMANCS/LPD per patient was 16 mg/injection. Multiple administrations of the oily anticancer agents were often required to fill the entire tumor with LPD (Figs. 27.1, 27.2, grade IV) [8]. The interval between each administration was usually 3–8 weeks. To detect the amount of residual oily anticancer agents in the tumor after administration of the drugs, CT scanning was carried out usually at 1 week and 1 month after the injection. When an adequate amount of LPD had accumulated, i.e., when the tumor retention had reached grade IV as observed by CT (Figs. 27.1,

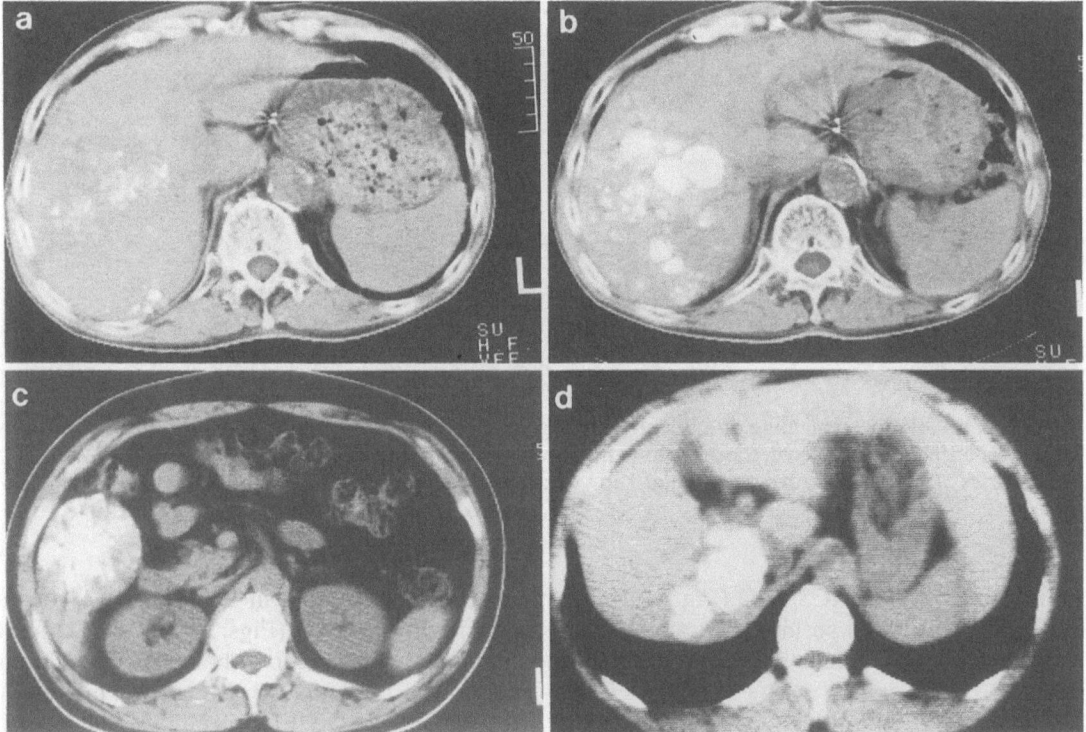

Fig. 27.2. a Grade II; LPD remains in less than 50% of the tumor (bright area). **b** Grade IV; after additional administration to the same patient as in **a**, LPD remains in the entire tumor as a bright area. **c** Grade III. **d** Grade IV

27.2), follow-up CT scanning was carried out every 1–2 months thereafter. For patients with a tumor in which the accumulation of LPD was inadequate as judged by CT (grades I–III; Figs. 27.1, 27.2), additional administration of the oily anticancer agents has been recommended [8].

The aforementioned treatment is not indicated in patients with a total bilirubin value greater than 3 mg/ml and uncontrollable ascites, because the results of therapy will be poor and unforeseen complications could occur.

5 Targeting by LPD-containing anticancer agents and drug release

Although LPD administered via the hepatic artery flows into both the neoplastic and the non-neoplastic areas of the liver, the LPD that has entered the nonneoplastic portion of the liver and other organs such as the spleen, stomach, and duodenum is cleared within a few days. In contrast, LPD that has entered the HCC remains for a much longer period (Fig. 27.3). It has been demonstrated that selective targeting to the HCC

could be assessed by a plain abdominal X-ray film (Fig. 27.3), CT [1, 8, 9], and, in the resected specimen, by Sudan III staining and soft X-rays (Fig. 27.5b, 27.10a).

The biological activity of SMANCS has been measured in both neoplastic and nonneoplastic areas of resected specimens [1, 6]. Its biological activity persists in the tumor even after 22 days and also in the immediately adjacent nonneo-plastic tissue where LPD had not been recognized on low-KVP X-ray films by the Softex instrument. By contrast, no biological activity has been detected in the nonneoplastic tissue away from the tumor (Table 27.1).

6 Differentiation of HCC from metastatic liver cancer and dose determination

Because of the selective retention of LPD, a low-density area in HCC on CT changes to a high-density area after administration of SMANCS/ LPD. Some lesions of HCC are not detectable on CT but become clearly visible after the ad-

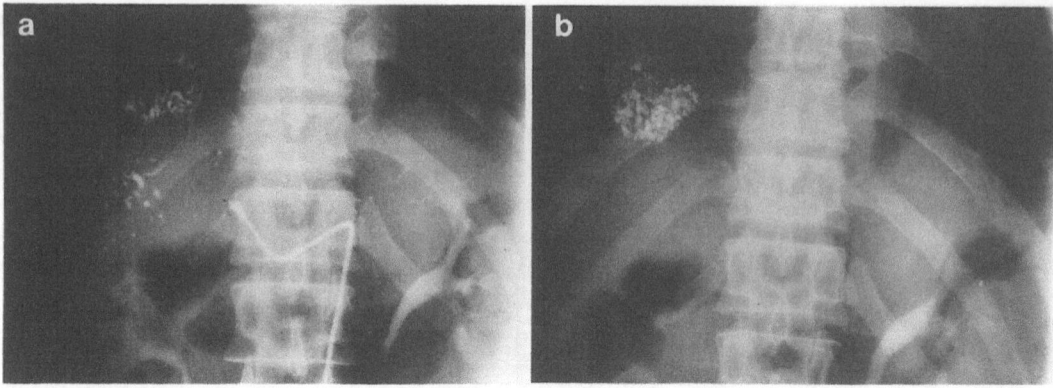

Fig. 27.3a, b. Selective remaining of oily anticancer agent. **a** Fluoroscopic view of the moment when the oily anticancer agent is administered; the drug flows into both the tumorous and nontumorous portions. White dots are particles of LPD. **b** Selective retention of LPD was clearly observed on a plain abdominal X-ray film

ministration of SMANCS/LPD (Fig. 27.4). The sensitivity of LPD is so high that an HCC as small as 3 mm in diameter can be detected (Fig. 27.5a, c).

The differentiation of HCC from metastatic liver cancer can also be made on the basis of the shape of the retained LPD. LPD retention in HCC occurs in the entire area of the tumor but is seen predominantly in the periphery of a metastasis, thus producing a ring-shaped appearance (Fig. 27.5d).

Dose determination of SMANCS/LPD can also be made on CT after the initial administration. The extent of the high-density area is clearly seen on the CT scan after the administration, and it may be classified into five grades (Figs. 27.1, 27.2). The degree of LPD retention in the tumor has been found to correlate well with tumor size and the amount of SMANCS/LPD administered [8, 10]. It has also been found to correlate well with chemotherapeutic effects [5, 8]. Thus, when a sufficient amount of LPD was retained or when the entire tumor was filled with SMANCS/LPD on CT (grade IV, Figs. 27.1, 27.2), the tumor never enlarged and regression was observed in the majority of cases. Therefore, administration of SMANCS/LPD should aim at attaining grade IV retention.

7 Antitumor effect of oily anticancer agents

The antitumor effect of targeting chemotherapy using oily anticancer agents can be evaluated by CT and angiography, as shown in Figs. 27.6 and 27.9. The serum alpha-fetoprotein level and tumor size decreased in 91% and 93% of the patients, respectively (Figs. 27.7, 27.8). Of the 98 tumors, 41 showed more than 50% reduction in size within 1–12 months. Recently, a mixture of MMC/LPD, ACR/LPD, and SMANCS/LPD was administered in patients with HCC that had enlarged despite SMANCS/LPD administration. This mixture of oily anticancer agent was injected into the proper hepatic or more distal arteries in five patients, and there was reduction of tumor size in all patients (Fig. 27.9).

Histological examination of resected specimens of 30 cases revealed extensive necroses of the tumor. In all but two cases, a single administration of 2–9 mg SMANCS/LPD was given 1–9 weeks before resection. In two cases, two administrations of total doses of 8 and 16 mg, respectively, were carried out. The degree of necrosis of the tumor tissue nearly paralleled the dose of SMANCS/LPD delivered [10]. In patients who received one dose of SMANCS, more than 0.25 mg/cm^2 of a maximal cut surface area of the liver, degeneration and necrosis of the entire tumor area were seen. More importantly, the nonneoplastic liver tissue was found to be unaffected (Fig. 27.10).

Although it is too early to evaluate the long-term effects of this method, we have compared our data with those of a group of patients with advanced HCC not treated with this protocol. The survival period of patients with advanced unresectable HCC treated with the present protocol was definitely longer than that of the control groups. The survival period obtained by the present method was as long as that of the group of patients in whom small HCC was resected and whose disease was at an early stage (Fig. 27.11).

Table 27.1. Biological activity of SMANCS in resected liver

Case	Dose of SMANCS (mg)	Administered hepatic artery	Period from administration to hepatectomy	Biological activity (μg SMANCS/g tissue)		
				Hepatoma	Nontumorous portion surrounding hepatoma	Nontumorous portion distant from hepatoma (over 10 cm)
62-yr. male	4	Common	15 days	0.94	1.06	0
54-yr. male	4	Common	22 days	5.4	1.06	0
53-yr. male	4	Proper	2 months	1.1	0.05	0
59-yr. male	4	Common	3 weeks	0.7	0.7	0

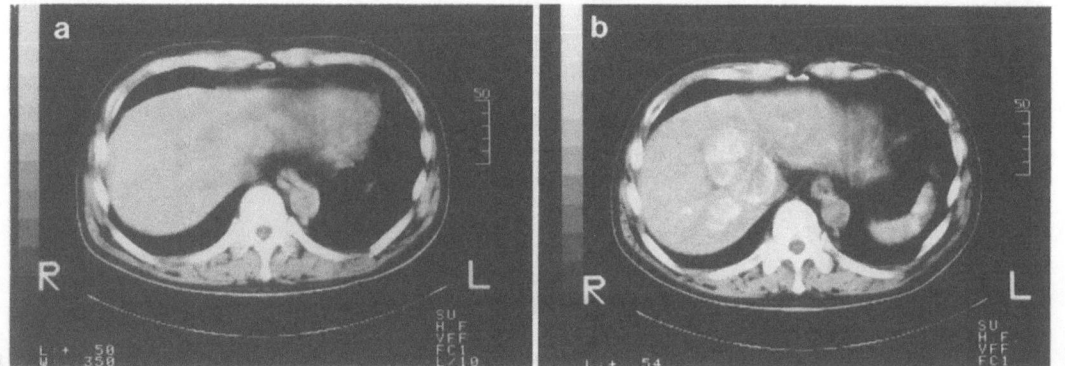

Fig. 27.4a, b. Demonstration of HCC by selective retention of LPD. **a** Lesion of hepatoma is not clear on CT before administration of SMANCS/LPD. **b** HCC is now clearly seen on CT after administration

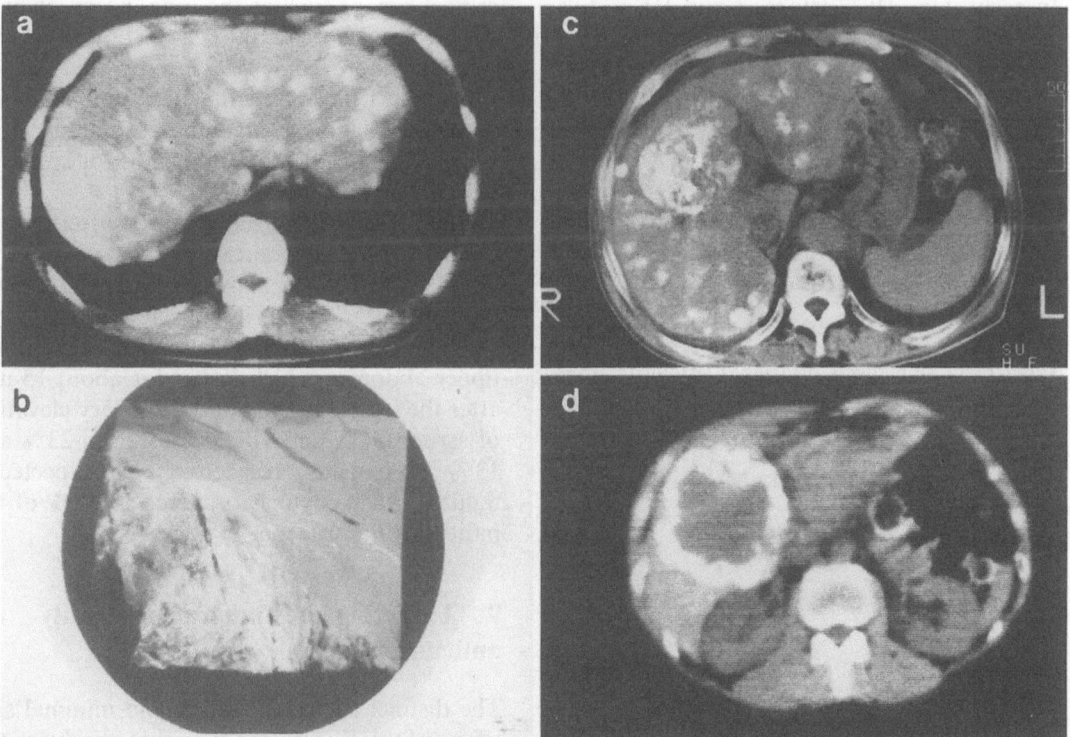

Fig. 27.5a–d. Selective retention of LPD on CT image and low-KVP X-ray film of a resected specimen. **a, c** Tumor size and number of HCC lesions became clearly detectable on CT after administration of SMANCS/LPD. **b** Low-KVP X-ray film of the resected specimen revealed selective retention of LPD. **d** Distinct pattern of LPD retention in metastatic liver cancer

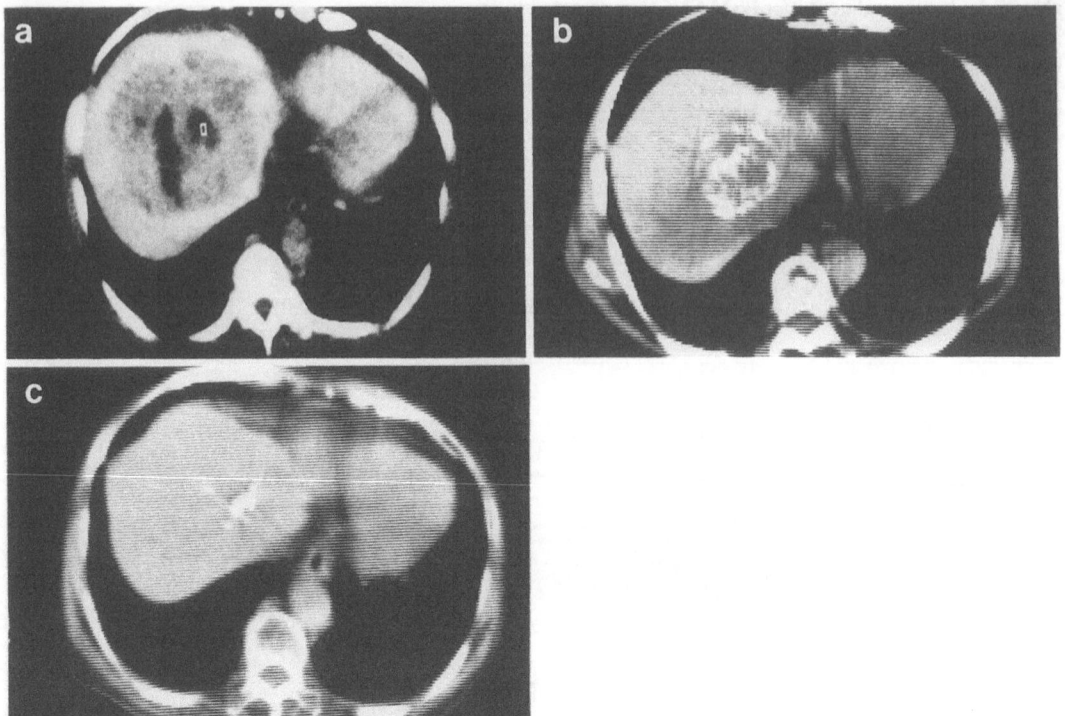

Fig. 27.6a–c. Demonstration of regression of HCC by CT scan. **a** Before administration of SMANCS/LPD. **b** Four months after administration. **c** Seventeen months after administration. After Konno et al. [1]

In early-stage HCC (stages I and II), a 2-year survival rate of 93% was achieved by this method combined with gelatin-gel embolization [11].

8 Side effects

After 371 selective arterial infusions with the oily anticancer agents, primarily with SMANCS/LPD, no adverse effect due to embolization of

Table 27.2. Side effects of arterial administration of SMANCS/LPD

	No. of patients	Percentage
Fever (38°–39°C)	167/322[a]	52
Pain	42/302[b]	14
Laboratory data		
GOT elevation	65/279[c]	23
GPT elevation	36/267[c]	13
WBC increase	85/191[c]	45
WBC decrease	34/191[c]	18

[a] Transitory, 7 days
[b] Transitory, 20 min
[c] Transitory and mild

critical organs such as the lung, heart, or brain has been noted. Untrapped LPD disappeared from the fluoroscopic view rapidly; we speculate that some LPD may circulate bound to serum albumin and lipoprotein and that some, although undetectable, may lodge in the lung or kidney or be excreted into the bile [12].

The major side effect observed after arterial infusion of the oily anticancer agent was fever of 38°–39°C (52%), as shown in Table 27.2; most patients became afebrile in a few days. About 14% of the patients experienced dull pain in the upper abdomen which lasted for about 15 min after the infusion. Mild and transitory elevation of serum GOT and GPT occurred in 23% and 13% of patients, respectively. Unexpectedly, moderate leukocytosis occurred in 45% of the patients after infusion.

9 Targeting chemotherapy with oily anticancer agents

The distinct anticancer effect and minimal side effects of this therapy are thought to be due to the following: (1) selective targeting by LPD (as a carrier), (2) long-lasting effect of the anticancer

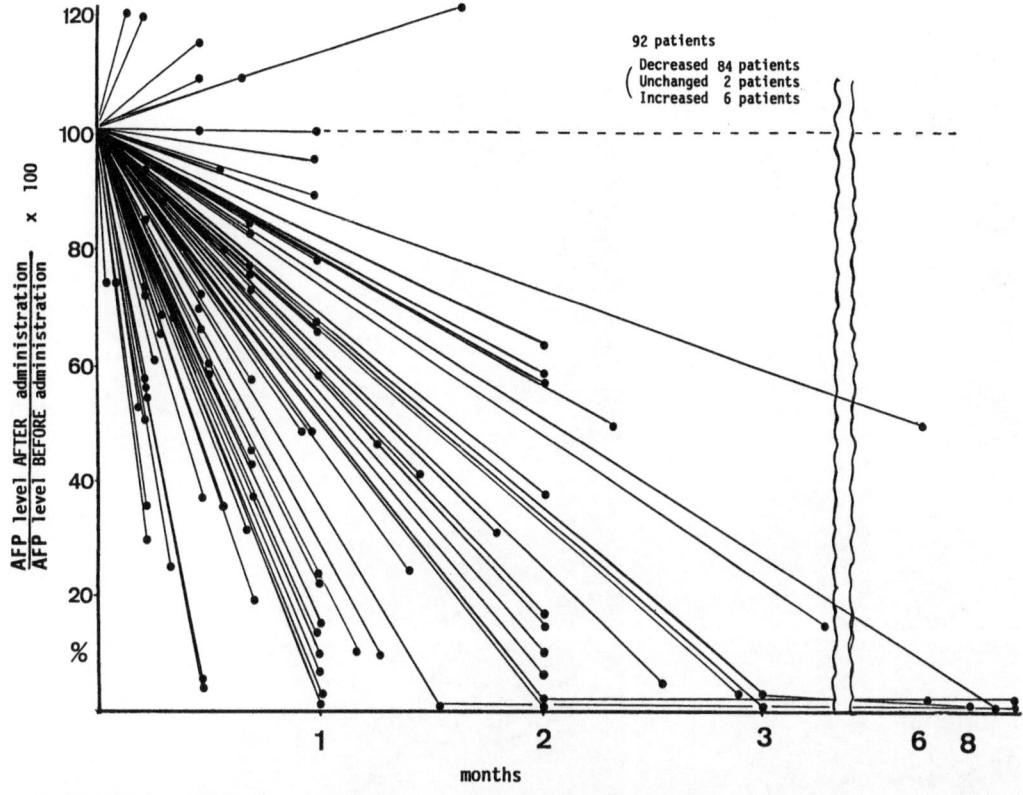

Fig. 27.7. Changes in alpha-fetoprotein value after administration of SMANCS/LPD in patients with HCC

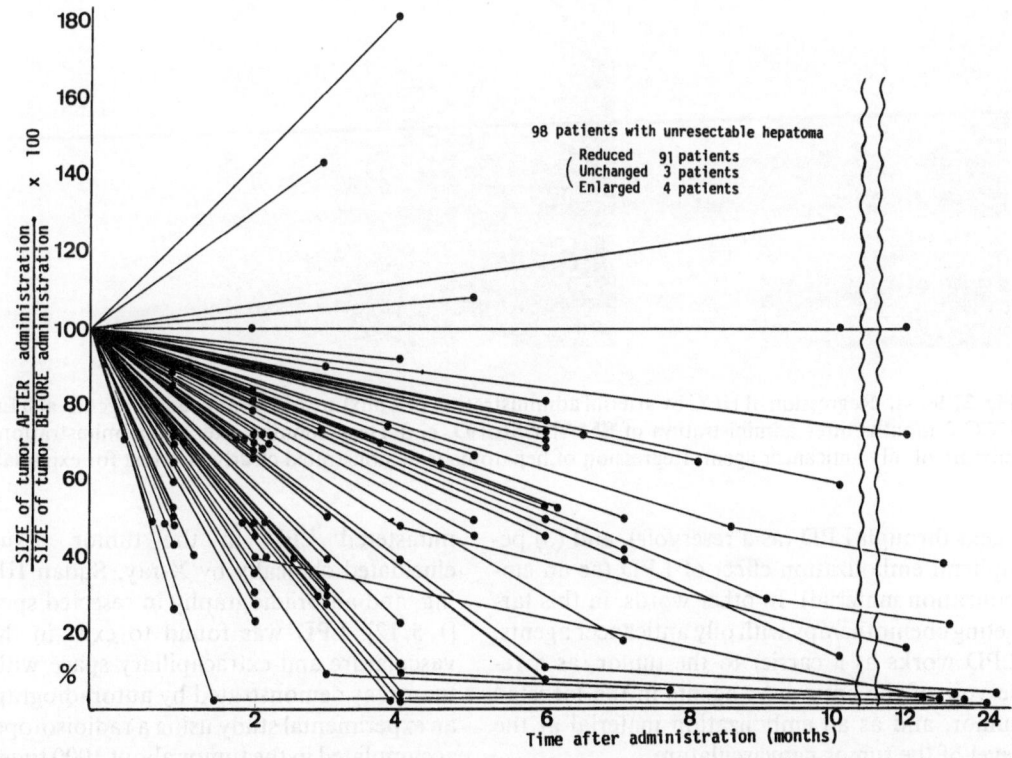

Fig. 27.8. Changes in tumor size after arterial administration of SMANCS/LPD in unresectable HCC

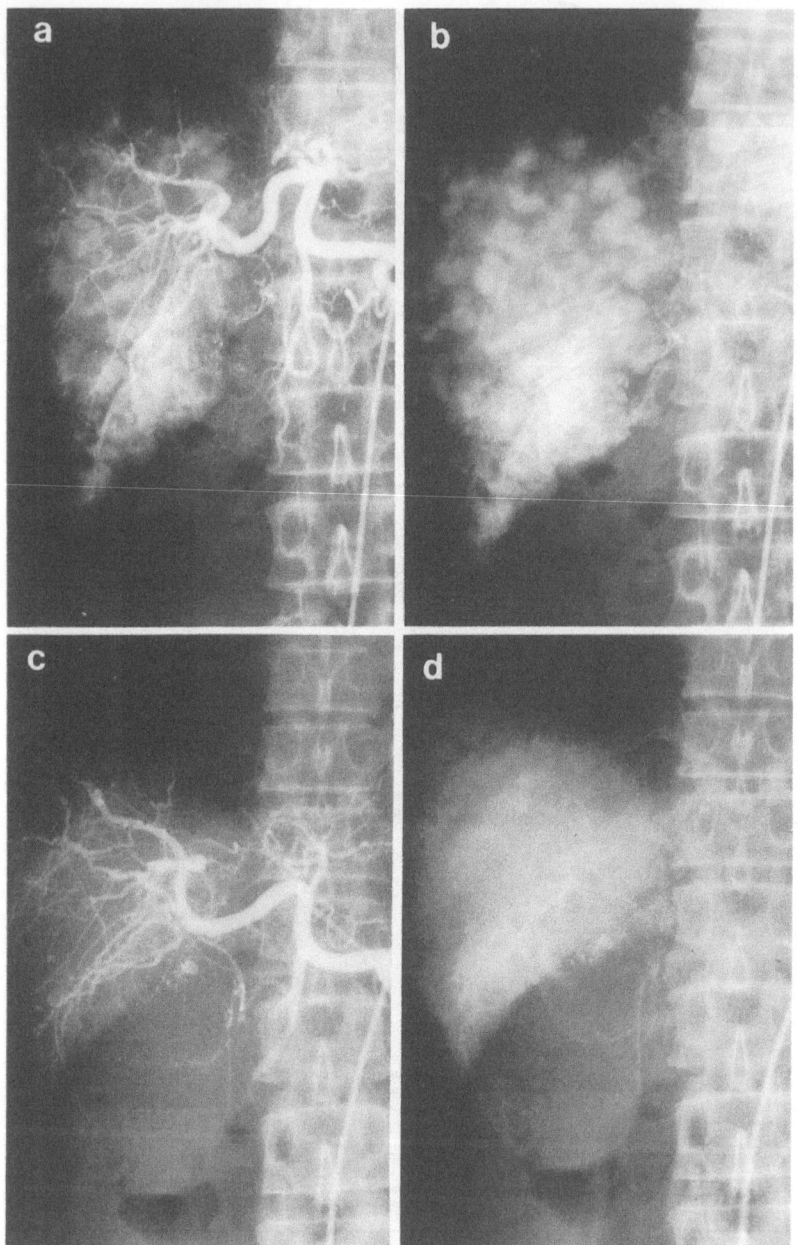

Fig. 27.9a–d. Regression of HCC by arterial administration of a mixture of oily anticancer agents. **a, b** Enlarged HCC 2 months after administration of SMANCS/LPD. **c, d** Three months after the administration of the mixture of oily anticancer agent. Regression of hepatoma is demonstrated clearly. See text for explanation

agent through LPD (as a reservoir), and (3) peripheral embolization effect of LPD (as an embolization material). In other words, in this targeting chemotherapy with oily anticancer agents, LPD works as a carrier to the tumor, as a reservoir of the anticancer agents in the targeted tumor, and as an embolization material at the level of the tumor neovasculature.

The selective accumulation of arterially ad-ministered LPD in the tumor tissue was elucidated clinically by X-ray, Sudan III staining, and autoradiography in resected specimens [1, 5, 12]. LPD was found to exist in the neo-vasculature and extracapillary space within the tumor, as demonstrated by autoradiography. In an experimental study using a radioisotope, LPD accumulated in the tumor about 1000 times more than in the blood [12].

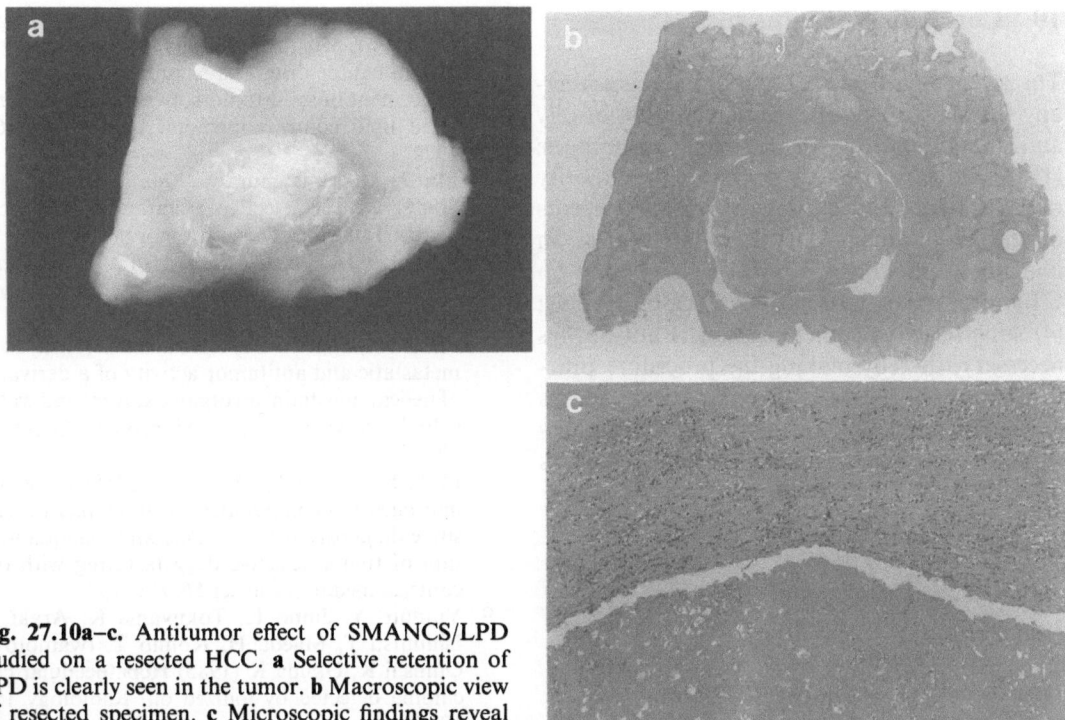

Fig. 27.10a–c. Antitumor effect of SMANCS/LPD studied on a resected HCC. **a** Selective retention of LPD is clearly seen in the tumor. **b** Macroscopic view of resected specimen. **c** Microscopic findings reveal complete necrosis of hepatoma

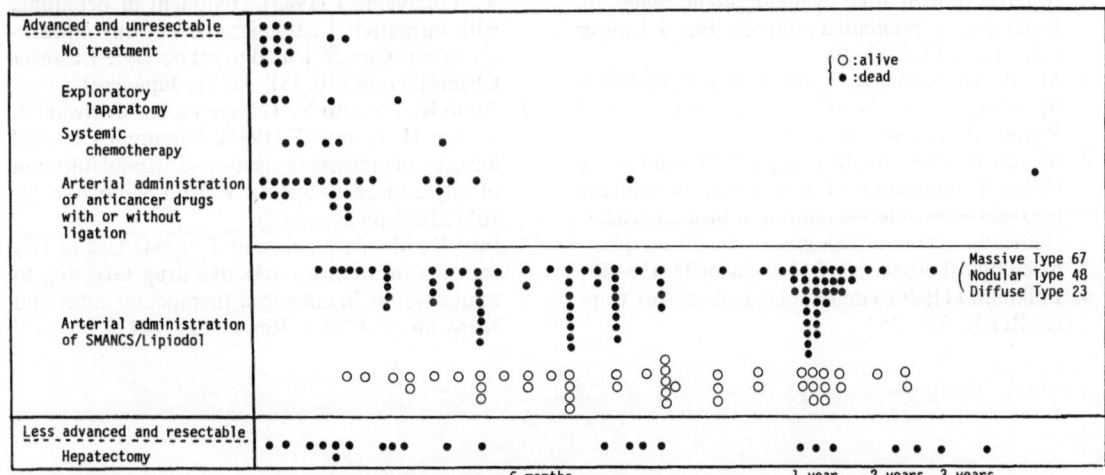

Fig. 27.11. Survival periods of patients with HCC after various methods of treatment

The anticancer agent dissolved in LPD is protected from degeneration by various hydrolytic enzymes in the aqueous phase which would otherwise inactivate or destroy it. Thus, an anticancer agent in LPD remains stable for a long period and LPD operates as a reservoir for the anticancer agent in the targeted tumor.

LPD itself may work as an embolizing agent in the neovasculature. Embolization due to LPD is not complete, and a small amount of blood flow was maintained even immediately after its administration. The growth of the tumor could not be controlled by embolization with LPD along, although a slight anticancer effect was observed [12]. It was speculated that a slight anticancer effect due to incomplete embolization by LPD was due to peripheral embolization at the level of the tumor neovasculature.

10   Concluding remarks

The recent development of targeting chemotherapy for HCC by arterial administration of oily anticancer agents has the following advantages: (1) The anticancer effect is definite in the majority of cases; (2) side effects due to anticancer agents appear to be minimal; (3) LPD is useful as an imaging agent which provides high contrast on CT and assists in the follow-up study of patients; (4) superselective catheterization is not always necessary, thereby making the procedure practical in most hospitals; (5) in many cases, patients can be discharged 1 week after arterial administration of the drugs and can be followed-up as outpatients; (6) the procedure is safe [1, 5, 10].

References

1. Konno T, Maeda H, Iwai K, Tashiro S, Maki S, Morinaga T, Mochinaga M, Hiraoka T, Yokoyama I (1983) Effect of arterial administration of high molecular-weight anticancer agent SMANCS with lipid lymphographic agent on hepatoma: a preliminary report. Eur J Cancer Clin Oncol 19: 1053–1065
2. Maeda H, Takeshita J, Konamaru R (1979) A lipophylic derivative of neocarzinostatin. Int J Peptide Protein Res 14: 81–87
3. Maeda H, Ueda M, Morinaga T, Matsumoto T (1985) Conjugation of poly (styrene-co-meleic acid) derivatives to the antitumor protein neocarzinostatin: Pronounced improvements in pharmacological properties. J Med Chem 28: 455–461
4. Folkman J (1974) Tumor angiogenesis. Adv Cancer Res 19: 331–359
5. Konno T, Maeda H, Iwai K, Maki S, Tashiro S, Uchida M, Miyauchi Y (1984) Selective targeting of anti-cancer drug and simultaneous image enhancement in solid tumors by arterially administered lipid contrast medium. Cancer 54: 2367–2374
6. Maeda H, Matsumura Y, Oda T, Sasamoto K (1986) Cancer selective macromolecular therapeusis: Tailoring of an antitumor protein drug. In: Whitaker JR, Feeney RE (eds) Protein tailoring for food and medical uses. Dekker, New York, pp 353–382
7. Maeda H, Takeshita J, Kanamaru R (1979) Antimetastatic and antitumor activity of a derivative of neocarzinostatin: an organic solvent and water-soluble polymer conjugated protein. Gann 70: 601–606
8. Maki S, Konno T, Maeda H (1985) Image enhancement in computerized tomography for sensitive diagnosis of liver cancer and semiquantitation of tumor selective drug targeting with oily contrast medium. Cancer 56: 751–757
9. Yumoto Y, Jinno K, Tokuyama K, Araki Y, Ishimitsu T, Maeda H, Konno T, Iwamoto S, Ohnishi K, Okuda K (1985) Hepatocellular carcinoma detected by iodized oil. Radiology 154: 19–24
10. Konno T, Tashiro S, Maeda H, Iwai K, Ogata K, Mochinaga M, Uemura K, Ishimaru Y, Miyauchi Y, Yokoyama I (1983) Treatment of hepatoma with intraarterial administration of oily anticancer agent. Gan to Kagakuryohoo (Jpn J Cancer Chemotherapy) 10: 351–357 (in Japanese)
11. Jinno K, Yumoto Y, Tokuyama K, Moriwaki S, Maeda H, Konno T (1985) Continuous arterial infusion of anticancer agents and arterial injection of oily anticancer agents. Rinsho Seijin Byo 15: 1657–1665 (in Japanese)
12. Iwai K, Maeda H, Konno T (1984) Use of oily contrast medium for selective drug targeting to tumor results in enhanced therapeutic effect and X-ray image. Cancer Res 44: 2115–2122

Chapter 28

Current Status of Hepatic Resection in the Treatment of Hepatocellular Carcinoma

Eizo Okamoto, Naoki Yamanaka, Akihiro Toyosaka, Nobutaka Tanaka, and Kohei Yabuki[1]

1 Introduction

Most patients suffering from hepatocellular carcinoma (HCC) in Japan have associated liver cirrhosis or a related liver disease. In the past, massive hepatic resection in these patients applied to cure the HCC frequently resulted in a fatal liver failure postoperatively. Preoperative assessment to determine a safe limit for resection is the most urgent problem for liver surgeons in Japan [1].

At the end of 1980, a multiple regression equation for prediction of posthepatectomy liver failure was established in our clinic [2]. The introduction of the prognostic index has successfully reduced operative mortality mainly caused by liver failure. In the past 5 years, our interests have been directed toward improving the long-term survival rate for HCC patients.

The recent use of advanced imaging modalities for high-risk patients has improved the detection of smaller carcinomas [3]. This has brought about revolutionary changes in the surgical techniques of hepatic resection in addition to better long-term survival [4–6]. Resection of a small part of the liver (segment or subsegment) recently has replaced the "classic" lobectomy or extended lobectomy. The current changing status in the treatment of HCC is documented in this chapter.

2 Review of surgical material

Three hundred and seventy-five adult patients were treated surgically from 1973 through 1985. The ages of the patients ranged from 22 to 83 years, with an average age of 64 years. There were 322 males (86%). Of 243 patients whose biopsy or resected specimens were examined his-

tologically, 195 (80%) had associated cirrhosis, while 31 of 243 (13%) had chronic hepatitis and/or fibrosis. Only 17 of 243 (7%) had normal liver tissue. Associated esophageal varices were seen in 139 of 307 (45.3%) patients who had been examined by esophagography and/or endoscopy; the varices were at an advanced stage in 45 (13.7%).

The operative procedures and the type of resections are documented in Table 28.1. Hepatic resection was carried out in 197 of the 375 patients, giving a resection rate of 52.5%. Four patients had additional resections for local recurrences. Currently, the types of resection that are increasingly used are wedge resection (referring to any kind of nonsegmental resection) and segmentectomy, accounting for 31% and 16% of 201 cases, respectively. The recent increase in the more limited resections is attributable to earlier detection of smaller sized HCCs, as shown in Fig. 28.1.

For patients with esophageal varices at risk for hemorrhage, nonshunting operations such as esophageal transection [7] or Hassab's procedure [8] were done simultaneously or metachronously with hepatectomy in 15 and with hepatic artery ligation (HAL)/hepatic artery cannulation (HAC) in 25. Endoscopic sclerotherapy [9] has been indicated, repeatedly if necessary, in advanced cirrhotic patients with varices for whom surgical intervention for HCC would have been risky.

3 Early prognosis after hepatectomy

Of 197 patients undergoing hepatectomy from 1973 to 1985, there were 17 operative deaths, giving a 30-day mortality of 8.6%; 34 patients who did not leave the hospital died, giving a hospital mortality of 17.3% (Table 28.2). When evaluating the mortality at the time of operation,

[1] First Department of Surgery, Hyogo College of Medicine, Nishinomiya, Hyogo, 663 Japan

Table 28.1. Surgical experience with HCC (April 1973–December 1985)

Procedure		Type of resection	
Hepatectomy	197 (53%)	Right lobectomy	69 (34%)
Rehepatectomy	4	Wedge resection	63 (31%)
HAL	120 (32%)	Segmentectomy	33 (16%)
HAL combined with hepatectomy	17	Left lobectomy	14
HAC	22	Trisegmentectomy	10
Others	15	Multiple resection	8
		Central bisegmentectomy	4
Total	375	Total	201

HAL hepatic artery ligation, *HAC* hepatic artery cannulation

the 30-day mortality was 21% (12/56) and hospital mortality 32% (18/56) during the first 8 years of 1973–1980. In the following 5 years (1981–1985), the mortality dropped to 3.5% and 11%, respectively.

The primary causes of hospital deaths (Table 28.2) were largely related to liver failure, accounting for 47% (16/34) of the total. The incidence of deaths due to liver failure was as high as 16% (9/56) during the early period and significantly dropped to 5.0% (7/141) during the later period, mainly accounting for the current decrease in the mortality. Therefore, a definite improvement in early prognosis results not only from advanced operative techniques but also from early detection of HCC and better selection of suitable candidates for surgery.

4 Prediction of a safe limit for hepatectomy

4.1 Quantified determination of the extent of resection

The operative or hospital deaths caused by hepatectomy are largely attributable to hepatic failure in both the Asian [10–12] and Western patients [13–15]. A critical question that needed to be answered was what percentage of liver tissue could be removed safely in patients suffering from various degrees of underlying liver disease. Before answering this question, it was essential to provide a method for exactly estimating the extent of the projected hepatectomy. The proportion of each segment in the human liver has been estimated as 35% for the right posterior, 30% for the right anterior, 20% for the left medial, and 15% for the left lateral segment [16]. Conventionally, surgeons assess the extent of hepatectomy by simply adding the percentage of the resected segments. For example, 65% has been

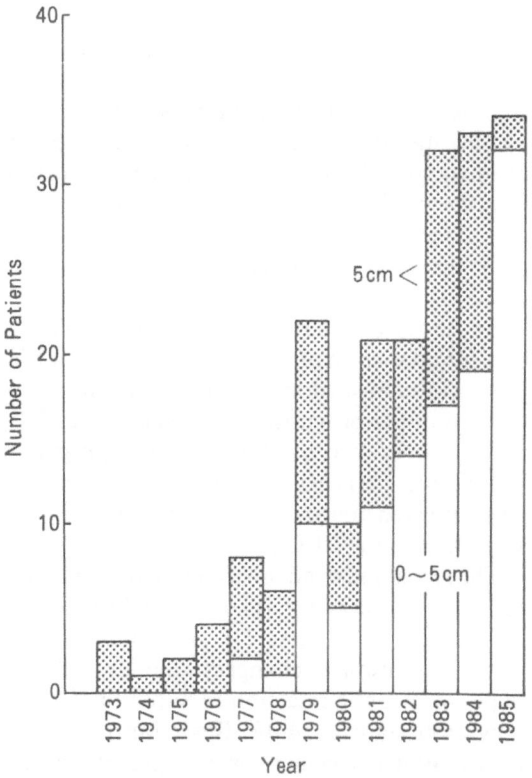

Fig. 28.1. Yearly size distribution of HCC. Small cancers less than 5 cm in diameter have been resected in increasing numbers since 1981

allocated to a right lobectomy and 85% to a right trisegmentectomy. However, these proportions are based on a normal liver and are not accurate in the pathological liver that is variably replaced by cancer. In addition, neoplastic tissue is not a functioning parenchyma, and there is usually compensatory hypertrophy in other areas of the liver.

We have developed a volumetric in vivo measurement using computed tomography (CT) [1].

Table 28.2. Primary causes of 30-day and hospital mortality following hepatectomy

	Apr. 1973–Dec. 1980 (n = 56)	Jan. 1981–Dec. 1985 (n = 141)	Total (n = 197)
Liver failure	5/56 8.9% (9/56 16%)	2/141 1.4% (7/141 5.0%)	7/197 3.6% (16/197 8.1%)
Cardiopulmonary	1 (2)	2 (2)	3 (4)
Intra-abdominal hemorrhage	3 (3)	0 (0)	3 (3)
Technical complication	3 (3)	0 (0)	3 (3)
GI bleeding	0 (0)	1 (3)	1 (3)
Recurrence	0 (0)	0 (3)	0 (3)
Others	0 (1)	0 (1)	0 (2)
Total	12/56 21% (18/56 32%)	5/141 3.5% (16/141 11%)	17/197 8.6% (34/197 17%)

Hospital mortality figures are given in parentheses. *GI* gastrointestinal

This study encouraged us to introduce the parenchymal hepatic resection rate (PHRR, percentage) as an indicator of what percentage of liver tissue, excluding the tumor, should be removed. It has been found that PHRR shows considerably different values among patients who had been subjected to the same anatomical extent of resection.

4.2 Factors predictive of posthepatectomy liver failure

There should be a good multifactorial system that combines several elements in terms of selection of patients who can survive hepatectomy without liver failure. We have applied a computer-generated multiple regression analysis to establish a formula for the preoperative prediction of posthepatectomy liver failure [2].

In a phase I retrospective study, those variables found to be statistically significant in distinguishing between the survivors and the nonsurvivors who died of liver failure are PHRR estimated by CT (percentage), indocyanine green dye (ICG) retention rate at 15 min (ICGR$_{15}$) [17], age, and ICG Rmax [18], in decreasing order of prognostic importance. The equations consisting of these three or four predictors are:

$$Y1 = -84.6 + 0.933X1 + 1.11X2 + 0.99X3 \quad \text{and}$$

$$Y2 = -110 + 0.9X1 + 1.36X2 + 1.17X3 + 5.94X4$$

where X1 is PHRR (%), X2 ICGR$_{15}$ (%), X3 patient's age, and X4 ICG-Rmax (mg/kg/min). Y1 and Y2 named as "prediction score" are operative risk scores for individuals who are to have hepatic resection. Prediction scores, computed by putting the selected predictor values of phase I patients into the equation, were found to distinguish between the survivors and nonsurvivors below and above approximately 50 points, respectively (Fig. 28.2).

A phase II prospective study was undertaken to analyze the predictive usefulness of the equations, using all the potential candidates for a major hepatectomy since the beginning of 1981. Of patients with HCC subjected to hepatic segmentectomy or lobectomy by the end of 1985, four of six (67%) with precalculated prediction scores of about 50 points or more died of liver failure 3–6 weeks after surgery. By contrast, 5 of 81 (6.1%) with scores of less than 50 points survived major hepatectomies without lethal liver failure. In patients with prediction scores much higher than 50 points, considered at high risk for major hepatectomy, treatment was switched to wedge resections for small favorably situated tumors and otherwise to HAL (4) or transcatheter arterial embolization (TAE) unless the main portal branch was obstructed with tumor thrombosis.

Hospital mortality caused by posthepatectomy liver failure dropped during the period from 1981 to 1985, using the prognostic index described above. The equations have provided us

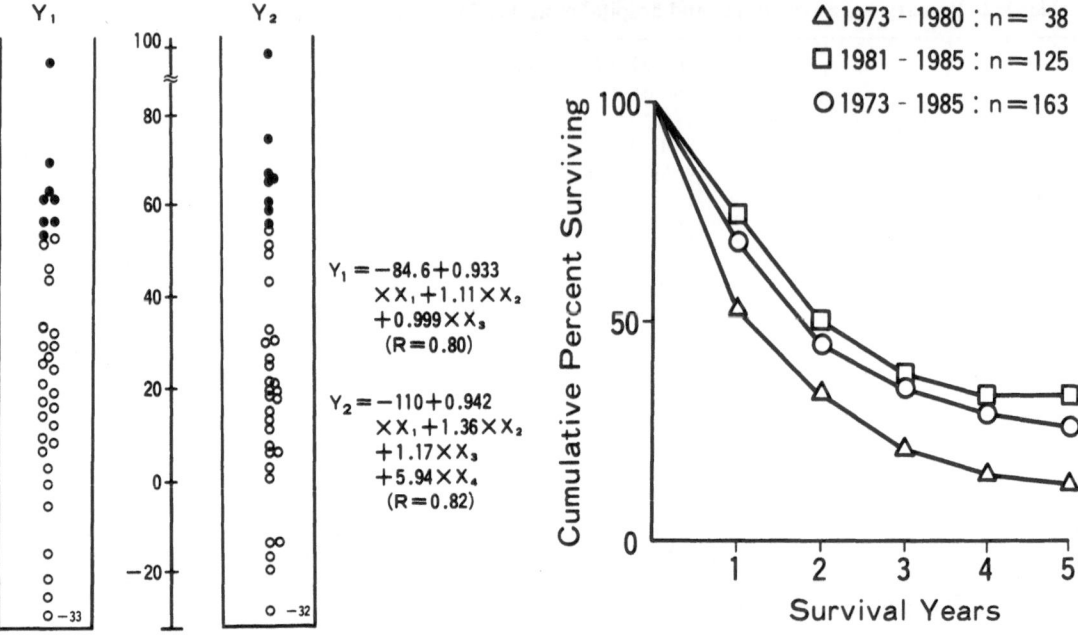

$$Y_1 = -84.6 + 0.933 \times X_1 + 1.11 \times X_2 + 0.999 \times X_3 \quad (R=0.80)$$

$$Y_2 = -110 + 0.942 \times X_1 + 1.36 \times X_2 + 1.17 \times X_3 + 5.94 \times X_4 \quad (R=0.82)$$

Fig. 28.2. Relationship between prediction score computed by the regression equation and early prognosis. *Closed circles* indicate the patients who died from hepatic failure and *open circles* indicate those who survived the hepatic resection

Fig. 28.3. Survival following resection by the time period of surgery

with an objective guideline for selection of the safest surgical treatment for individuals with HCC confined to either hepatic lobe.

5 Long-term results after hepatectomy

5.1 Current improvement in late survival

The early prognosis following hepatectomy has increasingly improved due to technical refinements and a preoperative assessment of the safe limits for hepatectomy. Further advances should include better selection of patients for long-term survival after hepatectomy.

In Asian countries where HCC is frequently associated with cirrhosis, worsening of the underlying liver disease must be considered as a possible cause of late deaths. However, 85% (74/87) of late deaths in the present series were primarily caused by local recurrences and/or distant metastases. On the other hand, late deaths caused by worsened cirrhosis accounted for only 6.9% (6/87) of total late deaths. This trend is similar to that reported in other series [10, 19] of patients treated by hepatectomy.

Overall the 1-, 3-, and 5-year cumulative survival rates in the 197 hepatectomized patients treated during the period 1973–1985 were 55%, 29%, and 21%, respectively, while those in the 163 patients excluding 34 hospital deaths were 68%, 35%, and 26%. In the present series, yearly survival figures were calculated by counting a cumulative percentage excluding hospital deaths. When the survival rates of the earlier period (1973–1980, n = 44) and the current period (1981–1985, n = 125) were compared, the latter had much better 1-, 3-, and 5-year survivals (74%, 38%, 33% vs 53%, 21%, 13%, respectively) than the former (Fig. 28.3). The long-term results of the current period are comparable with those reported in Western series [13, 14], although the incidence of associated cirrhosis with HCC is much higher in Japan [20] than in Western countries [13].

The percentage of patients with small tumors (less than 5 cm in diameter) increased from 32 (18/56) in the earlier period to 67 (94/141) in the current period (Fig. 28.1). Use of a screening program (alpha-fetoprotein test and imaging modalities such as ultrasonography and CT scan) for patients highly susceptible to HCC has made early detection and surgical removal of HCC possible, thus contributing to the current improvement in long-term survival.

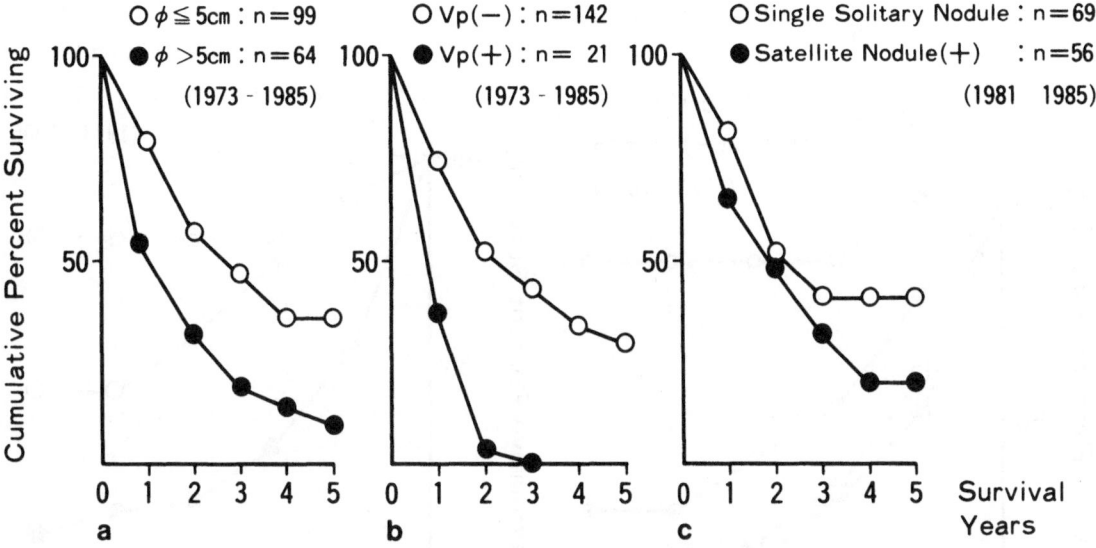

Fig. 28.4a–c. Survival following resection versus various prognostic factors. **a** Tumors size; **b** tumor thrombus; **c** tumor multiplicity. V*p* tumor thrombus in the main portal branches

5.2 Prognostic factors related to survival

5.2.1 Size of tumor

The 1-, 3-, and 5-year survival rates in the 79 patients with an HCC less than 5 cm in diameter were 79%, 47%, and 36% compared with 54%, 19%, and 10%, respectively, in the 64 patients with tumors larger than 5 cm (Fig. 28.4a). The significant influence of the smallness of the tumor on the prognosis after hepatectomy has also been noted in other Asian series [21]. But this does not seem to apply to Western patients [13], where size makes little difference in relation to survival. This discrepancy may be caused by a difference between growth patterns in Asian HCCs, which occur mostly in cirrhotic livers, and Western ones, which occur mainly in noncirrhotic livers.

5.2.2 Portal vein invasion

The tendency of an HCC to grow into the portal or hepatic vein is a widely accepted complication [6, 22]. The portal invasion of HCC is a causative factor of intrahepatic spread, leading to satellite lesions, as described below. Survival rates were compared between patients with and without tumor thrombi (Vp) located in the first and/or second order of the main portal branches (Fig. 28.4b). The 1- and 5-year survival rates of the Vp(+) group (*n* = 21) were much worse than those of the Vp(−) group (*n* = 142)—37% and 0 compared with 73% and 30%, respectively.

With regard to the presence of satellite nodules, the patients (*n* = 69) with a single isolated HCC had better prognoses of 81%, 41%, and

41% at 1, 3, and 5 years, respectively, than those with satellite nodules adjacent to the main tumor or multinodular growths (65%, 33%, and 20%, *n* = 56; Fig. 28.4c). These findings suggest that intraportal growth of an HCC, together with concomitant liver cirrhosis, are major limiting factors for cure by resection.

5.2.3 Cirrhosis and esophageal varices

There are conflicting reports [13, 23–25] on the influence of associated cirrhosis on the prognosis of patients with HCC. Some authors have concluded that it does correlate with natural [23] and treated survival [13, 24, 25]. In the present series of hepatectomized patients, a significant improvement in survival was not found in noncirrhotic patients compared with cirrhotic patients as in the other series in Japan [21]; 1-, 3-, and 5-year survival rates of noncirrhotics (*n* = 34) were 90%, 38%, and 31%, respectively, compared with 68%, 32%, and 20% of cirrhotics (*n* = 129). However, when we looked at patients with HCCs of less than 5 cm in size, the noncirrhotics (*n* = 9) had a much higher survival rate of 86% than the cirrhotics (*n* = 103) with a 29% survival rate at 5 years (Fig. 28.5). Less limited extent of resection in the noncirrhotic livers is more likely to provide a possible cure when compared with the limited extent of resection in the cirrhotic livers.

Fifteen of our patients underwent hepatectomy simultaneously or metachronously with nonshunting operations for concomitant esophageal varices. The survival rates at 1-, 3-, and 5-years were 74%, 66%, and 46%, respectively,

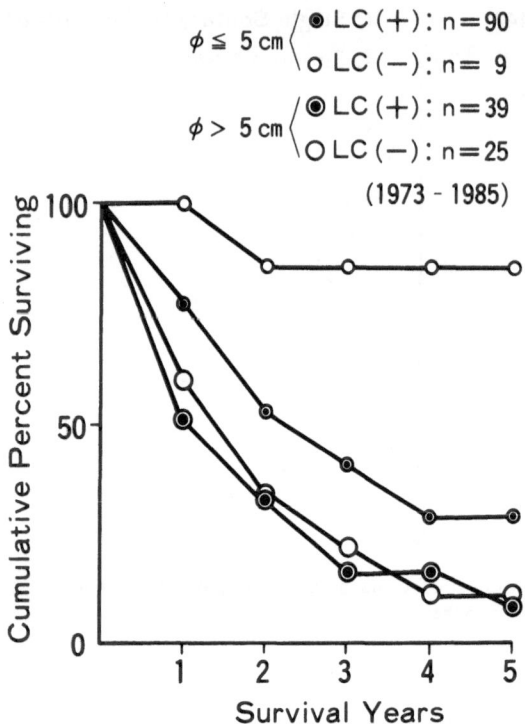

Fig. 28.5. Survival following resection versus tumor size and underlying liver cirrhosis (*LC*)

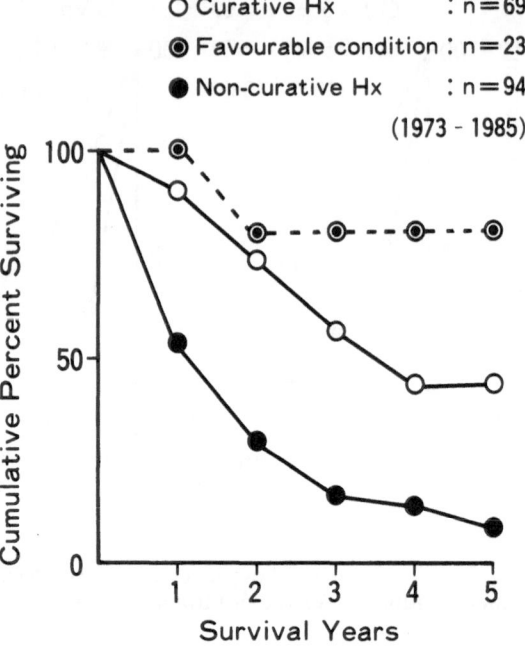

Fig. 28.6. Survival following resection (*Hx*) versus operative curability. Favorable conditions: tumor size ≦ 5 cm, no portal tumor thrombus, and no satellite nodule

with the longest survival of 61 months at the end of 1985. No bleeding from ruptured varices was seen after hepatectomy in these patients. The findings suggest that association of esophageal varices does not preclude acceptable survival as long as surgical management covers the varices as well as HCC within the safe limits of hepatectomy. For unresectable HCC with esophageal varices, HAL and endoscopic sclerotherapy were the treatments of choice.

5.2.4 Potential for cure by resection

Various clinical staging systems [26–28] that grade the extent of malignant involvement combined with clinical features have been proposed. In cases where resection is indicated, the potential for cure by surgery should be considered as a factor in survival. Our series has been tentatively divided into two categories—curative and noncurative resection groups, based on several distinguishing factors. The curative resection group refers to: (1) no involvement of margins of resection, (2) no macroscopic tumor invasion into the main vascular and biliary structures, and (3) all gross lesions confined to the resected portion.

The patients (*n* = 94) in our noncurative group had survival rates of 53%, 16%, and 8% at 1, 3, and 5 years, respectively (Fig. 28.6). These low

survival rates contrast sharply with 90%, 56%, and 43% for comparable years of our patients (*n* = 69) with curative resections. However, local recurrences have not infrequently been found in the patients for whom resection had been evaluated as curative.

The long-term results were reviewed for the selected patients of the curative resection group, who had favorable prognostic conditions as follows: tumor less than 5 cm in diameter, single solitary nodule, no tumor thrombi in the vascular structures, and no lesions at least 10 mm from the surgical margin. Twenty-three patients who met all four requirements showed a much better 5-year survival rate (79%) than the overall curative resection group (Fig. 28.6). The significant gap between the survival rates of the selected patients and the curative resection group indicates that latent intrahepatic metastatic foci possibly remain in the residual liver, even after gross curative surgery.

5.2.5 Hepatic resection versus hepatic artery ligation

The use of HAL for unresectable liver tumors has been pioneered by Scandinavian [29, 30] and Asian [31] surgeons. Since 1973, we have adopted ligation as the first choice of treatment for patients with unresectable HCCs. The proper hepatic artery was ligated provided that neither the right nor the left portal vein had been obstructed by cancer. Compensated liver cirrhosis is not a contraindication.

One hundred and twenty patients treated with HAL were divided into two groups. In group A, the cancer was confined to the liver, so that the ischemic effect of ligation covered all neoplastic lesions. In group B, the effect of ligation was limited because of extrahepatic spread or the presence of lesions in nonligated segments. In group A, 68 patients (excluding eight hospital deaths) achieved 1-, 3-, and 5-year survival rates of 60%, 22%, and 15% compared with 28%, 3%, and 0, respectively, of 32 patients in group B (excluding 12 hospital deaths; Fig. 28.7).

It is worth noting that there was no significant difference in the long-term survival rates between group A of HAL and noncurative resections (Figs. 28.6, 28.7). This suggests that ligation is preferable to an incomplete hepatic resection.

6 Early intrahepatic spread of HCC via portal vein

In the collective review by Foster in 1977 [13], the survival rate of patients undergoing hepatic resection was very low in Asian patients with cirrhosis compared with non-Asian patients without cirrhosis. Since there was no significant difference in the operative mortality rate between the two series, the much lower long-term survival of Asian patients was considered evidence that HCC might be multicentric in cirrhotic patients [13, 27]. However, in recent years, this concept has been modified. Thus, the introduction of mass screening in the high-risk areas of China [5] and follow-up using advanced imaging modalities of high-risk patients in Japan [3] have resulted in a remarkable increase in the number of patients detected with small and subclinical HCC. Early resection of these has substantially increased long-term survival in both countries [4–6].

Setting aside the question of whether HCC develops unicentrically or multicentrically, most pathologists and surgeons [6, 21, 32, 33] in Japan now agree that HCC has a tendency to invade portal branches, causing intraportal hepatic metastases. From the standpoint of surgical treatment, it is significant that this occurs at a very early stage of the disease.

We conducted a histological study on 34 re-

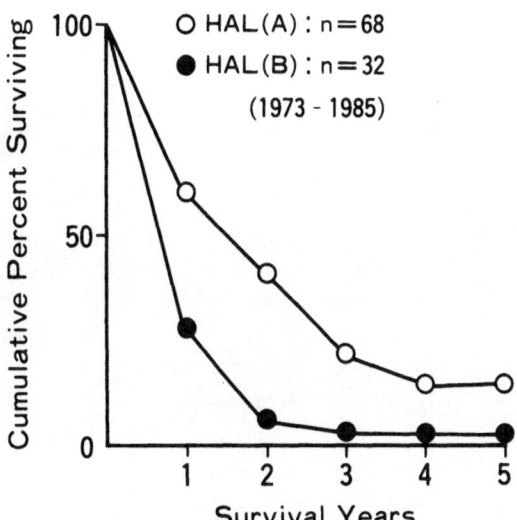

Fig. 28.7. Survival following hepatic artery ligation (*HAL*). *Open circles* signify cancer was confined to the liver and *closed circles* that there were extrahepatic spread or lesions in the nonligated segments

sected specimens of HCC of less than 3 cm in diameter (Fig. 28.8). The invasion of cancer cells into the portal branches was found in 50% (17/34) of the specimens and metastatic satellite nodules in 44.1% (15/34). When the study was confined to HCC of less than 2 cm, which is about the smallest clinically detectable size, the intraportal invasion and metastatic nodules were each seen in 20%.

With regard to the mechanism of intrahepatic metastasis of HCC, Nakashima [32] pointed out (from his study by means of barium injection into the blood vessels of an autopsied liver bearing HCC) that arterial branches act as the afferent vessels, while the capillarized sinusoids and portal branches act as the efferent channels for HCC. The same conclusion was arrived at in our study, in which a contrast material was injected directly into the tumor [33]. In 15 resected HCC specimens, barium sulfate solution was injected into the tumor and soft X-ray photographs were taken. In all but three noncirrhotic specimens, the portal branches were clearly visualized, while hepatic vein branches were not or only faintly stained. In the three noncirrhotic specimens, however, both portal and hepatic vein branches were opacified to the same extent.

In a patient with HCC (unresectable due to severe cirrhosis), the contrast material, mixed with Adriamycin, was injected directly into the tumor via a percutaneous transhepatic route and serial X-ray films were taken (Fig. 28.9). After

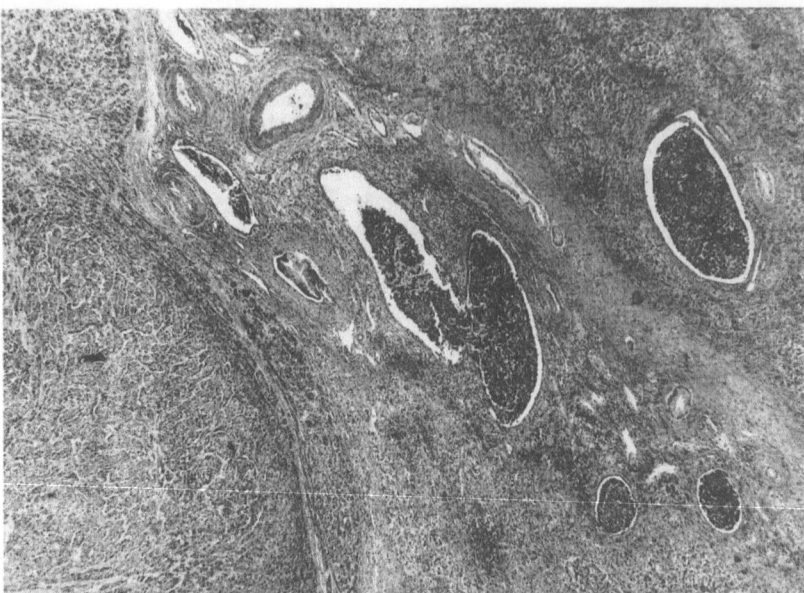

Fig. 28.8. Portal vein invasion of the HCC. Tumor cells, penetrating the pseudocapsule, grow into the small portal branches to form multiple tumor thrombi

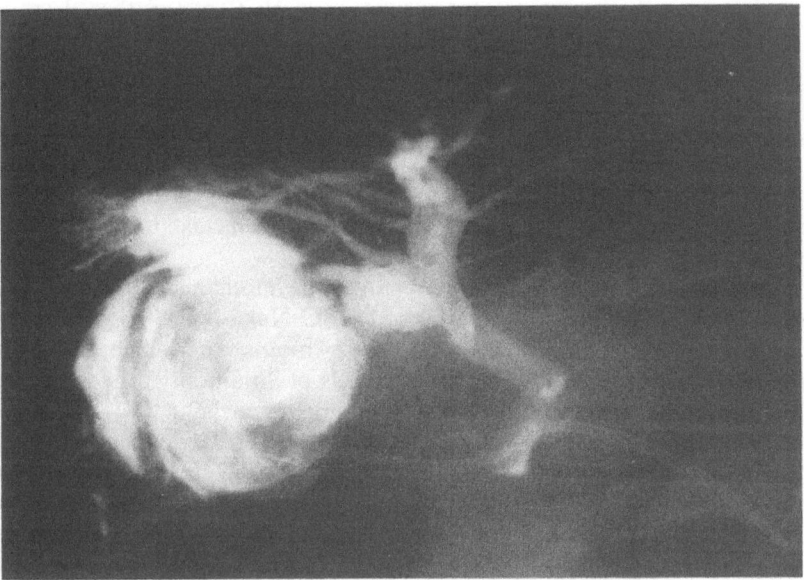

Fig. 28.9. Intrahepatic portagram obtained by direct injection of contrast material into an HCC through the percutaneous transhepatic route. Contrast medium entered the portal vein system only

filling the tumor, the injected contrast material immediately drained into portal branches and then all portal tributaries were visualized, while the hepatic vein was opacified later and only faintly. This reversal of the portal circulation in HCC, more marked in cirrhotic livers, seems to be responsible for the surprising early occurrence of intrahepatic metastases in cirrhotics.

One hundred and ninety-seven patients who underwent hepatic resection for HCC in our clinic had no evidence of lung or bone metastases, at least at the time of surgery. In contrast to other cancers, lymph node metastases were seldom encountered in these patients at laparotomy (less than 2%). Such an early occurrence of intrahepatic metastases via the portal vein is thus a distinct characteristic of this carcinoma as well as its most unfavorable aspect, precluding radical resection. Unfortunately, at present, HAL and TAE [34, 35] are not as effective for such metastatic satellite foci as they are for the encapsulated main tumor [36, 37].

Wider resection of the liver is indicated against the early intrahepatic spread of HCC, and yet in cirrhotic patients resection should be limited to minimize the operative risk. Further studies are needed to resolve this problem.

7 New method of controlled anatomical subsegmentectomy by suprahilar ligation

In recent years, with the rapid increase of cirrhotic patients with smaller HCCs detected by imaging, limited hepatectomies of less than one segment tend to outnumber regular and extended lobectomies. In view of the early intrahepatic spread of HCC through the portal bloodstream, anatomical segmental and subsegmental resections should be preceded by individual ligation of feeding and draining vessels. Until now, only the left lateral and medial segmentectomies have been established as anatomical segmentectomies. Anatomical resection of a segment or subsegment of the right lobe, with prior ligation of the hepatic pedicles at the level of the hilum, is considered difficult.

Segmentectomy or subsegmentectomy by an exclusive transparenchymatous approach to the vascular pedicles was reported by a team of French surgeons [38]. A method of ultrasonically guided subsegmentectomy was also reported by a surgical team of the National Cancer Center Hospital in Tokyo [39].

Very recently, we have devised a new technique for anatomical segmental or subsegmental resection of the right lobe by initial ligation at the suprahilar level of the Glisson's pedicles, going to the target areas in liver [40]. This method is based on the following anatomical facts: (1) The portal vein, hepatic artery, and bile duct reach the hilum of the liver by different routes, but thereafter the portal triads travel together in the common tunnels of Glisson's capsule into the segment and subsegment; (2) bifurcations of these Glissonian triads for each segment or subsegment are found surprisingly close to the hilum.

7.1 Selective and combined resection of right antero-inferior and -superior subsegments

In order to gain access to the Glisson's pedicles directed toward each subsegment, unroofing of the

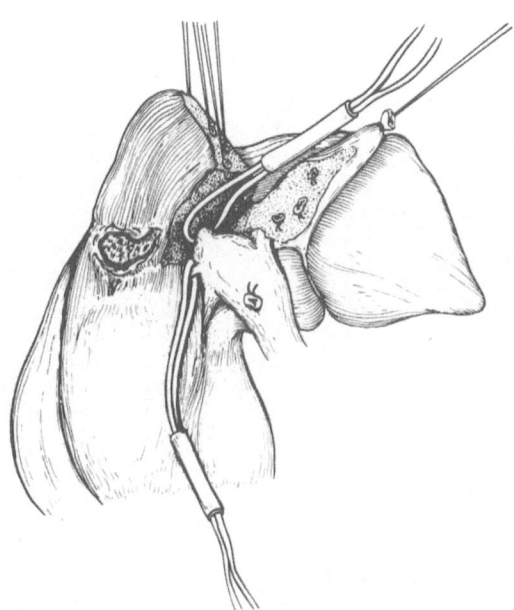

Fig. 28.10. Suprahilar mobilization of the caudate lobe. Roots of Glissonian pedicles toward the right anteroinferior and anteroposterior subsegments (Quinaud's segments V and VIII) are individually exposed

hilar plate, by mobilizing a part of the quadrate lobe that protrudes over the hilum, is often a useful method (Figs. 28.10, 28.11): The gallbladder is removed. The teres ligament is pulled upward and its peritoneum is opened longitudinally. Two or three portal pedicles directed toward the quadrate lobe are dissected on the right of the ligament. These pedicles are individually and sequentially ligated and divided in the liver parenchyma, and then the anteroinferior part of the middle segment becomes darkly discolored. When the discolored area covers enough of the protruding quadrate lobe, the dissection on the right of the teres ligament is discontinued.

The capsule of the quadrate lobe is incised transversely along the line just above the confluence of the right and left main lobar pedicles. The quadrate lobe is then dissected up from the main pedicles from left to right. One or two branches of the middle hepatic vein are usually encountered during this process, and they are ligated and divided.

At the end of this dissection, the pedicles of the anteroinferior and anterosuperior subsegments are exposed as a single confluent or separate trunks continuing from the right main pedicle. Meticulous dissection is continued around these

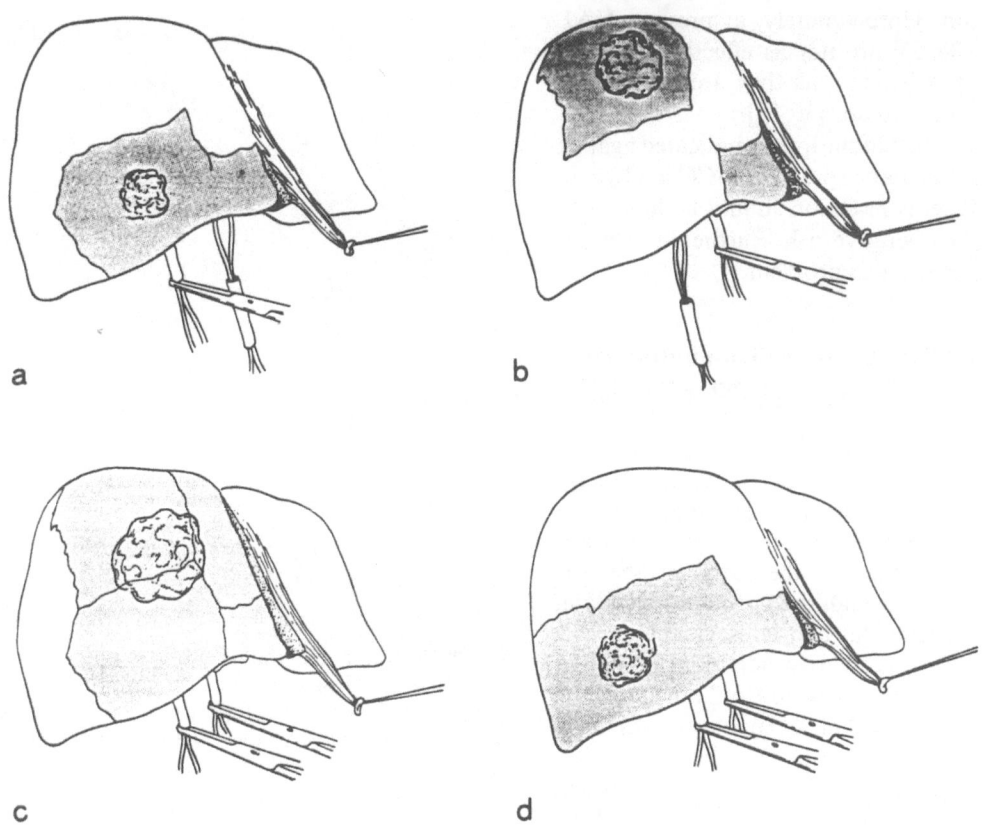

Fig. 28.11a–d. Various types of subsegmentectomy. **a** Single right anteroinferior subsegmentectomy (segment V); **b** single right anterosuperior subsegmentectomy (segment VIII); **c** central bisegmentectomy (segments IV, V, and VIII); **d** combined right anteroinferior and posteroinferior subsegmentectomy (segments V and VI)

structures without injuring Glisson's capsule in the liver parenchyma. The right main pedicle may be encircled by a thin Nelaton catheter, if necessary, to facilitate the dissection of the fine tributaries or to control bleeding if it occurs.

When the dissection proceeds ideally, not only the pedicles for the two anterior subsegments, but also those for the posteroinferior and posterosuperior subsegments are completely skeletonized at their roots. Branches of the right hepatic vein can also be identified between the anterior and posterior pedicles.

The intrahepatic routes of tributaries of the portal triads to each segment or subsegment frequently vary among patients. In addition, an HCC is not always located centrally but randomly in a segment or subsegment, in most cases with feeding vessels from adjacent segmental or subsegmental pedicles. Tentative clamping is thus essential to make sure that the isolated pedicle distributes only to the target area of the liver. If the discolored segment or subsegment does not include the entire target area of the liver that

needs resection, additional clamping of a pedicle or some of its tributaries of an adjacent subsegment is necessary until the appropriate area around the HCC becomes discolored.

After repeated testing, definitive ligation and division of a pedicle or pedicles and/or some of the tributaries is performed. The discolored area is then dissected out in a centroperipheral, or reverse, manner. In the course of dissection, three to five draining hepatic vein branches are found between the liver being resected and the right or middle hepatic vein trunks. After carefully ligating and dividing these vein branches, resection is finally accomplished.

7.2 Central bisegmentectomy

This combined resection of the right anterior segment and left medial segment is indicated most frequently for HCC located in the central dome of the liver (Fig. 28.11c). The first steps of this procedure are similar to those performed for the suprahilar resection technique for the right anterior segment. Thus, the quadrate lobe is

Fig. 28.12. Exposure of portal pedicles toward the right posteroinferior and posterosuperior subsegments (segments VI and VIII). The recess is widely opened anteriorly to the caudate lobe in the plane of the right lobar fissure

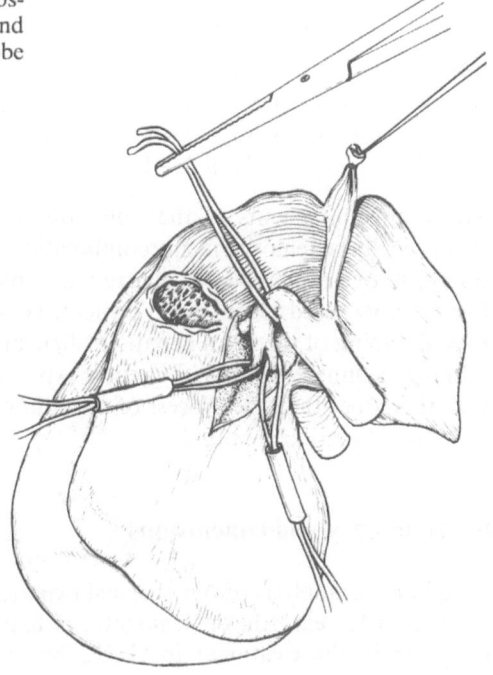

transected on the right of the teres ligament and mobilized suprahilarly, and the Glisson's pedicles for the right anterior segment are identified and divided after individual ligation.

The parenchymatous transection on the right of the teres ligament is then resumed, extending upward along the right side of the falciform ligament until the middle hepatic vein trunk is reached. The central bisegments that are now completely discolored are lifted and dissected up posteriorly toward the inferior vena cava. Several venous branches are ligated and divided on the left of the right hepatic vein trunk. The middle hepatic vein trunk is finally ligated and divided before it joins the left hepatic vein or the inferior vena cava, and the resection is completed.

7.3 Selective and combined resection of right postero-inferior and -superior subsegments

This procedure is indicated when the neoplastic lesion is located exclusively in the right posterior segment (Fig. 28.12). After laparotomy, the right lobe is completely mobilized by severing all the bands and ligaments, and the gallbladder is removed. The right lobe is gently rotated upward to expose clearly its visceral and posterior surfaces. The right main lobar pedicle is isolated anteriorly from the quadrate lobe by incising a part of the hilar plate and posteriorly from the

caudate lobe by lifting and dividing one or two short vascular pedicles. The right main pedicle is then encircled with tape. By manipulating this tape upward and downward, the dissection is more easily continued on the right side of the transverse fissure.

In the vicinity of the right main lobar pedicle, the roots of the pedicles for the right anterior segment are usually found in the plane between the right anterior and left median segments—main lobar fissure—just behind the base of the gallbladder bed; those for the posterior segment are in the plane between the anterior and posterior segments—right lobar fissure. The latter is not an anatomical fissure, but a recess is always found anterior to the base of the caudate process, where the roots of the posterior segment are widely exposed by dissecting the liver parenchyma anterior to the pedicles. The disclosed pedicles are individually and sequentially taped. By repeated test clamping, the segment or subsegment to be removed is determined. Definitive ligation is then performed and the discolored segment or subsegment is resected.

7.4 Results and comment

In the past two years up to the end of 1985, this type of subsegmentectomy was carried out in 18 patients with HCC. For convenience in comparison, the resected areas are listed below according to Couinaud's designation of liver segments [41]. Combinations of the segments resected are:

S5 − − − − − − − − 2   S5 + 6 − − − − − − − 2
S6 − − − − − − − 3   S5 + 8 − − − − − − − 2
S8 − − − − − − − 3   S6 + 7 − − − − − − − 3
S4 + 5 − − − − − − 3   S4 + 5 + 8 − − − − − 3

The four subsegments of the right lobe could theoretically be removed in any combination. No operative or hospital deaths ocurred, and blood loss did not exceed 600 ml in any patient. Temporary clamping of the main hepatic pedicle at the hilum was unnecessary. With greater experience with this procedure, the process of unroofing the caudate lobe can be omitted.

8 Summary and conclusions

Based on the analysis of our surgical experience of the past 13 years, the current status of hepatic resection in the treatment for HCC has been evaluated.

The association of HCC with liver cirrhosis, even though very frequent in Japan and other Asian countries, is not per se a contraindication for hepatic resection. The effect of the cirrhosis on the anatomical and functional aspects of the patient's liver should be carefully assessed in each case.

Our multiple regression equations consisting of PHRR by CT, ICG retention rate at 15 min, patient's age, and ICG Rmax, if available, are useful indicators for the preoperative prediction of posthepatectomy liver failure. These equations also give an objective guideline for selection of the safest treatment for patients with HCC.

Besides liver cirrhosis, the paradoxically early occurrence of intrahepatic metastasis via portal branches is the most unfavorable pathological feature of HCC that prevents radical resection and subsequently decreases long-term survival with this cancer. Early and curative resection of HCC before this occurs is highly desirable in treating the patient. On the other hand, the surgeon should realize that hepatic artery ligation or transcathether arterial embolization is highly preferable to an incomplete resection that leaves a part of the cancer or its metastasis behind.

A limited and yet curative approach toward hepatectomy is urgently required for the recently increasing number of small HCCs that are being detected. A new method of controlled anatomical subsegmentectomy by suprahilar ligation has been proposed.

References

1. Okamoto E, Kyo A, Yamanaka N, Tanaka N, Kuwata K (1984) Prediction of the safe limit of hepatectomy by combined volumetric and functional measurements in patients with impaired hepatic function. Surgery 95: 586–591
2. Yamanaka N, Okamoto E, Kuwata K, Tanaka N (1984) A multiple regression equation for prediction of posthepatectomy liver failure. Ann Surg 200: 658–663
3. Okuda K, Nakashima T (1979) Hepatocellular carcinoma: A review of the resent studies and development. In: Popper H, Schaffner F (eds) Progress in liver diseases: VI. Grune and Stratton, New York, pp 639–650
4. Okamoto E, Tanaka N, Yamanaka N, Toyosaka A (1984) Results of surgical treatments of primary hepatocellular carcinoma: some aspects to improve long-term survival. World J Surg 8: 360–366
5. Tang ZY, Ying YY, Gu TJ (1982) Hepatocellular carcinoma. Changing concepts in recent years. In: Popper H, Schaffner F (eds) Progress in liver diseases: VII. Grune and Statton, New York, pp 637–647
6. Yamasaki S, Hasegawa H, Makuuchi M (1981) Clinicopathological observation of minute liver cancer and the new method of hepatectomy: Analysis of 27 resected cases. Acta Hepatol Jpn 22: 1714–1724
7. Sugiura M, Futagawa S (1973) A new technique for treating esophageal varices. J Thorac Cardiovasc Surg 66: 677–685
8. Hassab MA (1964) Gastroesophageal deconection and splenectomy: A method of prevention and treatment of bleeding from esophageal varices associated with bilharzial hepatic fibrosis. Preliminary report. J Internal College Surg 41: 232–248
9. Shu A, Okamoto E, Toyosaka, Tanaka N, Yamanaka N, Eoden Y, Yabuki k (1986) Treatments for patients with hepatoma and esophageal varices. Nichigekaishi 86: 1231–1233 (in Japanese)
10. Lin TY (1979) Resection therapy for primary malignant hepatic tumors. Int Adv Surg Oncol 2: 25–54
11. Lee NW, Ong GB (1982) The surgical management of primary carcinoma of the liver. World J Surg 6: 66–75
12. Lin TY (1976) Recent advances in technique of hepatic lobectomy and results of surgical treatment for primary carcinoma of the liver. Prog Liver Dis 5: 668–682
13. Foster JH (1977) Liver resection-operative technique. In: Foster JH, Berman MM (eds) Solid liver tumors, vol. 23. Saunders, Philadelphia, pp 255–303
14. Fortner JG, Kim DK, Maclean BJ, Barrett MK, Iwatsuki S, Turnbull AD, Howland WS, Beattie EJ (1978) Major hepatic resection for neoplasia—personal experience of 108 patients. Ann Surg 188: 363–371
15. Iwatsuki S, Shaw BW, Starzl TE (1983) Expe-

rience with 150 liver resections. Ann Surg 197: 247–253

16. Stone HH, Long WD, Smith RB, Heynes CD (1969) Physiologic considerations in major hepatic resections. Am J Surg 117: 78–84

17. Nambu M (1966) Hepatic clearance of indocyanine green in liver diseases. Jpn Gastroenterol 63: 777–794 (in Japanese)

18. Moody FG, Leyton FR, Joagin SA (1974) Estimation of the functional reserve of human liver. Ann Surg 180: 592–598

19. Balasegaram M (1979) Hepatic resection for malignant tumors. Surg Round 2: pp14–26

20. The liver cancer study group of Japan (1984) Primary liver cancer in Japan. Cancer 54: 1744–1755

21. Kishi K, Shikata T, Hirohashi S, Hasegawa H, Yamazaki S, Makuuchi M (1983) Hepatocellular carcinoma—A clinical and pathologic analysis of 57 hepatectomy cases. Cancer 51: 542–548

22. Okuda K, Musha H, Nakajima Y, Kubo Y, Shimokawa Y, Jinnouchi S, Obata H, Okazak N, Kojiro M, Sakamoto K, Nakashima T (1977) Pathologic features of encapsulated hepatocellular carcinoma. A study of 26 cases. Cancer 40: 1240–1245

23. Johnson PJ, Melia WM, Palmer MK, Portmann B, Williams R (1981) Relationship between serum alpha-fetoprotein, cirrhosis and survival in hepatocellular carcinoma. Br J Cancer 44: 502–505

24. Lin TY (1976) Surgical treatment of primary liver cell carcinoma. In: Okuda K, Peters PR (eds) Hepatocellular carcinoma. Wiley, New york, pp 449–468

25. Cochrane AMG, Murray-Lyon IM, Brinkley DM, Williams R (1977) Quadruple chemotherapy versus radiotherapy in treatment of primary hepatocellular carcinoma. Cancer 40: 609–614

26. Primack A, Vogel CL, Kyalwazi SK, Ziegler JL, Simon R, Anthony PP (1975) A staging system for hepatocellular carcinoma: Prognostic factors in Ugandan patients. Cancer 35: 1357–1364

27. Fortner JG, MacLean BJ, Kim DK, Howland WS, Turnbull AD, Goldiner P, Carlon G, Beattie E (1981) The seventies evolution in liver surgery for cancer. Cancer 47: 2162–2166

28. El-Domeiri AA, Mojab K (1978) Intermittent occlusion of the hepatic artery and infusion chemotherapy for carcinoma of the liver. Am J Surg 135: 771–775

29. Nilsson LAV (1966) Therapeutic hepatic artery ligation in patients with secondary liver tumors

Rev Surg 23: 374–376

30. Plengvanit U, Limwonges K, Viranuvat V, Hitanat S, Chearanai O (1967) Treatment of primary carcinoma of the liver by hepatic artery ligation. Tijdschr Gastroenterol 106: 491–497

31. Balasegaram M (1972) Complete hepatic dearterialization for primary carcinoma of the liver: Report of twenty-four patients. Am J Surg 124: 340–345

32. Nakashima T (1976) Vascular changes and hemodynamics in hepatocellular carcinoma. In: Okuda K, Peters RL (eds) Hepatocellular carcinoma. Wiley, New York, pp 169–203

33. Okamoto E, Toyosaka A (1984) Portal vein invasion of hepatocellular carcinoma and longterm results. In: Development of hepatocellular carcinoma in patients with viral hepatitis. Hattori N (ed) Gun to Kagakuryohosha, Tokyo, pp 506–519 (in Japanese)

34. Goldstein HM, Wallace S, Anderson JH, Bree RL, Gianturco C (1976) Transcatheter occlusion of abdominal tumors. Radiology 120: 539–545

35. Yamada R, Sato M, Kawabata M, Nakatsuka H, Nakamura K, Takashima S (1983) Hepatic artery embolization in 120 patients with unresectable hepatoma. Radiology 148: 397–401

36. Tanaka N, Okamoto E, Toyosaka A, Fujiwara S (1985) Pathological evaluation of hepatic dearterialization in encapsulated hepatocellular carcinoma. J Surg Oncol 29: 256–260

37. Okamura J, Horikawa S, Fujiyama T, Monden M, Kambayshi, Sikujara O, Sakurai M, Kuroda C, Nakamura H, Kosai G (1982) An appraisal of transcatheter arterial embolization combined with transcatheter arterial infusion chemotherapeutic agent for hepatic malignancies. World J Surg 6: 352–357

38. Bismuth H, Houssin D, Castaing D (1982) Major and minor segmentectomies "reglees" in liver surgery. World J Surg 6: 10–24

39. Makuuchi M, Hasegawa H, Yamazaki S (1985) ultrasonically guided subsegmentectomy. Surg Gynec Obst 161: 346–350

40. Okamoto E (1986) Hepatic resection for primary hepatocellular carcinoma: new trials for controlled anatomic subsegmentectomies by an initial suprahilar Glissonian pedicular ligation method. Shokakigeka Seminar 23: 229–241 (in Japanese)

41. Couinaud C (1954) Lobes et segments hepatiques, notes sur l'architecture anatomique et chirurgicale du foie. Press Med 62: 709–712

Chapter 29
Surgical Treatment of Subclinical Cases of Hepatocellular Carcinoma

Zhao-you Tang[1]

Subclinical cases of hepatocellular carcinoma (subclin-HCC) are arbitrarily defined as those without obvious HCC symptoms and signs. They are detected principally by alphafetoprotein (AFP) serosurvey or by ultrasonography in asymptomatic subjects, particularly those with a background of liver disease. The early detection, diagnosis, and treatment of subclin-HCC has opened a new era in the clinical aspects of liver cancer research since the early 1970s. After long-term follow-up, the significance of the study of subclin-HCC has become clearer, especially in patients who have undergone surgical treatment.

1 Special features of subclin-HCC

From January 1958 to December 1984, a total of 879 cases with pathologically proven HCC were collected in Zhong Shan Hospital of Shanghai Medical University. Of the entire series, 121 cases were subclin-HCC while 758 cases were symptomatic clinical HCC (clin-HCC). The special features of subclin-HCC are compared with clin-HCC in Table 29.1; subclin-HCC had a much smaller median tumor size, much lower median serum AFP level, much lower gamma-glutamyl transpeptidase (GTP) values, and positive scintigraphy. Subclin-HCC was discovered by AFP serosurvey in the majority of cases, whereas clin-HCC was mainly discovered by the patient as a result of obvious symptoms or signs. However, the incidence of coexisting liver cirrhosis was similar in both groups.

[1] Liver Cancer Research Unit, Zhong Shan Hospital, Shanghai Medical University, Shanghai, People's Republic of China

2 Significance of surgical treatment of subclin-HCC

2.1 Long survival of HCC

Long survival of patients with HCC has rarely been encountered in the past several decades. Curutchet et al. [1] summarized the world literature from 1905 to 1970; only 45 cases with a 5-year survival were collected. However, there were 43 cases with a 5-year survival from 1958 to 1984 in Zhong Shan Hospital of Shanghai Medical University. Of the 43 cases, 23 were subclin-HCC after resection. The 5-year survival rate of subclin-HCC after resection was as high as 72.9% [2].

2.2 Improving overall 5-year survival of HCC

The overall 5-year survival rate of HCC was reported to be less than 3% for decades. However, a comparative study of the periods 1958–1966, 1967–1975, and 1976–1984 in Zhong Shan Hospital revealed that the overall 5-year survival rates dramatically increased from 1.7% through

Table 29.1. Special features of subclin-HCC

	Subclin-HCC (n = 121)	Clin-HCC (n = 758)
AFP serosurvey[a] (%)	97.5	8.4
Median size of tumor (cm)	4.0	10.0
Median AFP level (ng/ml)	2000	10 000
Positive scintigraphy (%)	42.1	90.5
Gamma-GTP > 10 units (%)	24.8	74.2
With cirrhosis (%)	86.3	81.3

[a] Discovered by AFP serosurvey or monitoring of subjects with liver disease

Table 29.2. Changing frequency of subclin-HCC and overall 5-year survival in different periods

	1958–1966 (n = 124)	1967–1975 (n = 277)	1976–1984 (n = 477)
Subclin-HCC in entire series (%)	0(0/124)	7.2(20/277)	21.2(101/477)
5-year survival rate of entire series (%)	1.7	7.1	19.5

Survival rates calculated by the life-table method

7.1% to 19.5%. These encouraging results were correlated to the increased number of cases of subclin-HCC (Table 29.2).

2.3 Early evolution of HCC

For decades, knowledge of human HCC was mainly derived from relatively late-stage patients. However, AFP serosurvey of asymptomatic subjects and, in particular, surgery of subclin-HCC have provided valuable clues to the study of the early evolution of HCC. Thus, a new concept of the natural history of HCC has been developed [3], and important data concerning its early evolution have accumulated [4].

3 Surgical indications for subclin-HCC

Surgery is recommended only in accordance with the following criteria.

3.1 Diagnostic criteria of AFP and localization measurements

Almost 70% of cases of HCC in China had an abnormal serum AFP level. The diagnostic criteria of AFP were AFP > 500 ng/ml persisting for 1 month or AFP > 200 ng/ml persisting for 2 months without coexistent active liver disease (i.e, without abnormal serum alanine aminotransferase (ALT), bilirubin, or prothrombin time) and with exclusion of pregnancy or teratoma of the gonads.

Although some other markers have been claimed to be of value in early diagnosis in about 30% of non-AFP-producing HCC, more reliable tests are needed. On the other hand, localization measurements have provided important diagnostic clues. The positivity of ultrasonography (US) in subclin-HCC was 75.4% (46/61) in our series. Small HCC usually showed a hypoechoic area with a capsule, whereas small hemangiomas were hyperechoic upon US examination. Strong positive filling after the injection of contrast medium might help in the diagnosis of subclin-HCC using computed tomography (CT). Hepatic angiography (HA) provided better informa-

tion in the diagnosis of subclin-HCC; the positivity in our series was 82.1% (32/39), with typical tumor vessels and tumor stain. The lowest limit for HA detection was around 1 cm, whereas it was about 1.5 cm by US and CT. Scintigraphy was less valuable in the diagnosis of subclin-HCC; the positivity was only 42.1% (48/114), with the lowest limit at about 2–3 cm. Complete absence of serum hepatitis B virus (HBV) markers can help to exclude HCC in China, since the positivity of HBV markers in the serum of patients with HCC was as high as 98.0% in our series.

3.2 Contraindications

Jaundice, ascites, distant metastases, or tumor emboli in the main trunk of the portal vein are contraindications to surgery. US is of great value in detecting emboli in the main trunk of the portal vein.

3.3 Subclin-HCC with compensated liver function

A reversed serum albumin/globulin ratio, impairment of prothrombin time (<50% of normal value), and/or bilirubin >2.0 mg/dl are contraindications to surgery.

4 Surgical procedure for Subclin-HCC

It has been repeatedly shown that surgical resection is the method of choice for the treatment of subclin-HCC [2, 5, 6]. No 5-year survival could be attained in subclin-HCC without resectional treatment. Therefore, every effort should be made to increase the resectability of HCC, decrease operative mortality, and improve survival after surgery.

4.1 Anesthesia and transfusion

When the abdominal approach is used, epidural anesthesia is recommended. However, general anesthesia remains the modality of choice for the transthoracic and abdominal approach. A sufficient oxygen supply is important. Transfusion with fresh blood through an upper extremity is superior to that with bank blood through the lower extremity.

4.2 Position and incision

The position of the patient is of prime importance for good operative exposure. US can help in determining the correct position according to the tumor site. A right subcostal incision is routinely used. An extension in a left subcostal direction is usually needed for resection of left lobe tumors. Interruption of one to two ribs without entering the chest might help the resection of a lesion in the lower part of the right lobe. However, the transthoracic and abdominal approach is routinely used for limited resection of cancer in the upper pole of the right lobe, especially in the bare area.

4.3 Selection of surgical treatment

As stated above, resection remains the method of choice for subclin-HCC. However, adequate cryosurgery (using $-196°C$ liquid nitrogen with repeated freeze-thawing cycles or high-power YAG laser vaporization) may lead to a similar result for small HCCs in the surface of the liver, especially those located near the hepatic hilum and inferior vena cava. Subclin-HCC with two nodules is not a contraindication to resection. However, patients with three or more tumor nodules are not good candidates for resection. Hepatic artery ligation and/or cannulation in the affected side is indicated for multiple or deep-seated nonresectable subclin-HCC. As shown in Table 29.3, the "therapeutic pattern" of subclin-HCC, as compared with clin-HCC, was characterized by a much higher resection rate (69.4% versus 29.2%) and a much lower conservative treatment (7.5% versus 36.2%) and no treatment rate (0% versus 11.1%). The rate of surgery other than resection was similar—23.1% and 23.5%, respectively. Thus, the effective treatment rate, including resection and surgery other than resection, in subclin-HCC was much higher than that in clin-HCC (92.5% versus 52.7%). For surgery other than resection, cryosurgery and lasers were more frequently employed in the treatment of subclin-HCC because of the smaller tumor size.

4.4 Resection

4.4.1 Resectability rate

Of the 121 cases with subclin-HCC, 115 (95.0%) underwent surgery, whereas in the clin-HCC

Table 29.3. Therapeutic pattern of subclin-HCC and clin-HCC

	Subclin-HCC ($n = 121$)	Clin-HCC ($n = 758$)
Resection	69.4	29.2
Cryosurgery	9.9	3.4
Laser vaporization	0.8	0.3
Hepatic artery ligation plus cannulation	4.1	6.7
Hepatic artery ligation	1.7	3.2
Hepatic artery cannulation	6.6	9.9
Exploration and conservative treatment	2.5	16.4
Conservative treatment without exploration	5.0	19.8
No treatment	0	11.1

All figures are percentages

group only 69.1% of patients were candidates for surgery. Furthermore, the resectability rate was much higher in the subclin-HCC group (73.1% versus 42.3%). The encouraging resectability rate for subclin-HCC was due to a smaller tumor size, less severe cirrhosis and liver dysfunction, and the resection technique selected. Analyses of the factors influencing the resectability rate of subclin-HCC revealed that resectability increased with younger age, lower levels of serum gamma-GTP and alkaline phosphatase, tumor location in the left lobe, and a single nodule.

4.4.2 Types of resection

As mentioned above, the associated liver cirrhosis in subclin-HCC patients was as high as 86.3%; 73.2% was macronodular in type. Therefore, limited resection was employed particularly in those cases with small HCC located in the right lobe of a cirrhotic liver. The types of limited resection include wedge-shaped resection or partial hepatectomy for a tumor in the peripheral part of the liver, round or spindle-shaped resection for a tumor in the central part of the liver, and enucleation for a tumor located close to the hepatic hilum or inferior vena cava. However, segmentectomy or lobectomy was not infrequently employed for a left lobe tumor when the cirrhosis was not severe and the remaining liver parenchyma seemed to be adequate in function (Fig. 29.1). Based on a long-term follow-up study, a resection margin of about 2 cm from the tumor capsule was accepted as providing curative resection for small HCC. Limited resection produced a high resectability rate and a low operative mortality for subclin-HCC. A similar

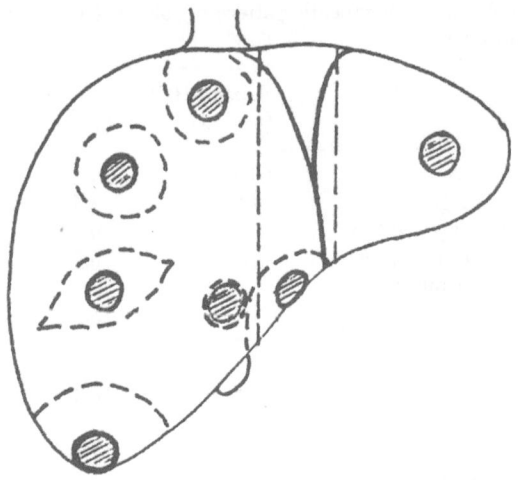

Fig. 29.1. Sites of limited resection. Tumors are *shaded* and resection lines are shown by interrupted lines

result was also noted in the literature [7]. The types of resection in our series are summarized in Table 29.4. It was clear that the principle of regular lobectomy, which was established in the 1950s, has remained true for clin-HCC with a relatively huge tumor, accounting for 74.6% of cases of clin-HCC. However, limited resection instead of classic lobectomy was the treatment of choice for resection of subclin-HCC with a relatively small tumor; it accounted for 64.3% of cases of subclin-HCC.

4.4.3 Procedure

Good exposure is of prime importance in facilitating the resection, minimizing blood loss, and shortening the occlusion time of the hepatic hilum. Careful assessment of the extent of resection is one of the key factors for a successful operation. The cutting line was routinely marked on the surface of the liver by a cautery. For control of bleeding during resection, a hepatic clamp or interrupted mattress suture was employed for tumors located in the peripheral part of the liver; temporal occlusion of the first hepatic hilar area using a rubber tube was employed for tumors located in the central part or near the hepatic hilum. The occlusion time should not exceed 10 min for severe cirrhosis and 15 min for a cirrhotic liver. Repeated occlusion was sometimes needed for a complicated resection. Finger fracture and careful ligation of all the vessels and ducts in the cut end is the technique of choice for resection. The raw surface was either approximated by suture without tension or covered by a thin layer of omentum or gel foam. Adequate drainage was important. In cases with satellite nodules or inadequate resection, hepatic artery cannulation in the affected side was routinely carried out for postoperative chemotherapeutic

perfusion. In previous years, bloodless operation with hypothermic perfusion was employed in five cases for resection of subclin-HCC situated close to the inferior vena cava in the second hepatic hilar area [8]. This has been discontinued since the routine hilar occlusion technique can fulfill the requirements of small HCC resection in different areas.

4.4.4 Operative mortality

A much lower operative mortality was observed for resection of subclin-HCC than with clin-HCC, being 1.2% (1/84) and 10.0% (22/221), respectively. The key points for a low operative mortality for resection of subclin-HCC were good exposure, limited resection instead of lobectomy of small HCC with cirrhosis in the right lobe, and shortened occlusion time of the porta hepatis.

4.5 Management of nonresectable subclin-HCC

Cryosurgery (with −196°C liquid nitrogen) can provide necrosis in the area of the ice ball that is formed. A cryoprobe 3.5 cm in diameter results in the formation of an ice ball with a surface diameter of 5–6 cm and a depth of 3.5–4 cm during 20 min of freezing. A double freeze-thawing cycle with temporal hilar occlusion could provide adequate necrosis of a 2- to 3-cm tumor on the surface of the liver [9]. The longest survival is 7 years after cryosurgery for a recurrent HCC of 2 cm in diameter; the patient was alive and free of disease at the last follow-up. High-power YAG laser is another alternative treatment of superficial nonresectable HCC. A small HCC nodule can be vaporized after irradiation of a nonfocused laser with good hemostatic action under temporary occlusion of the first

Table 29.4. Types of resection in subclin-HCC and clin-HCC

	Subclin-HCC		Clin-HCC	
	No. of cases	Percent	No. of cases	Percent
Limited resection	54	64.3	56	25.4
Left lateral segmentectomy	11	13.1	35	15.8
Left hemihepatectomy	5	6.0	75	33.9
Extended left hemihepatectomy	2	2.4	4	1.8
Right posterior lobectomy	5	6.0	2	0.9
Right hemihepatectomy	4	4.7	43	19.5
Extended right hemihepatectomy	0	0	4	1.8
Middle lobectomy	3	3.5	2	0.9
Total	84	100.0	221	100.0

hepatic porta vessels [10]. The longest survival after laser vaporization of small HCC is 6 years. Hepatic artery cannulation to the affected side is recommended for deeply seated nonresectable subclin-HCC. Insertion of the tube under direct visual control and injection of methylene blue can help to position the tube accurately. This technqiue can be combined with hepatic artery ligation in some patients.

4.6 Complications and postoperative care

Postoperative complications after resection of subclin-HCC was less frequently encountered than with clin-HCC. However, aggressive postoperative care focusing on noncompensated liver function is needed, particularly for resection of a right lobe subclin-HCC in a cirrhotic liver. An unexplained high pulse rate, marked increase of serum bilirubin exceeding 5 mg/dl, marked impairment of prothrombin time ($<20\%$ of normal level), and the early appearance of ascites (with 5–7 postoperative days) are poor prognostic findings. Careful attention to the extent of resection, minimization of blood loss, shortened occlusion time of the porta hepatis, transfusion with fresh blood, and sufficient oxygen inhalation were important preventive measures. Aggressive treatment with albumin, fresh plasma, glucose, vitamin K, antibiotics, and oxygen were needed. Aspiration of chest fluid and injection of *Corynebacterium parvum* could help to control loss of protein in patients with transthoracic and abdominal incisions. In 78.5% of patients who had an AFP-producing subclin-HCC, AFP normalized after resection, indicating that it was a radical resection. The median length of time for AFP to normalize was correlated to the original AFP level: <500 ng/ml, 20 days; 501–5000 ng/ml, 35 days; 5001–50 000 ng/ml, 50 days; $>50 000$ ng/ml, 100.5 days.

5 Early detection, diagnosis, and treatment of subclinical recurrence

5.1 Early detection

As reported previously, the 1-, 3- and 5-year recurrence rates after radical resection of HCC (including small and larger HCC) were 17.1%, 32.5%, and 61.5%, respectively [11]. Even in patients with small HCC, the recurrence rates were still as high as 6.5%, 25.7%, and 43.5%, respectively. Fortunately, AFP is also of value in the early detection of subclinical recurrences or metastases in AFP-producing HCC. The regeneration process induced by resection in humans never results in an elevated serum AFP value. Therefore, the reappearance of abnormal serum AFP levels (without evidence of chronic liver disease in an active stage) always indicates the recurrence of metastases. It is most important to follow up the serum AFP level and recheck by US every 2–3 months for more than 5 years. Generally, subclinical recurrence or metastases can be detected as early as 6–12 months before the development of symptoms.

5.2 Early diagnosis

Early diagnosis of subclinical recurrence was exactly the same as that of subclin-HCC. In AFP-producing HCC, determination of the location is necessary. In non-AFP-producing HCC, US is essential for diagnosis and localization of the tumor. A hypoechoic lesion with a capsule (particularly with a background of HBV infection) indicates the diagnosis of subclinical recurrence. A chest film is needed if US, CT, and HA fail to demonstrate the lesion in the liver.

Table 29.5. Pathology and operative findings

Finding	Subclin-HCC		Clin-HCC	
	Percent	No. of cases	Percent	No. of cases
Number of nodules				
One	67.0	77/115	46.6	206/442
Two	18.3	21/115	7.9	35/442
Three or more	14.8	17/115	45.5	201/442
Well-encapsulated	55.5	61/110	20.9	86/411
Tumor emboli in intrahepatic veins	3.4	3/87	41.3	111/269
Tumor site				
Left	19.1	22/115	24.7	113/458
Right	44.4	51/115	26.0	119/458
Portal	22.6	26/115	7.4	34/458
Bilateral	13.9	16/115	41.9	192/458
Differentiation				
Well	8.3	7/84	9/7	33/339
Moderate	79.8	67/84	72.3	245/339
Poor	11.9	10/84	18.0	61/339

5.3 Early treatment

Surgery was the modality of choice for treatment of subclinical recurrence or solitary lung metastasis. As previously reported, the median survival after diagnosis of recurrence was >31.5 months in patients who underwent reoperation, whereas it was only 11 months for conservative treatment; reoperation resulted in 20% improvement of 5-year survival in a group with radical resection (from 47.7% to 66.8%) [11]. The most important point, however, was still "early" and "radical." In this series, reoperation was performed in 14 patients in the subclin-HCC group and 16 patients in the clin-HCC group. Limited resection seemed to be the only choice, although cryosurgery or high-power laser vaporization were also frequently employed.

6 Pathology and operative findings

Surgery of subclin-HCC has provided valuable clues to the study of the early evolution of HCC. Comparison between subclin-HCC and clin-HCC clearly showed that (1) with progression of the disease, multiple tumor nodules and bilateral involvement increased, the incidence of well-encapsulated tumors decreased, and the incidence of tumor emboli in the intrahepatic veins increased. These findings suggested that spread of tumor to the blood vessels and through the capsule might play a more important role rather than multicentric tumor emergence as the cause of the multinodular tumor pattern. (2) The in-

cidence of poorly differentiated HCC in subclin-HCC was somewhat lower than in clin-HCC, indicating progressive change of tumor cell differentiation with advancing disease (Table 29.5). All of these findings strongly support early resection.

7 Prognosis of subclin-HCC

As shown in Table 29.6, the analysis of factors influencing prognosis of the entire series of subclin-HCC revealed that patients with a single tumor nodule, a tumor size of <4 cm (median size of subclin-HCC), without cirrhosis or with micronodular cirrhosis, and with normalization of AFP levels after operation had a much better prognosis than patients with multiple nodules, with a tumor size of >4 cm, macronodular cirrhosis, and without normalization of AFP after operation. Other factors including age, tumor site, and the preoperative AFP level did not clearly influence the prognosis. Therefore, it was essential to carry out early and radical resection for a better prognosis. The severity of the cirrhotic process may influence the resectability rate and, partly, the recurrence rate after operation.

8 Future prospects

It is concluded that surgery remains essential to secondary prevention and has dramatically altered the clinical outlook in HCC. Therefore, every effort should be made to eradicate subclin-HCC by the use of resection, cryosurgery, or laser vaporization, providing liver function is at a compensated stage. Briefly, the role of surgery has assumed greater significance in subclin-HCC, whereas it is of limited value in clin-HCC. However, early detection and early diagnosis of non-AFP-producing HCC, earlier resection of AFP-producing HCC (<2 cm), specific treatment of nonresectable subclin-HCC, treatment of noncompensated liver function, etc. are important goals in the near future.

Acknowledgments. The author wishes to express appreciation to Drs. YQ Yu, XD Zhou, BH Yang, ZY Lin, JZ Lu, and ZC Ma for their contribution in clinical work and to Dr. SL Ye for microcomputer analysis.

Table 29.6. Factors influencing prognosis of entire series of subclin-HCC

Factors	No. of cases	5-year survival rate (%)
Age		
<48 years	58	46.9
≥48 years	63	40.0
Tumor site		
Left	22	52.0
Others	93	42.8
Number of nodule		
Single	78	61.9
Multiple	37	17.1
Tumor size		
≤4 cm	59	64.0
>4 cm	54	30.8
Cirrhosis		
None or micronodular	43	62.7
Macronodular	74	35.7
AFP		
≤2000 ng/ml	79	44.7
>2000 ng/ml	42	41.0
Postoperative AFP		
≤20 ng/ml	67	70.1
>20 ng/ml	44	0

Survival rates calculated by the life-table method

Reference

1. Curutchet HP, Terz JJ, Kay S, Lawrence W Jr (1971) Primary liver cancer. Surgery 70: 467–479
2. Tang ZY (1985) Prognosis of hepatocellular carcinoma and factors influencing it. In: Tang ZY (ed) Subclinical hepatocellular carcinoma. China Acad Publ, Beijing; Springer, Berlin pp 179–188
3. Tang ZY (1981) A new concept on the natural course of hepatocellular carcinoma. Chin Med J 94: 585–588
4. Tang ZY (1985) The role of unicentric origin the subclinical hepatocellular carcinoma. In: Tang ZY (ed) Subclinical hepatocellular carcinoma. China Acad Publ, Beijing; Springer, Berlin, pp 162–170
5. Shanghai Coordinating Group for Research on Liver Cancer, China (1979) Diagnosis and treatment of primary hepatocellular carcinoma in early stage, report of 134 cases. Chin Med J 92: 801–806
6. Tang ZY, Yu YQ, Zhou XD, Zhou NQ (1983) Surgical treatment of subclinical hepatocellular carcinoma (HCC) and its ultimate outcome, a comparative study of 74 cases of subclinical HCC and 229 cases of clinical HCC undergone surgery. J Exp Clin Cancer Res 3: 261–268
7. Kanematsu T, Takenaka K, Matsumata T, Furuta T, Sugimachi K, Inokuchi K (1984) Limited hepatic resection effective for selected cirrhotic patients with primary liver cancer. Ann Surg 199: 51–56
8. Zhou XD, Tang ZY (1985) Bloodless hepatectomy and hepatic clamp in resection of small hepatocellular carcinoma. In: Tang ZY (ed) Subclinical hepatocellular carcinoma. China Acad Publ, Beijing; Springer, Berlin, pp 85–100
9. Zhou XD, Tang ZY, Yu YQ, Lu HX, Chen CG, Jiang YM, Xu YD (1979) Cryosurgery for liver cancer, experimental and clinical study. Chin J Surg 17: 480–483
10. Yu YQ (1985) High power Nd: YAG laser in the treatment of liver cancer, experimental study and clinical application. In: Tang ZY (ed) Subclinical hepatocellular carcinoma. China Acad Publ, Beijing; Springer, Berlin, pp 120–123
11. Tang ZY, Yu YQ, Zhou XD (1984) An important approach to prolonging survival further after radical resection of AFP positive hepatocellular carcinoma. J Exp Clin Cancer Res 3: 359–366

Chapter 30

Treatment of Primary Liver Cancer in Japan

A National Study

Yasuo Kamiyama and Takayoshi Tobe[1]

1 Introduction

Since 1965, the Liver Cancer Study Group of Japan [1–6] has been carrying out analyses of patients with primary liver cancer in Japan every 2 or 3 years. In the fist survey, 452 cases from 21 institutes were filed. The number of institutes participating and cases recorded has continuously increased (Table 30.1). In 1984, 5567 cases from 429 institutes throughout the country were filed and analyzed. The individual data were coded and fed into a computer for retrieval. Analysis of the data from the seventh survey is currently underway. This chapter will deal with the results obtained from the fifth and sixth surveys.

Histological diagnosis, male to female ratio, and number of cases are shown in Table 30.2. The peak incidence of hepatocellular carcinoma (HCC) and cholangiocarcinoma (CC) was in the fifth decade of life. The carcinoma cells of HCC were arranged most frequently in a trabecular pattern; those of CC were arranged mostly in a microtubular pattern. The grade of cancer cell differentiation according to Edmondson and Steiner [7] was most frequently described as grade II. The noncancerous portion of the liver showed cirrhosis in 78.0% and 83.2% of HCC cases in the fifth and sixth surveys, respectively (Table 30.3).

Metastasis of HCC was most frequent in the lung, followed by the lymph nodes. In CC, lymph node metastasis was the most frequent type, followed by metastasis to the lung. In the sixth report, angiography was the most frequently performed procedure for the diagnosis of HCC, being done in 35.7% of cases; scintiscanning was done in 18.3%, computed tomography in 16.2%, and ultrasonography in 15.2% of 1510 cases. The serum alpha-fetoprotein (AFP) level was mea- sured in 1738 cases of HCC and 117 cases of CC. AFP was less than 20 ng/ml in 18.9% of HCC cases, while it was over that level in 23.1% of 117 CC cases.

2 Hepatic resection

The surgical procedures for primary liver cancer are shown in Table 30.4. Laparotomies were performed in about half the HCC and CC cases. Almost all cases of hepatoblastoma were laparotomized. The frequency of laparotomy in these surveys is relatively high. One explanation for this high laparotomy rate is that this survey was based on histologically proven cases, which came more from surgical teams. Hepatic resection was performed in 55.8% and 69.2% of laparotomized HCC cases in the fifth and sixth reports, respectively (Table 30.4). Of the 619 resections of HCC in the sixth survey, 64 were extended lobectomies, 202 were lobectomies, 106 were segmentectomies, and 239 were partial resections (Table 30.5).

As shown in Table 30.3, in about 80% of HCC cases the noncancerous portion of the liver had liver cirrhosis or fibrosis. To prevent hepatic failure after massive resection in cirrhotic patients, partial resection was more frequently chosen for treatment. In the third survey, the ratio of extended lobectomies and lobectomies to all hepatic resections in HCC patients with cirrhosis was 0.63, and the ratio of partial resections to all resections was 0.18. However, the ratio of extended lobectomies and lobectomies to total resections in the sixth survey was 0.33, which is lower than that in the third and fifth reports.

Causes of death after hepatectomy are listed in Table 30.6; hepatic failure as the cause of death after hepatectomy was the most frequent. Death due to rupture of HCC was less frequent in hepatectomized patients than in all HCC patients.

[1] First Department of Surgery, Kyoto University School of Medicine, Kyoto, 606 Japan

Table 30.1. Details of national survey on primary liver cancer

	Survey no.						
	1	2	3	4	5	6	7
Period of survey	Up to 1969	1965–1972	1960–1974	1968–1977	1978–1979	1980–1981	1981–1983
No. of institutes	21	54	71	155	246	451	429
No. of cases filed[a]	452	1115	2716	4031	2727	4056	5567
No. of laparotomies[b]	452	1115	1734	1041	578	1000	1167
No. of resections[b]	125	289	332	361	319	679	952

[a] Cases with or without histological diagnosis
[b] Cases with histological diagnosis

Table 30.2. Histological diagnosis and number of cases

	Survey no.	Male	Female	M : F ratio	Total
Hepatocellular carcinoma	5	858	189	4.5	1047 (87.4%)[a]
	6	1700	330	5.2	2038 (89.2%)[b]
Cholangiocellular carcinoma	5	59	34	1.7	93 (7.8%)
	6	74	72	1.0	146 (6.4%)
Mixed	5	7	2	3.5	9 (0.8%)
	6	25	8	3.1	33 (1.4%)
Hepatoblastoma	5	10	6	1.7	16 (1.3%)
	6	23	7	3.3	30 (1.3%)
Unknown	5				1198
	6				2372
Total	5				2396
	6				4658

[a] Percentage of all cases with a histological diagnosis
[b] Eight cases of unknown sex are included

3 Chemotherapy

Of the various chemotherapeutic agents available, mitomycin C was employed most frequently followed by 5-flourouracil. Percutaneous intrahepatic arterial injection was the most frequently used route of administration (fifth survey).

4 Transcatheter arterial embolization

Operative or nonoperative transcatheter embolization was performed in 124 HCC cases. Gelfoam or gelfoam powder was the most frequently used embolizing substance. Transcatheter arterial embolization was evaluated as being effective for treatment in 79 of 124 HCC patients (sixth report).

5 Survival

Calculation of survival in patients in the fifth and sixth surveys is based on the mortality follow-up up to December 31, 1981, using the conventional lifetime table method of Cutler and Ederer [8]. The date of admission, diagnosis, or initial treatment is the starting point in calculating survival time.

Survival rates for HCC and CC with and without hepatic resection are shown in Figs. 30.1 and 30.2. In the HCC and CC resection groups, survival was much longer than in the group without resection. Among the HCC patients who underwent tumor resection, those without liver cirrhosis had a better prognosis than those with liver cirrhosis (Fig. 30.3). Figure 30.4 shows the survival rate for the HCC patients without cirrhosis in relation to the extent of hepatic resec-

Table 30.3. Accompanying changes in parenchyma at autopsy

	Survey no.	HCC	CC
Unremarkable	5	10.1%	61.5%
	6	8.7%	64.7%
Fibrosis	5	7.6%	7.6%
	6	5.1%	7.1%
Cirrhosis	5	78.0%	7.6%
	6	83.2%	14.1%
Others	5	4.1%	23.0%
	6	3.1%	14.1%
Total no. of cases	5	512	39
	6	1128	85

HCC hepatocellular carcinoma, *CC* cholangiocellular carcinoma

Table 30.4. Surgical procedures for primary liver cancer

	Survey no.	HCC	CC	MX	HB
Laparotomy Total filed	5	500/1022 (48.9%)	60/91 (65.9%)	3/9 (33.3%)	15/16 (93.8%)
	6	894/1760 (50.8%)	66/127 (52.0%)	12/25 (48.0%)	28/30 (93.3%)
Resection	5	279 (55.8%)	26 (43.3%)	3 (100%)	11 (73.3%)
	6	619 (69.2%)	30 (45.5%)	6 (50%)	24 (85.7%)
Ligation of hepatic artery	5	72 (14.4%)	5 (8.3%)	0	1 (6.7%)
	6	85 (9.5%)	4 (6.0%)	0	2 (7.0%)
Hepatic artery embolization	5	132 (26.4%)	7 (11.7%)	0	1 (6.7%)
	6	148 (16.5%)	5 (7.6%)	0	3 (10.7%)
Ligation of portal vein	5	7 (1.4%)	0	0	0
	6	6 (0.7%)	0	0	1 (3.6%)
Exploratory laparotomy	5	110 (22.0%)	22 (36.7%)	0	
	6	66 (7.4%)	18 (27.3%)	4 (33.3%)	1 (3.6%)

Figures in parentheses represent percentage of all laparotomies
HCC hepatocellular carcinoma, *CC* cholangiocellular carcinoma, *MX* mixed carcinoma, *HB* hepatoblastoma

Table 30.5. Extent of resection

	Survey no.	HCC	CC	MX	HB
Resection of liver (total)	5	279	26	3	11
	6	619	30	6	24
Extended lobectomy	5	43 (15.4%)	7 (26.9%)	0	4
	6	64 (10.3%)	8 (26.7%)	0	9
Lobectomy	5	111 (39.8%)	9 (34.6%)	3	4
	6	202 (32.6%)	12 (40.0%)	4	11
Segmentectomy	5	58 (20.8%)	4 (15.4%)	0	2
	6	106 (17.1%)	7 (23.3%)	1	1
Partial resection	5	67 (24.0%)	6 (23.1%)	0	1
	6	239 (38.6%)	3 (10.0%)	1	1

Figures in parentheses represent percentage of all resections
HCC hepatocellular carcinoma, *CC* cholangiocellular carcinoma, *MX* mixed carcinoma, *HB* hepatoblastoma

Table 30.6. Causes of death after hepatectomy

	Survey no.	HCC		CC	
		After hepatectomy	Overall	After hepatectomy	Overall
Hepatic failure	5	63 (37.2%)	309 (34.0%)	3 (18.8%)	20 (25.0%)
	6	81 (30.6%)	451 (27.8%)	3 (21.4%)	31 (24.6%)
Gastrointestinal bleeding	5	10 (5.9%)	102 (11.2%)	3 (18.8%)	13 (16.3%)
	6	15 (5.7%)	185 (11.4%)	0	11 (8.7%)
Rupture of esophageal varices	5	4 (2.4%)	64 (7.1%)	1 (6.3%)	1 (1.3%)
	6	15 (5.7%)	151 (9.3%)	0	0
Rupture of tumor	5	3 (1.8%)	101 (11.3%)	0	1 (1.3%)
	6	7 (2.6%)	163 (10.0%)	0	1 (1.3%)
Deterioration due to tumor growth	5	35 (20.7%)	204 (22.5%)	5 (31.3%)	29 (36.3%)
	6	74 (28.0%)	453 (28.0%)	9 (64.3%)	65 (51.6%)
Others	5	27 (16.0%)	80 (8.8%)	3 (18.8%)	10 (12.5%)
	6	29 (10.9%)	146 (9.0%)	0	12 (9.5%)
Unknown	5	27 (16.0%)	47 (5.2%)	1 (6.3%)	6 (7.5%)
	6	44 (16.6%)	69 (4.3%)	2 (14.2%)	8 (4.8%)
Total	5	169	907	16	80
	6	265	1618	14	126

Figures in parentheses represent percent of all deaths
HCC hepatocellular carcinoma, *CC* cholangiocellular carcinoma

Table 30.7. Transcatheter embolization of hepatic artery in primary liver cancer (sixth survey)

	HCC	CC	MX	HB
No embolization	776	62	13	14
Embolization with laparatomy	10 (1.1%)	0	0	1 (6.3%)
Without laparotomy	114 (12.7%)	2 (3.1%)	1 (5.9%)	1 (6.3%)

Figures in parentheses represent percent of all cases listed
HCC hepatocellular carcinoma, *CC* cholangiocellular carcinoma, *MX* mixed carcinoma, *HB* hepatoblastoma

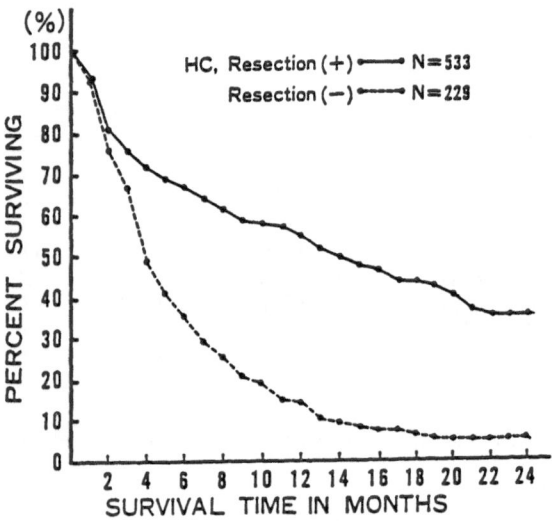

Fig. 30.1. Survival curves for laparotomized hepatocellular carcinoma patients with and without tumor resection

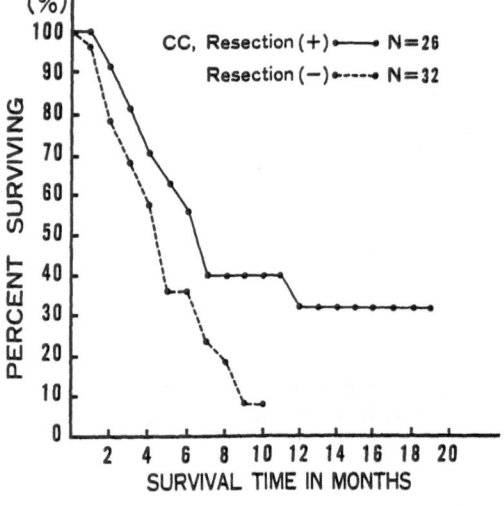

Fig. 30.2. Survival curves for laparotomized cholangiocellular carcinoma patients with and without tumor resection

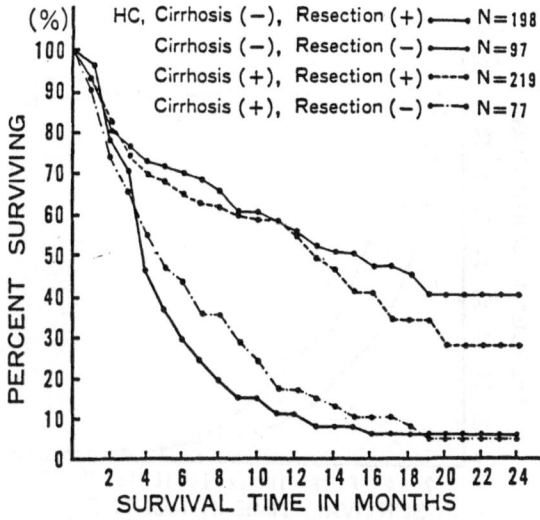

Fig. 30.3. Survival curves for cirrhotic and noncirrhotic hepatocellular carcinoma patients with and without tumor resection

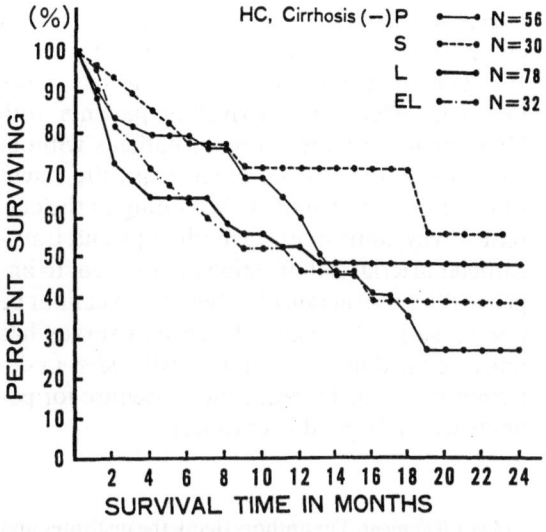

Fig. 30.4. Survival curves for hepatocellular carcinoma patients without liver cirrhosis according to extent of hepatic resection. *P* partital resection, *S* segmental resection, *L* lobectomy, *EL* extended lobectomy

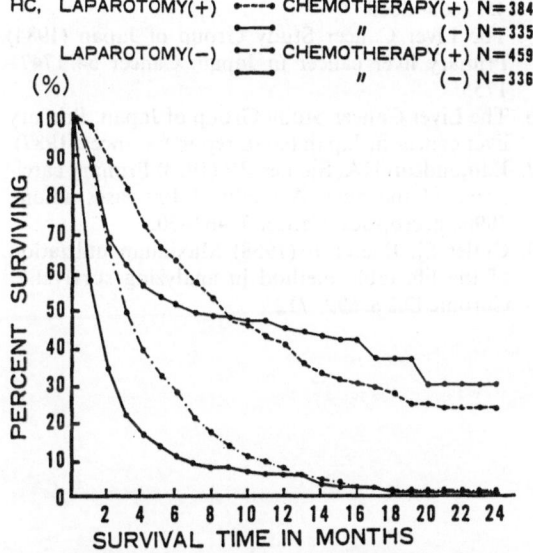

Fig. 30.5. Survival curves for hepatocellular carcinoma patients with and without laparotomy and with and without anticancer chemotherapy

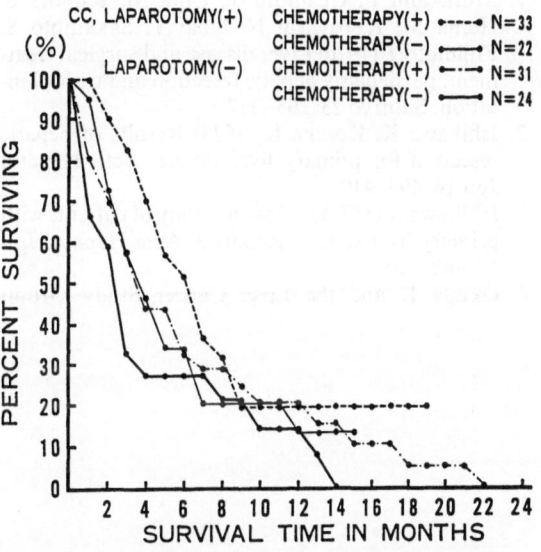

Fig. 30.6. Survival curves for cholangiocellular carcinoma patients with and without laparotomy and with and without anticancer chemotherapy

tion. It appears that HCC patients with segmental resection of the liver did better than those who had partial resection. Figures 30.5 and 30.6 show the survival curves for the patients with HCC and CC given anticancer chemotherapy with or without surgery, which includes all operative procedures: resection of the tumor, both radical and nonradical, arterial ligation, operative embolization of the hepatic artery, and exploratory laparotomy. Figure 30.7 shows the survival rate for patients with or without nonoperative transcatheter arterial embolization who did not undergo laparotomy. No significant difference in survival rate was observed between those with and those without arterial embolization in this survey.

Hepatic resection is obviously the treatment of choice of primary liver cancer in its early stage. It seems that segmental resection has more beneficial effects on survival in patients with HCC than partial resection in patients without cirrhosis; in the absence of cirrhosis, the extent of resection is not limited. According to the current survey, anticancer chemotherapy and transcatheter arterial embolization do not seem to improve the survival rate of patients who cannot be treated surgically. Thus, the current survey has failed to yield information that will assist in determining the best therapeutic procedure for patients with advanced liver cancer.

Acknowledgment. The authors thank the institutes and hospitals that participated in this study and those who kindly that supplied other necessary information.

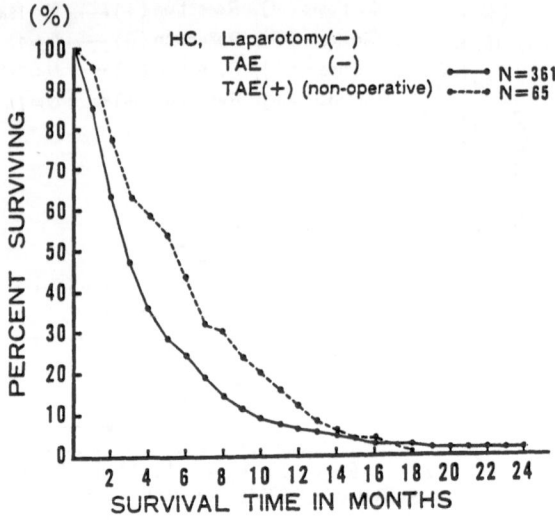

Fig. 30.7. Survival curves for hepatocellular carcinoma patients with and without transcatheter arterial embolization. No patients underwent laparotomy

References

1. Murakami F, Okamura T, Ohta M, Kubota S, Hama M, Kobayashi N, Ukai T, Sakamoto S, Fujimoto T (1970) Liver disease and surgical treatment, particularly hepatic resection and transplantation. Shinryo 23: 265–277
2. Ishikawa K, Kosaka K (1973) Results of hepatic resection for primary liver cancer. Acta Hepatol Jpn 14: 409–410
3. Ishikawa K (1976) Follow-up study of patients with primary liver cancer: Report 3. Acta Hepatol Jpn 17: 460–465
4. Okuda K and the Liver Cancer Study Group of Japan (1980) Primary liver cancer. Cancer 45: 2663–2669
5. The Liver Cancer Study Group of Japan (1984) Primary liver cancer in Japan. Cancer 54: 1747–1755
6. The Liver Cancer Study Group of Japan. Primary liver cancer in Japan (sixth report). Cancer (1987)
7. Edmondson HA, Steiner PE (1954) Primary carcinoma of the liver: A study of 100 cases among 48900 necropsies. Cancer 7: 462–503
8. Cutler Sj, Ederer F (1958) Maximum utilization of the life table method in analyzing survival. J Chronic Dis 8: 699–712

Chapter 31

Diagnosis and Treatment of Cholangiocarcinoma and Cystic Adenocarcinoma of the Liver

Ryuji Mizumoto and Yoshifumi Kawarada[1]

Primary carcinoma of the liver is usually classified into three types based on histological findings—hepatocellular carcinoma, cholangiocarcinoma, and a combined type. Of the many names applied to bile duct carcinoma of the liver, such as cholangioma, cholangiocarcinoma, malignant cholangioma, cholangiocellular carcinoma, alveolar carcinoma, and carcinoma adenomatosum, the International Association for the Study of the Liver adopted cholangiocarcinoma as the formal name.

Cholangiocarcinoma is relatively rare and constitutes only about 10% of all primary liver cancers. Because cholangiocarcinoma has a notable tendency to spread locally and to metastasize to the lymph nodes, resectability is generally limited, and the prognosis is so poor that very few long-term survivors have been described.

During the 9-year period from 1977 to 1985, 15 cases of cholangiocarcinoma were admitted to our clinic at Mie University Hospital, and 14 cases underwent surgery. Of the 14 cases, 11 (78.6%) had hepatectomies. There were no operative deaths. The 1-, 3-, and 5-year actuarial survival rates of these patients after hepatectomy have been 55.6%, 27.8%, and 27.8%, respectively. The longest survival is 6 years 10 months after surgery and the patient is still alive and well without recurrence at the time of writing. The second longest survival is 5 years 5 months, and this patient is also currently well without recurrence.

Cystic adenocarcinoma may originate from a cystadenoma, an intrahepatic bile duct itself, or a primary liver cyst. Cystic adenocarcinoma of the liver, including our four cases, will be described after a discussion of cholangiocarcinoma.

1 Cholangiocarcinoma

1.1 History and definition

In 1888, Hanot and Gilbert [1] suggested that primary liver cancers could be distinguished microscopically into carcinoma of the hepatic cells (cancer trabeculaire) and carcinoma of the bile duct (cancer alveolaire). In 1901, Eggel [2] collected 162 cases of primary liver cancer from the literature and added one case of his own; he divided the cases into carcinoma solidum and carcinoma adenomatosum. Goldzieher and von Bókay [3] in 1911 suggested that the tumor arising from the hepatic cells be called carcinoma hepatocellulaire and that arising from the epithelium of the small bile ducts be designated carcinoma cholangiocellulaire. In Japan, the terms hepatoma and cholangioma have been widely used since Yamagiwa [4] described these forms based on the morphology of primary hepatic tumors in 1911.

At present, primary carcinomas of the liver are histologically classified into hepatocellular carcinoma (malignant hepatoma), cholangiocarcinoma (malignant cholangioma), and the mixed type. However, there is confusion in terminology regarding the relationship of cholangiocarcinoma and tumor of the extrahepatic bile ducts. As the term "cholangioma" is a synonym for carcinoma of the bile duct, it may arise from any part of the biliary system. Therefore, it could be divided into three groups—intrahepatic, hilar, and extrahepatic—as in Murray-Lyon's classification, but in general cholangiocarcinoma or malignant cholangioma signifies a carcinoma of the intrahepatic bile duct.

Burdette [5] reported that cholangiocarcinoma in adults usually arose from the intrahepatic ducts. Hoyne and Kernohan [6] excluded any tumor arising from the common hepatic duct, either external to the liver at the porta hepatis or in the short course of this duct within

---

[1] First Department of Surgery, Mie University School of Medicine, Tsu, Mie, 514 Japan

the anatomical confines of the liver itself, from the class of primary carcinomas of the liver; they believed that such tumors should properly be classified as primary carcinomas of the hepatic duct. According to Hoyne and Kernohan [6], only carcinomas arising from bile ductules are to be termed cholangiocarcinomas. On the other hand, Okuda et al. [7] reported 57 autopsy subjects who had cholangiocarcinoma and divided them into two groups—the peripheral and hilar types. It is sometimes difficult to differentiate between a hilar-type small cholangiocarcinoma of the liver near the hilum and a carcinoma of the hepatic duct within the porta hepatis, as described by Klatskin [8] in 1965; the latter tumor should, however, be excluded from the term "cholangiocarcinoma."

1.2 Etiology

1.2.1 Thorotrast

Colloidal thorium dioxide (Thorotrast) was first utilized as a contrast medium in diagnostic radiology in 1928 [9] and was used all over the world in the 1930s and 1940s [9–11]. In 1957, MacMahon et al. [12] first reported the occurrence of an angiosarcoma as a late effect of Thorotrast administration. Battifora [13] reported that approximately 20% of hepatic malignancies induced by Thorotrast were hepatocellular carcinomas, 32% cholangiocarcinomas, 15% bile duct carcinomas, and 33% hemangiosarcomas as the predominant type.

The etiological association between Thorotrast and a variety of malignant hepatic neoplasms is well-known, and the simultaneous occurrence of two different hepatic neoplasms has recently been reported. In 1979, Winberg and Ranchod [14] described the simultaneous occurrence of hepatic angiosarcoma and cholangiocarcinoma in a 49-year-old man 22 years after the administration of Thorotrast. Kojiro et al. [15] reported a 64-year-old man who developed hepatic angiosarcoma and combined hepatocholangiocarcinoma 36 years after Thorotrast administration.

1.2.2 Oral contraceptives

Oral contraceptives are known to cause adenoma of the liver. Ellis et al. [16] reported a 29-year-old married woman with two normal children, who took the contraceptive pill for 22 months and developed adenocarcinoma of the liver. She died 3 months after diagnosis.

1.2.3 Polycystic disease

Cholangiocellular carcinoma may be related to polycystic disease, and it is known to have developed in two uremic patients with polycystic kidney and liver disease [17].

1.2.4 Chronic parasitic infestation

Chronic infestation by parasites such as Clonorchis sinensis has been proposed as a possible cause of cholangiocarcinoma. This parasite is known to damage the liver, and it is believed that irritation of the bile duct mucosa serves as a precursor to the development of the tumor.

Hou [18] demonstrated that chronic infestation of Clonorchis sinensis can ultimately lead to adenomatous hyperplasia of the bile duct epithelium and to cholangiocarcinoma. His study was based on the postmortem examination of 200 cases of primary carcinoma of the liver in Hong Kong, of which 30 cases were shown to be associated with Clonorchis infestation. However, the significance of parasitic infection in the development of primary carcinoma of the liver is still debatable [19, 20].

1.2.5 Hepatolithiasis

In Europe and North America, the incidence of hepatolithiasis in gallstone disease is below 1%. The incidence of intrahepatic stones is much higher in Japan (4%–15%) [21], Malaysia (10.2%) [22], and the Republic of Korea (17%) [23].

In 1942, Sanes and MacCallum [24] reported two cases of hepatic cholangiocarcinoma associated with hepatolithiasis. The epithelium of the dilated bile duct distal to the tumor showed occasional papillomatous and adenomatous proliferation with mitotic figures and atypical nuclei [24]. Falchuk et al. [25] found varying degrees of papillary or adenomatous hyperplasia with moderate atypia in some of the most severely inflamed areas of the bile duct. They suspected that chronic infection and hepatolithiasis played a pathogenetic role in the development of cholangiocarcinoma.

The first report by Sanes and MacCallum [24] of two cases in 1942 was followed by the paper of Shanmugaratnam [26] with three cases in 1956, Glenn and Moody [27] with one case in 1961, Longmire et al. [28] with ten cases in 1966, Koga et al. [29] with three cases in 1985, Nakanuma et al. [30] with 12 cases in 1985, ours with 15 cases of cholangiocarcinoma in this study, and others [31, 32].

Although the relationship between gallstones and carcinoma of the bile duct has long been debated, the etiological mechanism has not been clearly defined. It may be one of the causes of carcinoma in the liver or there may be no definite relationship since stones often are only incidental findings at surgery or autopsy. Therefore, a liver with hepatolithiasis should be evaluated carefully.

1.2.6 Cystic dilatation of bile duct

There are several different congenital cystic conditions affecting the liver and bile ducts. They include hepatic cysts and their precursors (Meyenburg complexes) and the lesions affecting the drainage system proper, such as congenital hepatic fibrosis, dilatation of the intrahepatic ducts, and choledochal cysts.

Idiopathic cystic dilatation of the common bile duct was reported for the first time by Todd in 1817 in the Dublin Hospital Reports [33]. Vachell and Stevens [34] wrote the earliest description of cystic dilatation of the intrahepatic bile ducts in 1906. In Japan, Sakuma [35] was the first to mention a case and thereafter reports of cases proved by operation or autopsy have increased. The theory that biliary cysts are congenital disorders caused by faulty epithelial proliferation and recanalization of the embryonic bile duct was first proposed by Yotsuyanagi in 1936 [36]. Cystic diseases of various types, namely, congenital fibrosis of the liver, Caroli's syndrome, choledochal cyst, and polycystic liver may be complicated by cholangiocarcinoma. The incidence of carcinoma arising from congenital bile duct cysts is reported to be between 2.5% and 15%. Longmire et al. [28] encountered four cases of carcinoma (8.2%) among 49 patients with congenital bile duct cysts.

According to a statistical analysis made by Bloustein [37], the frequency of neoplastic changes in congenital choledochal cysts is approximately 4% and the increased risk was in the order of 80 times that of the control value. When Alonso-Lej et al. in 1959 [38] classified dilated biliary tracts into three types, intrahepatic dilatation was not considered. Malignant changes in choledochal cysts usually occur in the extrahepatic bile duct. Kasai et al. [39] suggested that such patients have an increased risk of developing a neoplasm in the biliary tree and proposed that the cysts should be excised with a subsequent reconstructive hepaticojejunostomy. The report of Caroli and Couinaud [40] on intrahepatic cysts in 1958 was followed in 1964 by that of Engle and Salmon [41] on choledochal cysts combined with intrahepatic cysts. Ackerholm et al. [42] reported a case of a 15-year-old girl who had multiple neoplastic changes in the right and left lobes of the liver. Type IVa choledochal cyst of the classification of Todani et al. [43] is now recognized more often, and carcinomas arising from it also seem to be increasing in number. In 1978, Kagawa et al. [44] collected 47 cases in which congenital dilatation of the biliary tract was associated with carcinoma and stated that carcinoma may arise in any cystic portion of the bile duct, extrahepatic or intrahepatic. Bloustein [37] suggested that carcinoma arises with a frequency of approximately 7% in congenital cystic dilatation of the intrahepatic bile duct. In 1968, Schiewe et al. [45] described a cholangiocarcinoma developing in an intrahepatic cystic lesion. In 1983, Dayton et al. [46] reviewed the literature and found only six documented cases [43, 47–50] of carcinoma among 138 cases of Caroli's disease. They reported four more cases, making a total of ten which had had associated malignant growth among the 142 reported cases of Caroli's disease; this 7% incidence of associated malignant growth is similar to the one proposed by Bloustein [37].

1.2.7 Cyst

Primary malignant cystic lesions of the liver are very rare. In 1943, Willis [51] reported the first case, a 27-year-old female with primary carcinoma arising in the epithelium of a cystic malformation of the liver. A second case described by Richmond in 1956 [52] was a single woman of 41 years of age who survived resection of the primary growth for 15 months and eventually succumbed to widespread skeletal metastases. Subsequently, similar cases were reported by Dean and Bauer in 1963 [53], Cruickshank and Sparshott in 1971 [54], Ameriks et al. in 1972 [55], Kinami et al. in 1975 [56], Okuda et al. in 1977 [7], and Kasai et al. in 1977 [57].

In 1980, cholangiocarcinoma coexisting with developmental liver cysts was classified by Azizah and Paradinas [58] as a new entity different from cystadenocarcinoma. They described hepatic cystadenocarcinomas as solitary and multilocular with a mucinous or hemorrhagic content, although cholangiocarcinoma associated with a cyst is usually multiple and unilocular with a serous content lacking epithelium.

Imamura et al. in 1984 [59] reported a 46-year-old woman who had multiple liver cysts and underwent hepatectomy. The resected specimen contained one nonepithelialized cyst, which was invaded by cholangiocarcinoma, and three other epithelialized cysts, which were benign.

Attention has thus to be given to this category, which seems to be a different entity from cysta-

Table 31.1. Reports on cholangiocarcinoma

Author or series	Year	Reference	Total no. of primary liver tumors	No. of hepatocellular carcinoma cases	Cholangiocarcinoma cases	
					No.	Percentage
Hutt and Anthony (Uganda)	1963	63	556	528	19	3.4
Chan (Singapore)	1966	71	106	98	10	9.2
Anthony (Uganda)	1973	75	282	263	19	6.7
Al-Sarraf et al. (USA)	1974	87	65	53	9	13.8
Appleqvist (Finland)	1982	88	53	31	8	15.1
Oldenburg et al. (USA)	1982	77	192	152	40	20.0
Chearanai et al. (France)	1984	69	127	93	34	26.8
Ferenci et al. (Austria)	1984	89	73	67	5	6.8
Kingston et al. (Saudi Arabia)	1985	68	123	104	0	0
Li et al. (Guanzhon, China)	1985	85	114	100	8	7.0
Japanese series (1978–1979)	1984		1208	1047	93	7.7
Ours (Mie, Japan)	1986		171	149	15	10.1

denocarcinoma. In this chapter, carcinoma arising from liver cysts and cystadenocarcinoma will be described in Section 2.

1.3 Incidence, sex, age

Primary hepatic tumors are rare in the United States, being encountered in only 0.2%–0.7% of autopsies [60]. In Norway, the incidence was 3.0/100 000 men and 1.4/100 000 women/year during the period from 1972 to 1976 [61]. Cholangiocarcinoma is rare in northern Europe, and the overall frequency of primary malignant tumors of the liver is close to 0.5% [62]. However, the incidence of primary liver cancer is higher in Africa, the Orient, and South America. In Kyadondo County, Uganda, the annual incidence figures for liver cell carcinoma were 5.1/100 000 women and 11.1/100 000 men/year [63]. Primary liver cancer is one of the common malignancies in China, particularly Guangdong Province. According to retrospective surveys from 1973 to 1975, the standarized average annual mortality among primary liver cancer patients was 10.09/100 000, the third most common fatal malignancy in China [64,65]. In Japan, the Liver Cancer Study Group of Japan [66] statistically analyzed 2396 cases of primary liver cancer diagnosed from 1 January 1978 to 31 December 1979 in over 500 hospitals throughout the country. Histological data were available in 1198 cases (50%). There were 1047 cases of hepatocellular carcinoma, 93 of cholangiocarcinoma, 16 of hepatoblastoma, and 33 others. In our department, we had 171 cases of primary liver tumor, 149 cases of hepatocellular carcinoma, 15 cases of cholangiocarcinoma, one case of hepato-cholangiocarcinoma, two nonhepatocytic malignant mixed tumors [67], and four cases of cystadenocarcinoma, including one with carcinoma arising in a liver cyst.

The incidence of cholangiocarcinoma among primary liver cancers ranges from about 0% to 26.8% (Table 31.1). Kingston et al. [68] reviewed all cases of liver tumor referred to the King Faisal Specialist Hospital Research Center in Saudi Arabia during a period of 2 years 6 months. There were 104 cases of hepatocellular carcinoma but no cholangiocarcinomas. By contrast, 34 of 127 cases (26.8%) were cholangiocarcinoma in the series of Chearanai et al. in Thailand [69].

In 550 autopsies in a Japanese series [66], the noncancerous portion of the liver showed cirrhosis or fibrosis in 85.6% of hepatocellular carcinoma cases but only in 15.2% in cholangiocarcinomas. In a series of 16 303 necropsies at the Mayo Clinic, 20 had hepatocellular carcinoma and 11 cholangiocarcinoma; cirrhosis was present in 75% of the former and in 18.2% of the latter [70]. None of the patients with cholangiocarcinoma had concomitant cirrhosis in Chan's series [71], and cirrhosis was found in 5.8% of 34 cases of cholangiocarcinoma in the series of Chearanai et al. [69]. Therefore, cholangiocarcinoma is less frequently associated with cirrhosis than is hepatocellular carcinoma.

In general, the age of patients with hepatocellular carcinoma is 50–70 years, whereas cholangiocarcinoma is found in older patients, 60–70 years of age, especially in the 70s [72]. In our series, the youngest patient with cholangiocarcinoma was 26 years old and oldest 80 years, with an average age of 56.6 years, whereas in patients with hepatocellular carcinoma the ages ranged from 22 to 79 years, with an average of 51.2 years [73]. The majority of patients with primary carcinoma of the liver are men, especially those with hepatocellular carcinoma. In the study of Gall [74], the ratio of men to women was 6:1 in hepatocellular carcinoma and 2:1 in cholangiocarcinoma. In cholangiocarcinoma, the ratio of men to women was 1.7:1 in the Japanese series and 1.3:1 in Anthony's series [75], showing a male predominance. Hoyne and Kernohan [6], however, reported a female predominance for cholangiocarcinoma. In our series, the ratio of men to women was 6:9 (Table 31.2).

Table 31.2. Sex distribution of patients with cholangiocarcinoma

Author or series	Reference	No. of cases	Male	Female
Hoyne and Kernohan	6	11	5	6
MacDonald	90	24	13	11
Hutt and Anthony	63	19	6	13
Chan	71	10	4	6
Anthony	75	19	11	8
Ferenci et al.	89	5	5	0
Japanese series 1978–1979		93	59	34
Ours		15	6	6

1.4 Symptoms

There are no signs, symptoms, or physical findings that are characteristic of cholangiocarcinoma. The most common symptoms are upper abdominal pain, weight loss, hepatomegaly, an abdominal mass, jaundice, and ascites. However, symptoms of abdominal enlargement, pain, and jaundice were usually at the late stage of the disease. If cholangiocarcinoma arises from the intrahepatic duct close to the hilar area in the liver or a small cholangiocarcinoma invades the hilar area, jaundice may develop as an early symptom, just as in carcinoma of the extrahepatic bile duct. In the Japanese series [66], the objective signs were hepatomegaly in 62.2%, ascites in 26.7%, jaundice in 23.7%, splenomegaly in 2.3%, and esophageal varices in 2.3% of cases. In our series, the chief complaints were jaundice in six patients (40%), abdominal pain in six (40%), upper abdominal discomfort in one (6.7%), and an abdominal mass in one (6.7%).

1.5 Diagnosis

There are no specific laboratory studies diagnostic for cholangiocarcinoma. Alpha-fetoprotein is not produced by this tumor, but in some patients serum levels of total bilirubin and alkaline phosphatase are elevated. In our study, the serum alpha-fetoprotein level was elevated in only two patients (13.3%), but alkaline phosphatase levels were increased in ten (66.7%). Carcinoembryonic antigen (CEA) was elevated in 11 of 15 cases (73.3%).

Recently, tests for CA 19-9, a tumor marker, have been developed for the diagnosis of hepatobiliary malignancies as well as for pancreatic cancers. The CA 19-9 concentration in serum was above the upper normal limit in 73% of the patients with cholangiocarcinoma in the series of Jalanko [76], while it was most consistently increased in patients with pancreatic cancer (76%). In our series, the serum level of CA 19-9 was increased in all three cases in which this test was done; we feel that the serum level of CA 19-9 is a reliable tumor marker, especially in biliary or pancreatic malignancies.

Hypercalcemia may be observed in primary liver carcinoma. Oldenburg et al. [77] encountered hypercalcemia in 7.8% of patients with primary hepatic tumors, 5.3% in hepatocellular carcinoma, and 17.5% in cholangiocarcinoma. Therefore, primary hepatic tumors should be included in the differential diagnosis of hypercalcemia.

Table 31.3. Abdominal angiography and pathological findings in cholangiocarcinoma

	AAG finding	Gross type	Capsule	Growth pattern	Hilar invasion (%)	Periductal spread (%)
Hepatectomy (11 cases)						
Papillary adenocarcinoma 3 cases (27.3%)	Hypervascular 100% (3/3)	Nodular	+	Expansive	0	0
	Hypovascular 50% (4/8)	Massive				
Tubular adenocarcinoma 8 cases (72.7%)			−	Invasive	62.6 (5/8)	100 (8/8)
	Hypervascular 50% (4/8)	Nodular				

AAG abdominal angiography

Gallium uptake by hepatocellular carcinoma occurs in about 90% of all cases. In cholangiocarcinoma, Hamamoto et al. [78] reported the usefulness of this study for tumor detection in two cases, though Makhija [79] failed to show gallium uptake in the tumor area in two cases. Therefore, it seems that gallium scan is not really reliable in the diagnosis of cholangiocarcinoma.

Angiography in patients with cholangiocarcinoma reveals hypervascularity less often than in hepatocellular carcinoma. Chearanai et al. [69] reported that hypervascularity was observed in only 20.6% of cholangiocarcinoma cases, whereas it was seen in 77.4% of hepatoma patients. In a Japanese series [66], angiography demonstrated hypervascular lesions in 89.2% of 720 cases of hepatocellular carcinoma and in 37.7% of 61 cases of cholangiocarcinoma. In 21 (29%) of 720 cases of hepatocellular carcinoma and 7 (11.5%) of 61 cases of cholangiocarcinoma, hepatic tumors were not visualized in arteriograms. In the angiographic study by Chearani et al. in Thailand [69], the diagnostic accuracy was 91.4% for hepatocellular carcinoma and 70.6% for cholangiocarcinoma. In our series, the location of the tumor was diagnosed by ultrasonography (US), computed tomography (CT), and abdominal arteriography (AAG) with an accuracy of 90.9%, 85.7%, and 92.9%, respectively; it was 71.4% by percutaneous transhepatic cholangiography (PTC) or by endoscopic retrograde cholangiography (ERC) as well. On CT, a low-density mass was visualized in 12 of 14 cases (85.7%); on US, a hypoechoic mass was seen in 9 of 11 cases (81.8%) and a hyperechoic mass was seen in one (9.1%). Abdominal arteriography demonstrated hypervascular lesions in 7 (50%) of 14 cases and hypovascular lesions in 50%.

When we compared the pathological findings in 11 patients who had hepatectomy, three of the hypervascular tumors were papillary adenocarcinomas of a nodular type with a capsule; they were grossly expansive growths without invasion of the hilar area or periductal spread. However, of eight tubular adenocarcinomas, four were hypervascular tumors of the massive type. Invasive growth and periductal spread were seen in all eight cases of tubular adenocarcinomas. Hilar invasion was observed in five of these eight cases (Table 31.3).

When serum levels of carcinoembryonic antigen, CA 19-9, and/or alkaline phosphatase are elevated in the presence of a hypovascular tumor in the liver, a diagnosis of cholangicarcinoma is likely. Even when the tumor is hypervascular, cholangiocarcinoma should be considered if there is elevation of the serum level of CA 19-9.

1.6 Treatment and prognosis

A successful outcome depends on early diagnosis and prompt institution of surgical treatment. Hepatectomy should be considered at first as a curative procedure. Palliative surgery, such as internal or external biliary drainage, is necessary when a surgical cure is not achieved, because the patient frequently dies of biliary obstruction with cholangitis or liver abscess. In the Japanese series of 1968–1977 [72], 34.6% of all primary liver cancers were resectable and surgery for cholangiocarcinoma was performed in 19 (16.8%) of 113 cases. The increase in the number of resections is due partly to earlier diagnosis by improved diagnostic procedures and partly to the larger number of patients treated surgically in the 1978–1979 series. In the latter series [66], surgery for cholangiocarcinoma was carried out in 60 (65.9%) of 91 cases: 26 resections (28.6%), five ligations of the hepatic artery, seven intubations into the hepatic artery with chemotherapy, and 22 exploratory laparotomies (24.2%). Of the 26 hepatectomies, seven were extended lobectomies, nine were lobectomies, four were segmentectomies, and six were partial resections. In our series, 11 (73.3%) of all 15 cholangiocarcinoma cases had hepatectomies, which comprised 78.6% of 14 operated cases—three trisegmentectomies, three extended lobectomies, three lobectomies, and two lateral segmentectomies.

Total hepatectomy and transplantation as a form of treatment are not generally accepted at present. As of February 1986, there has as yet been no report of successful liver transplantation for cholangiocarcinoma.

Radiation therapy or chemotherapy for cholangiocarcinoma may also be considered with or without surgery. Of the 15 patients in our series, six underwent radiation therapy after surgery, but it had to be discontinued in three due to side effects or posttransfusion non-B hepatitis. However, one patient in our series is still alive 5 years 5 months after surgery that was followed by irradiation to the invaded left diaphragm. Therefore, radiation therapy should be considered as an additional treatment whenever possible.

Patton [80] found that the average survival from the time of diagnosis was 6.5 months with a range of 1–21 months. Lemmer [81] found the average time from onset of symptoms to death to be only 7 months.

In most cases, by the time the diagnosis is made the disease is usually inoperable due to metastasis. Cholangiocarcinoma metastasizes earlier and more frequently than does hepatocellular carcinoma. In the Japanese series [66], lymph node metastasis was the most frequent (62.5%), followed by metastasis to the peritoneum (46.3%), lung (41.4%), intraperitoneal organs (40.4%), adrenal (20.4%), bone (12.1%), skin (2.4%), and others (17.6%). In Cruickshank's 17 cases [82], lymph node involvement was noted in nine (52.9%), adrenals in seven (46.7%), lungs in three (20%), diaphragm, pleura, peritoneum, and bone in two each (13.3%), and kidney in one (0.7%).

Cholangiocarcinoma has a notable tendency toward lymph node metastasis and local spreading. Therefore, resectability of cholangiocarcinoma of the liver is very limited, and according to the English and Japanese literature there have been few survivors who lived more than 3 years

after surgery. Alpert et al. [83] reported a 52-year-old female who had a partial right hepatic resection for cholangiocarcinoma and remained in good health, free of evidence of tumor recurrence, 13 years later. Rockwell et al. [84] described a 67-year-old Caucasian woman who lived for 7 years after resection of the left lateral segment of the liver; they stressed that cholangiocarcinoma had a hopeless prognosis unless found at a very early stage. Li et al. [85] reported one 3-year and one 5-year survival among eight cases of cholangiocarcinoma. Sanguily et al. [86] described a 61-year-old woman in whom primary cholangiocarcinoma of the liver was diagnosed by liver scan and who was treated surgically by wedge resection of the right lobe of the liver. Two and a half years after surgery, the patients was still well and postoperative scans showed no sign of recurrence of the tumor.

In the previous Japanese series of 1968–1977 [72], surgery for cholangiocarcinoma was carried out in only 113 (42.2%) of 268 patients, and hepatic resection was performed in 19 (16.8%) of the patients. Of the 13 patients for whom follow-up data were complete, one died within 1 month and seven lived for more than 1 year, representing an actuarial 1-year survival rate of 58.8%, with the longest survival being 27 months after surgery. No patients survived more than 3 years.

The longest survival in our series at the time of the previous publication in 1984 [73] was 4 years 1 month, and the next longest survival was 2 years 8 months. Fortunately, both patients are still alive and well without recurrence 6 years 10 months and 5 years 5 months after surgery, respectively. Among the patients who underwent laparotomy for cholangiocarcinoma, survival was much longer after resection than after other surgical procedures [66].

The best treatment is, therefore, early diagnosis and early surgical removal.

1.7 Case report—longest survival in our series

A small 61-year-old woman (height 143 cm, weight 29 kg) was admitted to our unit at Mie University Hospital in February 1979. On admission, the liver was palpable 7 cm below the xyphoid process with a smooth surface and slight tenderness.

Laboratory studies revealed 32.5% hematocrit, a white blood cell count of 6000 cells/mm³, 0.6 mg/dl serum total bilirubin, 310 units alkaline phosphatase, and choline esterase of pH 0.6. Serum alpha-fetoprotein and carcinoembryonic antigen levels were within normal limits. Computed tomography and scintigraphy revealed a 7-cm mass in the right lobe of the liver. Percutaneous transhepatic cholangiography and endoscopic retrograde cholangiopancreatography revealed an obstruction of the bile duct at the hilum, and the left intrahepatic bile duct was markedly dilated compared with the right (Fig. 31.1). Selective celiac angiography of the liver showed a mass of 5 × 7 cm with a tumor stain in the right lobe (Fig. 31.2). With a diagnosis of hepatocellular carcinoma in the right lobe and hilar obstruction, a right trisegmentectomy was performed and the intrahepatic bile duct of the lateral segment was anastomosed to the jejunum by a Roux-en Y procedure. The resected liver weighed 456 g. There was a grayish white mass of 7 × 8 cm in the resected specimen (Fig. 31.3). The histological diagnosis was cholangiocarci-

noma. The patient received a total of 2400 mg 5-fluorouracil and 16 mg mitomycin C intravenously and was discharged on the 61st postoperative day. She is well without recurrence 6 years 10 months after surgery.

2 Cystic adenocarcinoma of liver

Biliary cystadenocarcinoma of the liver is extremely rare [91]. It usually consists of multilocular cystic masses lined by mucus-secreting epithelium with papillary infoldings and contains mucoid fluid; it arises from the intrahepatic bile ducts. The size of the tumor ranges from 3.5 to 25 cm in diameter [92]. There are approximately 50 cases reported in the English and Japanese literature [92–94].

Among 171 cases of primary liver cancer ad-

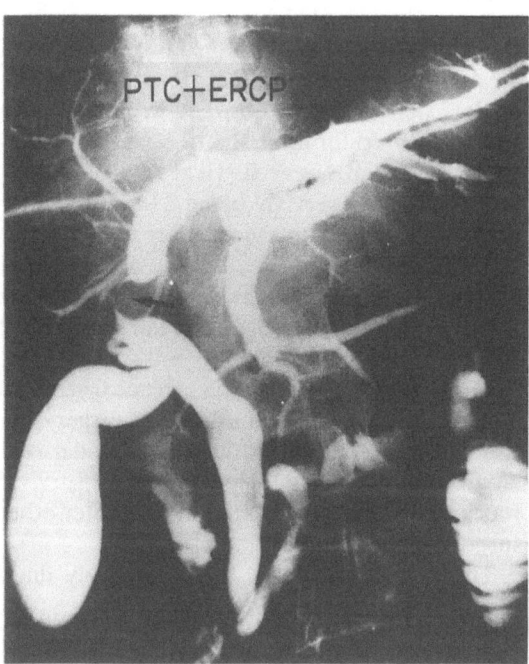

Fig. 31.1. A 61-year-old female with cholangiocarcinoma. Cholangiogram obtained by simultaneous PTC and ERCP demonstrating an obstruction of the bile duct at the hilum (*arrow*)

Fig. 31.2. Cholangiocarcinoma. Arteriography ▶ (above) shows a mass with an arterial encasement (arrow) in the right lobe of the liver which is hypervascular (arrows), especially in the venous phase (*below*)

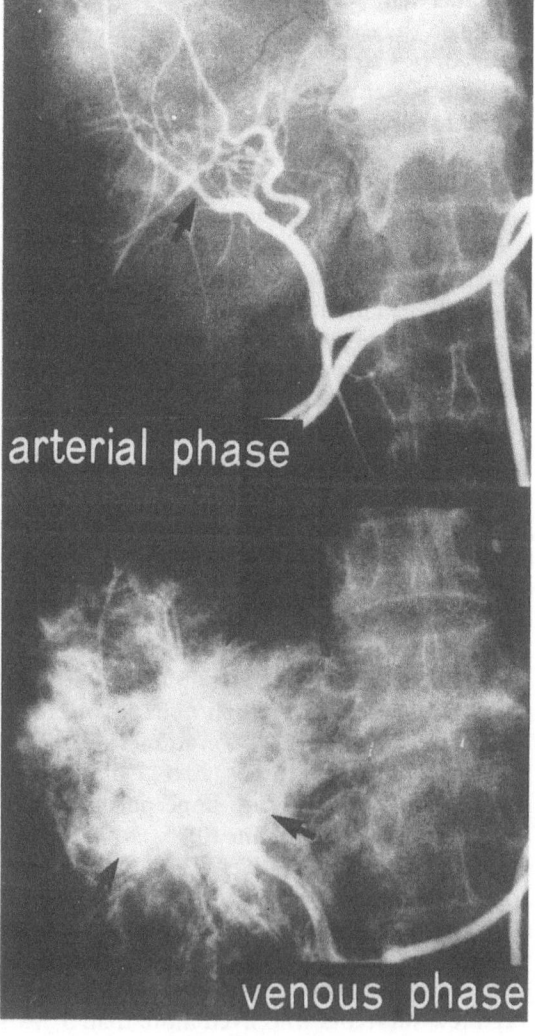

Fig. 31.3a, b. Cholangiocarcinoma. **a** The resected specimen of right trisegmentectomy. **b** Cut surface of the specimen. *C* common bile duct, *L* left hepatic duct, invaded, *R* right hepatic duct, invaded

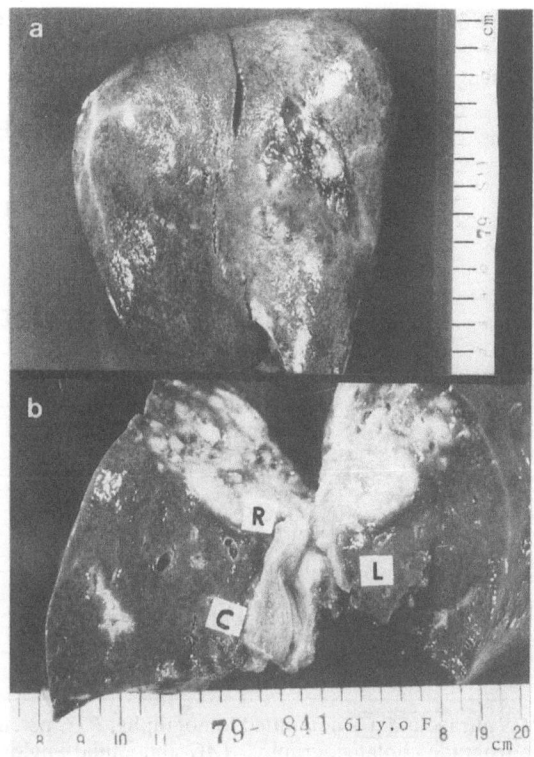

mitted to our unit during the past 9 years, there were four cases of cystic adenocarcinoma. including one with carcinoma arising in a liver cyst (Tables 31.4, 31.5).

Cystadenocarcinoma is more common in middle-aged women [92–94], but in our series males and females were equal in number, and the age ranged from 58 to 67 years with an average of 62.5 years. Chief complaints in our four patients were abdominal mass, jaundice, biliocutaneous fistula, and fever with abdominal pain, respectively.

On ultrasonography (US), the tumor is a globular or ovoid and thick-walled cystic mass, which often contains multiple septations or papillary infoldings. On computed tomography (CT), the tumor appears as a low-density intrahepatic mass which may contain mural nodules or internal septations. Angiographically, these tumors frequently reveal a hypovascular pattern, although abnormal clusters of vessels are frequently seen within the wall [92]. CT or US findings of these tumors have not yet been described in detail, because the diagnosis of the tumor was not considered preoperatively in the past. Currently, CT and US are good tools for detecting a tumor and defining its macroscopic features.

In our series, CT and US revealed multilocular, small intrahepatic cystic masses in three cases, as shown in Fig. 31.4, but a large cystic mass with papillary projections was observed in the other case as seen in Fig. 31.6. All four patients underwent surgery with resection (left hepatic lobectomies in cases 3 and 4 and left lateral segmentectomies in cases 1 and 2), followed by radiation and/or chemotherapy.

The prognosis seems to be much better than that of other hepatic tumors. In our series, case 1 is alive after 1 year 6 months and case 4 is also well without recurrence 2 years 7 months after the operation; case 3 died after 4 months and case 2 died 3 years 8 months after surgery (Table 31.5). In all four cases, the cyst fluid was mucinous. In cystadenocarcinoma, generally speaking, the cyst fluid may be mucinous or serous and contains hemosiderin, cholesterol, and necrotic or purulent material. The cysts rarely communicate with the bile duct, unlike our case 4 (Fig. 31.6).

Pathological study demonstrated cystadenocarcinoma of the liver in three cases (cases 1–3) and carcinoma arising in a liver cyst in case 4.

In 1958, Edmondson [95] outlined the criteria for the diagnosis of biliary cystadenoma. Diag-

Table 31.4. Imaging studies and tumor markers in serum in cystadenocarcinoma of the liver

Patient	Age (years), sex	Imaging studies				Tumor markers in serum (ng/ml)		
		US	CT	PTC and ERC	AAG	AFP	CEA	CA 19-9
TN	59, M			Compression of left intra-hepatic bile duct	Encasement of middle hepatic artery	3	2.1	280
NH	66, M	Hypoechoic, multilocular cystic pattern with septation	Well-defined, multilocular cyst with mural projection	Dilatation of common bile duct with compression of left hepatic duct	Hypovascular	2	2.3	—
SK	67, F			Obstruction of left hepatic duct	Hypervascular	2	56	16 400
OM	58, F	Unilocular, large cystic pattern with papillary projection	Unilocular, large cystic mass with papillary projection	Compression of left intra-hepatic bile duct	Hypovascular	2	1.5	—

US ultrasound, *CT* computed tomography, *PTC* percutaneous transhepatic cholangiography, *ERC* endoscopic retrograde cholangiography, *AAG* abdominal angiography, *AFP* alpha-fetoprotein, *CEA* carcinoembryonic antigen, *CA* carbohydrate antigen

Table 31.5. Treatment and results in cystadenocarcinoma of the liver

Patient	Age (years), sex	Chief complaints	Cystic appearance	Location	Operative procedure	Results after surgery
TN	59, M	Jaundice	Multilocular	Lateral segment	Left lateral segmentectomy	Well, 1 year 6 months
NH	66, M	Bile fistula			Left lateral segmentectomy	Died with recurrence, 3 years 9 months
SK	67, F	Upper abdominal pain, fever			Left hepatic lobectomy with caudate lobectomy	Died with recurrence, 4 months
OM	58, F	Hepatomegaly	Unilocular	Left lobe	Left hepatic lobectomy with cholecystectomy	Well, 2 years 7 months

nostic findings include a mutilocular hepatic cyst lined by mucin-producing columnar cells, with areas of papillary infoldings and a densely cellular stroma. According to the WHO classification, bile duct cystadenocarcinoma is a malignant epithelial tumor of the liver. The tumors are usually multilocular and contain mucoid fluid.

Cystadenocarcinoma may develop primarily in the liver and it may evolve from malignant transformation of cystadenoma (53, 54, 91, 96, 97). Some authors also reported adenocarcinoma developing within a dilated intrahepatic bile duct or a primary liver cyst (51, 98), as cystadenocarcinoma of the liver. Since Willis [51] reported a case of carcinoma arising in a congenital cyst of the liver, approximately ten such cases have been reported in the literature [51–59, 98].

We believe that cystadenocarcinoma and carcinoma arising in a primary liver cyst should be regarded as separate entities and that the classification of these tumors is necessary. However, in some advanced cases, it may be difficult or im-

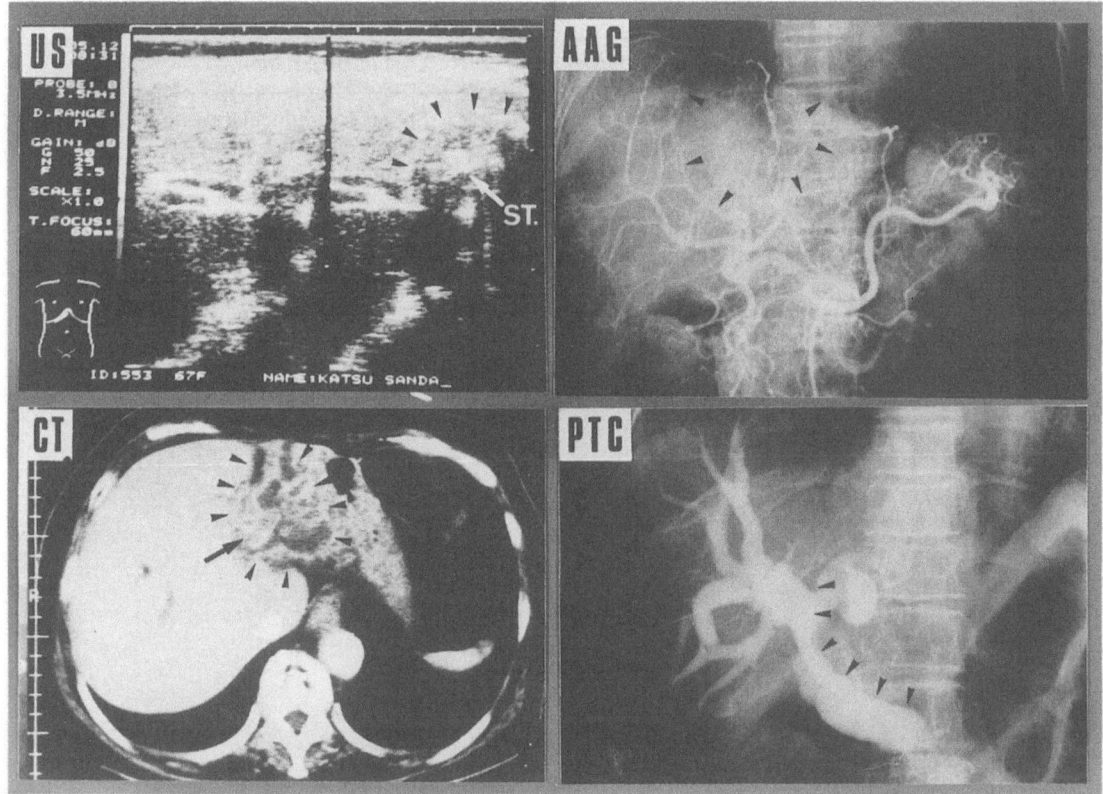

Fig. 31.4. Case 3, a 67-year-old female, cystadenocarcinoma of the liver. Left hepatic lobectomy was performed. CT and US revealed a multilocular, intrahepatic cystic mass. *US* ultrasonography, *CT* computed tomography, *AAG* abdominal angiography, *PTC* percutaneous transhepatic cholangiography

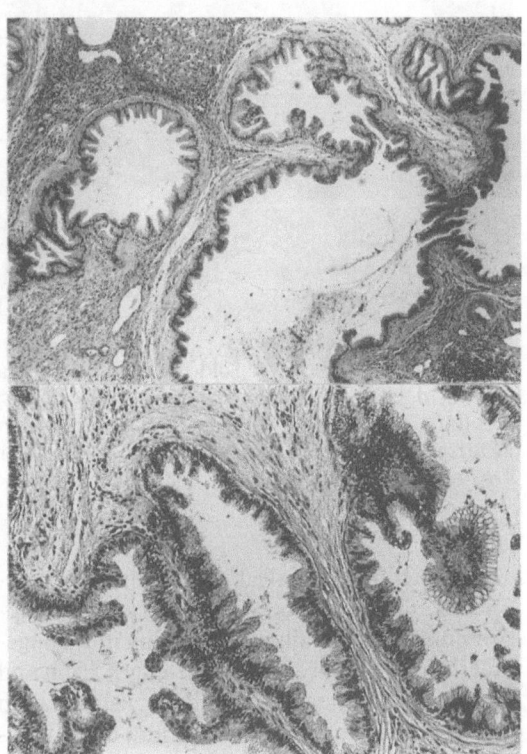

Fig. 31.5a, b. Case 3, cystadenocarcinoma of the liver. **a** 4 × 3.3, **b** 10 × 3.3. Microscopically, the loculi are lined by columnar mucus-secretory epithelia with an obvious proliferative papillary growth

Table 31.6. Differences between cystadenocarcinoma and cholangiocarcinoma with cysts

	Cholangiocarcinoma and cysts	Cystadenocarcinoma
Gross appearance	Usually multiple focal cysts	Solitary multilocular cyst
Contents of cyst	Serous; not bile stained	Mucinous or hemorrhagic
Cyst epithelium	Not flattened; papillary in areas of neo-plastic change	Columnar papillary
Tissue between cysts	Collagenized acellular stroma; hepatic remnants, including hamartomatous bile ducts	Spindle cell stroma; no hepatic remnants
Other area of liver	Other cysts and metastascs common	Other cysts and metastases rare
Distant metastases	Common	Rare
Cysts in kidneys	Common	Rare
Cysts in pancreas	Described	Described

After Azizah and Paradinas [58]

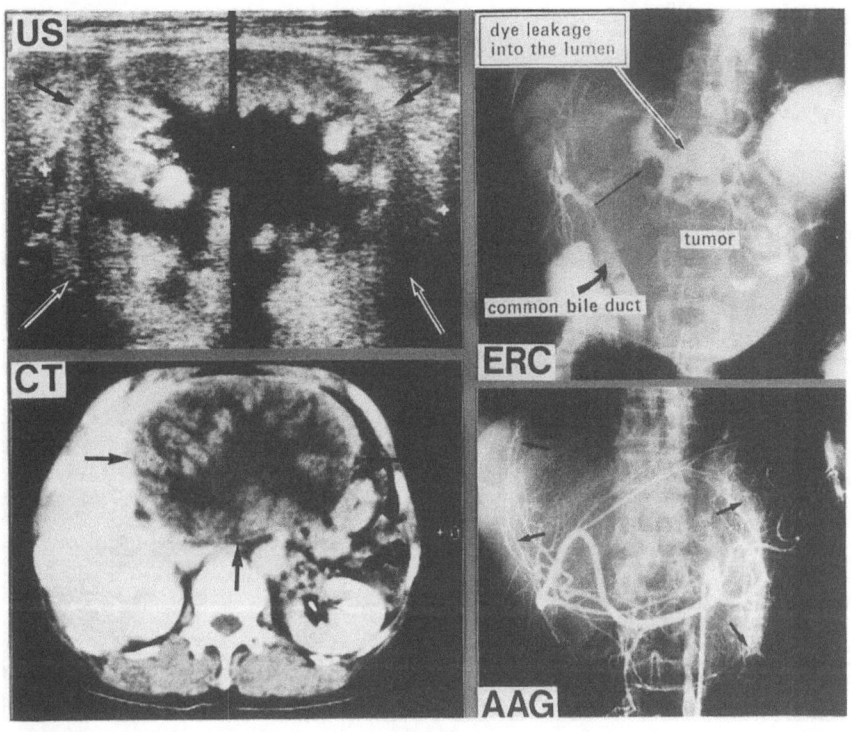

Fig. 31.6. Case 4, a 58-year-old female with carcinoma arising in a liver cyst. Left hepatic lobectomy was performed. US and CT show a large cyst with papillary projections (at arrows). ERC delineates the common bile duct (large arrow) and dye going into a lumen within the mass (thin arrows.) AAG demonstrates a large mass (at arrows). *US* ultrasonography, *CT* computed tomography, *ERC* endoscopic retrograde cholangiography, *AAG* abdominal angiography

possible to differentiate between them. Therefore, the distinction between biliary cystadeno-carcinoma and a malignancy arising in a congenital liver cyst is not always clear-cut. Azizah and Paradinas [58] attempted to distinguish between cholangiocarcinoma with a cyst and cystadeno-carcinoma, as seen in Table 31.6. It seems that biliary cystadenocarcinoma fulfills Edmondson's criteria and carcinomas arising from liver cysts usually reveal a solitary cystic mass. Therefore, some of the reported cases of cystadenocarci-noma may be reclassified as cholangiocarcinoma associated with liver cysts or a carcinoma arising from a liver cyst, e.g., our case 4.

Fig. 31.7 *1–5.* Case 4, carcinoma arising in a liver cyst. *1* Papillotubular adenocarcinoma with *2* large eosinophilic cells. *3* A transitional area between normal and malignant epithelia (at arrow). *4* The columnar-cuboidal epithelium layer of the liver cyst. *5* Abnormal malignant cell

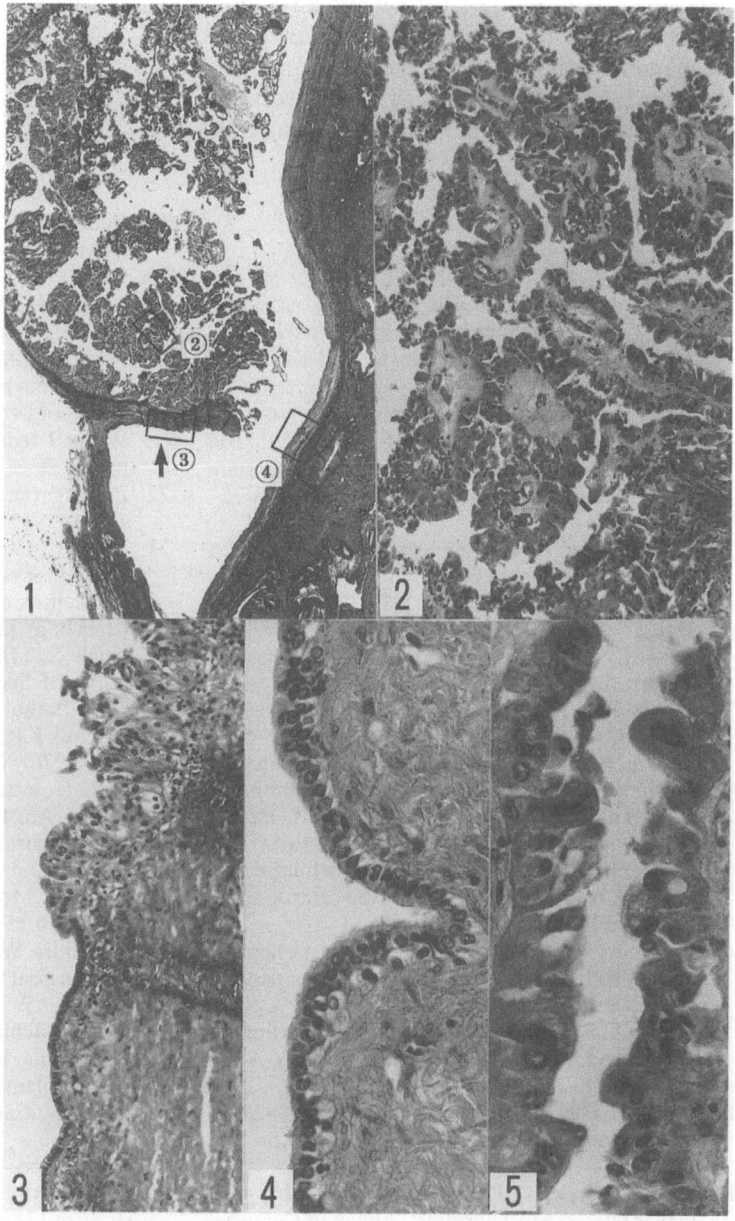

Hepatic abscess, intrahepatic hematoma, echinococcal cyst, simple congenital cyst, and cystadenoma should be differentiated from cystadenocarcinoma in the diagnosis. Aspiration of the cyst contents may be helpful for differential diagnosis. Kanamori et al. [99] reported that endoscopic aspiration of mucinous fluid via the major duodenal papilla should be tried as a diagnostic approach.

The case histories of two different cystic adenocarcinomas of the liver (discussed above) are briefly presented from our series (Tables 31.4, 31.5).

2.1 Cystadenocarcinoma (case 3)

A 67-year-old female presented with a chief complaint of upper abdominal pain and fever (Figs. 31.4, 31.5). A left hepatic lobectomy with caudate lobectomy was performed. Histological diagnosis was cystadenocarcinoma of the liver. She died of recurrence of the tumor 4 months after surgery.

2.2 Carcinoma arising from a liver cyst (case 4)

A 58-year-old female presented with hepatomegaly (Figs. 31.6, 31.7). A left hepatic lobectomy and cholecystectomy were carried out. Histological diagnosis was papillary adenocarcinoma arising from a large unilocular cyst of the liver. The patient is well 2 years and 7 months after surgery.

References

1. Hanot VC, Gilbert A (1888) Études sur les maladies du foie: Cancer (épithéliome): sarcome; cystes non-parasitaires; angiomas. Asselin and Houseau, Paris (cited by Hoyne and Kernohan [6])
2. Eggel H (1901) Ueber das primäre Carcinom der Leber. Beitr Z Path Anat u allg Path 30: 506–604
3. Goldzieher M, von Bókay Z (1911) Der primäre Leber Krebs. Virchows Arch f Path Anat 203: 75–131
4. Yamagiwa K (1911) Zur Kenntnis des primären parenchymatösen Leberkarzinoms (Hepatoma). Virchows Arch f Path Anat 206: 437–467
5. Burdette WJ (1956) Neoplasms of the liver. In: Shiff L (ed) Disease of the Liver, 4th edn. Lippincott, Philadelphia, 1051–1077
6. Hoyne RN, Kernohan JW (1947) Primary carcinoma of the liver. Arch Intern Med 79: 532–554
7. Okuda K, Kubo Y, Okazaki N, Arishima T, Hashimoto M, Jinnouchi S, Sawa Y, Shimokawa Y, Nakajima Y, Noguchi T, Nakano M, Kojiro M, Nakashima T (1977) Clinical aspect of intrahepatic bile duct carcinoma including hilar carcinoma. A study of 57 autopsy-proven cases. Cancer 39: 232–246
8. Klatskin G (1965) Adenocarcinoma of the hepatic duct at its bifurcation with the porta hepatis. Am J Med 28: 241–256
9. Dahlgren S (1967) Late effects of thorium dioxide on the liver of patients in Sweden. Ann NY Acad Sci 145: 718–723
10. Casper J (1967) The introduction in 1928–29 of thorium dioxide in diagnostic radiology. Ann NY Acad Sci 145: 527–529
11. Grampa G (1971) Radiation industry with particular reference to Thorotrast. Appleton-Century-Crofts, New York, p 147
12. MacMahon E, Murphy AS, Bates MI (1947) Endothelial cell sarcoma of the liver following thorotrast injection. Am J Pathol 23: 585–613
13. Battifora HA (1976) Thorotrast and tumors of the liver. In: Okuda K, Peters R (eds) Hepatocellular carcinoma. Wiley, New York, pp 83–93
14. Winberg CD, Ranchond M (1979) Thorotrast induced hepatic cholaniocarcinoma and angiosarcoma. Human Pathol 10: 108–112
15. Kojiro M, Kawano Y, Kawasaki H (1982) Thorotrast-induced hepatic angiosarcoma and combined hepatocellular and cholangiocarcinoma in a single patient. Cancer 49: 2161–2164
16. Ellis EF, Gordon PR, Gottlieb LS (1978) Oral contraceptives and cholangiocarcinoma. Lancet 1: 207
17. Landais P, Drünfeld J-P, Droz D, Drüeke T, Albouze G, Gogusev J, Chauveau D, Moynot A (1984) Cholangiocellular carcinoma in polycystic kidney and liver disease. Arch Intern Med 144: 2274–2276
18. Hou PC (1951) The relationship between primary carcinoma of the liver and infestation with clonorchis sinensis. J Pathol Bacteriol 72: 239–246
19. Berman (1951) Primary carcinoma of the liver. Lewis, London
20. Chen P-H, Lo H-W, Wang C-S, Tsai K-R, Chen Y-C, Lin K-Y, Siauw C-P, Hwang R-R, Liu M-H, Ko H-C, Chen T-Y (1984) Cholangiocarcinoma in hepatolithiasis. J Clin Gastroenterol 6: 539–547
21. Nakayama F (1984) Intrahepatic stones: epidemiology and etiology. In: Okuda K, Nakayama F, Wong J (eds) Hepatolithiasis. Liss, New York, pp 17–28
22. Balasegaram M (1972) Hepatic calculi. Ann Surg 175: 149–154
23. Min PC, Cho MH, Im HM et al. (1966) Biliary tract diseases among Koreans. Analysis of 100 consecutive cases. J Korean Surg Soc 8: 1 (cited by Chen et al. [20])
24. Sanes S, MacCallum JD (1942) Primary carcinoma of liver (cholangioma) in hepatolithiasis. Am J Pathol 18: 675–687
25. Falchuk KR, Lesser PB, Galdabini JJ, Isselbacher KJ (1976) Cholangiocarcinoma as related to chronic intrahepatic cholangitis and hepatolithiasis. Am J Gastroenterol 66: 57–61
26. Shanmugaratnam K (1956) Primary carcinoma of the liver and biliary tract. Br J Cancer 10: 232–246
27. Glenn F, Moody FG (1961) Intrahepatic calculi. Ann Surg 153: 711–724
28. Longmire WP, Passaro EP, Joseph WL (1966) The surgical treatment of hepatic lesion. Br J Surg 53: 852–859
29. Koga A, Ichimiya H, Yamaguchi K, Miyazaki K, Nakayama F (1985) Hepatolithiasis associated with cholangiocarcinoma, possible etiologic significance. Cancer 55: 2826–2829
30. Nakanuma Y, Terada T, Tanaka Y, Ohta G (1985) Are hepatolithiasis and cholangiocarcinoma aetiologically related? A morphological study of 12 cases of hepatolithiasis associated with cholangiocarcinoma. Virchows Archiv A 406: 45–58
31. Yoshimoto H, Ikeda S, Tanaka M, Matsumoto S (1985) Intrahepatic cholangiocarcinoma associated with hepatolithiasis. Gastrointestinal Endoscopy 31: 260–263
32. Kinami Y, Noto K, Miyazaki I, Matsubara F (1978) A study of hepatolithiasis associated with cholangioma. Acta Hepatol Jpn 19: 578–583 (in Japanese)
33. McConnel AA (1919–1920) Cyst of the common bile duct. Br J Surg 7: 520–524
34. Vachell HR, Stevens WM (1906) Case of intrahepatic calculi. Br Med J 1: 434–436
35. Sakuma S (1905) Retentionscyste des ductus choledochus. Okayama Med J 181: 49–73
36. Yotsuyanagi S (1936) Contributions to the aeti-

ology and pathogeny of idiopathic cystic dilatation of the common bile duct with report of 3 cases. A new aetiological theory, based on supposed unequal epithelial proliferation at the stage of the physiological epithelial occlusion of the primitive choledochus. Gann 30: 601–652

37. Bloustein PA (1977) Association of carcinoma with congenital cystic conditions of the liver and bile ducts. Am J Gastroenterol 67: 40–46

38. Alonso-Lej F, William BR Jr, Daniel JP (1959) Congenital choledochal cyst, with a report of 2, and an analysis of 94 cases. Int Abstr Surg 108: 1–30

39. Kasai M, Asakura Y, Taira Y (1970) Surgical treatment of choledochal cyst. Ann Surg 172: 844–851

40. Caroli J, Couinaud D (1958) Une affection nouvelle, sans doute congenitale, des voies biliares. La kilatation kystique unilobulaire des canaux hepatiques. Sem Hop Paris 34: 136–142

41. Engle J, Salmon PA (1964) Multiple choledochal cysts. Arch Surg 88: 354–356

42. Ackerholm P, Benediktsdotlir K, Lundell L, Thulin A (1981) Cholangiocarcinoma in a patient with biliary cysts. Acta Chir Scand 147: 605–607

43. Todani T, Watanabe Y, Naruse M, Tabuchi K, Okajima K (1977) Congenital bile duct cysts: Classification, operative procedures and review of thirty-seven cases including cancer arising from choledochal cyst. Am J Surg 134: 263–269

44. Kagawa Y, Kashihara S, Kuramoto S, Maetani S (1978) Carcinoma arising in a congenitally dilated biliary tract. Gastroenterology 74: 1286–1294

45. Schiewe R, Baudisch E, Erhhardt G (1968) Angeborene intrahepatishe Gallengangzyste mit Steinbildung und maligner Entartung. Bruns Beirt Klim Chir 216: 264–271

46. Dayton MT, Longmire WP, Tompkins RK (1983) Caroli's disease: A premalignant condition? Am J Surg 145: 41–48

47. Leroy JP, Charles JF, Diveres B, Bellet M (1979) Carcinome biliare developpe sur maladie de Caroli. Arch Anat Cyto Pathol 27: 121–125

48. Jones AW, Shreeve DR (1970) Congenital dilatation of intrahepatic biliary ducts with cholangiocarcinoma. Br Med J 2: 277–278

49. Gallagher PJ, Millis RR, Mitchinson MJ (1972) Congenital dilatation of the intrahepatic bile ducts with cholangiocarcinoma. J Clin Pathol 25: 804–808

50. Nasu S, Sakurai M, Miyagi T (1971) Cholangiocarcinoma arising in intrahepatic bile duct cyst. Nihonrinsho 29: 3075–3081 (in Japanese)

51. Willis RA (1943) Carcinoma arising in congenital cysts of the liver. J Pathol 4: 492–495

52. Richmond HG (1956) Carcinoma arising in congenital cysts of liver. J Pathology 72: 681–684

53. Dean DL, Bauer HM (1963) Primary cystic carcinoma of the liver. Am J Surg 117: 416–420

54. Cruickshank AH, Sparshott SM (1971) Malignancy in natural and experimental hepatic cysts: experiments with aflatoxin in rats and the malignant transformation of cysts in human livers. J Pathol 104: 183–190

55. Ameriks J, Appleman H, Frey C (1972) Malignant nonparasitic cyst of the liver. Ann Surg 171: 713–716

56. Kinami Y, Ohno S, Kawamura M, Furukawa S, Miyazaki I (1975) Surgical liver disease with cystic findings. Geka (Surg) 37: 813–818 (in Japanese)

57. Kasai Y, Sasaki E, Tamaki A, Koshino I, Kawanishi N, Hata Y (1977) Carcinoma arising in the cyst of the liver—Report of three cases Jpn J Surg 7: 65–72

58. Azizah N, Paradinas FJ (1980) Cholangiocarcinoma coexisting with developmental liver cyst: a distinct entity different from liver cystadenocarcinoma. Histopathology 4: 391–400

59. Imamura M, Miyashita T, Tani T, Naito A, Tobe T, Takahashi K (1984) Cholangiocellular carcinoma associated with multiple liver cysts. Am J Gastroenterol 79: 790–795

60. Silverberg E (1979) Cancer statistics 1979. Cancer J for clinicians 29: 6–21

61. Incidence of cancer in Norway 1972–1976. The cancer registry of Norway 1978, pp124–125

62. Anthony PP (1979) Hepatic neoplasms. In: MacSween RNM, Anthony PP, Scheuer PJ (eds) Pathology of the liver. Churchill Livingstone, Edinburgh, pp 387–413

63. Hutt MRS, Anthony P (1973) Tumors of liver, biliary system and pancreas. Rec Res Cancer 41: 57–78

64. LiBing et al. (1980) National survey of cancer mortality in China. Chin J Oncol 21: 1 (cited by Li et al. [85])

65. Editorial Committee for the Atlas of Cancer (1979) Mortality in People's Republic of China. China Map Press

66. The liver cancer study group of Japan (1984) Primary liver cancer in Japan. Cancer 54: 1747–1755

67. Kawarada Y, Uehara S, Noda M, Yatani R, Mizumoto R (1985) Nonhepatocytic malignant mixed tumor primary in the liver. Report of two cases. Cancer 55: 1790–1798

68. Kingston M, Ali MA, Lewall D (1985) Hepatic tumors in Saudi Arabia. A practical approach to diagnosis. Cancer 55: 1579–1585

69. Chearanai O, Plengvanit U, Damrongsak D, Tuchinda S, Damrongsak C, Viranuvatti V (1984) Primary liver cancer, angiographic study of 127 cases. J Med Assoc Thailand 67: 482–490

70. Hoyne RM, Kernohan JW (1974) Primary carcinoma of the liver. A study of thirty-one cases. Arch Intern Med 79: 532–554

71. Chan KT (1966) The management of primary liver carcinoma. Ann R Coll Surg 41: 253–282

72. Okuda K (1980) The liver cancer study group of Japan. Primary liver cancers in Japan. Cancer 45: 2663–2669

73. Kawarada Y, Mizumoto R (1984) Cholangiocellular carcinoma of the liver. Am J Surg 147: 354–359

74. Gall EA (1956) Tumor of the liver. In: Schiff L (ed). Disease of the liver. Lippincott, Philadel-

phia, pp 543–564

75. Anthony PP (1973) Primary carcinoma of the liver: A study of 282 cases in Ugandan Africans. J Pathol 110: 37–48

76. Jalanko H, Kuusela P, Roberts P, Sippone P, Haglung F, Mäkelä O (1984) Comparison of a new tumor marker, CA 19-9™, with alpha-fetoprotein and carcinoembryonic antigen in patients with upper gastrointestinal disease. J Clin Pathol 37: 218–222

77. Oldenburg WA, Van Heerden PA, Sizemore GW, Abbound CF, Sheedy PF (1982) Hypercalcemia and primary hepatic tumors. Arch Surg 117: 1363–1366

78. Hamamoto K, Torizuka K, Mukai T, Kosaka T, Suzuki T, Honjyo I (1972) Usefulness of computer scintigraphy for detecting liver with Ga-67 citrate and the scintillation camera. J Nucl Med 13: 667–672

79. Makhija MC (1981) Hepatic uptake of TC-99m MDP in a case of cholangiocarcinoma. Clin Nucl Med 6: 227–228

80. Patton RB (1964) Primary liver cancer—Autopsy study of 600 cases. Cancer 17: 757–768

81. Lemmer EK (1950) Primary cancer of the liver. Arch Surg 61: 599–609

82. Cruickshank AH (1961) The pathology of 111 cases of primary hepatic malignancy collected in the Liverpool region. J Clin Pathol 14: 120–131

83. Alpert LI, Zah FG, Wethamer S, Bochetto JF (1974) A cholangioma. Clinicopathologic study of five cases with ultrastructural observations. Human Pathol 5: 709–728

84. Rockwell G, Baker JW, Lasesohn JT (1966) Cholangiocarcinoma of the liver. Case report with seven-year survival, with review of the literature on primary liver tumors and hepatic resection. Cancer 19: 1178–1184

85. Li G, Wang C, Zhu S, Deng Z, Li G, Wan D, Li J, Zhan Y (1985) Hepatectomy for primary liver cancer in 114 cases. Chinese Med J 98: 377–383

86. Sanguily J, Calderin VO (1974) Partial resection of the liver for primary cholangiocarcinoma. Presentation of successful case. Am J Surg 128: 603–607

87. Al-Sarraf M, Go TS, Kithier K, Vaitkevicius K (1974) A review of the clinical features, blood groups, serum enzymes, therapy and survival of 65 cases. Cancer 33: 574–582

88. Appleqvist P (1982) Primary carcinoma of the liver: clinical course and therapeutic results. J Surg Oncol 21: 87–93

89. Ferenci P, Dragosics B, Marosi L, Kiss F (1984) Relative incidence of primary liver cancer in cirrhosis in Austria. Etiological considerations. Liver 4: 7–14

90. MacDonald RA (1956) Cirrhosis and primary carcinoma of the liver: Changes in their occurrence at the Boston City Hospital 1897–1954. New Engl J Med 255: 1179–1183

91. Ishak KG, Willis GW, Cummins SD, Bjjullock AA (1977) Biliary cystadenoma and cystadeno-carcinoma. Report of 14 cases and review of the literature. Cancer 38: 322–338

92. Stanley J, Vujic I, Schabel SI, Gobien RP, Reinjes HD (1983) Evaluation of biliary cystadenoma and cystadenocarcinoma. Radiology 8: 245–248

93. Woods GL (1981) Biliary cystadenocarcinoma. Case report of hepatic malignancy originating in benign cystadenoma. Cancer 47: 2936–2940

94. Berjian RA, Mime F, Douglass HO, Nava H (1981) Biliary cystadenocarcinoma. Report of a case presenting with osseous metastasis and a review of the literature. J Surg Oncol 18: 305–316

95. Edmondsen HA (1985) Tumors of the liver and intrahepatic bile ducts. In: Atlas of tumor pathology, fascicle 25, Armed Forces Institute of Pathology, Washington

96. More JRS (1966) Cystadenocarcinoma of the liver. J Clin Pathol 19: 470–474

97. Thompson JE, Wolff M (1965) Intra-hepatic cystadenoma of bile duct origin, with malignant alteration. Report of a case, treated with total left hepatic lobectomy. Military Med 130: 218–224

98. Devine P, Ucci AA (1985) Case studies, biliary cystadenocarcinoma arising in a congenital cyst. Human Pathol 16: 92–94

99. Kanamori H, Kawahara H, Oh S, Mine T, Osawa H, Murakami T, Ogata E (1985) A case of biliary cystadenocarcinoma with recurrent jaundice. Diagnostic evaluation of computed tomography. Cancer 55: 2722–2724

Chapter 32
Liver Transplantation in the Treatment of Liver Cancer

Shunzaburo Iwatsuki and Thomas E. Starzl[1]

The treatment of choice for hepatic malignancy has been total surgical removal of tumor(s). Extensive liver resection such as right and left trisegmentectomies can now be performed with an operative mortality of less than 5% [1]. Five-year survival of primary liver malignancy after subtotal liver resection has been as high as 46% [1]. On the other hand, the prognosis of liver cancer which cannot be treated with the conventional technique of subtotal liver resection because of extensive hepatic involvement of tumors or co-existing nonneoplastic liver disorders has been quite poor. Total hepatectomy with hepatic replacement (orthotopic liver transplantation) is, at least in concept, an ideal approach for the "unresectable" liver cancer.

The world's first attempt to treat "unresectable" liver cancer by total hepatectomy with hepatic replacement was made in Denver on May 5, 1963. The patient was a 48-year-old man with hepatocellular carcinoma in a cirrhotic liver. He died 22 days after transplant from pulmonary emboli and sepsis. The postmortem examination did not reveal any residual tumors. The first patient to live more than 1 year after liver transplantation also had hepatocellular carcinoma. This 1-year 7-month-old girl was the eighth recipient in Denver and lived 400 days after transplantation on July 23, 1967. Her tumor first recurred in the lungs 3 months after transplant and then disseminated into the liver homograft, other abdominal organs, and the brain. Despite efforts to control the tumor by chemotherapy, radiation therapy, and surgical debulking procedure, she died from carcinomatosis on August 26, 1968. These two early cases clearly illustrated the issues involved in liver transplantation for hepatic malignancies. By the time the early Den-ver experience in liver transplantation was reported in the monograph in 1969 [2], the enthusiasm for treating so-called unresectable liver cancer with orthotopic liver transplantation had been dampened because of the high incidence of aggressive tumor recurrence after potentially curative total hepatectomy with liver replacement. Nevertheless, the treatment of malignant tumors by liver transplantation has continued because of: (1) the lack of other effective therapy; (2) rare examples of cure of malignancy by total hepatectomy with hepatic replacement; and (3) the improved overall survival after liver transplantation with cyclosporine-steroid therapy in recent years.

The Denver-Pittsburgh experience in orthotopic transplantation in the presence of primary hepatic malignancy during the last 23 years from March 1963 to March 1986 will be summarized in this chapter. There have been several publications on this subject, reporting individual results in detail by the OT code numbers of the patients for interested readers to review [2–7]. Prof. Calne has provided a similar detailed account of his experience in England [8].

1 Selection of candidates

There are two different situations where patients who have primary hepatic malignancies require total hepatectomy with hepatic replacement (orthotopic liver transplantation). In the first, liver transplantation is needed primarily because of endstage nonmalignant liver disease, but a coincidental primary hepatic malignancy was also identified either before transplantation or after examination of the excised liver. Such tumors could have been totally removed by subtotal hepatectomy if the liver had not been so seriously diseased. Here, the selection of candidates is essentially the same as that of candidates with nonmalignant disease.

[1] Department of Surgery, University of Pittsburgh Health Center, University of Pittsburgh, Pittsburgh, PA 15261, USA

In the second situation, liver transplantation is needed because of a hepatic malignancy which cannot be removed by conventional techniques of subtotal hepatectomy. In such patients, an extensive search for extrahepatic metastases must be carried out before the patient is accepted as a candidate. Tumor metastases are investigated with chest X-ray, bone survey, CT scan of the chest, abdomen, and brain, bone marrow examination, and other sophisticated modern diagnostic procedures. A history of slow growth, of good response to chemotherapy or radiation therapy, and of known favorable histology may also play an important role in selecting a candidate. A final decision for or against hepatic replacement is often made after a donor liver graft becomes available, at which time definitive exploration is carried out. If a tumor is found outside the liver, long-term survival of the patient is so unlikely that the attempt usually is abandoned and the liver is given to a "backup" candidate.

The differentiation of primary hepatic malignancies (particularly cholangiocarcinoma) from liver metastases can be extremely difficult, even with adequate biopsy material for histological examination. There have been only a handful of examples of liver transplantation for metastatic liver tumors [2, 8, 9]. In general, patients with metastatic liver malignancies are not suitable candidates for liver transplantation, at least at the present time. However, there may be occasional patients who develop metastases only in the liver, years after complete local control of carcinomas or carcinoids of the intestinal tract. It is possible, but not proven, that such rare patients with metastatic liver disease can benefit by orthotopic liver transplantation.

2 Histological considerations

Hepatocellular carcinoma is the most common primary hepatic malignancy. It can develop in the normal liver. Many such tumors can be treated by subtotal hepatectomy. In many others, extrahepatic metastases have already developed by the time the diagnosis is made. Since hepatocellular carcinoma tends to metastasize relatively early in its clinical course, it is uncommon to find the disease in a stage where subtotal hepatectomy would not be curative, but where total hepatectomy would be successful.

In contrast, hepatocellular carcinomas in livers affected with some other disease may be much less advanced but not treatable by partial hepatectomy because of impaired hepatic function. Total hepatectomy with liver replacement may be the ideal treatment in such cases in which the primary diagnosis is macronodular or micronodular cirrhosis (posthepatitic cirrhosis, Laennec's cirrhosis), tyrosinemia, hemochromatosis, biliary atresia, Thorotrast liver disease, and other advanced liver diseases. Orthotopic liver transplantation has been effective in treating such coincidental hepatocellular carcinomas.

Although it develops in the normal liver, fibrolamellar carcinoma carries a better prognosis than other hepatocellular carcinomas. This tumor is a histological subtype of hepatocellular carcinoma and is composed of large polygonal eosinophilic cells dispersed throughout a fibrolamellar stroma. It is characterized by its prevalence in young patients, its indolent growth, and an increased resectability rate and survival in comparison with other types of hepatocellular carcinoma [10–14]. Because metastases occur late in its clinical course, fibrolamellar carcinomas which cannot be resected (even by the most extensive subtotal hepatectomy, such as right or left trisegmentectomy) may be treated effectively by total hepatectomy and replacement.

Cholangiocarcinoma is the second most common primary hepatic malignancy. It usually arises in the normal liver and, like hepatocellular carcinoma, it metastasizes relatively early in its course. Therefore, it is rare to find this tumor in a stage suitable for liver transplantation.

Hepatoblastoma is the most common hepatic malignancy in early childhood. It grows rapidly and spreads outside the liver early in its clinical course. It is rare for hepatoblastoma to be effectively treated by liver transplantation, unless the tumor has been under good chemotherapeutic control.

There are other unusual primary hepatic malignancies, such as hemangiosarcoma, rhabdomyosarcoma, and leiomyosarcoma. These sarcomas, like hepatoblastoma, grow rapidly and metastasize early. It is exceptional that these sarcomas can be effectively treated by liver transplantation.

Although classified as sarcomas, epithelioid hemangioendotheliomas or epithelioid hemangioendothelial sarcomas of the liver possess distinct clinical and pathological features. This type of tumor was originally described as intravascular bronchioloalveolar tumor (IVBAT) of the lung by Dail and Liebow in 1975 [15]. The angiogenic nature of IVBAT was subsequently confirmed by light-microscopic and ultrastructural observations. Factor VIII-related antigen, an endothelial cell marker, was first identified in tumor cells of IVBAT by Weldon-Linne et al. [16]. In 1982, the term "epithelioid hemangioendothelioma" was proposed by Weiss and Enzinger [17]. Involvement of the liver was first thought to be metastatic from IVBAT of the lung or its soft tissue counterpart, but later it was confirmed that this tumor can originate in the liver as well. Ishak et al. [18] reported 32 cases of epithelioid hemangioendothelioma of the liver in 1984. The clinical course of this tumor is between that of hemangioma and conventional angiosarcoma. Nine of the 32 patients in this report survived 5 years or longer regardless of the treatment, but the same number of patients developed metastases during follow-up. This tumor may be effectively treated by total hepatectomy and liver replacement when conventional techniques of subtotal hepatectomy cannot be applied.

A carcinoma arising from the junction of the right and left hepatic ducts is called Klatskin's tumor. Because of the location, signs of obstructive jaundice appear when the tumor is still small, usually less than a few centimeters in diameter, and the diagnosis of malignancy can be made relatively early. This tumor usually grows slowly and metastasizes late in its clinical course. It can often be resected, with or without partial hepatectomy, and the bile duct can be reconstructed. However, in many cases, the tumor is located too high in the liver tissue and complete resection is not possible. In such patients, the bile duct can be intubated surgically or under radiological control to relieve obstructive jaundice, followed by radiation therapy. This palliative measure has been successful both in prolonging life and in improving the quality of life for 1–2 years on average [19]. Although this Klatskin's tumor would appear to be an excellent indication for orthotopic liver transplantation because of its small size, slow growth, and relatively late metastasis, the survival after transplantation has been disappointing and not significantly better than that after palliative procedures, as will be discussed later in this chapter.

3 Denver-Pittsburgh experience with transplantation

During the 23-year period from March 1963 to March 1986, 750 patients received orthotopic liver transplantation at the University Health Sciences Center of Colorado (1963–1980) and

Table 32.1. Histological diagnosis of 63 primary liver malignancies

	Group				Total
	1A	1B	2A	2B	
Hepatocellular carcinoma	2	11	13	16	42
(fibrolamellar type)		(1)	(1)	(7)	(9)
Bile duct cancer (Klatskin's tumor)	0	0	5	5	10
Epithelioid hemangio-endothelioma	0	0	2	3	5
Cholangiocarcinoma	0	0	1	1	2
Hepatoblastoma	1	0	0	0	1
Angiosarcoma	0	0	0	1	1
Adenocarcinoma of unknown primary site	0	0	0	1	1
Epithelioid tumor, histology undetermined	0	0	0	1	1
Total	3	11	21	28	63

the University Health Center of Pittsburgh (1981–1986). The first 170 patients were treated by azathioprine and steroids with or without antilymphocyte globulin, and the following 580 patients were treated by cyclosporine and steroids with or without monoclonal anti-T-lymphocyte antibody. Of the 750 patients, 63 (8.4%) had transplantation in the presence of a primary hepatic malignancy. For analysis, the 63 patients were divided into two groups.

Group 1 consisted of 14 patients who had liver replacement primarily to treat an endstage nonmalignant liver disease, but who were found to have a coincidental primary hepatic malignancy either before transplantation or after examination of the excised whole liver. The tumor could have been totally removed by the conventional technique of partial hepatectomy if the liver had not been so seriously diseased.

Group 2 consisted of 49 patients whose sole or principal reason for liver replacement was a malignancy which could not be removed by partial hepatectomy. The patients in both groups 1 and 2 were further classified according to whether immunosuppression was with azathioprine and corticosteroids (subgroup A) or cyclosporine and corticosteroids (subgroup B).

3.1 Histological diagnosis

The histological diagnoses of 63 primary liver malignancies treated with orthotopic liver transplantation are listed in Table 32.1. There were 42 hepatocellular carcinomas (HCCs), of which nine were of the fibrolamellar variant. The other tumors were ten bile duct carcinomas (Klatskin's tumors), five epithelioid hemangioendotheliomas, two cholangiocarcinomas, and one each of hepatoblastoma, angiosarcoma, adenocarcinoma of unknown primary site, and epithelioid tumor of undetermined histology.

Of the 14 primary liver malignancies in group 1 (coincidental tumors), 13 were HCCs and one was a hepatoblastoma. These coincidental hepatic malignancies were found in tyrosinemia (four cases), biliary atresia (three cases), alpha-1-antitrypsin deficiency disease (two cases), posthepatitic cirrhosis (two cases), Laennec's cirrhosis (one case), Neville's disease (one case), and familial cholestatic syndrome (one case).

Of the 49 primary liver malignancies in group 2 (unresectable tumors), 14 developed in livers that had underlying serious hepatic diseases. Six HCCs were in livers that had postnecrotic cirrhosis. The underlying disease in two cases was tyrosinemia, and in one case each the diagnoses were Thorotrast liver and biliary atresia. Three patients with bile duct carcinoma (Klatskin's tumor) had sclerosing cholangitis. One case of cholangiocarcinoma had developed against a background of postnecrotic cirrhosis. The remaining 35 malignancies had developed in an apparently normal liver.

3.2 Residual tumor

No patient with primary liver malignancy who underwent liver transplantation was known preoperatively to have had extrahepatic involvement. However, five patients of group 2 (unresectable tumor) were found to have metastases at the time of transplantation. One patient with epithelioid hemangioendothelioma had fine metastases to the lung and peritoneum. This patient is still alive and well without any sign of tumor regrowth more than 9 years later. The second patient with hemangiosarcoma had metastases to the lungs and the omentum at the time of emergency transplantation for intra-abdominal bleeding, which was thought to be from ruptured multiple hemangiomas. When this patient died 3 months after operation as a result of pneumonia and liver graft failure, the autopsy also revealed metastases to the bone marrow. The third patient had adenocarcinoma of unknown primary site and was found to have metastases to many abdominal lymph nodes during surgery; some were not removed. This patient developed radiological evidence of bone metastases at 11 months but is still alive with a tumor

15 months after transplantation. The fourth patient with fibrolamellar HCC had tumor invasion of the diaphragm. Microscopic examination of the excised whole liver also revealed tumor-positive hilar lymph nodes. This patient died 1 month after transplantation from liver failure and infectious complications. The autopsy revealed no residual fibrolamellar HCC, but there was an incidental small adenocarcinoma of the lung. The fifth patient had bile duct carcinoma and primary sclerosing cholangitis. Several regional lymph nodes were involved at the time of surgery. This patient is alive without evidence of tumor regrowth 3 months after transplantation.

Eleven other patients in group 2 (unresectable tumor) died within 2 months from various complications of liver transplantation. Preoperatively and at the time of operation, all 11 were thought to be free of extrahepatic tumor. At autopsy, only one had gross or microscopic evidence of residual neoplasm. This patient, who survived only 5 days after liver transplantation, had metastatic cholangiocarcinoma in the lungs, vertebrae, kidneys, and some abdominal lymph nodes. The remaining ten patients were free of tumor insofar as this could be determined from complete postmortem examination, indicating that screening for candidacy had been grossly accurate in the great majority of cases.

3.3 Tumor recurrence

3.3.1 Incidental malignancies

In group 1, there have been no tumor recurrences among the 14 patients whose excised liver contained incidental primary liver malignancies. Thirteen patients had HCC and one had hepatoblastoma. Two patients died after liver transplantation—one on the 1st postoperative day from hyperkalemia and the other almost 2 years after the operation from lung cancer. The remaining 12 patients are alive and free of tumor recurrence from 3 months to more than 16 years after liver transplantation (median 24 months).

3.3.2 Unresectable malignancies

In group 2, 36 of 49 patients whose main reason for liver transplantation was primary liver malignancy survived for at least 3 months after transplantation and thus became suitable for meaningful observations with respect to recurrence. The 36 patients included four of the five who were found at the time of transplantation to have extrahepatic involvement as described in the preceding section. The other 32 were all considered

Table 32.2. Incidence of tumor recurrence and 1-year tumor-free survival among the patients in group 2 who survived over 3 months after liver transplant; all gross tumors were removed by total hepatectomy

	Tumor recurrence		1-year tumor-free	
	No.	Percent	No.	Percent
Hepatocellular carcinoma	12/20	60	7/15	47
Nonfibrolamellar	(8/13)	62	(1/9)	11
Fibrolamellar	(4/7)	57	(6/6)	100
Bile duct cancer	4/7	57	2/4	50
Epithelioid hemangioendothelial sarcoma	2/4	50	1/3	33
Cholangiocarcinoma	1/1	100	1/1	100
Total	20/32	63	11/23	48

to have had a gross tumor removed by total hepatectomy.

In 20 (63%) of the 32 patients who were made potentially tumor-free by liver transplantation, the original tumor recurred after 1–42 months (median 9 months). HCC that was not fibrolamellar in type recurred in 8 (62%) of 13 patients, all within 1 year (median 4 months; Table 32.2). Recurrence of fibrolamellar HCC was also seen in five (71%) of seven patients (Table 32.2), but all after 1 year (median 16 months). Four of the seven bile duct carcinomas recurred, two before and two after 1 year; the exceptional patient who did not have a recurrence died of other causes 3 months after operation. Two of the four epithelioid hemangioendotheliomas recurred within 1 year. One patient with cholangiocarcinoma developed a tumor recurrence in the 15th postoperative month. One-year tumor-free rates are also shown in Table 32.2.

3.4 Location of recurrences

The first location of tumor recurrence and the organs ultimately involved by tumors were examined in the 20 patients of group 2 who rendered potentially tumor-free at the time of transplantation but who later developed metastases. The grafted liver and the lung were the two organs most commonly affected by tumor recurrences (Table 32.3).

The liver was the first site of recurrence in eight patients, the lung in six patients, both the liver and the lung simultaneously in two patients, the bone in two patients, and the skin and the pelvic peritoneum in one patient each.

The liver was ultimately involved by recurrent tumors in 12 patients. Other locations within the abdomen, such as the abdominal lymph nodes and the peritoneum, were affected in 13 patients.

Table 32.3. Location of recurrence of original primary liver malignancy in 20 patients

	First location of recurrence	Organ ultimately involved
Liver	10 (2)[b]	12
Abdomen other than liver[a]	1	13
Lung	8 (2)	11
Bone	2	3
Brain	0	3
Skin	1	1

[a] Abdominal lymph nodes, peritoneum
[b] Two patients had recurrences both in the liver and the lung discovered simultaneously

The lung became ultimately involved in 11 patients, and the brain and bone in three patients each.

3.5 Patient survival

The overall survivals after liver transplantation have greatly improved since the introduction of cyclosporine-steroid therapy in March 1980 [6]. Since that time, the survival rate at 1 year after operation and each year thereafter for at least 5 years has more than doubled compared with that previously obtained with azathioprine and steroid therapy (Fig. 32.1). The actuarial 5-year survival in all patients treated since 1980 is slightly better than 60%.

3.5.1 Survival of patients with group 1 tumors
Of the 14 patients who had incidental hepatic malignancies, 12 are still alive and free of tumor from 3 months to 16 years after operation. Two patients died after transplantation. One patient with biliary atresia and an incidental HCC

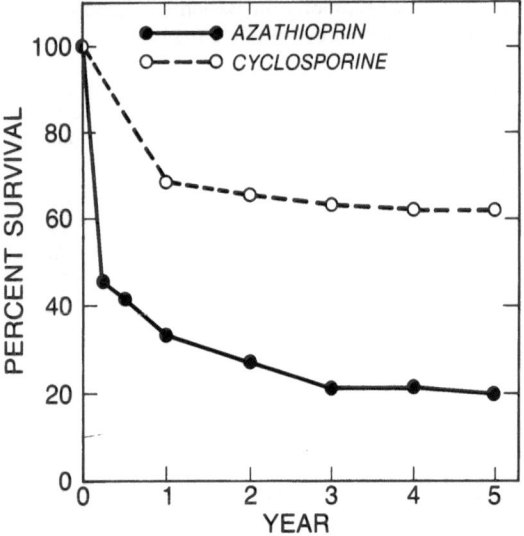

Fig. 32.1. The survivals after liver transplantation have more than doubled since the introduction of cyclosporine in 1980

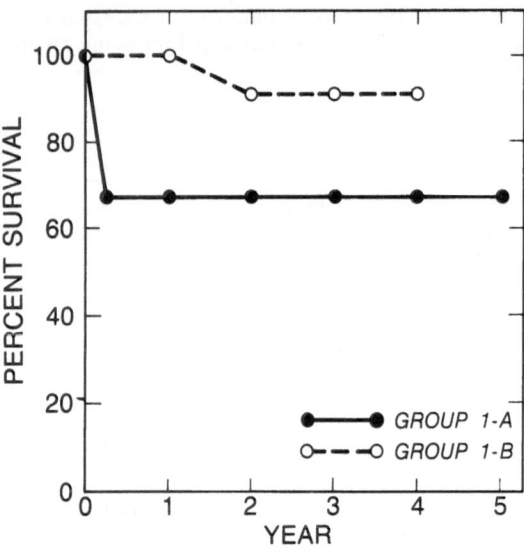

Fig. 32.2. The survivals of patients with incidental primary malignancy. Group 1A—incidental tumor treated by azathioprine and steroids; group 1B—incidental tumor treated by cyclosporine and steroids

died on the 1st postoperative day from hyperkalemia. Another patient with a micronodular (Laennec's) cirrhosis and incidental HCC died 23 months after transplantation from disseminated oat cell cancer of the lung, which was discovered 16 months after transplantation. Actuarial survival curves of patients with incidental primary liver malignancy are shown in Fig. 32.2.

3.5.2 Survival of patients with group 2 tumors (unresectable tumors)

Of the 20 patients of subgroup A who were treated with azathioprine and steroids, 13 (65%) had died by the end of the first 6 months. At the end of the year, only six (30%) remained alive, of whom all but one have subsequently died (Fig. 32.3). The single survivor, now 9½ years after transplantation, had epithelioid hemangioendothelioma with peritoneal and pulmonary metastases at the time of transplantation.

The patients of subgroup B who were treated with cyclosporine and steroids had greatly improved early postoperative results with a 6-month actuarial survival of 80%. This reflected the better overall prognosis for early recovery using cyclosporine-steroid therapy. However, after the half-year mark, survival continued to decline, primarily because of the recurrent malignancies, as will be described in the following sections. The actuarial 1- and 3-year survivals of patients with unresectable tumors after liver transplantation with cyclosporine-steroid ther-

apy (group 2B) are projected at 58% and 24%, respectively (Fig. 32.3). As of April 1986, only 12 (41%) of the original 29 recipients in group 2B are still alive after 2 months to 4½ years. Three of the surviving patients at 2, 3, and 13 months, respectively, had tumor-positive regional lymph nodes at the time of transplantation, and five others are living with known recurrences.

3.6 Main causes of deaths in group 2

Of the 49 patients whose principal reason for liver transplantation was the presence of unresectable primary liver malignancy (group 2), 36 had died before April 10, 1986. Of the 36 deaths, 26 were within 1 year after transplantation. Seven of the 26 deaths were due to nonneoplastic complications such as liver graft failure of infections or both: The majority of these nonneoplastic deaths occurred among the patients transplanted before 1970 [2–7]. Of the ten deaths that occurred a year or more after transplantation, nine were directly caused by tumor recurrence. Thus, the shape of the survival curves both before and after the introduction of cyclosporine was dominated from the 6th month onward by the fatal effects of tumor recurrence (Fig. 32.3).

3.7 Histology, recurrence, and survival in group 2

Of the eight patients with fibrolamellar HCC, two died of nonneoplastic transplant complica-

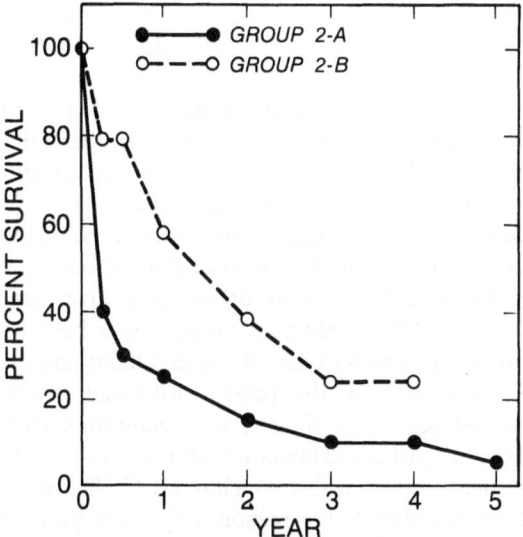

Fig. 32.3. The survivals of patients with unresectable primary liver malignancy. Group 2A—unresectable tumor treated by azathioprine and steroids; group 2B—unresectable tumor treated by cyclosporine and steroids

tions in the 2nd and 7th months without any evidence of residual or recurrent tumors. The remaining six patients lived for at least 1 year. These six 1-year survivors were thought to be free of tumor when they passed the 12-month mark. However, metastases subsequently developed in four of the six patients, two of whom died 21 and 36 months after operation. The other two are living with known metastases after more than 2 and 4 years. A fifth patient died from liver graft failure and infectious complications just less than 3 years after operation. The sixth patient is alive, free of tumor recurrence more than 4 years after transplantation.

In contrast, patients with nonfibrolamellar HCC had earlier and more lethal metastases. Of 21 such patients, eight died within 3 months, too soon to allow meaningful evaluation for recurrence. Of the 11 patients with a longer follow-up, eight developed a recurrent tumor within a year and subsequently died from tumor recurrence within 18 months after transplantation; two more patients died from nonneoplastic causes 3 and 6 months after transplantation. As of April 1986, only three patients are alive and free of tumor recurrence 3, 11, and 27 months after transplantation; the follow-ups of two of these three are too short to be meaningful. Thus, the conventional HCCs carried a far poorer prognosis than the fibrolamellar variant.

Of the ten patients with bile duct cancer

(Klatskin's tumor), four died from nonneoplastic causes within 3 months after transplantation. Two patients died directly from recurrent tumors within a year, and two others developed tumor recurrences after a year and died from recurrent malignancy 25 and 54 months after liver transplantation. Two others who are alive and free of tumor after 3 and 6 months have too short a follow-up to be considered.

Of the five patients with epithelioid hemangioendothelioma, two developed recurrent tumors 2 and 11 months after transplantation and died directly from a recurrent tumor 3 and 16 months after transplantation, respectively. Three others are alive and free of tumor more than 6 months, 2 years, and 9 years after transplantation.

Of the five patients with other primary liver malignancies, two lived more than a year. One with cholangiocarcinoma developed tumor recurrence 15 months after transplantation and died directly from a recurrent tumor 5 months afterward. Another with adenocarcinoma of unknown primary site developed a recurrence 11 months after transplantation, but he is alive more than 5 months later.

4 Past reflections and future prospects

Remarkable progress has been made in the field of organ transplantation since the introduction of cyclosporine in the late 1970s. More than 70% of liver recipients now survive at least a year after operation, and approximately 60% overall are expected to live for 5 years after liver transplantation. However, the survival of patients who received liver transplantation because of unresectable primary hepatic malignancies has been poor and less than a quarter of these patients will survive 3 years after liver transplantation even with cyclosporine therapy. Two-thirds of the patients developed tumor recurrence even though they were thought to have been rendered tumorfree after total hepatectomy. Recurrent tumors were the most frequent cause of death among these patients, and nearly all of the deaths after a year were directly caused by or attributed to recurrent neoplasms.

The high recurrence rate after liver transplantation for unresectable tumors reflects in part the advanced development of the neoplasms by the time a decision was made to attempt therapy with transplantation. However, the immunosuppression necessary to prevent graft rejection might actually have expedited the growth of residual nests of malignant cells left after the total hepatectomy, as was suggested a number of years ago [2] and has since been supported by many recent investigations of host factors promoting tumor metastases [20–22].

The tendency of the metastases from hepatic malignancies to recur in the liver grafts is of particular interest in reflecting on the mechanisms of tumor metastasis. One possible explanation is that the malignant cells of primary hepatic tumors may find the best microenvironment to be in the liver itself. Another explanation could be that the grafted liver, which is itself under constant attack from the host immune system, may provide the location of the weakest antitumor defense where circulating neoplastic cells can nest and grow. Further investigations are needed to explain this peculiar and dangerous phenomenon.

Of all the tumors with which experience has been accumulated so far, fibrolamellar HCC has emerged as the best for treatment with transplantation. This tumor is known to behave less aggressively than most other malignant hepatic neoplasms [10–14]. Although it recurred in more than half the patients after transplantation, the metastases tended to appear late and to grow relatively slowly. Two of our patients with recurrence have been in good condition for more than 1 and 3 years after multiple pulmonary metastases were first proved.

Epithelioid hemangioendothelioma is a peculiar malignant neoplasm which can originate in the lung, soft tissue, and liver [15–18]. Our experience in this tumor has been mixed with aggressive recurrences and potential cures. Two of the five patients died from aggressive recurrent tumors. The remaining three, including one with distant metastases at the time of transplantation, are alive and well without any clinical evidence of tumor more than 6 months, 2 years, and 9 years after transplantation.

With all other kinds of tumor, metastases tended to appear early and led to death promptly. The prognosis with nonfibrolamellar HCC has been very poor. None of our patients with proximal duct cell carcinomas (Klatskin's tumors) have lived 5 years and, to our knowledge, this has not been accomplished in any other center [8, 23].

It is sometimes tempting during the acquisition of this experience to conclude that liver transplantation for malignant hepatic malignancy is conceptually unsound, except for coinci-dental malignancies and probably for fibrolamellar HCC, and to abandon such efforts. However, the most encouraging aspect of this experience was the almost uniform survival of patients with coincidental hepatic malignancy. The fact that none of these patients developed a recurrence during the follow-up proved that the mere presence of a hepatic malignancy is not an absolute contraindication for liver transplantation.

Even in the patients of group 2, arrest and control of the malignant process have been accomplished under some of the least likely circumstances, as with the patient who had distant metastases at the time of transplantation from hepatic epithelioid hemangioendothelioma and a patient with nonfibrolamellar HCC. There has been no identifiable reason why some patients were spared recurrence and why others were not.

The poor results so far have made it clear that liver transplantation for unresectable cancer will have to be tied to some other kind of therapeutic effort in future trials. The usual approach of giving adjuvant chemotherapy or radiation therapy will not be sufficient to prevent tumor recurrence for a long time as was experienced in two of our four recent patients who developed aggressive recurrences of nonfibrolamellar HCC within a few months in spite of prophylactic treatment with adriamycin and other chemotherapeutic agents. Huber et al. [9] have described a novel approach in which patients with metastatic liver malignancies had liver replacement as well as total body irradiation and ultradose chemotherapy, followed by autotransplantation of stored bone marrow. One of their patients whose original disease was a carcinoma of the breast was alive, free of tumor, more than 3 years after liver transplantation (personal communication).

Further experiences and more effective adjuvant therapies are required for liver transplantation to establish a firm role in the treatment of hepatic malignancies.

References

1. Iwatsuki S, Shaw BW Jr, Starzl TE (1982) Experience with 150 liver resections. Ann Surg 197: 247–253
2. Starzl TE (with the assistance of Putnam CW) (1969) Experience in hepatic transplantation. WB Saunders Company, Philadelphia
3. Starzl TE, Porter KA, Putnam CW, et al. (1976) Orthotopic liver transplantation in 93 patients. Surg Gynecol Obstet 142: 487–505

4. Starzl TE, Koep LJ, Halgrison CG, et al. (1979) Fifteen years of clinical liver transplantation. Gastroenterology 77: 375–388

5. Iwatsuki S, Klintmalm GBG, Starzl TE (1982) Total hepatectomy and liver replacement (orthotopic liver transplantation) for primary hepatic malignancy. World J Surg 6: 81–85

6. Starzl TE, Iwatsuki S, Van Thiel DH, Gartner JC, Zitelli BJ, Malatack JJ, Schade RR, Shaw BW Jr, Hakala TR, Rosenthal JT, Porter KA (1982) Evolution of liver transplantation. Hepatology 2: 614–636

7. Iwatsuki S, Gordon RD, Shaw BW Jr, Starzl TE (1985) Role of liver transplantation in cancer therapy. Ann Surg 202: 401–407

8. Calne RY (ed) (1983) Liver transplantation: The Cambridge/King's College Hospital Experience. Grune and Stratton, London/New York

9. Huber C, Niederwieser D, Schonitzer D, et al. (1984) Liver transplantation followed by high-dose cyclosphosphamide, total-body irradiation, and autologous bone marrow transplantation for treatment of metastatic breast cancer. Transplant 37: 311–312

10. Edmondson HA (1956) Differential diagnosis of tumors and tumor-like lesions of the liver in infancy and childhood. Am J Dis Child 91: 168–186

11. Peters RL (1975) Pathology of hepatocellular carcinoma. In: Okuda K, Peters R (eds) Hepatocellular carcinoma. Wiley, New York, pp 107–168

12. Craig JR, Peters RL, Edmondson HA, Omata M (1980) Fibrolamellar carcinoma of the liver; a tumor of adolescents and young adults with distinctive clinicopathologic features. Cancer 46: 372–379

13. Berman MM, Libbey NP, Foster JH (1980) Hepatocellular carcinoma: Polygonal cell type with fibrous stroma—an atypical variant with a favorable prognosis. Cancer 46: 1448–1455

14. Starzl TE, Iwatsuki S, Shaw BW Jr, Nalesnik MA, Farhi DC, Van Thiel DH (1986) Treatment of fibrolamellar hepatoma with partial hepatectomy or with total hepatectomy and liver transplantation. Surg Gynecol Obstet 162: 145–148

15. Dail DH, Liebow AA (1975) Intravascular bronchioloalveolar tumor. Am J Pathol 78: 61a

16. Weldon-Linne CM, Victor TA, Christ ML, et al. (1981) Angiogenic nature of the "intravascular bronchioloalveolar tumor" of the lung: an electron microscopic study. Arch Pathol Lab Med 105: 174

17. Weiss SW, Enzinger FM (1982) Epithelioid hemangioendothelioma: a vascular tumor even often mistaken for a carcinoma. Cancer 50: 970

18. Ishak KG, Sesterheen IA, Goodman JD, Rabin L, Stromeyer FW (1984) Epithelioid hemangioendothelioma of the liver: a clinicopathologic and follow-up study of 32 cases. Human Pathol 15: 839–852

19. Alexander F, Rossi RL, O'Bryan M, Khettry U, Braasch JW, Watkins E Jr (1984) Biliary carcinoma: a review of 190 cases. Am J Surg 147: 503–509

20. Alexander P, Eccles SA (1983) Host mediated mechanisms in the elimination of circulating cancer cells. Symp Foundam Cancer Res 36: 293–308

21. Hanna N (1983) Role of natural killer cells in host defense against cancer metastasis. Symp Foundam Cancer Res 36: 309–320

22. Milas L, Peters TJ (1983) Conditioning of tissues for metastasis formation by radiation and cytotoxic drugs. Symp Foundam Cancer Res 36: 321–336

23. Pichlmayr R, Brolsch CH, Wonigiet K, et al. (1984) Experiences with liver transplantation in Hannover. Hepatology 4: 56S–60S

Chapter 33
Prognosis of Hepatocellular Carcinoma

KUNIO OKUDA and KUNIHIKO OHNISHI[1]

Of the various types of solid cancer, hepatocellular carcinoma (HCC) is perhaps the most difficult to treat because of the frequently associated cirrhosis [1–5]. Although there are large differences in its global incidence and in the frequency of coexisting cirrhosis that varies with the ethnic group [6–9], the basic clinical features and the generally poor prognosis are the same regardless of race and place. The survival times of patients with HCC as a whole have been estimated to be several months at most [10–13] with rare exceptions of long survival [14–16] and spontaneous regression [17, 18].

With the progress in diagnostic procedures in recent years, small HCCs have come to be detected and considered for surgery [19–26]. Surgical techniques have improved along with the development of new chemotherapeutic agents and improvement in the way of delivering drugs against the cancer. Therefore, the prognosis of these patients may have changed from what was experienced in the past [27, 28].

In this chapter, we will discuss the new staging scheme and natural history and survival of patients in different stages of HCC in relation to various therapeutic modalities currently used.

1 Proposed staging scheme for evaluation of survival

There are many factors that will influence the prognosis. The best documented staging scheme for HCC is perhaps the Kampala scheme [29] and its modification made by Primack et al. [11]. They analyzed various factors proposed by the Kampala Symposium and concluded that ascites, weight loss, portal hypertension, and

serum bilirubin (with a dividing level at 2 mg/dl) be used for staging. They divided 72 untreated patients in Uganda into three stages and demonstrated differences in survival among these stages. The median survival of their entire series was only 1 month. In contrast, patients with HCC in Japan live much longer due in part to early diagnosis and relatively slow growth, as shown in Fig. 33.1. Thus, the Kampala scheme is not applicable to patients in the Far East.

Berman wrote in his monograph in 1951: "In my own series of 75 cases, duration of the disease was never more than 4 months from the first appearance of symptoms, and the stay in hospital varied from 1 to 81 days, the average being 20 days" [27]. It seems that young Black gold miners in South Africa who come down with HCC rarely have preceding advanced liver cirrhosis as we see in Japan. In fact, a number of reports suggest a less frequent incidence of cirrhosis and a more malignant course of the disease among the Bantu race [12, 30–32]. Outside South Africa, the majority of patients with HCC have a progressive underlying cirrhosis and already have symptoms attributable to cirrhosis at the time of cancer diagnosis [14, 32, 33]. For this reason, the use of the signs of portal hypertension and weight loss suggested by Primack et al. [11] seems inappropriate for staging of the Japanese HCC cases. On the other hand, a simple staging scheme based on tumor size only [34] could not be applied to HCC because of varying degrees of cirrhosis, which more often determines the prognosis. Many of the patients with HCC in Japan die from hepatic failure rather than from the cancer itself, as observed by Idhe et al. [35] in the USA; a different staging scheme was, therefore, required.

It was believed that staging should be as simple and practical as possible and that the consideration of many functional parameters and division of tumor sizes into many groups would

---

[1] The First Department of Medicine, Chiba University School of Medicine, Inohana, Chiba, 280 Japan

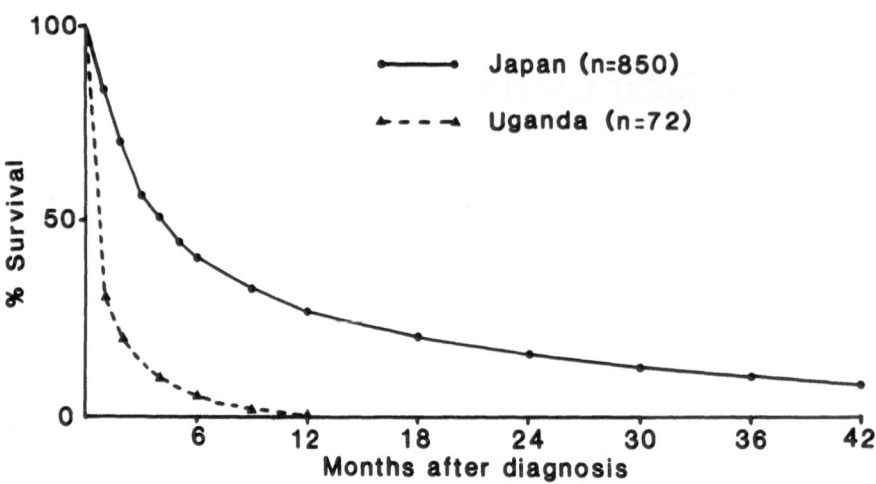

Fig. 33.1. Life-table analysis of survival of patients with HCC. Comparison between patients in Uganda [11] and Japan [36]

result in a staging scheme that was too complicated. Therefore, in addition to tumor size, we considered only ascites, jaundice, and serum albumin, which indirectly assess the functioning hepatic mass and the degree of cirrhosis. The two-dimensional size of the tumor was estimated from the radionuclide colloid scintiscan, X-ray computed tomography (CT) scan, and celiac angiogram. A preliminary study in which all values of albumin and bilirubin were plotted against survival suggested that 50% tumor size, 3 g/dl albumin, and 3 mg/dl bilirubin would provide a practical separation for long and short survivals. Thus, the following new staging scheme (Table 33.1) was adopted: Stage 1—not advanced, tumor size is smaller than 50%, there is no ascites, albumin is greater than 3 g/dl, and bilirubin 3 mg/dl; stage II—moderately advanced, one or two of the signs of advanced disease are present; and stage III—very advanced, three or four (all) of the advanced signs are present.

2 Natural history of HCC and prognosis in relation to treatment

A total of 850 unequivocal cases of HCC seen from 1975 to 1983 were analyzed [36]. Surgery, ranging from partial resection or enucleation to extended lobectomy, was carried out in 157 patients, systemic chemotherapy was given in 122, intra-arterial chemotherapy using a bolus dose of mitomycin C with or without systemic 5-fluorouracil (5-FU) in 222, transcatheter arterial embolization using Gelfoam [37–39] and/or mitomycin C microcapsules [40, 41] in 112,

radiation in three, mitomycin C needles in five; no specific cancer treatment was given to 229 patients (Table 33.2). The median survival of 229 patients who received no specific treatment was 1.6 months: 0.7 month for stage III patients, 2.0 months for stage II, and 8.3 months for stage I (Fig. 33.2).

Survival in stage I cases in Uganda was 3 months; in our series, it was 8.3 months, which may be either due to early diagnosis or to a slower growth of tumor up to stage II in Japan, which in turn may be related to differences in frequency of the various gross patterns of HCC. Hepatic resection was carried out in 157 patients (18.5%) in our series. The prognosis of surgically treated patients in stages I and II was considerably better than in the nonsurgical cases (Figs. 33.3, 33.4). The difference is explained in part by the fact that only highly selected patients had surgery. Nonetheless, these results are encouraging for liver surgeons and suggest that many of the long survivors had unicentrically evolved HCC. Furthermore, the absence of intrahepatic metastases or nonmultifocal tumorigenesis was correctly diagnosed preoperatively. That hepatic resection, if successful, prolongs survival has already been amply documented [42–46]. In practice, however, resection is not always possible even though the detected cancer is small because of the coexistent cirrhosis. Obviously, early deaths that occurred in stage I patients with resection in our study were due to underestimation of cirrhosis.

Various modalities of medical treatment and a number of chemotherapeutic agents have been recommended and used. However, i.v. or oral systemic chemotherapy has been rather dis-

Table 33.1. The staging scheme

Stage	Tumor size		Ascites		Albumin		Bilirubin	
	>50% (+)	<50% (−)	(+)	(−)	<3 g/dl (+)	>3 g/dl (−)	>3 mg/dl (+)	<3 mg/dl (−)
I		(−)		(−)		(−)		(−)
II 1 or 2 are (+)								
III 3 or 4 are (+)								

+ Sign of advanced disease

Table 33.2. The stages of disease and treatment given in 850 patients with HCC

Treatment	No. of patients	Stage of disease		
		I	II	III
Surgery	157	115	42	0
Medical	693	157	424	112
Intra-arterial chemotherapy	222	55	141	26
Systemic chemotherapy	122	23	82	17
Transcatheter arterial embolization[a]	112	41	64	7
Others[b]	8	5	3	0
No treatment	229	33	134	62
Total	850 (100%)	272 (32%)	466 (55%)	112 (13%)

[a] Includes mitomycin C microcapsule chemoembolization
[b] Includes radiation and insertion of mitomycin C needles

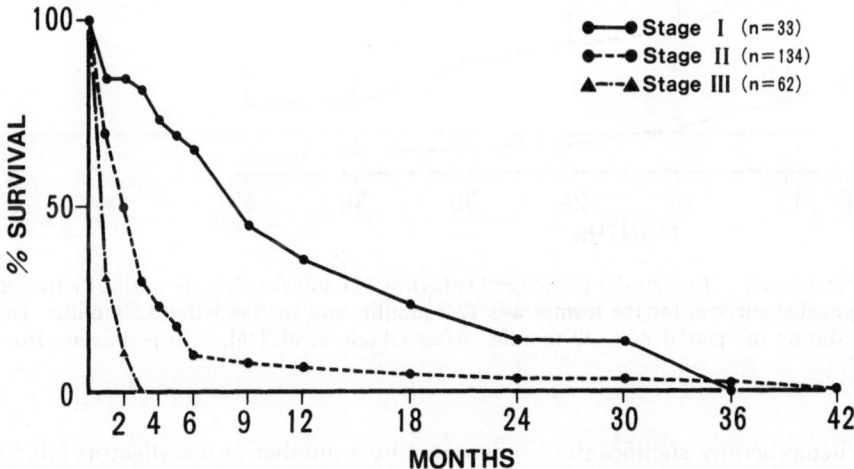

Fig. 33.2. Survival curves for 229 patients who received no specific treatment. The median survival was 0.7 months for 62 stage III patients, 2.0 months for 134 stage II patients, and 8.3 months for 33 stage III patients. Survival is clearly dependent on the stage of disease. After Okuda et al. [36], with permission from Lippincott Co.

appointing in HCC patients [47, 49] except for Adriamycin (doxorubicin), which gives a relatively high response rate [50–52]. In Japan, mitomycin C has been preferred by many to other agents, and its use by intrahepatic arterial bolus injection has been advocated [53, 54].

Furthermore, it can be performed at the time of celiac angiography, an important diagnostic procedure for HCC. In fact, our study clearly supported this preference up to several years ago, with a total of 222 patients treated with intra-arterial bolus injection of mitomycin C. It was

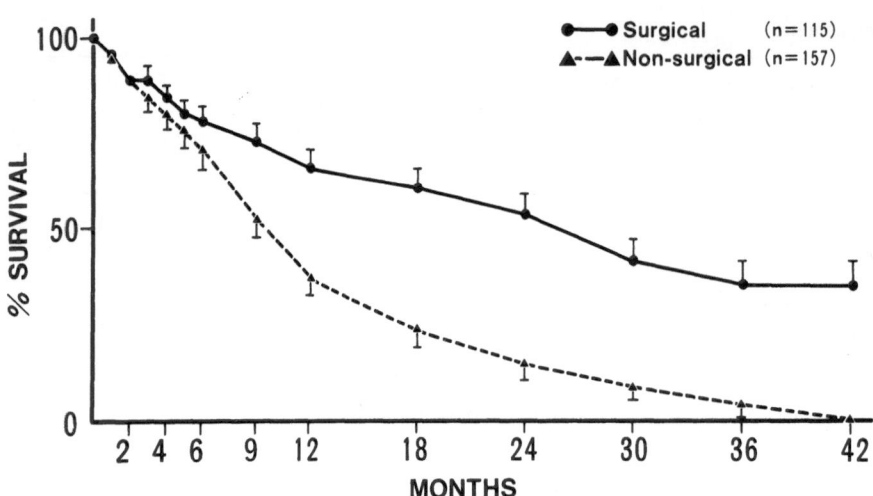

Fig. 33.3. Survival of stage I surgical cases ($n = 115$) in comparison with that of stage I nonsurgical (including the untreated) cases ($n = 157$). The median survival for the former was 25.6 months and for the latter 9.4 months. The difference is survival is significant after 9 months. After Okuda et al. [36], with permission from Lippincott Co.

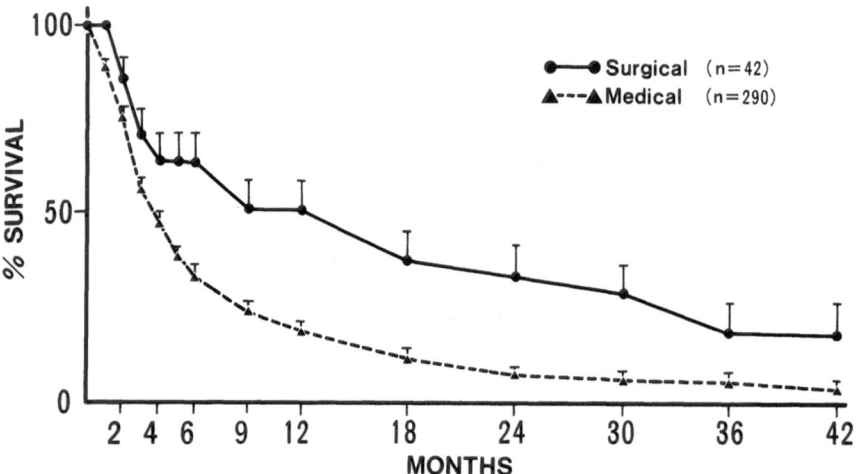

Fig. 33.4. Survival curves for stage II surgically treated patients ($n = 42$) and for stage II medically treated patients ($n = 290$). The medial survival for the former was 12.2 months and for the latter 3.5 months. The difference is significant during the period of 6–30 months. After Okuda et al. [36], with permission from Lippincott Co.

found that arterial chemotherapy significantly improved survival in stage II and stage III patients (Figs. 33.5, 33.6). Systemic chemotherapy also showed some effect in stage III patients, but it was not significant in stage II. In stage I patients, these chemotherapeutic modalities did not demonstrate a definitive benefit compared with untreated stage I patients (Fig. 33.7). Perhaps the deleterious effects of chemotherapeutic agents on liver cells counteracted the anticancer effects.

Intra-arterial infusion chemotherapy has been advocated by a number of investigators [10, 55, 56], but our past experience with this procedure was not very favorable and it was not used during the current study. Transcatheter arterial embolization [37–39] and chemoembolization [40, 41] have been increasingly used during the last several years in Japan. Cancer cells in an expanding type of HCC [3, 32], particularly in an encapsulated HCC [57], are almost totally necrotized by this procedure. It significantly prolongs survival in stage II patients, and when compared with the results obtained by surgery in

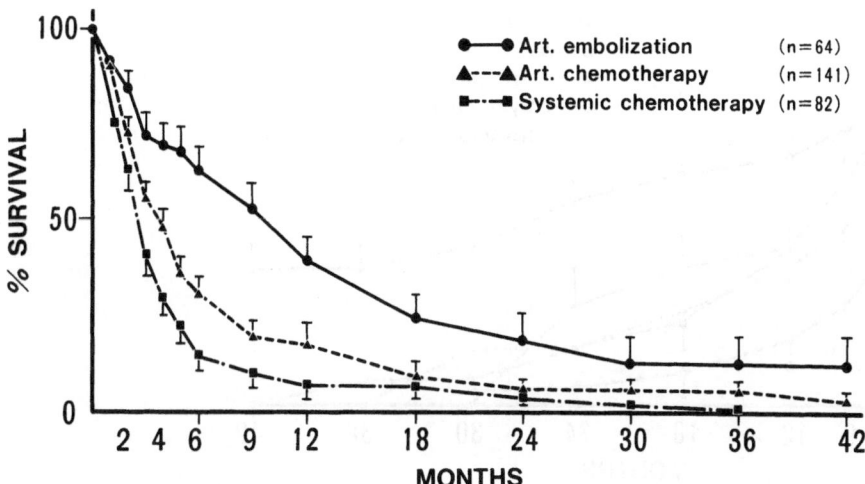

Fig. 33.5. Comparison of survival curves for arterial embolization ($n = 64$), arterial chemotherapy ($n = 141$), and systemic chemotherapy ($n = 82$) in stage II patients. The median survival for embolization was 9.5 months, for arterial chemotherapy 3.7 months, and for systemic chemotherapy 2.5 months. Differences are significant between embolization and arterial chemotherapy (3–18 months) but not between the two chemotherapeutic modalities. After Okuda et al. [36], with permission from Lippincott Co.

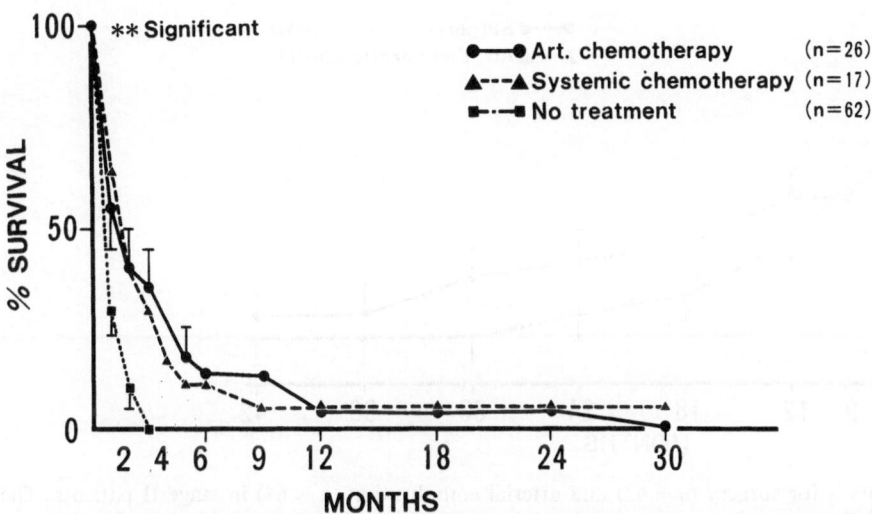

Fig. 33.6. Survival curves for arterial chemotherapy ($n = 26$) and systemic chemotherapy ($n = 17$) in comparison with no treatment ($n = 62$) in stage III patients. The chemotherapeutic groups were significantly better than the no treatment group. After Okuda et al. [36], with permission from Lippincott Co.

the same stage patients, no significant differences are found (Fig. 33.8). In other words, arterial embolization is almost as good as resection in stage II patients and should be considered seriously in inoperable stage II patients at the present time. However, it does not improve survival in stage I patients. The reason is perhaps the same as that for the lack of effects with chemotherapy in stage I patients, namely that embolization damages the noncancerous hepatic parenchyma and cancels the anticancer effects.

In the study of Cochrane et al. [33], quadruple chemotherapy improved survival in stage A patients. Their results are not comparable with ours since we only used one or two drugs.

Liver transplantation [58, 59], if successful, may be the ideal treatment for cirrhosis-based HCC, but it is costly and its contribution is very limited on a global scale. Our efforts are directed to early detection and early resection, but progress is hampered by the coexisting cirrhosis.

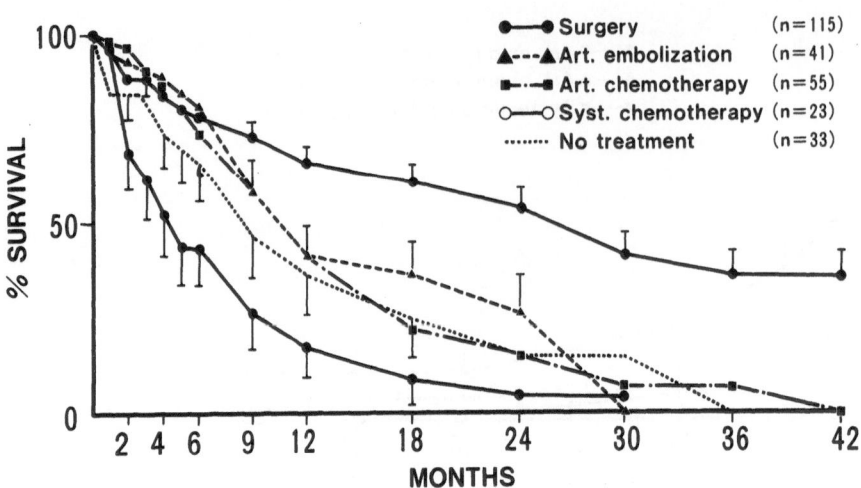

Fig. 33.7. Survival curves for different therapeutic modalities in stage I patients. The median survival was 25.6 months for the surgical group ($n = 115$), 10.4 months for embolization ($n = 41$), 10.3 months for arterial chemotherapy ($n = 55$), 4.3 months for systemic chemotherapy ($n = 23$), and 8.3 months for no treatment ($n = 33$). Both embolization and arterial chemotherapy were better than systemic chemotherapy during the period of 2–12 months. After Okuda et al. [36], with permission from Lippincott Co.

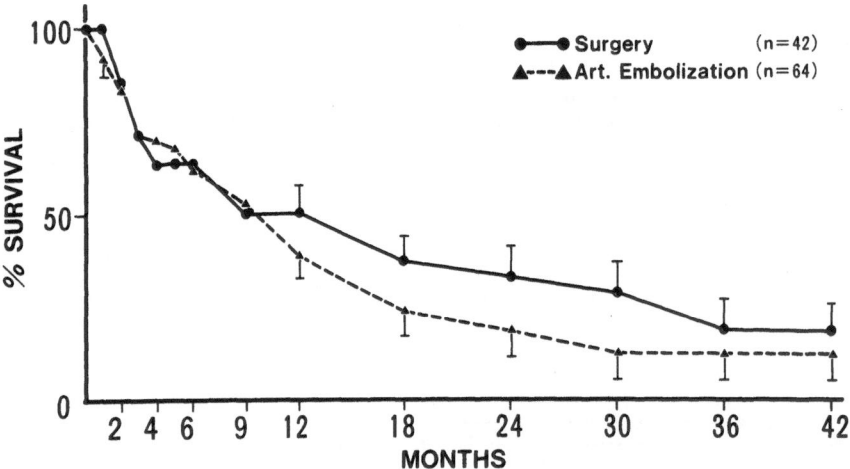

Fig. 33.8. Survival curves for surgery ($n = 42$) and arterial embolization ($n = 64$) in stage II patients. The difference is not significant

2.1 Causes of death

In our study with 850 cases of HCC, the cause of death could be determined in 613 of 659 fatal cases (Table 33.3). It is noteworthy that cancer death was rather uncommon and that hepatic failure and gastrointestinal bleeding were the two leading causes of death. Of the surgically treated patients, 45.0% died from hepatic failure, whereas 38.5% of nonsurgically treated patients died from hepatic failure. Gastrointestinal bleeding was the direct cause of death in 23.3% of the nonsurgical cases and in 13.8% of those surgically treated, but the difference was not significant.

3 Natural history of minute HCC and prognosis in relation to surgical treatment

In our analysis of 166 patients with HCC smaller than 25% of the two-dimensional area of the liver, the median survival of 88 patients treated surgically was 29 months and that of 78 treated nonsurgically was 13 months ($P < 0.05$; Fig. 33.9). The median survival of 27 patients with an HCC occupying 25%–50% of the liver area after surgery was about 8 months. Thus, the results of hepatic resection are definitely better if the tumor is small and if the surgery does not lead to postoperative hepatic failure.

Table 33.3. The causes of death in 659 patients with HCC

Treatment	Cause of death (%)					
	Hepatic failure	GI bleeding	Intra-abdominal bleeding	Cancer death	Others	Unclear
Surgery (n = 80)	45.0	13.8	8.8	8.8	7.5	16.3
No surgery (n = 579)	38.5	23.3	13.8	10.9	7.9	5.7

GI gastrointestinal

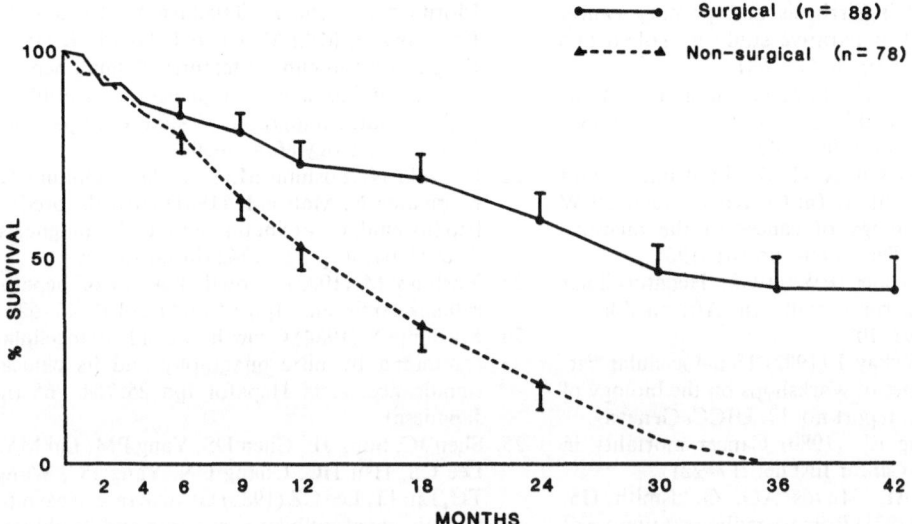

Fig. 33.9. Survival curves for surgically and nonsurgically treated stage I patients with a cancer smaller than 25% of the liver size. The median survival for the former was 29.0 months and for the latter 13.0 months. After Okuda et al. [36], with permission from Lippincott Co.

In the last several years, HCCs smaller than 5 cm have been detected more frequently [20–25]. Some of these patients were followed without treatment in Japan [22–24, 26] and Taiwan [25]. The reasons for lack of treatment are usually the patient's refusal of anticancer treatment, very advanced cirrhosis, delay in definitive diagnosis, and severe complicating diseases in other organs. These unfavorable situations enabled us and others to determine the doubling time of minute HCC, natural course, and causes of death of patients with minute HCC.

In our observations of 22 patients with cirrhosis and minute HCC <3 cm in diameter, the growth speed (calculated from the doubling time from tumor volume) varied considerably from case to case, with an average of 6.5 ± 5.7 months; it was able to change and become faster during the course of growth. Similar observations have been made by Okazaki et al. [22] in seven cases

of HCC, Yoshino [23] in 19 HCCs (diameter 30 ± 15 mm) discovered in 13 patients, Mashima [24] in 27 HCCs including 20 minute HCCs <3 cm in diameter in 27 patients, and Sheu et al. [25] in 31 asymptomatic HCCs (diameter <5 cm) in 28 patients. The mean doubling time of HCC was 119 ± 96 days according to Yoshino [23], 75 days Mashima [24], and 117 days Sheu et al. [25].

Conclusion

Despite the progress in early diagnosis and treatment of HCC, a complete cure is very rare, and room for further improvement in survival is limited. Prevention of hepatocarcinogenesis through curtailment of vertical transmission of hepatitis B virus, the major etiological factor in HCC [8], is the most practical global strategy in the overall management of HCC.

References

1. Edmondson HA, Steiner PE (1954) Primary carcinoma of the liver. A study of 100 cases among 48 900 necropsies. Cancer 7: 462–503
2. Peters RL (1976) Pathology of hepatocellular carcinoma. In: Okuda K, Peters RL (eds). Hepatocellular carcinoma. Wiley, New York, pp 107–158
3. Nakashima T, Okuda K, Kojiro M, Jimi A, Yamaguchi K, Sakamoto S, Ikari T (1983) Pathology of hepatocellular carcinoma in Japan. 232 consecutive cases, autopsied in 10 years. Cancer 51: 863–877
4. Mori W (1967) Cirrhosis and primary cancer of the liver. Comparative study in Tokyo and Cincinnati. Cancer 20: 627–631
5. Anthony PP (1973) Primary carcinoma of the liver. A study of 282 cases in Ugandan Africans. J Pathol Bacteriol 110: 37–49
6. Munoz N, Linsell A (1982) Epidemiology of primary liver cancer. In: Correa P, Haenszel W (eds) Epidemiology of cancer of the digestive tract. Nijhoff, The Hague, pp 161–195
7. Kew MC, Geddes EW (1982) Hepatocellular carcinoma in rural southern African blacks. Medicine 61: 98–108
8. Okuda K, Mackay I (1982) Hepatocellular carcinoma. A series of workshops on the biology of human cancer, report no. 17. UICC, Geneva
9. Li FP, Shiang EL (1980) Cancer mortality in China. J Natl Cancer Inst 65: 217–221
10. EL-Domeiri AL, Huvos AG, Goldsmith HS, Foote FW Jr (1971) Primary malignant tumors of the liver. Cancer 27: 7–11
11. Primack A, Vogel CL, Kyalwazi SK, Ziegler JL, Simon R, Anthony PP (1975) A staging system for hepatocellular carcinoma: Prognostic factors in Ugandan patients. Cancer 35: 1357–1364
12. Falkson G, Moertel CG, Lavin P, Pretorius FJ, Carbone PP (1978) Chemotherapy studies in primary liver cancer. A prospective randomized clinical trial. Cancer 42: 2149–2156
13. Lai CL, Lam KC, Wong KP, Wu PC, Todd D (1981) Clinical features of hepatocellular carcinoma: Review of 211 patients in Hong Kong. Cancer 47: 2746–2755
14. Okuda K (1976) Clinical aspects of hepatocellular carcinoma: Analysis of 134 cases. In: Okuda K, Peters RL (eds) Wiley, New York, pp 387–436
15. Berman MM, Libbey NP, Foster JH (1980) Hepatocellular carcinoma: Polygonal cell type with fibrous stroma. An atypical variant with a favorable prognosis. Cancer 46: 1448–1455
16. Yoshida T, Okazaki N, Yoshino M, Kitaoka H, Hirohashi S, Shimozato Y (1982) Minute hepatocellular carcinoma without appreciable change in size for 7 years: A case report. Cancer 49: 1491–1495
17. Gottfried E, Steller R, Paronetto F, Lieber CS (1982) Spontaneous regression of hepatocellular carcinoma. Gastroenterology; 82: 770–774
18. Lam KC, Ho JCI, Yeung RTT (1982) Spontaneous regression of hepatocellular carcinoma. Cancer 50: 332–336
19. Okuda K, Nakashima T, Obata H, Kubo Y (1977) Clinicopathological studies of minute hepatocellular carcinoma: Analysis of 20 cases, including 4 with hepatic resection. Gastroenterology 73: 109–115
20. Chen DS, Sheu JC, Sung JL, Lai MY, Lee CS, Su CT, Tsang YM, How SW, Wang TH, Yu JY, Yang TH, Wang CY Hsu CY (1982) Small hepatocellular carcinoma: A clinicopathological study in thirteen patients. Gastroenterology 83: 1109–1119
21. Shinagawa T, Ohto M, Kimura K, Tsunetomi S, Morita M, Saisho H, Tsuchiya Y, Saotome N, Karasawa E, Miki M, Ueno T, Okuda K (1984) Diagnostic and clinical features of small hepatocellular carcinoma with emphasis on the utility of real-time ultrasonography: A study of 51 patients. Gastroenterology 86: 496–502
22. Okazaki N, Yoshino M, Yoshida T, Ohkura H, Moriyama N, Matsue K (1981) Growth speed of hepatocellular carcinoma and early diagnosis. Acta Hepatol Jpn 22: 1742 (in Japanese)
23. Yoshino M (1983) Growth kinetics of hepatocellular carcinoma. Jpn J Clin Oncol 13: 45–52
24. Mashima Y (1984) Growth rate of hepatocellular carcinoma by ultrasonography and its clinical significance. Acta Hepatol Jpn 25: 754–765 (in Japanese)
25. Sheu JC, Sung JL, Chen DS, Yang PM, Lai MY, Lee CS, Hsu HC, Chang CN, Yang PC, Wang TH, Lin JT, Lee CZ (1985) Growth rate of asymptomatic hepatocellular carcinoma and its clinical implications. Gastroenterology 89: 259–266
26. Ebara M, Ohto M, Shinagawa T, Sugiura N, Kimura K, Matsutani S, Morita M, Saisho H, Tsuchiya Y, Okuda K (1986) Natural history of minute hepatocellular carcinoma smaller than three centimeters complicating cirrhosis. A study in 22 patients. Gastroenterology 90: 289–298
27. Berman C (1951) Primary carcinoma of the liver. Lewis, London, pp 46–48
28. Halpert B, Erickson EE (1955) Carcinoma of the liver. A study of twenty-eight cases. Cancer 8: 992–1002
29. Vogel CL, Linsell CA (1972) International symposium on hepatocellular carcinoma, Kampala, Uganda (July 1971). J Natl Cancer Inst 48: 567–571
30. Steiner PE (1960) Cancer of the liver and cirrhosis in trans-Saharan Africa and the United States of America. Cancer 13: 1085–1166
31. Kew MC (1981) Clinical, pathologic, and etiologic heterogeneity in hepatocellular carcinoma: Evidence from southern Africa. Hepatology 1: 366–369
32. Okuda K, Peters RL, Simson I (1984) Gross anatomical features of hepatocellular carcinoma from three disparate geographic areas: Proposal of new classification. Cancer 54: 2165–2173
33. Cochrane AMG, Murray-Lyon IM, Brinkley DM, Williams R (1977) Quadruple chemotherapy

versus radiotherapy in treatment of primary hepatocellular carcinoma. Cancer 40: 609–614

34. Almersjo, O, Bengmark S, Rudenstam CM, Hafstrom L, Nilsson LAV (1972) Evaluation of hepatic dearterialization in primary and secondary cancer of the liver. Am J Surg 124: 5–9

35. Idhe DC, Sherlock P, Winaxer SJ, Fortner JG (1974) Clinical manifestations of hepatoma: A review of 6 years' experience at a cancer hospital. Am J Med 56: 83–91

36. Okuda K, Ohtsuki T, Obata H, Tomimatsu M, Okazaki N, Hasegawa H, Nakajima Y, Ohnishi K (1985) Natural history of hepatocellular carcinoma and prognosis in relation to treatment. Study of 850 patients. Cancer 56: 918–928

37. Nakamura H, Tanaka T, Hori S, Yoshioka H, Kuroda C, Okamura J, Sakurai M (1983) Transcatheter embolization of hepatocellular carcinoma: Assessment of efficacy in cases of resection following embolization. Radiology 147: 401–405

38. Yamada Y, Sato M, Kawabata M, Nakatsuka H, Nakamura K, Takashima S (1983) Hepatic artery embolization in 120 patients with unresectable hepatoma. Radiology 148: 397–401

39. Takayasu K, Moriyama N, Muramatsu Y, Suzuki M, Yamada T, Kishi K, Hasegawa H, Okazaki N (1984) Hepatic arterial embolization for hepatocellular carcinoma: Comparison of CT scans and resected specimens. Radiology 150: 661–665

40. Kato T, Nemoto R, Mori H, Takahashi M, Tamakawa Y, Harada M (1981) Arterial chemoembolization with microencapsulated anticancer drug: An approach to selective cancer chemotherapy with sustained effects. JAMA 245: 1123–1127

41. Ohnishi K, Tsuchiya S, Nakayama T, Hiyama Y, Iwama S, Goto N, Takashi M, Kono K, Nakajima Y, Okuda K (1984) Arterial chemoembolization of hepatocellular carcinoma with mitomycin C microcapsules. Radiology 152: 51–55

42. Iwatsuki S, Shaw BW, Starzl TE (1983) Experience with 150 liver resections. Ann Surg 197: 247–253

43. Tang Z, Yu Y, Zhou X (1981) Factors influencing primary liver cancer resection survival rate. Chin Med J 94: 749–754

44. Adson MA, Weiland LH (1981) Resection of primary solid hepatic tumors. Am J Surg 141: 18–21

45. Lin TL (1976) Surgical treatment of primary liver cell carcinoma. In: Okuda K, Peters RL (eds) Wiley, New York, pp 449–468

46. Kanematsu T, Takenaka K, Matsumata T, Furuta T, Sugimachi K, Inokuchi K (1984) Limited hepatic resection effect for selected cirrhotic patients with primary liver cancer. Ann Surg 199: 51–56

47. Nelson RS, DeElizalde R, Howe CD (1966) Clinical aspects of primary carcinoma of the liver. Cancer 19: 533–537

48. Okazaki N (1976) Systemic chemotherapy of hepatocellular carcinoma. In: Okuda K, Peters RL (eds) Wiley, New York, pp 469–475

49. Link JS, Batemen JR, Paroly WS, Durkin WJ, Peters RL (1977) 5-Fluorouracil in hepatocellular carcinoma: Report of 21 cases. Cancer 39: 1936–1939

50. Vogel CL, Bayley AC, Borrker RJ, Anthony PP, Ziegler JL (1977) A phase II study of Adriamycin (NSC 123127) in patients with hepatocellular carcinoma from Zambia and the United States. Cancer 39: 1923–1929

51. Johnson PJ, Williams R, Thomas H, Sherlock S, Murray-Lyon IM (1978) Induction of remission in hepatocellular carcinoma with doxorubicin. Lancet 1: 1006–1009

52. Olweny CLM, Katongole-Mbidde E, Bahendeka S, Otim D, Mugersa J, Kyalwazi SK (1980) Further experience in treating patients with hepatocellular carcinoma in Uganda. Cancer 46: 2717–2722

53. Kubo Y, Shimokawa Y (1976) Arterial injection chemotherapy. In: Okuda K, Peters RL (eds). Wiley, New York, pp 477–490

54. Kinami Y, Miyazaki I (1978) The superselective and the selective one shot methods for treating inoperable cancer of the liver. Cancer 41: 1720–1727

55. Provan JL, Stokes JF, Edward D (1968) Hepatic artery infusion chemotherapy in hepatoma. Br Med J 3: 346–349

56. Al-Sarraf M, Go TS, Kithier K, Vaikevicius VK (1974) Primary liver cancer: A review of the clinical features, blood groups, serum enzymes, therapy, and survival of 65 cases. Cancer 33: 574–582

57. Okuda K, Musha H, Nakajima Y, Kubo Y, Shimokawa Y, Nagasaki Y, Sawa Y, Jinnouchi S, Obata H, Hisamitsu T, Okazaki N, Kojiro M, Sakamoto K, Nakashima T (1977) Clinicopathological features of encapsulated hepatocellular carcinoma: A study of 26 cases. Cancer 40: 1240–1245

58. Starzl TE, Iwatsuki S, Shaw BW Jr, Van Thiel DH, Gartner JC, Zitelli BJ, Malatack JJ, Schade RR (1984) Analysis of liver transplantation. Hepatology 4: 47S–49S

59. Rolles K, Williams R, Neuberger J, Calne R (1984) The Cambridge and King's College Hospital experience of liver transplantation, 1968–1983. Hepatology 4: 50S–55S

Subject Index